DARSE NISWAN

Simplifying Syllabus. Amplifying Success.

A Comprehensive Textbook of Unani GYNECOLOGY
Based on NCISM Final Year Syllabus

Dr. Misba Naim

notionpress.com

INDIA • SINGAPORE • MALAYSIA

ISBN
Hardcase 979-8-90362-5-130
Paperback 979-8-90362-5-123

Dedication

"For the voices that shaped me—and the learners I write for."

To the students of Unani medicine—
whose resilience and curiosity are the lifeblood of our tradition.
This book is for you.
To my teachers and mentors—
whose wisdom lit every page I wrote.
Thank you for your guidance.
To my family and loved ones—
who offered unwavering support, faith, and patience.
Your love gave me the strength to complete this mission.
And finally,
to the Unani system itself—
a science of healing that continues to enrich humanity.

Dr. Misba Naim
Author | Educator | Guide

Contents

A Message to My Readers

"To every student who asked: 'Where do I begin?' — this book is your answer."

As both a student and teacher of Unani medicine,
I have witnessed the challenges that arise from fragmented resources,
especially in the subject of *Amraze Niswan*.
To prepare for exams, I referred to multiple texts,
compared topics across volumes, and compiled personal notes.
As a teacher, I saw my students struggle with the same scattered syllabus—
and I knew something had to change.
That is why this book is written:
To bring the entire NCISM syllabus of *Amraze Niswan* into one unified guide.
To honor the dedication of students and support educators
who strive every day to make this subject clearer, stronger and more accessible.
This is not just a textbook. It is a labor of love—
crafted with sincerity, purpose and the hope that
every reader feels more confident, more equipped and more empowered.
I welcome you to learn, revise, teach and succeed—
with every page, you are not alone.

With gratitude,
Dr. Misba Naim
Author | Educator | Guide

Acknowledgements

"With gratitude to the hands that lifted me, and to the legacy I carry forward."

All praise and gratitude belong to **ALMIGHTY**— the source of knowledge, mercy and inspiration. It is by **H**is will that this book came into existence, and through **H**is guidance that I was able to persevere in its creation.

To my beloved parents and family, whose prayers built my foundation, whose sacrifice gave me strength, and whose unwavering love continues to shape the educator and student within me .

To my loving husband and children, who walked this journey with me—patiently, lovingly and with faith—

your presence gave me strength when I was weary and purpose when I felt lost.

I extend heartfelt appreciation to my teachers and mentors, both in Aligarh Muslim University and National Institute of Unani Medicine,Bengaluru, whose wisdom and patience illuminated my academic path. You shaped my understanding of *Amraze Niswan* and instilled in me the reverence for our timeless Unani heritage.

To my students, past and present — your curiosity, your questions and your hunger, to learn pushed me to make this book a reality. You reminded me that every complicated topic deserves clarity, every question deserves compassion and every classroom deserves structure.

To my friends, colleagues and the Unani academic community, thank you for championing educational innovation, for keeping tradition alive through teaching, and for welcoming the idea of reform and reorganization in our shared curriculum.

To NCISM for shaping the future of Unani medical education through a unified syllabus — this textbook is my contribution toward that vision.

And finally, to every student who struggled to make sense of this subject and to every teacher who longed for a consolidated book— *AMRAZE NISWAN* is written for you.

Dr. Misba Naim
Author | Educator | Guide

01

Anatomy and Physiology of Female Genital Tract and its Variations

(Zanana A'da' Tanasuliyya ki tashrih wa Manafi' aur Ghayr Tabi'I shaklen)

1.1 *Bairooni A'da' Tanasul* (External Genitalia)
1.2 *Androoni A'da' Tanasul* (Internal Genitalia)
1.3 *Thadi* (Breast)
1.4 *Zanan Majra-i-Bawl* (Female Urinary Tract)
1.5 *Am'a' mustaqeem wa Qanat shrjiya* (Rectum and Anal Canal)
1.6 *Farsh-i- Ana ke Adalat aur Ribatat* (Perineum, Pelvic Floor Muscles & Ligaments)
1.7 *Khilqi nqayes* (Developmental Anamolies)
1.8 *Bayn al-jinsiyat ka byan* (Description of intersex)

Learning Objective (At the end of the session, the students should be able to)

Discuss the anatomy and physiology of External & Internal Genital organs.
Describe the perineum Pelvic Floor Muscles & Ligaments.
Describe the Female Urinary Tract, Rectum & Anal Canal.
Demonstrate the anatomy of the Breast .

1.1 External Genitalia

(*Bairooni A'da' Tanasul*)

The female external genitalia, collectively known as the vulva or pudendum, comprises a group of structures located external to the vagina, having role in sexual function, reproduction and urinary excretion.

Anatomy of the Female External Genitalia

The vulva includes the following structures mons pubis, labia majora, labia minora, clitoris, vestibule and the perineum. They are all visible on external examination.

1. Mons Pubis

A rounded, fatty prominence located over the pubic symphysis. Composed of subcutaneous adipose tissue covered by skin with coarse pubic hair after puberty. (Hair pattern is called euscatcheon or inverted triangle)

Function: Provides cushioning and protects the underlying pubic bone.

Clinical Note: Excessive fat accumulation or hair distribution changes may indicate hormonal imbalances.

2. Labia Majora

Two longitudinal folds of skin extending from the mons pubis to the perineum, forming the lateral boundaries of the vulva. Lined by squamous epithelium. Contain adipose tissue, sebaceous and sweat glands, and are covered with pubic hair on their outer surfaces. The inner surfaces are smooth and hairless.

Embryological Origin: Homologous to the scrotum in males, derived from the genital swellings. Round ligaments terminate at its anterior third.

Function: Protect the inner structures of the vulva and contribute to sexual arousal due to sensitivity.

Clinical Note: May be affected by conditions like Bartholin's gland cysts or abscesses due to proximity to gland ducts.

3. Labia Minora

Two thin, hairless folds of skin located medial to the labia majora, surrounding the vaginal and urethral orifices. Anteriorly they enclose the clitoris and unite with each other in front and behind the clitoris to from the prepuce and frenulum, respectively. Lower portion unites to form forchette. Labia minora do not contain hair follicle. Fossa navicularis is situated between fourchette and the vaginal orifice. Homologous to ventral aspect of penis. Composed of connective tissue, erectile tissue and sebaceous glands, with a rich vascular supply, giving them a pinkish appearance.

Function: Contribute to the closure of the vaginal introitus and provide sensory feedback during sexual activity.

Clinical Note: Prone to irritation, infections or trauma; hypertrophy may lead to discomfort or cosmetic concerns.

4. Clitoris

A highly sensitive erectile organ, about 2.5 cm, located at the anterior junction of the labia minora, partially covered by a prepuce (clitoral hood). It is attached to the undersurface of the symphysis pubis by the suspensory ligament.

Structure: Glans Clitoris: The visible, external portion, approximately 0.5–1 cm in diameter.

Body (Corpus): Internal, composed of two corpora cavernosa, which are erectile tissues.

Crura: Paired extensions of the corpora cavernosa anchoring to the pubic arch.

Bulbs of the Vestibule: Erectile tissues adjacent to the vaginal opening, homologous to the bulb of the penis.

Embryological Origin: Homologous to the penis, derived from the genital tubercle.

Function: Primary organ for sexual pleasure due to its dense concentration of sensory nerve endings.

Clinical Note: Clitoromegaly (enlargement) may indicate hyperandrogenism or congenital adrenal hyperplasia.

5. Vestibule

The triangular area bounded anteriorly by the clitoris, posteriorly by the fourchette and on either side by labia minora. There are four openings into the vestibule.

Components:

a. **Vaginal Orifice (Introitus):** The external opening of the vagina, partially covered by the hymen in prepubertal females or virgins.
b. **Urethral Orifice**: Located anterior to the vaginal orifice, approximately 1.5 cm below the clitoris, for urinary excretion.
c. **Skene's Glands**: Paraurethral glands with ducts opening near the urethral orifice, homologous to the prostate.
d. **Bartholin's Glands**: Paired glands located posterolaterally to the vaginal orifice, secreting lubricating mucus during arousal. They are pea sized, of about 0.5 cm and yellowish white in color. The glands are of racemose variety. And lined by columnar epithelium. Each gland has a duct of about 2 cm and opens into the vestibule, at the junction of anterior two third and posterior one third in the groove between the hymen and labium minora. The duct is lined by columnar epithelium but at its opening by stratified squamous epithelium.

   Function: Facilitates urination, sexual intercourse and childbirth.
   Clinical Note: Infections (e.g., Bartholin's gland abscess) or vestibular pain (e.g., vulvodynia) may affect this region.

e. **Hymen:** A thin, elastic membrane partially covering the vaginal orifice in prepubertal or non-sexually active females.

   Variations: Shape varies (e.g., annular, crescentic, imperforate); may be absent or rupture naturally due to physical activity or tampon use.
   Function: No definitive physiological function; cultural significance in some societies.
   Clinical Note: Imperforate hymen can cause hematocolpos (menstrual blood accumulation), requiring surgical intervention.

Blood Supply

Arterial Supply: Internal pudendal artery: Primary supply to the vulva, with branches including the perineal artery, dorsal clitoral artery, and deep arteries to erectile tissues.

External pudendal artery: Supplies the labia majora and mons pubis.

Venous Drainage: Veins follow arterial paths, draining into the internal pudendal veins and ultimately the internal iliac veins.

Lymphatic Drainage: Superficial structures (mons pubis, labia) drain to superficial inguinal lymph nodes.

Deep structures (clitoris, vestibule) drain to deep inguinal or internal iliac nodes.

Clinical Note: Lymphatic spread is critical in vulvar cancers, guiding staging and treatment.

Nerve Supply

Sensory Innervation: Derived primarily from the pudendal nerve (br. of post cut. nerve of thigh (S2–S4), which branches into: Dorsal nerve of the clitoris: Supplies the clitoris, responsible for sexual sensation. Perineal nerve: Innervates the labia and vestibule.

Additional innervation from the genitofemoral nerve L1 and L2 (mons pubis) and ilioinguinal nerve (anterior vulva).

Autonomic Innervation: Sympathetic and parasympathetic fibers regulate blood flow and glandular secretions (e.g., Bartholin's glands).

Clinical Note: Pudendal nerve damage (e.g., during childbirth) may lead to sensory loss or sexual dysfunction.

Functions of the Female External Genitalia

a. **Sexual Function:** The clitoris, labia minora and vestibular bulbs are highly sensitive and engorge during arousal, facilitating sexual pleasure.

   Bartholin's and Skene's glands secrete lubricating fluids to reduce friction during intercourse.

b. **Reproductive Function:** The vulva protects the vaginal opening, which serves as the entry for sperm and the exit for childbirth.
c. **Urinary Function:** The urethral orifice allows for controlled urination.
d. **Protective Function:** The labia majora and minora shield internal structures from trauma and pathogens.

Developmental and Embryological Notes

The external genitalia develop from the genital tubercle, genital folds and genital swellings under the influence of sex hormones. In the absence of androgens, the genital tubercle forms the clitoris, genital folds become the labia minora and genital swellings form the labia majora.

Applied Anatomy

Anomalies (e.g., ambiguous genitalia) may occur due to hormonal imbalances or genetic conditions (e.g., congenital adrenal hyperplasia).

1. **Congenital Anomalies**: Imperforate hymen, clitoromegaly, or labial fusion may require medical or surgical management.
2. **Candidiasis**: Fungal infection causing itching and discharge.
3. **Bartholin's gland cysts/abscesses**: Obstruction or infection of gland ducts.
4. **Herpes simplex virus**: Painful ulcers on the vulva.
5. **Trauma**: Common during childbirth (e.g., perineal tears) or sexual assault; may require surgical repair.
6. **Vulvar Pain Syndromes**: Vulvodynia: Chronic pain without clear etiology, often affecting the vestibule.
7. **Vaginismus**: Involuntary muscle spasms complicating intercourse.
8. **Neoplasms**: Vulvar intraepithelial neoplasia (VIN): Precancerous lesion linked to HPV.
9. **Squamous cell carcinoma**: Most common vulvar cancer, often presenting as a lump or ulcer.

Development of female genitalia

Fertilization (XX Chromosome)
↓
Genital Ridge Formation (~5th week)
↓
Indifferent Gonad (can form testis/ovary)
↓
Absence of SRY → Ovary Development (6-8 weeks)
↓

↓ Internal Genitalia
↓
Mullerian Ducts
(Fallopian tubes, uterus, cervix, upper vagina)

↓ External Genitalia
↓
Genital Tubercle(→ Clitoris)
Urogenital folds (→ Labia minora)
Labioscrotal swellings (→ Labia majora)

1.2 Internal Genitalia

(*Androoni A'da' Tanasul*)

The female internal genitalia comprise the vagina, uterus, fallopian tubes and ovaries. These organs are located within the pelvic cavity and require special instruments for visualization. These organs are essential for reproductive and sexual functions, including menstruation, fertilization and pregnancy.

1. Vagina

A fibromuscular tube connecting the external genitalia (vulva) to the uterus, serving as the copulatory organ, birth canal and passageway for menstrual discharge.

Dimensions and Location: Approximately 7–10 cm long, extending from the vestibule to the cervix. The anterior wall (7 cm) is shorter than the posterior wall (9 cm) due to the cervix's projection into the vagina. It lies posterior to the bladder and urethra and anterior to the rectum. (D.C. Dutta, p. 16)

Structure: The vagina is inclined at a 45° angle to the vertical plane in the standing position. The fornices are recesses around the cervix: anterior (shallowest), posterior (deepest) and two lateral fornices, clinically significant for pelvic examinations and culdocentesis. The diameter of canal is about 2.5 cm. The vaginal wall is rugated (transverse folds or rugae), allowing distension during intercourse or childbirth.

Relations: Anterior: Upper one third with bladder and lower one third with urethra.

Posterior: Rectum, rectouterine pouch (of Douglas) and anal canal.

Lateral: Levator ani, pelvic fascia and ureters.

Superior: Cervix.

Inferior: Vestibule and hymen (partially present in virgins).

Histology: Mucosa: Non-keratinized stratified squamous epithelium, resistant to mechanical stress. No glands; thus no secretion, lubrication comes from cervical mucus and Bartholin's glands.

Submucosa: Loose connective tissue with elastic fibers and a rich venous plexus.

Muscular Layer: Inner circular and outer longitudinal smooth muscle layers, blending with the uterine myometrium superiorly.

Adventitia: Fibrous connective tissue anchoring the vagina to surrounding structures.

Epithelium: The vaginal epithelium is under the action of hormones. At birth and upto 10-14 days, the epithelium is stratified squamous under the influence of maternal estrogens circulating in the new born. Upto puberty and postmenopause, the epithelium becomes thin.

From puberty till menopause, the epithelium is stratified squamous and devoid of any gland.

Secretion: The vaginal secretion is very scanty, making the vagina moist only. The secretion is mainly derived from the glands of cervix, uterus, transudation of the vaginal epithelium and Bartholin glands (during sexual excitement). The pH is acidic (4-5.5). The pH is highest in upper vagina because of contaminated cervical secretions.

Embryology Origin: The upper two-thirds arise from the fused Mullerian (paramesonephric) ducts, and the lower third from the urogenital sinus.

Development: By the 12th week of gestation, the Müllerian ducts fuse to form the uterovaginal canal, which canalizes to form the vagina. The hymen marks the junction of these embryonic structures.

Anomalies: Vaginal agenesis (Mayer-Rokitansky-Kuster-Hauser syndrome), transverse vaginal septa, or imperforate hymen.

Blood Supply

Arterial: Vaginal branches of the internal iliac artery, with contributions from the uterine and middle rectal arteries. Cervicovaginal branch of the uterine artery.

Venous: Vaginal venous plexus drains into the internal iliac veins.

Lymphatics: Upper two-thirds to internal iliac nodes; lower third to superficial inguinal nodes.

Nerve Supply

Autonomic: Sympathetic (T12–L2) and parasympathetic (S2–S4) fibers via the hypogastric and pelvic plexuses regulate blood flow and smooth muscle tone. Somatic: The lower vagina is sensitive to touch and pain via the pudendal nerve (S2–S4).

Clinical Correlations

Infections: Bacterial vaginosis, candidiasis, and trichomoniasis alter vaginal pH and flora.

Prolapse: Weakness of pelvic floor muscles (e.g., levator ani) leads to cystocele, rectocele, or vaginal vault prolapse.

Fistulae: Vesicovaginal or rectovaginal fistulae cause incontinence, often post-obstetric trauma.

Cancer: Primary vaginal carcinoma is rare, often squamous cell type; secondary spread from cervical or endometrial cancer is more common (Shaw's, p. 56).

2. Uterus

A hollow, muscular organ that supports implantation, fetal development and labor. Pear-shaped, approximately 7.5 cm long, 5 cm wide, and 2.5 cm thick in nulliparous women (larger in multiparous). Located in the pelvis between the bladder anteriorly and rectum posteriorly, normally in an anteverted and anteflexed position.

Parts: Fundus: Dome-shaped portion above the fallopian tube openings.

Body (Corpus): Main portion, the body is triangular and lies between the openings of the tubes and the isthmus. The superolateral angle of the body are called cornua of the uterus. The fallopian tube (uterine tube), round ligament and ligament of the ovary are attached to each cornu.

Isthmus: Constricted part, measures about 0.5 cm between the body of uterus and the cervix. It is limited above by the anatomical internal os and below by the histological internal os.

Cervix: The cervix is the lowermost part of the uterus. Cylindrical shape (2.5 cm), partially projecting into the vagina. It is divided into a supravaginal part -the part lying above the vagina and the vaginal part which lies within the vagina, each measuring 1.25 cm.

In nulliparous, vaginal part of the cervix is conical and the external os is circular. In parous the cervix is cylindrical with external os having bilateral slits, giving rise to anterior and posterior lips of the cervix.

Cavity: Triangular in the body, measures about 3.5 cm (uterine body), communicating with fallopian tubes via cornua and cavity is spindle-shaped in the cervix (endocervical canal) measuring 2.5 cm.

Relations: Anterior: Vesico uterine pouch and bladder.

Posterior: Rectouterine pouch (Pouch of Douglas) and rectum.

Lateral: Broad ligaments, uterine arteries, and ureters.

Superior: Fallopian tubes and ovaries (via ligaments).

Inferior: Vagina.

Histology

The wall consists of 3 layers from outside inwards:

Endometrium: The mucus lining of the cavity is called endometrium. No submucosa, so endometrium is directly apposed to myometrium. The surface epithelium is a single layer of ciliated columnar epithelium.

Functional Layer: Simple columnar epithelium with tubular glands, shed during menstruation.

Basal Layer: Regenerates the functional layer post-menstruation.

Varies with menstrual cycle: Proliferative (estrogen-driven, thin, glandular) and secretory (progesterone-driven, thick, edematous). The endometrium is changed to decidua during pregnancy.

Myometrium: Three layers of smooth muscle (outer longitudinal, middle oblique, inner circular), thickest in the fundus, with interstitial connective tissue.

Perimetrium: Peritoneal covering (serosa) on the posterior surface and fundus.

Cervix

Composed of fibrous stroma with minimal smooth muscle (10-15%).

Endocervix: Simple columnar epithelium with mucus-secreting glands.

Ectocervix: Also called portio vaginalis. Stratified squamous epithelium, extends right upto the external os where there is abrupt change to columnar type.

The transitional zone (transformation zone) may be of 1-10 mm. It is not static but changes with hormone level of estrogen. The site is constantly irritated by hormones, infection and trauma. Thus there is chance of severe dysplasia, carcinoma in situ or even invasive carcinoma at this zone.

Secretion

The endometrial secretion is scanty and watery. The physical and chemical properties of the cervical secretion change with menstrual cycles and with pregnancy. The cervical glands secrete an alkaline mucus with pH 7.8. The mucus is rich in fructose, glycoprotein and mucopolysaccharides. It also contains sodium chloride. The fructose has got nutritive function to spermatozoa.

Under estrogenic stimulation- glycoprotein network is arranged parallel to each other so as to ease sperm entry.

Progesterone produces interlacing bridges thus prevent sperm entry.

Cervical mucus forms the mucus plug which blocks the canal and also has bacteriolytic action.

Embryological origin: Formed by the fusion of Mullerian ducts (8–12 weeks gestation), creating the uterovaginal canal.

Development: The fundus, body, and cervix differentiate by the 20th week. The cervix develops a fibrous stroma distinct from the muscular body.

Anomalies: Bicornuate uterus, septate uterus, or unicornuate uterus due to incomplete fusion or resorption (D.C. Dutta, p. 19).

Blood Supply

Arterial: Uterine arteries (branches of internal iliac) anastomose with ovarian arteries, forming arcuate arteries in the myometrium.

Venous: Uterine veins drain into the internal iliac veins.

Lymphatics: Fundus to para-aortic nodes; body to external iliac nodes; cervix to internal iliac and sacral nodes.

Nerve Supply

Autonomic: Sympathetic (T12–L2) and parasympathetic (S2–S4) fibers via the superior hypogastric and pelvic plexuses. Pain (e.g., dysmenorrhea) travels via sympathetics.

Somatic: Cervix has limited somatic innervation via the pudendal nerve.

The cervix is insensitive to touch, heat and instrument handling. The uterus also is insensitive to handle during surgery.

Changes of the uterus with age

At birth, the cervix is much larger than the body of uterus. In childhood, the cervix to body ratio is 2:1. At puberty, the body of uterus grows faster under the action of hormones (estrogen), and the proportion is reversed to 1:2. After childbirth, it becomes 1:3 and after menopause uterus atrophies and the overall length is reduced.

Position of uterus

The normal position of uterus is anteversion and anteflexion.

Anteversion relates the long axis of cervix to the long axis of vagina which is about 90 degree. Anteflexion relates the long axis of the body to the long axis of the cervix and is about 120 degree. In about 15-20 %, normally the uterus remains in retroverted position.

Clinical Correlations

1. **Agenesis/Hypoplasia**: Absent or underdeveloped uterus (e.g., Mayer-Rokitansky-Kuster-Hauser syndrome).
2. **Retroversion/Retroflexion:** Posterior tilting, often asymptomatic but may complicate pregnancy.
3. **Endometriosis**: Ectopic endometrial tissue causing pelvic pain and infertility.
4. **Fibroids (Leiomyomas):** Benign myometrial tumors causing menorrhagia or pressure symptoms.
5. **Adenomyosis:** Endometrial glands within the myometrium, leading to dysmenorrhea.
6. **Cervical Dysplasia/Cancer:** Detected via Pap smear; human papillomavirus (HPV) is a major risk factor.

3. Fallopian Tubes (Uterine tubes)

Paired tubular structures that transport ova from the ovaries to the uterus and serve as the site of fertilization. 10–12 cm long (4 inch), extending from the uterine cornua to the ovaries, lying within the broad ligament's superior border. Each tube has two openings, one communicate with the uterine cavity called the uterine opening and other on the lateral part of the tube, called pelvic opening or abdominal ostium.

There are four parts of fallopian tube:

1. Intramural (Interstitial): 1 cm in length and 1 mm in diameter, within the uterine wall, narrowest portion.
2. Isthmus: 2.5 cm in length and 2.5 mm inch, almost straight, and thick-walled, adjacent to the uterus.
3. Ampulla: tortuous part, about 5 cm in length, widest portion, site of fertilization.
4. Infundibulum: about 1.25 cm long with diameter of 6 mm. Funnel-shaped, with fimbriae (finger-like projections) that capture the ovum; one fimbria (ovarian) attaches to the ovary.

Relations: Medial: Uterus.
Lateral: Ovary and pelvic wall.
Superior: Peritoneal cavity.
Inferior: Broad ligament.

Histology

Mucosa: Simple columnar epithelium with ciliated cells (beat toward uterus) and secretory (peg) cells (nourish ovum). Longitudinal mucosal folds increase in complexity toward the ampulla.

Muscular Layer: Inner circular and outer longitudinal smooth muscle, facilitating peristalsis.

Serosa: Peritoneal covering continuous with the broad ligament.

Embryology

Origin: Derived from the unfused cranial portions of the Müllerian ducts.

Development: By the 10th week, the tubes form as hollow structures with fimbriae developing near the ovaries.

Anomalies: Accessory tubes or tubal atresia, though rare.

Functions: 1) transport of gametes,

2) to facilitate fertilization

3) survival of zygote through its secretion (D. C. Dutta)

Blood Supply

Arterial: Tubal branches of uterine and ovarian arteries.

Venous: Drains into uterine and ovarian veins.

Lymphatics: Para-aortic and internal iliac nodes.

Nerve Supply

Sympathetic (T10–L2) and parasympathetic (S2–S4) via the ovarian and hypogastric plexuses. Pain from tubal distension (e.g., ectopic pregnancy) is referred to the abdomen.

Clinical Correlations

Accessory Ostia: Additional openings in the tube, potentially increasing ectopic pregnancy risk.

Tubal Diverticula: Outpouchings, which may predispose to ectopic implantation.

Ectopic Pregnancy: Implantation in the ampulla (most common), risking rupture and hemorrhage.

Salpingitis: Infection (e.g., Chlamydia) causing infertility due to tubal occlusion.

Tubal Ligation: Surgical contraception by occlusion of the isthmus or ampulla.

Hydrosalpinx: Fluid-filled tube due to distal obstruction (Shaw's, p. 64).

4. Ovary

Paired organs responsible for oogenesis and hormone production (estrogen, progesterone and androgens) in females.

Dimensions and Location: Almond-shaped, pinkish in colour, later it changes to greyish, 3 cm long, 2 cm wide, 1 cm thick, located in the ovarian fossa (lateral pelvic wall). Attached to the broad ligament via the mesovarium and to the uterus via the ovarian ligament. Each ovary has two ends- tubal and uterine, two borders- mesovarium and free posterior and two surfaces- medial and lateral.

Structure

Covered by a thin germinal epithelium (simple cuboidal). Divided into a cortex (follicles and stroma) and medulla (vascular core).

Relations:
Anterior: Broad ligament.
Posterior: Rectum and pelvic wall.
Lateral: Obturator vessels and nerves.
Medial: Fallopian tube fimbriae.

Histology

Cortex: During reproductive years, it contains follicles at various stages: primordial (oocyte with flat granulosa cells), primary, secondary and Graafian (mature, with antrum and cumulus oophorus) and corpus luteum. Atresia of these follicles results in formation of atretic follicles or corpus albicans. These are related to sex hormone production and ovulation.

Stroma: Spindle-shaped cells resembling connective tissue, producing androgens.

Medulla: Loose connective tissue with blood vessels, lymphatics, and nerves. Hilus cells are present which are homologous to the interstitial cell of the testis.

Surface Epithelium: Simple cuboidal (germinal epithelium), prone to malignant transformation.

Embryology

Origin: Develop from the gonadal ridge (mesoderm) on the posterior abdominal wall.

Development: Primordial germ cells migrate to the ridge by the 6th week, forming oogonia. By the 20th week, primordial follicles form, peaking at 6–7 million (declining to 1–2 million at birth).

Anomalies: Gonadal dysgenesis (e.g., Turner syndrome) or accessory ovaries.

Blood Supply

Arterial: Ovarian arteries (direct branches of the aorta), anastomosing with uterine arteries.

Venous: Right ovarian vein drains into the inferior vena cava; left into the left renal vein.

Lymphatics: Para-aortic nodes near the renal vessels.

Nerve Supply

Autonomic: Sympathetic (T10–T11) and parasympathetic (vagus) via the ovarian plexus. Pain (e.g., ovarian cyst rupture) is referred to the lower abdomen.

Clinical Correlations

Polycystic Ovary Syndrome (PCOS): Multiple follicular cysts, hyperandrogenism and anovulation.

Ovarian Cysts: Functional (follicular, corpus luteum) or neoplastic (dermoid, serous cystadenoma).

Ovarian Cancer: Often epithelial (serous/mucinous), with poor prognosis due to late detection.

Torsion: Twisting of the ovarian pedicle, causing acute pain and ischemia.

Supporting Structures

Ligaments

Broad Ligament: Peritoneal fold enclosing the fallopian tubes, ovaries, and parametrium, supporting lateral stability.

Round Ligament: Maintains uterine anteversion, extending from the cornua to the labia majora.

Cardinal Ligament: Supports the cervix and upper vagina, containing uterine vessels. Major support.

Uterosacral Ligament: Anchors the cervix posteriorly to the sacrum.

Pelvic Floor: Levator ani and coccygeus muscles support the vagina and uterus, preventing prolapse.

Functions

Vagina: Facilitates intercourse, childbirth, and menstrual flow.

Uterus: Prepares for implantation (endometrial cycling), supports pregnancy and contracts during labor.

Fallopian Tubes: Transport ova and sperm, enabling fertilization in the ampulla.

Ovaries: Produce ova and hormones regulating the menstrual cycle and secondary sexual characteristics.

1.3 Breast

(*Thadi)*

Anatomy of the Female Breasts

The breasts, or mammary glands, are paired structures located on the anterior thoracic wall, primarily over the pectoral muscles. They are modified sweat glands specialized for milk production and delivery in females, though present in rudimentary form in males. The breasts vary in size, shape and position among individuals, influenced by genetics, hormones and body composition.

External Anatomy

Location: Extend from the 2nd to 6th ribs vertically and from the sternal edge to the midaxillary line horizontally. Lie superficial to the pectoralis major, serratus anterior and external oblique muscles.

Components

Nipple: A cylindrical projection at the centre of the breast, typically at the 4th intercostal space in non-pendulous breasts. Contains smooth muscle fibres for erection and 15–20 lactiferous duct openings.

Areola: A pigmented circular area surrounding the nipple (2–6 cm in diameter). Contains sebaceous (Montgomery) glands that secrete oily secretions for lubrication during lactation.

Skin: Thin, elastic skin covers the breast, with increased pigmentation in the areola.

Blood Supply

Arterial: Internal thoracic artery (perforating branches). Lateral thoracic and thoracoacromial arteries (branches of the axillary artery). Posterior intercostal arteries (branches of the aorta).

Venous Drainage: Axillary, internal thoracic and intercostal veins, with potential anastomosis to vertebral veins (relevant in breast cancer metastasis).

Lymphatic Drainage: Primarily to axillary lymph nodes (75%). Parasternal (internal mammary) nodes (20%). Interpectoral (Rotter's) nodes and supraclavicular nodes (5%).

Nerve supply

Sensory: Anterior and lateral cutaneous branches of the 2nd–6th intercostal nerves (T2–T6).

Sympathetic: Innervates smooth muscle of the nipple/areola for erection response.

Function: Aesthetic, sexual (sensory stimulation), and protective (covering underlying muscles).

Internal Anatomy

Structure: Composed of glandular, adipose and connective tissues within a superficial fascial covering.

Glandular Tissue: Lobes: 15–20 lobes per breast, each drained by a lactiferous duct. Lobules: Smaller units within lobes, containing alveoli (milk-producing acini). Lactiferous Ducts: Converge toward the nipple, dilating into lactiferous sinuses beneath the areola for milk storage.

Connective Tissue: Suspensory Ligaments (Cooper's Ligaments): Fibrous bands anchoring glandular tissue to the dermis and pectoral fascia, providing structural support.

Stroma: Fibrous and adipose tissue surrounding glandular elements, determining breast size and shape.

Adipose Tissue: Varies in proportion, located between lobes and beneath the skin, contributing to breast volume.

Blood Supply (Internal): Same as external, with perforating branches supplying glandular tissue.

Innervation (Internal): Sensory innervation to glandular tissue via intercostal nerves; autonomic innervation regulates ductal smooth muscle and vascular tone.

Function: Glandular tissue produces and delivers milk; adipose tissue provides volume and contour.

Microscopic Anatomy

Alveoli: Lined by cuboidal epithelial cells (secretory) surrounded by myoepithelial cells (contractile, oxytocin-responsive for milk ejection).

Ducts: Lined by columnar epithelium, transitioning to stratified squamous near the nipple.

Stroma: Collagen, elastin and adipocytes, with scattered lymphocytes and macrophages.

Hormonal Receptors: Estrogen and progesterone receptors in epithelial cells drive development and cyclical changes.

Physiology of the Female Breasts

The breasts undergo dynamic changes across the lifespan, driven by hormonal, reproductive and aging processes. Their primary physiological role is lactation, with secondary roles in sexual arousal and aesthetics.

1. Developmental Physiology

Embryology: Breasts arise from ectodermal milk lines (4th week of gestation). By birth, rudimentary ducts and nipples form.

Puberty: Estrogen stimulates ductal proliferation and adipose deposition; progesterone promotes lobuloalveolar development. Growth typically completes by age 16–18.

Menstrual Cycle: Cyclical oestrogen and progesterone cause mild glandular proliferation and edema, leading to tenderness or swelling premenstrually.

Pregnancy: Estrogen, progesterone and prolactin induce lobuloalveolar maturation, ductal branching and colostrum production.

Menopause: Estrogen decline leads to glandular atrophy, increased adipose tissue and reduced elasticity.

2. Lactation: During pregnancy, prolactin and human placental lactogen stimulate alveolar development. Progesterone inhibits milk secretion until delivery.

Milk Production: Postpartum progesterone drop and prolactin surge initiate lactogenesis. Oxytocin triggers myoepithelial contraction for milk ejection (let-down reflex).

Composition: Colostrum (days 1–5) is rich in immunoglobulins; mature milk contains water, lactose, proteins and fats.

Regulation: Suckling stimulates prolactin (milk synthesis) and oxytocin (milk ejection) via hypothalamic-pituitary reflexes.

Cessation: Weaning reduces prolactin, leading to involution of glandular tissue.

3. Sexual Function: The nipple and areola are highly sensitive due to dense sensory innervation (T4 dermatome). Stimulation triggers nipple erection (smooth muscle contraction) and sexual arousal via neural pathways to the hypothalamus. Breast tissue responds to tactile stimulation, contributing to sexual pleasure.

4. Protective and Immunological Role: Montgomery glands lubricate the nipple/areola, preventing cracking during lactation. Colostrum and milk provide passive immunity to neonates via immunoglobulins and immune cells.

Normal Variations in Female Breasts

Breast anatomy exhibits significant variation, influenced by genetics, ethnicity, hormonal status and lifestyle.

Clinical Note: Asymmetry is common (up to 25% volume difference). Extreme macromastia may cause physical discomfort (e.g., back pain).

1. Nipple Variation: Size (4–10 mm diameter), projection (flat, protruding, inverted) and number (supernumerary nipples along milk line in 1–6% of individuals).

Clinical Note: Inverted nipples are congenital in 10% of women but may indicate pathology (e.g., ductal carcinoma) if newly acquired.

2. Areola Variation: Diameter (2–6 cm), pigmentation (pink to dark brown) and Montgomery gland prominence. Pigmentation darkens with pregnancy or hormonal changes.

Clinical Note: Asymmetry in areolar size or irregular pigmentation may need evaluation.

3. Position and Symmetry Variation: Breasts situated at different position (e.g., due to scoliosis or rib cage asymmetry). Ptosis (sagging) varies with age, parity and skin elasticity.

Clinical Note: Significant ptosis may require surgical correction (mastopexy) for functional or aesthetic reasons.

4. Glandular vs. Adipose Proportion Variation: Dense (glandular) breasts are common in younger women or nulliparous individuals; fatty breasts predominate post-menopause or in higher BMI.

Clinical Note: Dense breasts reduce mammographic sensitivity, increasing reliance on ultrasound or MRI for screening.

Age-Related Changes

Puberty: Asymmetry during growth is common and usually resolves.

Pregnancy/Lactation: Hypertrophy, increased vascularity and areolar darkening occur. Post-lactation involution may cause ptosis.

Menopause: Glandular atrophy, increased adiposity and skin laxity lead to flattening or ptosis.

Congenital Anomalies

Amastia: Complete absence of breast tissue, nipple and areola. (rare, often unilateral).

Amazia: Absence of breast tissue with a normal nipple and areola.

Polymastia: Supernumerary breasts along the milk line (functional or vestigial).

Polythelia: Extra nipples (1–6% prevalence).

Tuberous Breasts: Constricted base, herniated areola and underdeveloped lower pole, often requiring surgical correction.

Poland Syndrome: Unilateral hypoplasia of breast and pectoralis major.

1.4 Female Urinary Tract

(*Zanana Majra-i-Bawl*)

The female urinary tract is a complex system responsible for the production, storage and elimination of urine. It comprises the kidneys, ureters, urinary bladder and urethra, each with distinct anatomical and physiological roles.

Anatomy of the Female Urinary Tract

Kidney

Paired retroperitoneal organs located at T12-L3 vertebral levels, with the right kidney slightly lower due to liver displacement. Each kidney measures ~10-12 cm long, 5-6 cm wide, and 3-4 cm thick, weighing ~120-150 g in females. Encased in a fibrous renal capsule, perirenal fat and renal fascia, anchored within the retroperitoneum. The renal hilum, on the medial aspect, contains the renal artery, vein and ureter.

Internal Anatomy: Divided into the cortex (outer) and medulla (inner).The medulla contains 8-12 renal pyramids, with apices forming papillae that project into minor calyces. Minor calyces merge into 2-3 major calyces, draining into the renal pelvis.

Blood Supply

Renal arteries (branches of the abdominal aorta) supply ~20-25% of cardiac output.

Venous drainage via renal veins to the inferior vena cava. Microcirculation includes glomerular capillaries for filtration and peritubular capillaries for reabsorption.

Nerve supply

Sympathetic (T10-L1) and parasympathetic (vagus nerve) inputs via the renal plexus regulate blood flow and ureteral peristalsis.

Variations

Accessory renal arteries (~20-30% of individuals).

Horseshoe kidney (1 in 500): Fused kidneys at the lower poles, often asymptomatic but prone to obstruction.

Congenital solitary kidney (1 in 1000): One kidney absent, with compensatory hypertrophy.

Pelvic kidney: Ectopic kidney in the pelvis due to failed ascent during embryogenesis.

Ureter

Three anatomical constrictions: Ureteropelvic junction, pelvic brim (where it crosses the common iliac vessels) and vesicoureteral junction.

Histology: Mucosa: Transitional epithelium with a lamina propria.

Muscularis: Inner longitudinal and outer circular smooth muscle layers (reverse in the lower third).

Adventitia: Connective tissue anchoring the ureter.

Blood Supply: Segmental supply from renal, gonadal, common iliac and vesical arteries.

Venous drainage correspond to arterial supply.

Nerve supply: Sympathetic (T10-L2) and parasympathetic (S2-S4) fibres via the ureteric plexus.

Variations

Duplicated ureter (1 in 125): Complete or partial duplication, increasing risk of vesicoureteral reflux (VUR) or obstruction.

Retrocaval ureter: Right ureter passes behind the inferior vena cava, potentially causing hydronephrosis.

Ectopic ureter: Insertion outside the bladder trigone (e.g., urethra, vagina), leading to incontinence or infection.

Urinary Bladder

A hollow, muscular organ in the pelvis, posterior to the pubic symphysis and anterior to the uterus and vagina. Shape varies with filling: tetrahedral when empty, ovoid when full.

Capacity: ~300-500 mL in females, with urge to void at ~200-250 ml.

Anatomical regions: Apex, body, fundus and neck (containing the internal urethral orifice).The trigone, a smooth triangular area between the ureteral orifices and internal urethral orifice, is relatively fixed.

Histology: Mucosa: Transitional epithelium (5-7 layers, thinning when stretched) with a lamina propria.

Muscularis (detrusor muscle): Three smooth muscle layers (inner longitudinal, middle circular, outer longitudinal).

Adventitia (partial serosa superiorly): Connective tissue with peritoneum on the superior surface.

Blood Supply

Arterial: Superior and inferior vesical arteries (branches of the internal iliac artery).

Venous drainage via the vesical venous plexus to the internal iliac veins.

Nerve Supply

Parasympathetic (S2-S4, pelvic splanchnic nerves): Detrusor contraction, internal sphincter relaxation.

Sympathetic (T11-L2, hypogastric nerves): Detrusor relaxation, internal sphincter contraction. Somatic (S2-S4, pudendal nerve): External urethral sphincter control.

Variations

Congenital diverticula: Outpouchings of the bladder wall, predisposing to stasis and infection.

Urachal anomalies: Persistent urachus (e.g., patent urachus, urachal cyst) from incomplete closure of the allantois.

Exstrophy: Bladder exposed externally due to anterior abdominal wall defect (rare, ~1 in 50,000).

Urethra

A short muscular tube (~3-5 cm long, 6-8 mm diameter) extending from the bladder neck to the external urethral meatus. Located anterior to the vagina, embedded in the anterior vaginal wall. Passes through the urogenital diaphragm, surrounded by the external urethral sphincter (striated muscle). External meatus opens in the vestibule, between the clitoris and vaginal orifice.

Histology

Mucosa: Transitional epithelium near the bladder, transitioning to stratified squamous epithelium distally. Submucosa: Vascular spongy tissue with mucous glands (paraurethral glands).

Muscularis: Inner longitudinal and outer circular smooth muscle, plus the external sphincter.

Blood Supply

Arterial: Internal pudendal and vaginal arteries; **venous drainage** to the internal pudendal veins.

Nerve Supply

Somatic (pudendal nerve, S2-S4): External sphincter control. Autonomic: Sympathetic (T11-L2) and parasympathetic (S2-S4) for smooth muscle.

Variations

Urethral diverticulum: Outpouching of the urethral wall, often causing dysuria or dribbling.

Hypospadias (rare in females): Urethral meatus opens on the anterior vaginal wall.

Urethral duplication: Extremely rare, with a second urethral channel.

Physiology of the Female Urinary Tract

Kidney Functions

1. Filtration

Glomeruli filter ~180 L/day of plasma, producing a glomerular filtrate (GFR ~120 mL/min in females). Filtration barrier: Fenestrated endothelium, basement membrane and podocyte slit diaphragms.

2. Reabsorption and Secretion

a. Proximal tubule: Reabsorbs ~65% of filtrate (water, glucose, Na+, K+, amino acids).
b. Loop of Henle: Establishes medullary osmotic gradient for urine concentration.
c. Distal tubule and collecting duct: Fine-tune electrolyte and water balance under hormonal control (aldosterone, ADH). Secretion of H+, K+ and organic compounds (e.g., drugs) into the filtrate.

3. Hormonal Regulation

a. Renin-angiotensin-aldosterone system (RAAS): Regulates blood pressure and Na+ reabsorption.
b. Antidiuretic hormone (ADH): Increases water reabsorption in collecting ducts.
c. Erythropoietin: Stimulates red blood cell production.1,25-dihydroxyvitamin D3: Enhances calcium absorption.

Ureteral Function

Peristalsis: Smooth muscle contractions (1-5/min) propel urine from the renal pelvis to the bladder. Initiated by pacemaker cells in the renal pelvis, modulated by autonomic innervation.

Anti-reflux mechanism: Oblique entry of ureters into the bladder and intramural compression prevent vesicoureteral reflux (VUR).

Bladder function

Storage Phase: Detrusor muscle relaxes (sympathetic dominance, β-adrenergic receptors), and the internal sphincter contracts (α-adrenergic receptors). External sphincter remains tonically contracted (somatic control). Bladder compliance allows filling without significant pressure rise.

Voiding Phase: Parasympathetic stimulation (M3 receptors) causes detrusor contraction and internal sphincter relaxation. Somatic inhibition relaxes the external sphincter, allowing micturition. Coordination via the pontine micturition centre and sacral spinal reflexes (S2-S4).

Hormonal Influence: Estrogen enhances urethral mucosal integrity and sphincter tone; progesterone may reduce detrusor tone, increasing residual volume during pregnancy.

Urethral Function

Continence: Coaptation of the urethral mucosa, submucosal vascular cushion and sphincter tone maintain closure. Intra-abdominal pressure (e.g., coughing) compresses the urethra against the anterior vaginal wall, aiding continence.

Micturition: Relaxation of the external sphincter and smooth muscle allows urine flow. Short length and proximity to the vagina increase susceptibility to bacterial ascension (e.g., E. coli).

Shorter urethra (3-5 cm vs. 18-20 cm in males) increases risk of urinary tract infections (UTIs), with ~50% of females experiencing a UTI in their lifetime. Proximity of the urethral meatus to the vagina and anus facilitates bacterial contamination. Pelvic organs (uterus, vagina) influence bladder position and function, especially during pregnancy or prolapse.

Physiological Variations

Pregnancy: Increased renal blood flow (+50-80%), GFR (+50%), and ureteral dilation (right > left due to dextrorotation of the uterus), predisposing to hydronephrosis and UTIs.

Menopause: Estrogen deficiency reduces urethral mucosal thickness and sphincter tone, increasing risk of incontinence and UTIs.

Clinical Implications

1. Stress urinary incontinence (SUI): Common in females (~25-45% prevalence), due to weakened pelvic floor muscles or urethral hypermobility (e.g., post-childbirth).
2. Overactive bladder (OAB): Detrusor overactivity, affecting ~15-20% of women, often idiopathic or post-menopausal.
3. Vesicovaginal fistula: Rare but significant, often post-surgical or obstetric, causing continuous incontinence.

Developmental and Congenital Variations

Embryology

Kidneys develop from the metanephros, with ascend from the pelvis to the lumbar region by the 8th week of gestation. Ureters form from the ureteric bud, and the bladder develops from the urogenital sinus and allantois. Urethra derives from the urogenital sinus, with female differentiation driven by the absence of androgens.

Common Anomalies

1. Multicystic dysplastic kidney: Non-functional kidney with cysts, often unilateral.
2. Ureterocoele: Cystic dilation of the distal ureter, potentially obstructing urine flow.
3. Posterior urethral valves (rare in females): Membranous obstruction causing bladder outlet obstruction.

Clinical Relevance and Diagnostic Imaging

1. Ultrasound: First-line for detecting hydronephrosis, stones or congenital anomalies.
2. CT/MRI: Detailed anatomy for complex variations (e.g., ectopic ureter).

3. Voiding cystourethrogram (VCUG): Assesses VUR or urethral pathology.
4. Functional Tests: Urinalysis and culture: Diagnose UTIs or hematuria.
5. Urodynamics: To evaluate bladder pressure, capacity and sphincter function in incontinence or overactive bladder.
6. Cystoscopy: Visualizes urethra and bladder mucosa for structural abnormalities.
7. Antibiotics for UTIs; prophylaxis in recurrent cases.
8. Pelvic floor exercises or surgery (e.g., mid-urethral sling) for SUI. Anticholinergics or β3-agonists for OAB. Surgical correction for congenital anomalies (e.g., ureteral reimplantation for VUR).

1.5 Rectum and Anal Canal

(*Am'a' mustaqeem wa Qanat shrjiya*)

The rectum and anal canal form the terminal segments of the gastrointestinal tract, playing critical roles in the storage and controlled expulsion of feces. Their anatomical and physiological adaptations ensure effective defecation while maintaining continence.

Anatomy of the Rectum

The rectum is the final 12–15 cm of the large intestine, extending from the sigmoid colon to the anal canal. It serves as a temporary storage site for feces before defecation.

Gross Anatomy

Location: The rectum lies in the posterior pelvis, anterior to the sacrum and coccyx and posterior to the bladder (in males) or uterus and vagina (in females).

Boundaries

Proximal: Begins at the rectosigmoid junction (approximately at the level of the S3 vertebra or the sacral promontory), where the sigmoid mesocolon ends.

Distal: Terminates at the anorectal junction, where it transitions into the anal canal, marked by the passage through the pelvic diaphragm.

Structure

The rectum lacks taeniae coli, omental appendices and haustra, distinguishing it from the sigmoid colon. It has a wider lumen than the sigmoid colon, with three lateral flexures corresponding to the valves of Houston (transverse folds of mucosa and submucosa).

The rectum is divided into:

1. Upper third: Intraperitoneal, covered by peritoneum anteriorly and laterally.
2. Middle third: Retroperitoneal, with peritoneum covering only the anterior surface.
3. Lower third: Extraperitoneal, below the peritoneal reflection.
4. Curvatures: Sacral flexure: A posterior curve following the concavity of the sacrum.
5. Perineal flexure: An anterior curve at the anorectal junction, maintained by the puborectalis muscle, forming the anorectal angle (approximately 90° at rest).

Relations

1. Anterior: Rectouterine pouch (pouch of Douglas), uterus, cervix and vagina.
2. Posterior: Sacrum, coccyx, sacral plexus and median sacral vessels.
3. Lateral: Pararectal fossae, iliac vessels, ureters and levator ani muscles.

Microscopic Anatomy -The rectal wall consists of four layers:

Mucosa: Epithelium: Simple columnar with goblet cells, producing mucus for lubrication. Lamina propria: Contains lymphoid nodules and crypts of Lieberkühn (no villi). Muscularis mucosae: Thin layer of smooth muscle.

Submucosa: Loose connective tissue with blood vessels, lymphatics and Meissner's plexus. **Muscularis externa**: Two layers of smooth muscle (inner circular, outer longitudinal) without taeniae coli. The inner circular layer thickens at the anorectal junction to form the internal anal sphincter.

Serosa/Adventitia: Peritoneum covers the upper rectum (serosa); the lower rectum has adventitia blending with surrounding connective tissue.

Blood Supply

Arterial: Superior rectal artery: From the inferior mesenteric artery, supplies the upper and middle rectum. Middle rectal arteries: From the internal iliac arteries, supply the lower rectum (variable). Inferior rectal arteries: From the internal pudendal arteries, supply the anorectal junction.

Venous: Superior rectal vein: Drains into the portal system via the inferior mesenteric vein. Middle and inferior rectal veins: Drain into the systemic circulation via the internal iliac veins.

Portosystemic anastomoses: Occur between superior and middle/inferior rectal veins, clinically significant in portal hypertension (forming haemorrhoids).

Lymphatic Drainage: Upper rectum: Drains to inferior mesenteric and para-aortic nodes.

Lower rectum: Drains to internal iliac and inguinal nodes.

Nerve Supply

Sympathetic: From the inferior mesenteric and hypogastric plexuses (L1–L2), inhibits peristalsis and contracts the internal anal sphincter.

Parasympathetic: From pelvic splanchnic nerves (S2–S4), promotes peristalsis and relaxes the internal anal sphincter.

Enteric: Auerbach's (myenteric) and Meissner's (submucosal) plexuses coordinate local motility and secretion.

Anatomy of the Anal Canal

The anal canal is a 3-4 cm muscular tube extending from the anorectal junction to the anus, responsible for maintaining continence and facilitating defecation.

Gross Anatomy

Boundaries

Proximal: Anorectal junction, where the rectum passes through the levator ani (puborectalis sling). Distal: Anus, the external opening surrounded by perianal skin.

Divisions

1. Anatomical anal canal: From the anorectal junction to the anus.
2. Surgical anal canal: From the dentate (pectinate) line to the anus.
3. Dentate (Pectinate) Line: A critical landmark at the midpoint of the anal canal (1.5–2 cm from the anus). Marks the transition between endodermal (above) and ectodermal (below) derivatives. Site of anal valves and crypts, where anal glands may open.
4. Anal Columns (of Morgagni): Longitudinal mucosal folds above the dentate line, containing terminal branches of the superior rectal vessels.
5. Anal Sinuses: Recesses between anal columns, draining into anal glands.
6. Anorectal Angle: Formed by the puborectalis muscle, maintained at 90° to promote continence.

Sphincters

Internal Anal Sphincter (IAS): Involuntary smooth muscle, a thickened continuation of the rectal circular muscle layer. Extends from the anorectal junction to just above the dentate line. Maintains resting tone (70-85% of continence).

External Anal Sphincter (EAS): Voluntary striated muscle, composed of three parts (subcutaneous, superficial, deep). Surrounds the lower anal canal, blending with the puborectalis superiorly. Provides voluntary control during defecation.

Puborectalis Muscle: Part of the levator ani, forms a U-shaped sling around the anorectal junction. Maintains the anorectal angle and contributes to continence.

Microscopic Anatomy

1. Above the Dentate Line: Epithelium: Simple columnar, continuous with the rectum. Submucosa: Contains terminal branches of superior rectal vessels and nerves.
2. Below the Dentate Line: Epithelium: Stratified squamous (non-keratinized above the anal opening, keratinized at the perianal skin).
3. Submucosa: Dense connective tissue with inferior rectal vessels and nerves.
4. Transitional Zone: A 0.5–1 cm region above the dentate line with stratified columnar or cuboidal epithelium.

Blood Supply

Arterial: Above dentate line: Superior rectal artery (inferior mesenteric). Below dentate line: Inferior rectal arteries (internal pudendal).

Venous: Above dentate line: Superior rectal vein (portal system).

Below dentate line: Inferior rectal veins (systemic circulation).

Portosystemic anastomoses: At the dentate line, contributing to haemorrhoid formation.

Lymphatic Drainage: Above dentate line: Internal iliac and inferior mesenteric nodes.

Below dentate line: Superficial inguinal nodes.

Nerve Supply

1. Above Dentate Line: Autonomic: Sympathetic (hypogastric plexus) and parasympathetic (pelvic splanchnic nerves). Insensitive to pain (visceral innervation).

2. Below Dentate Line: Somatic: Inferior rectal nerves (from pudendal nerve, S2–S4). Sensitive to pain, touch, and temperature.
3. Internal Anal Sphincter: Autonomic (sympathetic contracts, parasympathetic relaxes).
4. External Anal Sphincter and Puborectalis: Somatic (pudendal nerve, voluntary control).

Physiology of the Rectum and Anal Canal

The rectum and anal canal coordinate the storage, sensation and expulsion of feces while maintaining continence through a complex interplay of muscular, neural and sensory mechanisms.

Rectal Functions Storage: The rectum acts as a compliant reservoir, accommodating feces until defecation is appropriate. The valves of Houston slow faecal descent, allowing gradual distension.

Sensation: Stretch receptors in the rectal wall detect distension, triggering the recto anal inhibitory reflex (RAIR) and the urge to defecate. The RAIR causes transient relaxation of the internal anal sphincter in response to rectal distension, allowing sampling of rectal contents by the anal mucosa.

Motility: Weak peristaltic contractions move feces toward the anal canal. Retrograde contractions may return feces to the sigmoid colon to delay defecation.

Anal Canal Functions

1. Continence: Resting Tone: Primarily maintained by the internal anal sphincter (70–85%), with contributions from the external anal sphincter and puborectalis.
2. Anorectal Angle: The puborectalis sling creates a 90° angle, mechanically obstructing faecal passage.
3. Hemorrhoidal Cushions: Vascular plexuses above and below the dentate line act as a seal, preventing leakage.
4. Anal Sampling: The RAIR allows the anal mucosa to distinguish between solid, liquid, and gas, enabling selective passage (e.g., flatus).
5. Defecation: Initiation: Rectal distension stimulates the RAIR, relaxing the internal anal sphincter, and signals the urge to defecate via pelvic splanchnic nerves.
6. Voluntary Control: The external anal sphincter and puborectalis can contract to delay defecation or relax to permit it.
7. Expulsion: The squatting position or Valsalva manoeuvre straightens the anorectal angle (to ~120°). Relaxation of the external anal sphincter and puborectalis, combined with rectal contraction and increased intra-abdominal pressure, expels feces. The levator ani elevates to widen the pelvic outlet.
8. Neural Coordination
    a. Intrinsic (Enteric): Myenteric and submucosal plexuses regulate local reflexes (e.g., RAIR).
    b. Extrinsic: Parasympathetic: Pelvic splanchnic nerves promote rectal contraction and sphincter relaxation. Sympathetic: Inhibits motility and maintains sphincter tone.
    c. Somatic: Pudendal nerve controls voluntary sphincter contraction.
    d. Cortical Control: The brain modulates the urge to defecate, allowing voluntary inhibition via the external anal sphincter.

9. Mucus Secretion: Goblet cells in the rectal mucosa and anal glands secrete mucus to lubricate feces, reducing trauma during defecation. Mucus also protects the anal epithelium from abrasion and infection.

Clinical Correlations

Understanding the anatomy and physiology of the rectum and anal canal is essential for diagnosing and managing related disorders:

1. **Haemorrhoids:** Engorgement of portosystemic venous plexuses due to increased intra-abdominal pressure or portal hypertension.
2. **Anal Fissures:** Tears in the anal mucosa below the dentate line, causing pain due to somatic innervation.
3. **Rectal Prolapse:** Weakness of pelvic floor muscles or ligaments allowing rectal protrusion.
4. **Faecal Incontinence:** Dysfunction of the internal/external anal sphincters or puborectalis, often due to trauma, neuropathy, or surgery.
5. **Anorectal Abscess/Fistula**: Infection of anal glands at the dentate line, leading to abscess formation or fistulous tracts.
6. **Colorectal Cancer:** Commonly arises in the rectum, requiring knowledge of lymphatic drainage for staging and treatment.

1.6 Perineum, Pelvic Floor Muscles & Ligaments

(*Farsh-i- Ana ke Adalat aur Ribatat*)

Perineum

The perineum is the superficial region located between the thighs, extending from the pubic symphysis anteriorly to the coccyx posteriorly. It is the inferior boundary of the pelvis and contains structures critical for urogenital and anorectal functions.

Anatomical Boundaries

The perineum is diamond-shaped and divided into two triangles by an imaginary transverse line connecting the ischial tuberosities:

Anterior (Urogenital) Triangle: Boundaries: Pubic symphysis (anterior), ischial tuberosities (lateral), transverse line (posterior).

Contents: External genitalia, urethra and superficial pelvic floor muscles.

Posterior (Anal) Triangle: Boundaries: Transverse line (anterior), coccyx (posterior), ischial tuberosities (lateral).

Contents: Anus, anal sphincter complex and ischioanal fossae.

Perineal Body

A fibromuscular structure at the midline junction of the urogenital and anal triangles.

Location: Between the vaginal opening (or posterior scrotum in males) and the anus.

Attachments: Serves as an anchor for muscles of the perineum, including the external anal sphincter, superficial and deep transverse perineal muscles, and bulbospongiosus.

Clinical Significance: The perineal body is critical for pelvic floor integrity. Damage (e.g., during childbirth) can lead to pelvic organ prolapse or incontinence.

Layers of the Perineum

1. Skin: Thin and sensitive, with hair in adults.
2. Subcutaneous Tissue: Contains fat and connective tissue, with the superficial perineal pouch.
3. Perineal Fascia:
    a. Superficial Perineal Fascia: Continuous with Colles' fascia; covers the superficial perineal pouch.
    b. Deep Perineal Fascia: Forms the inferior boundary of the deep perineal pouch (urogenital diaphragm).
4. Muscles and Pouches:
    a. Superficial Perineal Pouch: Contains ischiocavernosus, bulbospongiosus and superficial transverse perineal muscles.
    b. Deep Perineal Pouch: Contains the external urethral sphincter, deep transverse perineal muscles.

Pelvic Floor Muscles

The pelvic floor is a muscular diaphragm that supports pelvic viscera, maintains continence and facilitates childbirth, urination and defecation. It consists of the levator ani and coccygeus muscles, collectively termed the pelvic diaphragm.

Levator Ani

The levator ani is a broad, funnel-shaped muscle group forming the majority of the pelvic floor. It arises from the pelvic sidewalls and converges toward the midline to support pelvic organs.

Components of Levator Ani

1. Pubococcygeus

Origin: Posterior surface of the pubis and anterior tendinous arch of the pelvic fascia.

Insertion: Coccyx, anococcygeal ligament and perineal body (via midline raphe).

Subdivisions: Pubovaginalis (females): Supports the vagina.

2. Iliococcygeus

Origin: Tendinous arch of the pelvic fascia and ischial spine.

Insertion: Coccyx and anococcygeal raphe.

Function: Provides a broad supportive platform for pelvic viscera.

3. Puborectalis

Origin: Pubic bone (bilaterally).

Insertion: Forms a U-shaped sling around the rectum, with no bony insertion. Forms a sling around the anorectal junction, maintaining the anorectal angle (90°) for faecal continence.

Function: Elevates the pelvic floor, compresses the urethra and vagina, and maintains the anorectal angle. Pulls the rectum anteriorly, maintaining faecal continence .

Nerve Supply

Pudendal nerve (S2–S4): Supplies the puborectalis and external anal sphincter. Nerve to levator ani (direct branches from S3–S5): Supplies pubococcygeus and iliococcygeus.

Blood Supply

Internal pudendal artery and branches of the inferior gluteal artery.

Coccygeus (Ischiococcygeus)

Origin: Ischial spine and sacrospinous ligament.

Insertion: Lateral margins of the coccyx and lower sacrum.

Blood Supply: Inferior gluteal and internal pudendal arteries.

Nerva Supply: Branches of S4–S5.

Function: Supports the pelvic floor and stabilizes the sacroiliac joint

Perineal Muscles (Superficial and Deep)

Superficial Perineal Muscles

1. Ischiocavernosus: Covers the crura of the penis/clitoris.

Function: Maintains penile/clitoral erection by compressing venous outflow.

2. Bulbospongiosus: In females: Surrounds the vaginal introitus, supporting the perineal body.

(In males: Surrounds the bulb of the penis, aiding in ejaculation)

3. Superficial Transverse Perinea: Stabilizes the perineal body.

Nerve supply: Pudendal nerve (S2–S4).

Blood Supply: Internal pudendal artery.

Deep Perineal Muscles

1. Deep Transverse Perineal: Supports the perineal body and stabilizes the urethra.
2. External Urethral Sphincter: Compresses the urethra to maintain urinary continence.

Nerve Supply: Pudendal nerve.

Blood Supply: Internal pudendal artery.

Ligaments of the Pelvic Floor

Ligaments provide passive support to the pelvic viscera and reinforce the pelvic floor muscles. They are condensations of pelvic fascia or connective tissue.

Tendinous Arch of Pelvic Fascia: A thickened band of fascia extending from the pubis to the ischial spine. Serves as the origin for parts of the levator ani (pubococcygeus and iliococcygeus).

Function: Anchors the pelvic floor muscles to the pelvic sidewall.

Sacrospinous Ligament: Location: Extends from the ischial spine to the sacrum and coccyx. Relation: Lies deep to the coccygeus muscle. Function: Stabilizes the sacrum and coccyx, divides the greater and lesser sciatic foramina.

Sacrotuberous Ligament: Location: Extends from the sacrum and coccyx to the ischial tuberosity. Function: Stabilizes the sacroiliac joint and supports the pelvic floor indirectly.

Anococcygeal Ligament: Location: Extends from the anus to the coccyx. Function: Supports the pelvic floor and anchors the levator ani.

Pubovesical Ligament: Anchors the bladder to the pubis.

Transverse Cervical (Cardinal or Mackenrodt) Ligament: Supports the uterus and vagina. This is the most important of all the ligaments.

Uterosacral Ligament: Anchors the uterus to the sacrum.

Perineal Membrane (Urogenital Diaphragm): A fibromuscular layer spanning the urogenital triangle. Contains the deep transverse perineal muscles and external urethral sphincter.

Function: Supports the urethra and vagina, maintaining continence.

Physiology of the Perineum and Pelvic Floor

The perineum and pelvic floor function as an integrated unit to support pelvic organs, maintain continence and facilitate reproduction and excretion.

Support of Pelvic Viscera

The levator ani and coccygeus muscles form a dynamic sling that supports the bladder, uterus (in females), prostate (in males), and rectum. The perineal body and perineal membrane provide additional passive support. Ligaments (e.g., sacrospinous, sacrotuberous) stabilize the bony pelvis, indirectly supporting the pelvic floor.

Continence

Urinary Continence: The external urethral sphincter (voluntary) and internal urethral sphincter (involuntary) control urine flow. The pubococcygeus and puborectalis compress the urethra during increased intra-abdominal pressure (e.g., coughing).

Faecal Continence: The puborectalis maintains the anorectal angle, preventing involuntary defecation. The external anal sphincter (voluntary) and internal anal sphincter (involuntary) regulate anal closure.

Defecation and Urination

Relaxation of the puborectalis straightens the anorectal angle, facilitating defecation.

Relaxation of the external urethral sphincter allows urination, coordinated with detrusor muscle contraction.

Reproduction

The pelvic floor relaxes during childbirth to allow passage of the fetus. The perineal body and bulbospongiosus support vaginal integrity.

The pelvic floor muscles contribute to vaginal tone and sexual sensation in females.

Clinical Correlations

1. Pelvic Organ Prolapse: Weakening of the levator ani or perineal body (e.g., due to childbirth or aging) can lead to prolapse of the bladder (cystocele), uterus, or rectum (rectocele).

2. Episiotomy: Surgical incision of the perineum during childbirth to facilitate delivery and prevent severe tearing may weaken the perineal body, increasing prolapse risk.

3. Incontinence:

Stress Urinary Incontinence: Weak pelvic floor muscles fail to compress the urethra during increased intra-abdominal pressure.

Faecal Incontinence: Damage to the puborectalis or external anal sphincter impairs the anorectal angle or sphincter function.

4. Pudendal Nerve Injury: Trauma or compression (e.g., during prolonged labor) can weaken perineal muscles, leading to incontinence or prolapse.

5. Perineal Tears: Obstetric trauma can damage the perineal body or anal sphincter, requiring surgical repair.

1.7 Developmental Anomalies

(*Khilqi nqayes*)

Congenital anomalies of the female genital tract arise from abnormal embryonic development of the Mullerian (paramesonephric) ducts, urogenital sinus or associated structures. These anomalies vary widely in presentation, ranging from asymptomatic variations to severe defects causing infertility, pain or obstetric complications.

Embryological Basis

The female genital tract develops primarily from the Mullerian ducts and the urogenital sinus between the 6th and 12th weeks of gestation:

Mullerian Ducts: Originate as paired structures in the intermediate mesoderm. Cranial portions form the fallopian tubes. Caudal portions fuse to form the uterus, cervix and upper two-thirds of the vagina. Fusion and subsequent canalization are needed for normal anatomy.

Urogenital Sinus: Contributes to the lower third of the vagina and parts of the external genitalia. The sinovaginal bulbs and vaginal plate are key structures in vaginal development.

External Genitalia: Develop from the genital tubercle, urogenital folds and labioscrotal swellings under the influence of hormonal signals (or lack of).

Key Processes

1. Fusion: The Mullerian ducts fuse midline to form a single uterovaginal canal.
2. Canalization: The fused ducts form a lumen.
3. Septal Resorption: The midline septum between the ducts resorbs to create a single uterine cavity and vagina.
4. Regression of Male Structures: In females, the Wolffian (mesonephric) ducts regress due to the absence of anti-Mullerian hormone (AMH) and testosterone.

Disruptions in these processes (e.g., incomplete fusion, failed resorption, or abnormal signaling) lead to congenital anomalies. Genetic, environmental and hormonal factors may contribute, though many cases are idiopathic.

Classification of Anomalies

Congenital anomalies are classified based on anatomical defects and embryological origins. The American Society for Reproductive Medicine (ASRM) classification (updated 2021) is widely used, supplemented by the European Society of Human Reproduction and Embryology (ESHRE)/European Society for Gynaecological Endoscopy (ESGE) system for detailed subtyping.

Anomalies are grouped as follows:

1. Uterine Anomalies: Result from defective fusion, canalization or septal resorption of Mullerian ducts. Examples: Septate uterus, bicornuate uterus, unicornuate uterus, uterine didelphys.
2. Cervical Anomalies: Often associated with uterine or vaginal anomalies. Examples: Cervical agenesis, cervical duplication.
3. Vaginal Anomalies: Arise from defective canalization or fusion of Mullerian ducts and urogenital sinus. Examples: Vaginal agenesis, transverse vaginal septum, longitudinal vaginal septum.
4. External Genitalia Anomalies: Less common; often linked to disorders of sexual differentiation or urogenital sinus anomalies. Examples: Ambiguous genitalia, clitoral hypertrophy.
5. Complex Anomalies: Involve multiple structures (e.g., Mullerian agenesis syndromes like Mayer-Rokitansky-Kuster-Hauser syndrome).

Specific Anomalies: Anatomy and Physiology

Uterine Anomalies

a. Septate Uterus

Anatomy: Partial or complete failure of septal resorption after Mullerian duct fusion, resulting in a fibrous or muscular septum dividing the uterine cavity. Subtypes include partial (subseptate) or complete septum extending to the cervix.

Physiology: The septum may impair implantation or placental development, increasing risks of miscarriage, preterm birth and malpresentation. Endometrial function is typically normal, but the septum's avascular nature can reduce viable implantation sites.

Prevalence: Most common uterine anomaly (~35–50% of uterine malformations).

Clinical Implications: Recurrent pregnancy loss, infertility, or asymptomatic presentation. Diagnosed via hysterosalpingography (HSG), 3D ultrasound or MRI.

b. Bicornuate Uterus

Anatomy: Incomplete fusion of Mullerian ducts, leading to a heart-shaped uterus with two horns and a partial fundal indentation. Subtypes include bicornuate unicollis (single cervix) or bicollis (two cervices).

Physiology: The endometrial cavity is divided, potentially reducing functional space for gestation. Cervical competence may be compromised, increasing preterm delivery risk.

Prevalence: ~10–25% of uterine anomalies.

Clinical Implications: Obstetric complications (e.g., preterm labor, malpresentation) or asymptomatic. Surgery (e.g., metroplasty) is rarely indicated.

c. Unicornuate Uterus

Anatomy: Unilateral Mullerian duct development with agenesis or hypoplasia of the contralateral duct. May have a rudimentary horn (communicating or non-communicating).

Physiology: Reduced uterine capacity limits fetal growth, increasing risks of preterm birth and intrauterine growth restriction (IUGR). Rudimentary horns may cause pain or ectopic pregnancy if functional.

Prevalence: ~5–20% of uterine anomalies.

Clinical Implications: Infertility, ectopic pregnancy, or rupture of rudimentary horn. Associated with renal anomalies (e.g., unilateral renal agenesis).

d. Uterine Didelphys

Anatomy: Complete failure of Mullerian duct fusion, resulting in two separate uteri and cervices, often with a longitudinal vaginal septum.

Physiology: Each uterus functions independently, but obstetric complications (e.g., preterm delivery, malpresentation) are common due to reduced uterine volume.

Prevalence: ~5–10% of uterine anomalies.

Clinical Implications: May be asymptomatic or present with dyspareunia, dysmenorrhea or obstetric issues. Vaginal septum resection may improve outcomes.

e. Arcuate Uterus

Anatomy: Mild indentation at the uterine fundus due to incomplete septal resorption. Considered a normal variant by some classifications.

Physiology: Minimal impact on reproductive function; endometrial and myometrial function are typically normal.

Prevalence: Common (~15–25% of women in some studies).

Clinical Implications: Rarely associated with adverse outcomes; often incidental finding.

Cervical Anomalies

a. Cervical Agenesis/Dysgenesis

Anatomy: Complete absence (agenesis) or hypoplasia (dysgenesis) of the cervix, often with a functional uterus. May be isolated or associated with vaginal agenesis.

Physiology: Menstrual outflow obstruction leads to hematometra, causing cyclic pelvic pain or amenorrhea. Fertility is compromised unless surgical reconstruction is feasible.

Clinical Implications: Primary amenorrhea, endometriosis due to retrograde menstruation, or infertility. Hysterectomy may be required in severe cases.

b. Cervical Duplication

Anatomy: Two cervices, typically associated with uterine didelphys or septate uterus.

Physiology: Each cervix may function normally, but obstetric risks (e.g., cervical incompetence) are elevated.

Clinical Implications: Often asymptomatic but may complicate labor or delivery.

Vaginal Anomalies

a. Vaginal Agenesis (Mayer-Rokitansky-Kuster-Hauser Syndrome, MRKH)

Anatomy: Absence of the vagina and variable uterine development (often rudimentary uterine remnants). Ovaries are typically normal.

Physiology: Normal ovarian function results in secondary sexual characteristics but primary amenorrhea due to absent uterus/vagina. Sexual function is impaired without intervention.

Prevalence: ~1 in 4,500–5,000 females.

Clinical Implications: Diagnosed in adolescence with primary amenorrhea.

Treatment includes vaginal dilators or surgical neovagina creation. Associated with renal (30–40%) and skeletal anomalies.

b. Transverse Vaginal Septum

Anatomy: Fibrous or muscular septum across the vaginal canal, resulting from incomplete canalization. May be complete (obstructing) or partial.

Physiology: Complete septa cause menstrual outflow obstruction, leading to hematocolpos or hematometra. Partial septa may allow menstruation but cause dyspareunia.

Clinical Implications: Cyclic pelvic pain, primary amenorrhea, or infertility. Surgical resection is curative.

c. Longitudinal Vaginal Septum

Anatomy: Midline septum dividing the vagina, often associated with uterine didelphys.

Physiology: May cause no symptoms or lead to dyspareunia, obstructed labor, or difficulty with tampon use.

Clinical Implications: Resection improves sexual and obstetric outcomes.

External Genitalia Anomalies

Anatomy: Malformations of the clitoris, labia, or vaginal introitus, often linked to urogenital sinus anomalies or disorders of sexual differentiation.

Physiology: Functional impact depends on severity; severe cases may affect urination, sexual function or fertility.

Clinical Implications: May require surgical correction for functional or cosmetic reasons. Associated with syndromes like congenital adrenal hyperplasia.

Complex Anomalies

a. Mullerian Agenesis Syndrome

Include MRKH and other rare conditions with combined uterine, cervical and vaginal agenesis.

Physiology: Normal ovarian function but absent menstrual and reproductive capacity.

Clinical Implications: Psychological counselling and fertility options (e.g., surrogacy) are critical.

b. Obstructed Hemivagina and Ipsilateral Renal Anomaly (OHVIRA) Syndrome

Anatomy: Uterine didelphys with an obstructed hemivagina and ipsilateral renal agenesis.

Physiology: Menstrual blood accumulates in the obstructed hemivagina, causing pain and potential endometriosis.

Clinical Implications: Early surgical intervention prevents complications like infection or infertility.

Variations and Normal Findings

Some findings, previously considered anomalies, are now recognized as normal variations:

1. Arcuate Uterus: Minimal fundal indentation with negligible clinical impact.
2. Vaginal Rugae Variations: Differences in vaginal wall texture or length within normal ranges.
3. Hymenal Variants: Imperforate, microperforate or septate hymens may be congenital but are often managed easily.

Diagnostic Approach

Diagnosis relies on a combination of history, physical examination and imaging:

History: Primary amenorrhea, cyclic pelvic pain, infertility or recurrent miscarriage.

Physical Exam: Assess external genitalia, vaginal patency and palpable masses (e.g., hematocolpos).

Imaging:

1. Ultrasound (2D/3D): First-line for uterine and vaginal anomalies.
2. MRI: Gold standard for complex anomalies, especially MRKH or OHVIRA. 3. Hysterosalpingography (HSG): Evaluates uterine cavity and tubal patency. 4.Laparoscopy/Hysteroscopy: Confirms diagnosis and allows therapeutic intervention (e.g., septum resection).

Physiological and Clinical Implications

1. Reproductive Impact: Anomalies like septate or unicornuate uterus increase miscarriage and preterm birth risks due to reduced uterine capacity or poor implantation sites.
2. Vaginal/cervical obstructions cause infertility if untreated.
3. Menstrual Dysfunction: Outflow obstructions (e.g., transverse septum, cervical agenesis) lead to hematometra/ hematocolpos, causing pain and endometriosis.
4. Obstetric Complications: Malpresentation, preterm labor and cesarean delivery are more common with uterine anomalies.
5. Psychosocial Impact: Diagnoses like MRKH can cause significant emotional distress, requiring counselling and support.

Management and Treatment

Observation

Asymptomatic anomalies (e.g., arcuate uterus, partial septate uterus) often require no intervention.

Surgical Management

1. Septate Uterus: Hysteroscopic septum resection improves pregnancy outcomes.
2. Vaginal Septum: Surgical excision for transverse or longitudinal septa.

3. MRKH Syndrome: Vaginal dilators or neovagina creation (e.g., McIndoe procedure).
4. OHVIRA: Resection of obstructed hemivagina.

Fertility Options: Assisted reproductive technologies (ART) for women with unicornuate uterus or post-surgical infertility. Surrogacy for MRKH or severe uterine anomalies.

Multidisciplinary Care: Involves gynaecologists, reproductive endocrinologists, urologists and psychologists for complex cases.

Associated Anomalies

Congenital genital tract anomalies are often associated with other systems due to shared embryological origins.

Renal Anomalies: Unilateral renal agenesis (common in unicornuate uterus, MRKH, OHVIRA).

Skeletal Anomalies: Vertebral defects in MRKH .

Cardiac/Other: Rare, but seen in syndromes like MURCS (Mullerian duct aplasia, renal aplasia, and cervicothoracic somite dysplasia).

Key References

American Society for Reproductive Medicine. (2021). Mullerian anomalies classification. ESHRE/ ESGE. (2013).

Consensus on the classification of female genital tract congenital anomalies. Chan, Y. Y., et al. (2011).

Reproductive outcomes in women with congenital uterine anomalies: A systematic review. Ultrasound in Obstetrics & Gynaecology. Grimbizis, G. F., et al. (2016).

Clinical implications of congenital uterine anomalies: A meta-analysis. Human Reproduction Update.

1.8 Description of intersex

(*Bayn al-jinsiyat ka byan*)

Intersex

Intersex may be defined as the presence of both male and female external and /or internal genital organs in the same individual causing confusion in the diagnosis of true sex. These conditions result in variations in internal or external genitalia, gonadal structure or sex chromosomes, leading to a spectrum of phenotypic presentations.

Epidemiology: Estimates vary widely, ranging from 0.05% to 1.7% of the population, depending on the criteria used. Broader definitions, including milder variations like hypospadias, increase prevalence.

Geographic and Ethnic Variation: No significant geographic or ethnic predisposition is noted, though certain genetic conditions (e.g., Congenital Adrenal Hyperplasia) may be more prevalent in specific populations due to consanguinity or founder effects.

Classification of Intersex

Intersex conditions are classified based on the underlying etiology, including chromosomal, gonadal or anatomical differences. The 2006 Consensus Statement on Management of DSD categorizes them into three main groups:

1. 46, XX DSD

Individuals with a 46, XX karyotype but atypical genital or reproductive development due to excessive androgen exposure, gonadal anomalies or other factors.

a. Congenital Adrenal Hyperplasia (CAH)

Etiology: Most common cause: 21-hydroxylase deficiency (autosomal recessive, CYP21A2 gene mutations). Other enzyme defects: 11β-hydroxylase deficiency, 3β-hydroxysteroid dehydrogenase deficiency (rarer). Leads to impaired cortisol and aldosterone synthesis, causing adrenal hyperplasia and excess adrenal androgens.

Pathophysiology: Reduced cortisol feedback increases ACTH, stimulating adrenal androgen production. Androgens virilize external genitalia during fetal development, while Mullerian structures (uterus, fallopian tubes) remain intact due to absent anti-Mullerian hormone (AMH).

Clinical Features

Neonatal: Ambiguous genitalia (e.g., clitoromegaly, labial fusion, urogenital sinus). Severity graded by Prader scale (I–V).

Salt-Wasting CAH: Hypotension, hyponatremia, hyperkalemia and dehydration due to aldosterone deficiency (life-threatening if untreated).

Non-Salt-Wasting CAH: Milder virilization, may present later with precocious puberty or hirsutism.

Adolescence/Adulthood: Menstrual irregularities, infertility or polycystic ovary syndrome (PCOS)-like features due to persistent hyperandrogenism.

Diagnosis

Lab Tests: Elevated 17-hydroxyprogesterone, androstenedione and ACTH; low cortisol. Electrolyte imbalances in salt-wasting forms.

Genetic Testing: CYP21A2 mutation analysis.

Imaging: Ultrasound to confirm Mullerian structures and adrenal hyperplasia. Newborn Screening: Routine in many countries to detect 21-hydroxylase deficiency early.

Management

Medical: Glucocorticoids (e.g., hydrocortisone) to suppress ACTH and adrenal androgens. Mineralocorticoids for salt-wasting CAH. Monitoring for adequate suppression and growth velocity.

Surgical: Vaginoplasty or clitoroplasty for severe virilization, ideally delayed until informed consent unless medically necessary (e.g., urogenital sinus causing obstruction).

Psychosocial: Counseling for gender identity, family support and patient education.

Long-Term Considerations: Risk of adrenal crisis during stress (e.g., illness, surgery). Fertility challenges due to anovulation or anatomical issues; assisted reproductive technologies may be required. Osteoporosis risk from long-term glucocorticoid use. Psychological support for body image and gender identity concerns.

b. Maternal Androgen Exposure

Etiology: Exposure to exogenous androgens (e.g., anabolic steroids, progestins) or endogenous androgens (e.g., maternal adrenal or ovarian tumors) during pregnancy.

Pathophysiology: Androgens cross the placenta, virilizing the fetus's external genitalia while Mullerian structures remain unaffected.

Clinical Features: Ambiguous genitalia at birth (e.g., clitoromegaly, labial fusion). Normal internal female reproductive structures. No adrenal or gonadal dysfunction postnatally.

Diagnosis: Maternal history of medication use or tumors. Normal 46,XX karyotype and hormonal profile. Ultrasound to confirm Mullerian structures.

Management: Address maternal condition (e.g., tumor resection, cessation of offending drugs). Surgical correction of genitalia, if desired, typically delayed. Psychosocial support for family and patient.

Long-Term Considerations: Generally good prognosis with no ongoing hormonal issues. Fertility unaffected.

c. Ovotesticular DSD (46, XX)

Etiology: Presence of both ovarian and testicular tissue, often due to mosaicism, chimerism, or SRY gene translocation to an X chromosome.

Pathophysiology: Mixed gonadal tissue leads to variable hormone production (estrogens, androgens, AMH), causing ambiguous genitalia or atypical pubertal development.

Clinical Features: Ambiguous genitalia at birth (e.g., ovotestis, urogenital sinus). Variable pubertal development (e.g., breast development with virilization). May present with primary amenorrhea or infertility.

Diagnosis: Karyotyping (46,XX or mosaic).Hormonal testing: Mixed estrogen, testosterone, and AMH levels. Imaging and biopsy to confirm ovotesticular tissue.

Management: Hormonal therapy to align with gender identity or address deficiencies.

Surgical options: Gonadectomy (due to malignancy risk in testicular tissue), genital reconstruction based on patient preference. Multidisciplinary care with psychosocial support.

Long-Term Considerations: High risk of gonadal tumors (e.g., gonadoblastoma). Infertility common; fertility preservation may be explored. Ongoing psychological support for gender identity and social integration.

2. 46, XY DSD

Individuals with a 46, XY karyotype but incomplete masculinization due to defects in androgen production, action or gonadal development.

a. Androgen Insensitivity Syndrome (AIS)

Etiology: Mutations in the AR gene (X-linked) impair androgen receptor function.

Complete AIS (CAIS): Complete receptor dysfunction.

Partial AIS (PAIS): Partial receptor function.

Pathophysiology

CAIS: Androgens (testosterone, DHT) produced by testes are ineffective, leading to female external genitalia. AMH causes Müllerian duct regression (no uterus).

PAIS: Partial androgen action results in ambiguous genitalia (e.g., micropenis, hypospadias).

Clinical Features

CAIS: Female external genitalia, blind-ending vagina. Absent uterus and fallopian tubes; intra-abdominal testes. Presents with primary amenorrhea in adolescence or incidental inguinal hernias (containing testes). Normal breast development due to aromatized estrogens.

PAIS: Ambiguous genitalia at birth (e.g., clitoromegaly, hypospadias).Variable pubertal development (e.g., partial virilization, gynecomastia).

Diagnosis: Karyotype: 46, XY. Hormonal profile: Elevated testosterone and LH (in CAIS); variable in PAIS. Genetic testing: AR gene mutations.

Imaging: Ultrasound/MRI to locate testes and confirm absent Mullerian structures.

Management

CAIS: Estrogen replacement post-pubertal gonadectomy to prevent osteoporosis and support feminization. Gonadectomy due to malignancy risk (e.g., seminoma, ~2–5% risk). Vaginoplasty or dilation for sexual function, if needed.

PAIS: Hormonal therapy (e.g., testosterone for masculinization or estrogen for feminization, based on gender identity).

Surgical correction of genitalia, delayed until informed consent. Psychosocial support for gender identity and family.

Long-Term Considerations: Infertility universal in CAIS; possible in PAIS with assisted reproductive techniques. Psychological support for gender dysphoria or social stigma. Monitoring for gonadal tumors if testes retained.

b. 5-alpha-Reductase Deficiency

Etiology: Autosomal recessive mutations in SRD5A2 gene, impairing conversion of testosterone to DHT.

Pathophysiology: DHT is critical for external genital masculinization; its deficiency leads to undervirilized genitalia despite normal testicular testosterone production. Mullerian structures absent due to AMH action.

Clinical Features: Ambiguous genitalia at birth (e.g., micropenis, hypospadias, cryptorchidism). Virilization at puberty due to high testosterone levels (e.g., deepening voice, muscle development). May be raised as female but identify as male at puberty.

Diagnosis: Karyotype: 46,XY.Hormonal profile: High testosterone, low DHT, elevated testosterone/DHT ratio. Genetic testing: SRD5A2 mutations. Imaging: Testes present, no Mullerian structures.

Management: Hormonal therapy: Testosterone or DHT analogs for masculinization, if aligned with gender identity. Surgical options: Genital reconstruction (e.g., hypospadias repair) based on patient preference. Psychosocial support for gender identity transitions, especially at puberty. Long-Term Considerations: Fertility possible with assisted reproductive technologies. Psychological support for potential gender role changes. Monitoring for testicular malignancy if cryptorchidism untreated.

c. Gonadal Dysgenesis (e.g., Swyer Syndrome)

Etiology: Mutations in genes critical for testicular development (e.g., SRY, SOX9, DMRT1).

Swyer syndrome: 46, XY with nonfunctional or streak gonads.

Pathophysiology: Failure of testicular differentiation leads to absent testosterone and AMH, resulting in female external genitalia and persistent Mullerian structures.

Clinical Features: Female external genitalia, normal uterus and fallopian tubes. Streak gonads, leading to primary amenorrhea and lack of spontaneous puberty. Tall stature, minimal secondary sexual characteristics.

Diagnosis: Karyotype: 46, XY. Hormonal profile: Low testosterone, estrogen and AMH; elevated FSH/LH. Genetic testing: SRY or related gene mutations.

Imaging: Ultrasound/MRI to confirm Mullerian structures and streak gonads.

Management: Hormonal therapy: Estrogen and progesterone replacement for pubertal induction and maintenance. Gonadectomy due to high risk of gonadoblastoma (>30%). Fertility options: Uterus present, allowing pregnancy via donor oocytes and assisted reproduction. Psychosocial support for gender identity and infertility.

Long-Term Considerations: Osteoporosis risk without estrogen replacement. Psychological support for infertility and gender identity. Regular monitoring for hormone therapy side effects.

3. Sex Chromosome DSD

Conditions involving atypical sex chromosome configurations (e.g., 45X, 47XXY, mosaicism).

a. Turner Syndrome (45, XO or Mosaic)

Etiology: Partial or complete absence of one X chromosome (45X or mosaic, e.g., 45X/46XX).

Pathophysiology: Loss of X-linked genes (e.g., SHOX) leads to streak gonads, ovarian failure and systemic features (e.g., short stature).

Clinical Features: Female phenotype, short stature, webbed neck, lymphedema, cardiac anomalies (e.g., coarctation of aorta). Primary amenorrhea, absent puberty due to ovarian dysgenesis. Normal external genitalia, underdeveloped uterus.

Diagnosis: Karyotype: 45X or mosaic. Hormonal profile: Elevated FSH/LH, low estrogen. Imaging: Ultrasound to confirm streak ovaries and Mullerian structures. Screening for comorbidities (e.g., cardiac, renal anomalies).

Management: Growth hormone therapy for height optimization. Estrogen and progesterone replacement for pubertal induction and bone health. Fertility options: Oocyte donation for pregnancy. Multidisciplinary care for comorbidities (e.g., cardiology, endocrinology).

Long-Term Considerations: Infertility without assisted reproduction. Increased risk of osteoporosis, cardiovascular disease, and hypothyroidism. Psychosocial support for body image and infertility.

b. Klinefelter Syndrome (47, XXY)

Etiology: Extra X chromosome (47,XXY or mosaic).

Pathophysiology: Testicular dysfunction due to additional X chromosome leads to hypogonadism and impaired spermatogenesis.

Clinical Features: Male phenotype, tall stature, small testes, gynecomastia. Delayed or incomplete puberty, infertility. Learning disabilities or behavioral challenges in some cases.

Diagnosis: Karyotype: 47,XXY or mosaic.

Hormonal profile: Low testosterone, elevated FSH/LH, variable estradiol.

Semen analysis: Azoospermia or severe oligospermia.

Management: Testosterone replacement for pubertal development, muscle mass, and bone health. Fertility options: Sperm retrieval (e.g., testicular sperm extraction) for assisted reproduction. Psychosocial support for body image, infertility, and learning difficulties.

Long-Term Considerations: Increased risk of osteoporosis, metabolic syndrome, and breast cancer. Regular monitoring for testosterone therapy side effects. Psychological support for social and fertility concerns.

c. Mixed Gonadal Dysgenesis (e.g., 45,X/ 46,XY Mosaicism)

Etiology: Mosaicism or chimerism involving 45,X and 46,XY cell lines.

Pathophysiology: Variable gonadal development (e.g., streak gonad on one side, dysgenetic testis on the other), leading to asymmetric hormone production and genital ambiguity.

Clinical Features: Ambiguous genitalia at birth (e.g., unilateral cryptorchidism, hypospadias). Variable Mullerian structures (e.g., hemi-uterus). May present with short stature or Turner-like features.

Diagnosis: Karyotype: Mosaic 45,X/46,XY. Hormonal profile: Variable testosterone, estrogen, and AMH levels. Imaging and biopsy: To assess gonadal structure and Mullerian remnants.

Management: Hormonal therapy based on gender identity (estrogen or testosterone). Gonadectomy due to high gonadoblastoma risk (>30%). Surgical correction of genitalia, if desired, delayed until informed consent. Psychosocial support for gender identity and family.

Long-Term Considerations: Infertility common; fertility preservation explored if feasible.

Monitoring for gonadal tumors and hormone-related complications.

Psychological support for gender dysphoria and social integration.

General Diagnostic Approach History

Prenatal exposures, family history, developmental milestones.

Physical Exam: Genital assessment (Prader/Quigley scale), secondary sexual characteristics, dysmorphic features.

Lab Tests: Karyotype, hormonal profiles (testosterone, DHT, AMH, FSH, LH, 17-hydroxyprogesterone), genetic testing.

Imaging: Ultrasound/MRI for internal genitalia and gonadal location.

Biopsy: For ovotesticular or dysgenetic gonads, if indicated.

Psychosocial Assessment: Gender identity, family dynamics, and mental health.

General Management

Hormonal therapy tailored to condition and gender identity; monitoring for complications (e.g., adrenal crisis, gonadal malignancy).

Surgical: Deferred until informed consent unless medically urgent (e.g., malignancy risk, urinary obstruction). Procedures include gonadectomy, vaginoplasty, or hypospadias repair.

Psychosocial: Counseling for patients and families, addressing gender identity, fertility, and societal stigma. Support groups enhance patient empowerment.

Fertility: Discuss preservation options early (e.g., oocyte/sperm banking, assisted reproduction).

Complications and Long-Term Outcomes

Medical: Gonadal tumors, osteoporosis, cardiovascular risks, adrenal crisis (in CAH).

Psychosocial: Gender dysphoria, stigma, mental health challenges.

Fertility: Infertility common; assisted reproductive technologies may be viable in select cases.

Long Answer Questions (LAQs)

1. Describe the anatomy of the female genital tract, including the external structures in details.
2. Describe the anatomical features of the internal genital organs and explain their physiological functions in detail. .
3. Discuss the embryological development of female genitalia, highlighting internal and external differentiation.
4. Explain the phases and hormonal regulation of the menstrual cycle with suitable diagrams.
5. Explain the term intersex in details and its classifications.

Short Answer Questions (SAQs)

1. What are the different parts of the external genitalia?
2. Describe the various developmental anomalies of uterus
3. Write a short note on the structure and function of the breast.
4. What is the role of the pelvic floor ligaments and name them?
5. Explain turner syndrome and Klinefelter syndrome in short.

Multiple Choice Questions (1 Mark Each)

1. Which hormone triggers ovulation?

a) Estrogen b) FSH c) LH d) Progesterone

Ans: c) LH

2. The uterus develops embryologically from:

a) Wolffian duct b) Müllerian duct c) Genital tubercle d) Mesonephros

Ans: b) Mullerian duct

3. Average duration of a menstrual cycle is:

a) 24 days b) 28 days c) 32 days d) 36 days

Ans: b) 28 days

4. The clitoris develops from:

a) Urogenital sinus b) Genital tubercle c) Labioscrotal swelling d) Müllerian duct

Ans: b) Genital tubercle

5. Corpus luteum secretes:

a) FSH b) LH c) Estrogen d) Progesterone

Ans: d) Progesterone

6. Which organ is the site of fertilization?

a) Ovary b) Uterus c) Vagina d) Fallopian tube

Ans: d) Fallopian tube

7. What is the average length of the fallopian tubes?

a) 5-7 cm b) 10-12 cm c) 15-20 cm d) 25-30 cm

Ans: b) 10-12 cm

8. The innermost layer of uterus is called:

a) Myometrium b) Endometrium c) Perimetrium d) Parametrium

Ans: b) Endometrium

9. Hormone responsible for endometrial proliferation:

a) Progesterone b) Estrogen c) LH d) Testosterone

Ans: b) Estrogen

10. Which of the following is a part of the internal genitalia?

a) Labia minora b) Vagina c) Clitoris d) Mons pubis

Ans:b)Vagina

02

History Taking & Gynecological Examination

(Rudad-i-marad aur nesayee imtehan)

2.1 *Amrad-i-Niswan ke ilaj wa Mu'alaja se mutalliq akhlaqiyyat aur usul wa zawabit* (Moral Values & Ethics in gynecology practice)
2.2 *Ruduad-i-marad* (History taking)
2.3 *Imtehan-i-Umumi wa Nizami* (General and systemic examination)
2.4 *Imtehan-i-ana* (Pelvic Examination)
2.5 Imtehan-i-thadyayn (Breast Examination)

Learning Objective (At the end of the session, the students should be able to)

Describe the Moral Values & justify the importance of Ethics in Gynaecology & Obstetrics Practices.
Describe & create a document for the Informed consent.
Discuss the detailed History-taking in Gynaecology & Obstetrics.
Illustrate the General & Systemic Examination.
Perform & explain the Breast examination and Breast self- examination.
Observe & assist in the performance of Pelvic Examination.
Document & present 10 Complete Case Report of Gynaecology with Provisional Diagnosis.
Document & present 10 Complete Case Report of Obstetrics with Provisional Diagnosis.
Document & present Patient's Discharge summary.

2.1 Moral Values and Ethics in Gynecology Practice

(*Amrad-i-Niswan ke ilaj wa Mu'alaja se mutalliq akhlaqiyyat aur usul wa zawabit*)

Gynecology is a medical specialty that focuses on women's reproductive health, including menstruation, pregnancy, childbirth and diseases of the reproductive system. Because gynecology involves sensitive, personal and sometimes life-altering decisions, moral values and ethics play a critical role in ensuring patients are treated with respect, dignity and fairness.

Moral Values: These are beliefs about what is right and wrong. They guide how doctors interact with patients, colleagues and society. Examples include honesty, respect, compassion and fairness.

Ethics: Ethics in medicine are rules and principles that help doctors make decisions that are morally right. Medical ethics provide a framework to balance patient needs, medical science and societal values.

In gynecology, moral values and ethics ensure that doctors provide care that respects patient rights, maintains trust and promotes well-being.

Core Ethical Principles in Gynecology

Four main ethical principles guide medical practice, including gynecology. These principles help doctors make decisions when faced with complex situations:

1. Autonomy

Respecting a patient's right to make decisions about their own body and health.

In gynecology: Gynecologists must ensure patients understand their health conditions and treatment options so they can make informed choices. For example, a woman deciding whether to have a hysterectomy (removal of the uterus) should be given clear information about risks, benefits, and alternatives and her decision should be respected, even if the doctor disagrees.

Example: A 30-year-old woman refuses a recommended cesarean section for childbirth, preferring a normal vaginal delivery. The gynecologist should respect her choice, provided she understands the risks and benefits.

2. Beneficence

Acting in the best interest of the patient to promote their health and well-being.

In gynecology: Gynecologists should recommend treatments that are likely to benefit the patient based on medical evidence. For instance, prescribing medication to manage heavy menstrual bleeding or performing surgery to remove ovarian cysts can improve a patient's quality of life.

Example: A gynecologist recommends regular cervical cancer screenings for a patient to catch any issues early, even if the patient feels healthy.

3. Non-Maleficence

"Do no harm." Doctors must avoid causing harm to patients through their actions or decisions.

In gynecology: This means carefully weighing the risks of procedures or treatments. For example, a gynecologist should avoid unnecessary surgeries that could lead to complications like infections or infertility.

Example: Before prescribing a hormonal treatment for menopause symptoms, the gynecologist checks the patient's medical history to avoid risks like blood clots.

4. Justice

Treating all patients fairly and ensuring equal access to care, regardless of their background, income or beliefs.

In gynecology: Gynecologists should provide the same quality of care to all patients, whether they are rich or poor, young or old, or from different cultural backgrounds. This also includes advocating for resources, like access to contraception or cancer screenings, for underserved communities.

Example: A gynecologist ensures that a low-income patient receives free or subsidized mammograms through a community health program.

Importance of Ethics in Gynecology

Gynecology deals with sensitive issues like reproduction, sexuality and personal health choices, which can deeply affect a patient's life. Ethical practice is essential for the following reasons:

Building Trust: Patients share personal and private information with gynecologists. Ethical behavior, such as maintaining confidentiality, ensures patients feel safe and respected.

Respecting Diversity: Women come from different cultures, religions and backgrounds. Ethical gynecologists respect these differences when discussing treatments, such as contraception or fertility options.

Protecting Vulnerable Patients: Some patients, like teenagers or survivors of abuse, may feel scared or powerless. Ethical care ensures their voices are heard and their rights are protected.

Balancing Conflicting Interests: Gynecologists often face situations where patient wishes, family expectations and medical guidelines conflict. Ethics help navigate these challenges fairly.

Key Ethical Issues in Gynecology

Gynecologists often encounter unique ethical challenges. Below are common issues and how to address them ethically:

1. Informed Consent

Patients must fully understand their diagnosis, treatment options, risks and benefits before agreeing to any procedure.

Example: Before performing a tubal ligation (sterilization), the gynecologist explains that it is permanent method and discusses reversible contraception options also. The patient should sign a consent form only after understanding all details.

Ethical tip: Use simple language, avoid medical terms and give patients time to ask questions.

2. Confidentiality

Gynecologists must keep patient information private unless the patient gives permission to share it or there is a legal requirement (e.g., reporting abuse).

Example: A teenager seeks birth control but doesn't want her parents to know. The gynecologist respects her privacy, provided it's legally allowed in that region.

Ethical tip: Always explain to patients how their information will be protected and when it might need to be shared (e.g., for insurance purposes).

3. Cultural Sensitivity

Patients may have cultural or religious beliefs that affect their healthcare choices, such as refusing certain treatments or preferring female doctors.

Example: A Muslim patient requests a female gynecologist for a pelvic exam due to religious beliefs. The clinic arranges for a female doctor to respect her preferences.

Ethical tip: Learn about the cultural practices of your patient population and avoid judgment.

4. Reproductive Choices

Gynecologists often counsel patients on sensitive topics like abortion, contraception or infertility treatments. They must remain neutral and respect the patient's decisions.

Example: A woman considering abortion is given unbiased information about her options, including continuing the pregnancy, adoption or termination, without the doctor pushing their personal beliefs.

Ethical tip: Focus on the patient's needs and values, not your own opinions.

5. Dealing with Minors Teenagers

It may seek care for issues like contraception or pregnancy without parental consent. Laws vary by country, but ethical practice prioritizes the minor's autonomy and safety.

Example: A 16-year-old requests an STI test. The gynecologist provides the test confidentially, following local laws and counsels her on safe practices.

Ethical tip: Know the legal guidelines in your area regarding minors and healthcare.

6. End-of-Life and Palliative Care

In cases of advanced gynecological cancers, gynecologists may need to discuss end-of-life care or palliative options to reduce suffering.

Example: A patient with terminal ovarian cancer is offered palliative care to manage pain and improve quality of life, respecting her wishes to avoid aggressive treatments.

Ethical tip: Involve the patient and family in discussions and focus on comfort and dignity.

7. Resource Allocation

In areas with limited healthcare resources, gynecologists must decide how to fairly distribute care, such as prioritizing patients for surgery or screenings.

Example: A hospital has limited slots for free cervical cancer screenings. The gynecologist prioritizes high-risk patients, like those with a family history of cancer, while advocating for more resources.

Ethical tip: Advocate for equitable access to care for all patients.

Ethical Gynecology Practice

1. Communicate Clearly: Use simple language to explain medical conditions and treatments. Encourage patients to ask questions and express concerns.

2. Listen Actively: Pay attention to patient's fears, preferences and values. This builds trust and helps individualize care to their needs.
3. Stay Updated: Follow the latest medical guidelines and ethical standards to provide evidence-based care.
4. Seek Consent: Always obtain informed consent before procedures, ensuring patients understand all aspects of their care.
5. Respect Privacy: Protect patient information and discuss sensitive topics in private settings.
6. Avoid Bias: Treat all patients equally, regardless of their background and avoid letting personal beliefs influence care.
7. Collaborate: Work with other healthcare professionals, like counselors or social workers, to address complex ethical issues.
8. Reflect on Decisions: Regularly think about your actions and whether they align with ethical principles. Seek guidance from ethics committees if needed.

Ethical Dilemmas and How to Handle Them

Sometimes, gynecologists face situations where ethical principles conflict.

For example:

1. Dilemma: A pregnant patient refuses a life-saving treatment for religious reasons, but it could harm the fetus.

Approach: Respect the patient's autonomy while explaining the risks to both her and the fetus. Offer counseling and involve an ethics committee if needed to balance autonomy and beneficence.

2. Dilemma: A patient requests a procedure (e.g., cosmetic genital surgery) that the doctor believes is unnecessary or risky.

Approach: Discuss the patient's reasons for wanting the procedure, provide evidence-based information about risks, and explore alternatives. If the patient insists, consider referring them to another provider while respecting their autonomy.

To resolve dilemmas: Gather all relevant facts about the patient's condition and wishes. Consult ethical guidelines, such as those from medical associations (e.g., FIGO or ACOG). Discuss with colleagues or an ethics committee for complex cases. Document your decision-making process clearly.

The Role of Professional Guidelines

Many organizations, like the International Federation of Gynecology and Obstetrics (FIGO) and the American College of Obstetricians and Gynecologists (ACOG), provide ethical guidelines for gynecologists. These guidelines cover topics like informed consent, confidentiality and reproductive rights. Gynecologists should familiarize themselves with these standards and local laws to ensure ethical practice.

Conclusion

Moral values and ethics are the foundation of good gynecology practice. By respecting patient autonomy, acting in their best interest, avoiding harm, and ensuring fairness, gynecologists can provide care that is compassionate and trustworthy. Ethical practice not only improves patient outcomes but also strengthens the doctor-patient relationship and upholds the integrity of the medical profession.

2.2 History Taking in Gynecology

(Ruduad-i-marad)

History taking is a critical first step in gynecology, as it helps doctors understand a patient's health concerns, diagnose conditions and plan appropriate treatments. Gynecology focuses on women's reproductive health, including menstruation, pregnancy, childbirth and disorders of the reproductive system. Since many gynecological issues are personal and sensitive, taking a thorough and empathetic history is essential to build trust and provide patient-centered care.

History Taking

History taking involves asking a patient specific questions about their health, symptoms and life circumstances to gather information that guides diagnosis and treatment. In gynecology, the history helps identify issues related to the reproductive system, such as menstrual problems, pelvic pain, infertility or pregnancy-related concerns. A well-taken history can provide up to 80% of the information needed for an accurate diagnosis, making it a cornerstone of gynecological care.

Importance of History taking

Identifies the Problem: The patient's description of symptoms (e.g., abnormal bleeding, pain) helps diagnosing potential conditions like endometriosis or fibroids.

Guides Examinations and Tests: The history determines which physical exams or diagnostic tests (e.g., ultrasound, Pap smear) are needed.

Builds Trust: Listening carefully and showing empathy makes patients feel comfortable discussing sensitive topics like sexual health or miscarriage.

Personalizes Care: Understanding the patient's lifestyle, medical history and preferences allows doctors to individualize treatments to their needs.

Prevents Errors: A thorough history reduces the chance of missing critical details that could lead to misdiagnosis or inappropriate treatment.

Key Components of a Gynecological History

A gynecological history is structured to cover all relevant aspects of a patient's health. Below are the main components, with explanations and examples:

Patient Identification and Demographics

Record the patient's name, age, occupation and marital status.

Age and lifestyle can influence gynecological conditions. For example, younger women may have irregular periods due to hormonal changes, while older women may face menopausal symptoms.

Example: A 25-year-old single woman may have different concerns (e.g., contraception) compared to a 55-year-old married woman (e.g., menopausal symptoms).

Chief Complaint

"What brought you here today?" or "What problem are you experiencing?" Ask about the main symptom in the patient's own words.

The chief complaint focuses the history and examination.

Example: A patient says, 'I've been having heavy periods for the last three months.' This guides the doctor to explore menstrual history and possible causes like fibroids.

History of Present Illness

Explore the chief complaint in detail using the "OPQRST" framework:

Onset: When did the symptom start? Was it sudden or gradual?

Position/Location: Where is the problem (e.g., pelvic pain)?

Quality: What does it feel like (e.g., sharp, dull, burning)?

Radiation: Does the symptom spread to other areas?

Severity: How bad is it (e.g., on a scale of 1–10)?

Timing: When does it happen? Is it constant or intermittent? Any triggers (e.g., menstruation, intercourse)?

This helps narrow down possible diagnoses. For example, pelvic pain during periods may suggest endometriosis, while pain during intercourse could indicate infections or ovarian cysts.

Example: A patient reports pelvic pain (chief complaint). On questioning, she says it started six months ago, is sharp, occurs during periods, and rates it 7/10 in severity. This prompts further questions about menstrual history and possible endometriosis.

Menstrual History

Age at menarche (first period).

Regularity, duration and flow of periods (e.g., cycle length, days of bleeding, heavy or light flow).

Any pain during periods (dysmenorrhea).

Last menstrual period (LMP) date.

Symptoms like clotting, spotting, or irregular bleeding.

Menopause status (if applicable) and symptoms like hot flashes.

Menstrual history is central to gynecology, as abnormalities can indicate conditions like polycystic ovary syndrome (PCOS), fibroids or hormonal imbalances.

Example: A 30-year-old woman reports irregular periods (every 40–60 days) and heavy bleeding with clots. This suggests possible PCOS or fibroids, prompting further investigation.

Obstetric History

Number of pregnancies (gravida) and outcomes (para), including live births, miscarriages, abortions or ectopic pregnancies.

Details of each pregnancy: Delivery method (vaginal or cesarean), complications or preterm births.

Current pregnancy status (if relevant).

Obstetric history can affect current gynecological health. For example, multiple cesarean sections may increase the risk of placenta previa in future pregnancies.

Example: A patient is “G3P2,” meaning three pregnancies and two live births. She had one miscarriage, which may prompt questions about recurrent pregnancy loss.

Gynecological History

Previous gynecological conditions (e.g., endometriosis, ovarian cysts, fibroids).

Past gynecological surgeries (e.g., hysterectomy, tubal ligation).

History of sexually transmitted infections (STIs). Cervical cancer screening (e.g., Pap smear results, HPV testing).

Use of contraception (e.g., pills, IUD, condoms).

Past conditions or surgeries can influence current symptoms or treatment options. For example, a history of abnormal Pap smears may indicate a higher risk of cervical cancer.

Example: A patient with a history of ovarian cysts reports new pelvic pain, suggesting a possible recurrence.

Sexual History

Sexual activity status (active or not). Number of partners and sexual orientation (if relevant). Any pain during intercourse (dyspareunia). History of sexual abuse or trauma (asked sensitively). Use of contraception or protection against STIs.

Sexual history can reveal risks for STIs, infertility, or conditions like vaginismus. It also guides counseling on safe practices.

Example: A patient reports pain during intercourse and irregular periods. This could suggest endometriosis or an infection, prompting further questions and tests.

Medical History

Chronic conditions (e.g., diabetes, hypertension, thyroid disorders).

Past surgeries (not just gynecological). Allergies to medications or other substances. Current medications (including over-the-counter drugs or supplements).

Medical conditions can affect gynecological health. For example, diabetes increases the risk of recurrent vaginal infections.

Example: A patient with hypothyroidism reports irregular periods, which may be linked to her thyroid condition.

Family History

Family history of gynecological conditions (e.g., breast or ovarian cancer, endometriosis). Genetic conditions or hereditary diseases. A family history of ovarian or breast cancer may indicate a need for genetic testing (e.g., BRCA mutations).

Example: A patient’s mother had ovarian cancer, prompting the doctor to recommend earlier or more frequent screenings.

Socioeconomic History

Lifestyle factors: smoking, alcohol, drug use, exercise, diet.

Occupation and stress levels. Living situation and support system (e.g., partner, family).

Cultural or religious beliefs affecting healthcare choices.

Social factors can influence health. For example, smoking increases the risk of cervical cancer and stress may affect menstrual regularity.

Example: A patient who smokes and uses oral contraceptives is at higher risk for blood clots, requiring counseling on alternative contraception.

Review of Systems

Ask about symptoms in other body systems, such as weight changes, fatigue, urinary issues or bowel problems.

Gynecological conditions can affect or be affected by other systems. For example, urinary symptoms may suggest a gynecological issue like a prolapsed uterus.

Example: A patient with pelvic pain also reports urinary urgency, which could indicate a urinary tract infection or pelvic organ prolapse.

Taking a gynecological history

Taking a gynecological history requires skill, empathy and sensitivity.

First create a comfortable environment

Ensure privacy (e.g., close the door, draw curtains).

Use a calm and friendly tone to put the patient at ease.

Explain that all information is confidential unless legally required to be shared.

Document clearly

Write or type the history in an organized format, including all components (chief complaint, menstrual history, etc.). Use clear, concise language for other healthcare providers to understand.

Special Considerations in Gynecology History

1. Taking Adolescent Patients

Teenagers may feel shy or scared. Build trust by explaining confidentiality and involving parents only if necessary (based on local laws). Focus on issues like irregular periods, contraception or STI prevention.

Example: A 15-year-old seeks contraception. Ask about her sexual activity sensitively and explain options like pills or condoms.

2. Elderly Patients

Older women may have menopausal symptoms, incontinence or cancer risks. Ask about postmenopausal bleeding, which could indicate endometrial cancer.

Example: A 65-year-old reports vaginal bleeding.

Explore the duration and amount, as this is a red flag requiring urgent investigation.

3. Cultural Sensitivity

Respect cultural beliefs that may affect care, such as preferences for female providers or avoidance of certain treatments.

Example: A patient refuses a pelvic exam due to cultural discomfort. Offer alternatives like imaging or a female provider.

4. Patients with Trauma

Survivors of sexual abuse or trauma may find gynecological visits distressing. Ask permission before discussing sensitive topics and avoid triggering language.

Example: Say, "Is it okay if I ask about your sexual history? You can skip any questions that make you uncomfortable."

5. Language Barriers

Use interpreters if the patient doesn't speak your language. Avoid relying on family members, as this may compromise confidentiality.

Example: A non-native language-speaking patient needs an interpreter to discuss her irregular periods accurately.

Example of a Gynecological History

Patient: 28-year-old female, married, teacher.

Chief Complaint: Heavy menstrual bleeding for 4 months.

History of Present Illness: Bleeding lasts 8 days (normal: 5 days), with large clots. Rates severity 8/10. No pain, but feels tired. No triggers identified.

Menstrual History: Menarche at 13, cycles every 28–30 days, usually moderate flow. LMP: 10 days ago. No dysmenorrhea.

Obstetric History: G1P1 (one vaginal delivery, no complications).

Gynecological History: No prior surgeries or STIs. Normal Pap smear 1 year ago. Uses condoms for contraception.

Sexual History: Sexually active with husband, no dyspareunia.

Medical History: No chronic conditions, no allergies, no medications.

Family History: Mother had fibroids. No cancer history.

Social History: Non-smoker, occasional alcohol, no drug use. Moderate stress from work.

Review of Systems: Fatigue, no urinary or bowel issues.

Summary: 28-year-old woman with heavy menstrual bleeding and fatigue, possibly due to fibroids given family history. Plan: Physical exam, ultrasound, blood tests for anemia.

Conclusion

History taking in gynecology is both an art and a science. It requires medical knowledge to ask the right questions and interpersonal skills to make patients feel heard and respected. By systematically covering all components—chief complaint, menstrual history, obstetric history and more—gynecologists can gather the information needed to diagnose and treat conditions effectively.

2.3 General and systemic examination

(*Imtehan-i-Umumi wa Nizami*)

A general and systemic examination in gynecology is a critical component of a comprehensive patient assessment, aimed at evaluating the overall health of the patient and identifying any gynecological or systemic conditions that may influence reproductive health.

General and Systemic Examination in Gynecology

The general and systemic examination in gynecology is performed to assess the patient's overall health status and to identify any underlying medical or systemic conditions that may impact gynecological health. It complements the specific gynecological examination (e.g., pelvic examination) and is essential for formulating a diagnosis and treatment plan. The examination is conducted systematically, with attention to detail, and noted in sequence, the patient's presenting complaints, medical history and clinical context.

1. General Examination

The general examination begins with a thorough observation and evaluation of the patient's overall appearance, vital signs and physical condition. This helps identify systemic conditions that may manifest with gynecological symptoms or affect reproductive health.

A. General Appearance

1. **Built and Nutrition:** Assess the patient's body habitus (e.g., thin, average, obese) and nutritional status. Obesity may be associated with conditions like polycystic ovary syndrome (PCOS), while cachexia may suggest malignancy or chronic illness.
2. **Posture and Gait:** Observe for abnormalities in posture or gait that may indicate musculoskeletal or neurological conditions affecting pelvic structures.
3. **Pallor:** Check for signs of anemia (e.g., pale conjunctiva, nail beds, or tongue), which may be related to menorrhagia or chronic disease.
4. **Icterus:** Look for jaundice in the sclera, skin or mucous membranes, which may indicate liver dysfunction or hemolytic conditions.
5. **Cyanosis:** Assess for central or peripheral cyanosis, which may suggest cardiorespiratory issues.
6. **Clubbing:** Examine fingers for clubbing, which could indicate chronic hypoxia or underlying malignancy.
7. **Edema:** Check for pedal edema or generalized edema, which may point to cardiac, renal or hypoproteinemic states.
8. **Lymphadenopathy:** Palpate for enlarged lymph nodes (e.g., cervical, axillary, inguinal), which may suggest infection, inflammation or malignancy.
9. **Skin and Hair:** Note skin texture, pigmentation (e.g., acanthosis nigricans in PCOS), or hirsutism (indicative of hyperandrogenism). Assess hair for thinning or alopecia, which may be related to hormonal imbalances.

B. Vital Signs

Pulse: Record the rate, rhythm, and volume. Tachycardia may indicate anemia, infection or anxiety.

Blood Pressure: Measure in both arms to detect hypertension (e.g., in preeclampsia) or hypotension (e.g., in hypovolemia due to heavy menstrual bleeding).

Respiratory Rate: Note any abnormalities, as respiratory conditions may impact surgical or pregnancy outcomes.

Temperature: Assess for fever, which may indicate infection (e.g., pelvic inflammatory disease).

C. Anthropometric Measurements

Height and Weight: Calculate the body mass index (BMI) to assess obesity or undernutrition. Obesity is a risk factor for endometrial cancer, PCOS and infertility.

Waist-to-Hip Ratio: Useful in assessing central obesity, which is linked to metabolic syndrome and gynecological disorders.

D. Specific Observations

Facial Features: Look for signs of hormonal disorders, such as acne, hirsutism or moon facies (Cushing's syndrome).

Thyroid Examination: Palpate the thyroid gland for enlargement or nodules, as thyroid dysfunction can affect menstrual cycles and fertility.

Breast Examination: Inspect and palpate for masses, nipple discharge or skin changes (e.g., peau d'orange in breast cancer). Breast tenderness may be associated with hormonal changes or pregnancy.

Secondary Sexual Characteristics: Assess breast development, pubic hair and axillary hair for signs of delayed or precocious puberty, or hormonal imbalances.

2. Systemic Examination

The systemic examination involves a detailed assessment of all major organ systems to identify conditions that may contribute to or complicate gynecological complaints. Each system is examined systematically, with specific attention to findings relevant to gynecology.

A. Cardiovascular System

Inspection: Look for jugular venous distension, precordial pulsations or signs of heart failure.

Palpation: Check the apex beat and assess for thrills or heaves.

Auscultation: Listen for heart sounds, murmurs or added sounds. Cardiovascular diseases may impact pregnancy outcomes or surgical fitness.

Relevance to Gynecology: Conditions like hypertension or heart disease are critical in managing pregnancy, especially in cases of preeclampsia or eclampsia.

B. Respiratory System

Inspection: Observe chest symmetry, respiratory rate and use of accessory muscles.

Palpation: Assess for chest expansion and tactile vocal fremitus.

Percussion and Auscultation: Check for abnormal breath sounds or areas of dullness. Respiratory conditions may affect anesthesia or pregnancy management.

Relevance to Gynecology: Chronic respiratory diseases can complicate pregnancy or surgical interventions.

C. Gastrointestinal System

Inspection: Look for abdominal distension, scars or visible peristalsis.

Palpation: Assess for tenderness, organomegaly (e.g., liver or spleen), or masses. Differentiate between gynecological masses (e.g., ovarian cysts) and gastrointestinal masses (e.g., appendiceal mass).

Percussion: Evaluate for ascites (e.g., shifting dullness in ovarian malignancy) or tympany.

Auscultation: Listen for bowel sounds to rule out obstruction or ileus.

Relevance to Gynecology: Gastrointestinal symptoms (e.g., bloating, pain) may overlap with gynecological conditions like ovarian tumors or endometriosis.

D. Central Nervous System

Higher Mental Functions: Assess consciousness, orientation and cognitive function.

Cranial Nerves: Evaluate for any deficits, especially in cases of suspected intracranial pathology (e.g., pituitary tumors affecting menstrual cycles).

Motor and Sensory System: Check muscle tone, power, reflexes and sensation. Neurological deficits may indicate spinal or pelvic nerve involvement.

Relevance to Gynecology: Neurological conditions may affect pelvic floor function or sexual health.

E. Endocrine System

Thyroid: Palpate for goiter or nodules. Hypothyroidism or hyperthyroidism can cause menstrual irregularities or infertility.

Adrenal: Look for signs of hyperandrogenism (e.g., hirsutism, acne) or Cushing's syndrome (e.g., striae, buffalo hump).

Pituitary: Assess for signs of prolactinoma (e.g., galactorrhea) or other pituitary dysfunctions affecting reproductive hormones.

Relevance to Gynecology: Endocrine disorders are closely linked to menstrual disorders, infertility and PCOS.

F. Musculoskeletal System

Spine and Pelvis: Inspect for deformities (e.g., scoliosis, kyphosis) that may affect pregnancy or delivery.

Joints: Assess for arthritis or joint pain, which may indicate autoimmune conditions like systemic lupus erythematosus (SLE), which can complicate pregnancy.

Relevance to Gynecology: Musculoskeletal abnormalities may impact labor or pelvic organ support.

G. Renal System

Inspection and Palpation: Check for costovertebral angle tenderness or renal enlargement.

Relevance to Gynecology: Renal dysfunction may be associated with preeclampsia or urinary tract infections, which are common in gynecological practice.

H. Hematological System

Signs of Anemia: Pallor, fatigue or koilonychia may indicate iron deficiency due to menorrhagia.

Bleeding Tendencies: Look for bruising, petechiae or ecchymosis may suggest coagulopathies.

Relevance to Gynecology: Hematological disorders can contribute to abnormal uterine bleeding or complicate pregnancy.

3. Specific Considerations in Gynecological Examination

While the general and systemic examination provides a holistic assessment, certain findings are particularly relevant in the context of gynecology:

1. Hormonal Imbalances: Signs like hirsutism, acne or galactorrhea may point to PCOS, hyperprolactinemia or adrenal disorders.
2. Systemic Diseases: Conditions like diabetes mellitus, hypertension or autoimmune diseases (e.g., SLE) can affect menstrual cycles, fertility or pregnancy outcomes.
3. Malignancy: Cachexia, lymphadenopathy or ascites may suggest gynecological malignancies like ovarian or endometrial cancer.
4. Infections: Fever, lymphadenopathy or skin lesions may indicate pelvic inflammatory disease or sexually transmitted infections.

4. Documentation

All findings from the general and systemic examination should be meticulously documented, including:

- Positive findings (e.g., pallor, thyroid enlargement, abdominal mass).
- Negative findings (e.g., no lymphadenopathy, normal heart sounds).
- Relevant measurements (e.g., BMI, blood pressure).
- Any abnormalities requiring further investigation (e.g., imaging, laboratory tests).

5. Clinical Correlation

The findings from the general and systemic examination must be correlated with the patient's history and specific gynecological examination (e.g., pelvic, speculum or bimanual examination). For example:

A patient with menorrhagia and pallor may require a complete blood count to confirm anemia.

A patient with hirsutism and obesity may need hormonal assays to diagnose PCOS.

A patient with ascites and weight loss may require imaging to rule out ovarian malignancy.

Conclusion

The general and systemic examination in gynecology is a cornerstone of patient evaluation, providing critical insights into the patient's overall health and its impact on gynecological conditions. By systematically assessing each organ system and correlating findings with the patient's history and gynecological examination, clinicians can formulate accurate diagnoses and effective management plans.

2.4 Pelvic Examination in Gynecology

(Imtehan-i-ana)

Pelvic examination is a cornerstone of gynecological clinical practice. It allows the physician to evaluate the external and internal female genitalia and related pelvic organs. It is essential for diagnosing a wide range of gynecological disorders and for routine health screening.

I. Indications for Pelvic Examination

Pelvic pain

Abnormal vaginal bleeding

Abnormal vaginal discharge or itching

Menstrual irregularities

Infertility evaluation

Routine gynecologic check-up

Suspected pelvic mass

Screening for cervical cancer (Pap smear)

Postmenopausal bleeding

Sexual dysfunction

II. Contraindications

Absolute: None

Relative: Severe pain or anxiety (may require sedation or delay), acute infections (perform gently or defer if needed)

III. Components of Pelvic Examination

Pelvic examination includes the following:

1. Preparation and Consent

Informed Consent: Explain the purpose, steps and possible discomfort. Gain verbal consent.

Privacy & Comfort: Ensure privacy, chaperone presence (especially for male examiners), use of drapes.

Bladder: Ask the patient to empty the bladder before the examination.

Position: Lithotomy position on examination table with feet in stirrups.

2. Inspection of External Genitalia (Vulval Examination)

Structures examined: Mons pubis, Labia majora and minora, Clitoris, Urethral meatus, Vaginal introitus, Perineum, Anus.

Look for: Skin lesions (warts, ulcers, pigmentation), Discharge (color, odor, amount), Inflammation, edema, Signs of trauma or abuse, Bartholin's gland swelling, female genital mutilation (FGM)

3. Speculum Examination (Vaginal and Cervical Inspection)

Types of Specula:

Cusco's speculum (self-retaining; used for non-pregnant women)

Sims' speculum (non-self-retaining; used with posterior vaginal wall retractor)

Procedure:

Warm and lubricate speculum (avoid lubricant if Pap smear is planned)

Gently insert speculum closed and angled downward

Open blades to visualize cervix and vaginal walls

Evaluate:

Vagina: Discharge, atrophy, lesions, foreign body

Cervix: Color, size, shape (nulliparous = round os, multiparous = slit-like os), ectopy, erosions, polyps, growths, bleeding

Discharge: Nature (white, curdy, green, foul-smelling, purulent)

Pap Smear/Biopsy: Collect samples if indicated

Wet mount or High Vaginal Swab (HVS): For infection.

4. Bimanual Examination

Purpose: To assess uterus, cervix, adnexa (ovaries and fallopian tubes)

Steps: Lubricate gloved index and middle fingers of the dominant hand. Gently insert into the vagina and place the non-dominant hand on the lower abdomen (just above pubic symphysis).

Finding

Cervix

Position (central, anterior, posterior)

Mobility (freely mobile or fixed)

Tenderness (cervical motion tenderness – seen in PID)

Consistency (firm or soft – soft in pregnancy)

Uterus

Size (normal, enlarged – fibroid, pregnancy)

Shape (globular in pregnancy, irregular in fibroids)

Position (anteverted, retroverted)

Mobility (mobile or fixed – adhesions, endometriosis)

Tenderness (suggests infection or inflammation)

Adnexa (Ovaries and Tubes)

Normally non-palpable

Palpable mass – ovarian cyst, tubo-ovarian abscess

Tenderness – PID

Fixity or irregularity – malignancy or endometriosis

5. Rectovaginal Examination (if indicated)

Indications:

To assess posterior pelvic structures (e.g., uterosacral ligaments, pouch of Douglas)

Suspected endometriosis, retroverted uterus, rectal involvement in malignancy.

Procedure: One finger in the vagina and one in the rectum

Assess: Thickness, nodularity or tenderness of uterosacral ligaments

Posterior uterine wall

Masses in the pouch of Douglas

Rectal masses or lesions

IV. Special Considerations

1. Pediatric and Adolescent Patients: External genital inspection only unless absolutely necessary, use smallest speculum if needed and psychological support and consent.
2. Virgin Patients: Avoid vaginal speculum and bimanual examination. Consider transabdominal or transrectal ultrasound and recto-abdominal exam if necessary
3. Pregnant Patients: Use appropriate-sized speculum. Be gentle during bimanual exam to avoid bleeding and cervical length, consistency, and os should be evaluated.

V. Documentation of Findings

Always record: Date and time of examination, Informed consent obtained, Presence of chaperone.

Findings: External genitalia, vaginal walls, cervix, discharge, uterine size/shape/position, adnexa.

Any samples taken (Pap smear, HVS, biopsy)

Patient response (pain, anxiety)

Conclusion

Pelvic examination remains a vital tool in gynecological diagnosis and screening. A systematic, gentle and respectful approach, with clear communication and patient comfort as priority, ensures accurate diagnosis and strengthens doctor–patient trust.

2.5 Breast Examination in Gynecology

(Imtehan-i-Thadyayn)

Breast examination is an essential component of a gynecologic evaluation as breast health is closely linked with reproductive and hormonal status. Early detection of breast pathology, particularly cancer, significantly improves prognosis and outcomes.

I. Importance of Breast Examination

Early detection of breast cancer

Evaluation of breast pain, lumps or discharge

Assessment of hormonal changes (e.g., puberty, pregnancy, lactation, menopause)

Routine check-up

Evaluation of gynecomastia or breast development abnormalities

II. Indications

Palpable breast lump

Breast pain (mastalgia)

Nipple discharge

Changes in breast shape, size, or skin

Follow-up of previously detected lesions

High-risk screening (family history, BRCA mutation)

Part of routine gynecologic or obstetric examination

III. Preparation and Patient Considerations

Ensure privacy and comfort

Explain the procedure thoroughly to the patient

Obtain informed consent

Use a female chaperone during the exam, especially if the examiner is male

Position: Sitting and supine positions required for complete evaluation

IV. Components of Breast Examination

Breast examination includes inspection and palpation, performed in two positions:

1. Sitting (upright)
2. Supine (lying down)

1. Inspection

Position: Patient seated upright, arms relaxed and then in raised positions.

Observe for: Symmetry (slight asymmetry is normal).

Size and shape of both breasts

Skin changes: Dimpling or puckering (suggests malignancy involving Cooper's ligaments), Redness or peau d'orange (edema of skin overlying cancer), Ulceration or eczematous changes (esp. Paget's disease)

Nipples

Position: Inversion, deviation

Discharge: Color, spontaneous or expressed

Retraction or ulceration

Areola: Pigmentation, scaling

Inspection in Different Arm Positions:

Arms at sides, arms raised above head, Hands pressed on hips (contracts pectoral muscles – brings out dimpling) or leaning forward (for pendulous breast evaluation)

2. Palpation

Performed in both seated and supine positions.

Seated palpation (if indicated): For axillary tail of Spence and axilla (esp. if large or pendulous breasts)

Supine Palpation

Position: Patient lies down with one arm raised above head (to flatten breast tissue) and examiner uses the pads of fingers of the opposite hand.

Techniques: Systematic approach is crucial.

Palpate each quadrant using one of these patterns:

Radial spoke pattern (from nipple outward)

Vertical strip pattern (up and down in rows)

Concentric circle pattern (circular motion from outer to inner)

Assess for: Lumps or masses, location (clock position & distance from nipple)

Size (in cm), shape (round, irregular)

Consistency (soft, firm, hard)

Margins (well-defined vs. ill-defined)

Mobility (mobile or fixed)

Tenderness

Nipple discharge

Expressed from each duct and note color, quantity, spontaneous vs. provoked

Skin or temperature changes: Overlying redness, warmth (suggests inflammation or abscess)

3. Axillary and Regional Lymph Node Examination

Position: Seated or semi-reclining.

Nodes to examine: Axillary lymph nodes: Central, Lateral (along humerus), Anterior (pectoral), Posterior (subscapular) and Apical.

Supraclavicular and infraclavicular nodes.

Internal mammary chain (not palpable directly but assessed indirectly).

Note: Size, Consistency (soft, firm, hard), Mobility (mobile or fixed) and Tenderness

V. Special Considerations

1. Pregnancy and Lactation

Breasts are enlarged, nodular and tender.

Montgomery tubercles more prominent

Colostrum may be expressed

Be gentle during palpation

2. Adolescents

Tanner staging to assess pubertal development

Fibroadenomas are most common lumps

Avoid unnecessary imaging (use ultrasound if needed)

3. Elderly Women

Breast tissue atrophies; easier palpation

Higher risk for malignancy; even small changes must be investigated

VI. Investigations Following Breast Exam (if indicated)

Ultrasound: For younger women or to differentiate solid vs cystic lesions

Mammography: Screening and diagnostic tool in women >40 years

MRI breast: High-risk cases, dense breasts or unclear mammograms

FNAC/Core needle biopsy: To assess any suspicious lump

Nipple discharge cytology

Hormonal assays: In galactorrhea

VII. Documentation

Clearly note:

Breast symmetry and skin findings

Lump characteristics (location, size, shape, mobility)

Lymph node status

Type and nature of any discharge

Investigations advised

Conclusion

Breast examination is a critical, low-cost and high-yield diagnostic skill in gynecology. A meticulous, respectful approach with proper technique ensures early detection of pathology, especially breast cancer and improves clinical outcomes.

03

Menstruation & Related Disorders

(Idrar-i-tamth aur mutalliqa Ghayr Tabi-I Taghayyurat)

3.1 *Nizam-i-taulidi laqnati* (Reproductive Endocrinology)
3.2 *Dauray-i-Tamth ka mekaniya* (Physiology of Menstruation)
3.3 *Ihtibas al- tamth* (Amenorrrhoea)
3.4 *Usr al- Tamth* (Dysmenorrhoea)
3.5 *Mutalazema sabiq -al-Hayd* (Pre Menstrual Syndrome)
3.6 *Qillat-i-Tamth* (Oligomenorrhoea)
3.7 *Taht al-Tamth* (Hypomenorrhoea)
3.8 *Ta'addud -i-Tamth* (Polymenorrhoea)
3.9 *Kathrat -i- Tamth* (Menorrhagia)
3.10 *Istihaza* (Metrorrhagia)
3.11 *Nazf al -Rahim Ghayr Tabi'I* (Abnormal Uterine Bleeding)
3.12 *Shuraniat* (Hirsutism)

Learning Objective (At the end of the session, the students should be able to)

Summarise the reproductive endocrinology.
Describe in detail physiology of Menstruation.
Describe & discuss the causes of primary and secondary *Ahtabaas-e-Tams* (Amenorrhoea), its investigations and principles of management.
Define hirsutism and enumerate its causes.
Describe, classify & discuss the causes, diagnosis and management of *Usar-e-Tams* (Dysmenorrhoea).
Describe Pre-Menstrual Syndrome & its management.
Define *Qillat Tams* (Oligomenorrhoea), *Tahtut Tams* (Hypomenorrhoea), *Kasrat-e-Tams* (Menorrhagia) & *Istehaza* (Metrorrhagia).
Define *Taadud-e-Tams* (Polymenorrhoea), discuss *Ghair Tabaiee Idrar-e-Tams* (Abnormal Uterine Bleeding) its etiology, diagnosis, complications & management

3.1 Reproductive Endocrinology

(Nizam-i-taulidi laqnati)

Reproductive endocrinology is a subspecialty of obstetrics and gynecology that focuses on the hormonal regulation of reproduction, including the diagnosis and management of disorders affecting the reproductive system. It integrates the study of endocrine glands, hormones and their effects on reproductive processes, comprising puberty, menstrual cycles, fertility, pregnancy, menopause and associated disorders.

Introduction to Reproductive Endocrinology

Reproductive endocrinology examines the interplay of hormones produced by the hypothalamic-pituitary-gonadal (HPG) axis, adrenal glands, thyroid and other endocrine systems in regulating reproductive function. It addresses both male and female reproductive physiology, and this chapter focuses primarily on female reproductive endocrinology.

Key Objectives

Understand the hormonal regulation of the female reproductive system.

Identify disorders of reproductive endocrinology and their clinical implications.

Apply diagnostic and therapeutic strategies for managing endocrine-related reproductive disorders.

Anatomy and Physiology of the Reproductive Endocrine System

Hypothalamic-Pituitary-Ovarian (HPO) Axis

The HPO axis is the cornerstone of reproductive endocrinology, coordinating the release of hormones that regulate ovarian function, menstrual cycles and fertility.

Hypothalamus: Secretes gonadotropin-releasing hormone (GnRH) in a pulsatile manner, stimulating the anterior pituitary.

GnRH pulse frequency and amplitude vary across the menstrual cycle, influencing follicle-stimulating hormone (FSH) and luteinizing hormone (LH) release.

Dysregulation (e.g., excessive stress, low body weight) can disrupt GnRH pulsatility, leading to amenorrhea or infertility.

Anterior Pituitary: Produces FSH and LH in response to GnRH.

FSH stimulates follicular growth and estrogen production in the ovaries.

LH triggers ovulation and supports the corpus luteum, which produces progesterone.

Ovaries: Produce estrogens (estradiol, estrone), progesterone and androgens (testosterone, androstenedione).

Estrogens promote endometrial proliferation and secondary sexual characteristics.

Progesterone prepares the endometrium for implantation and maintains pregnancy.

Ovarian feedback (negative and positive) regulates hypothalamic and pituitary activity.

Other Endocrine Glands

Adrenal Glands: Produce androgens (e.g., dehydroepiandrosterone [DHEA], androstenedione) and cortisol, which can influence reproductive function.

Excess adrenal androgens (e.g., in congenital adrenal hyperplasia) can cause hyperandrogenism.

Thyroid Gland: Thyroid hormones (T3, T4) affect metabolism and reproductive function.

Hypothyroidism can lead to irregular menstruation, while hyperthyroidism may cause oligomenorrhea.

Adipose Tissue: Produces leptin, which signals energy availability to the hypothalamus, influencing GnRH secretion.

Placenta (during pregnancy): Secretes human chorionic gonadotropin (hCG), estrogens and progesterone to maintain pregnancy.

Menstrual Cycle

The menstrual cycle (average 28 days) is divided into three phases, driven by hormonal fluctuations:

1. Follicular Phase (Days 1–14):

FSH stimulates follicular growth, leading to a dominant follicle.

The dominant follicle secretes estradiol, which promotes endometrial proliferation.

Rising estradiol triggers a positive feedback loop, causing an LH surge.

2. Ovulation (Day 14):

The LH surge induces follicular rupture and release of the oocyte.

3. Luteal Phase (Days 15–28):

The corpus luteum forms, secreting progesterone and estradiol to maintain the endometrium.

If implantation does not occur, the corpus luteum regresses, leading to menstruation.

Hormones in Reproductive Endocrinology

Hormone	**Source**	**Function**
GnRH	Hypothalamus	Stimulates FSH and LH release
FSH	Anterior Pituitary	Promotes follicular growth and estrogen production
LH	Anterior Pituitary	Triggers ovulation, supports corpus luteum
Estradiol	Ovaries	Endometrial proliferation, secondary sexual characteristics
Progesterone	Ovaries, Corpus Luteum	Endometrial maintenance, pregnancy support
Testosterone	Ovaries, Adrenals	Libido, follicular development (precursor to estrogen)
Inhibin	Ovaries	Inhibits FSH secretion
hCG	Placenta	Maintains corpus luteum in early pregnancy

Feedback Mechanisms

Negative Feedback: Estradiol and progesterone inhibit GnRH, FSH and LH to prevent overstimulation.

Positive Feedback: High estradiol levels in the late follicular phase trigger the LH surge, leading to ovulation.

Disorders of Reproductive Endocrinology

1. Puberty Disorders

a. Precocious Puberty

Onset of puberty before age 8 in girls.

Causes: Central (GnRH-dependent, e.g., hypothalamic tumors) or peripheral (GnRH-independent, e.g., ovarian tumors).

Diagnosis: GnRH stimulation test, imaging (MRI, ultrasound).

Treatment: GnRH agonists for central precocious puberty; address underlying cause for peripheral one.

b. Delayed Puberty

Absence of pubertal development by age 13 in girls.

Causes: Constitutional delay, hypogonadotropic hypogonadism (e.g., Kallmann syndrome), hypergonadotropic hypogonadism (e.g., Turner syndrome).

Diagnosis: Karyotyping, hormone levels (FSH, LH, estradiol), imaging.

Treatment: Hormone replacement therapy (HRT), address underlying conditions.

2. Menstrual Disorders

a. Amenorrhea

i) Primary Amenorrhea: No menarche by age 15 with normal secondary sexual characteristics or by age 13 without secondary sexual characteristics.

Causes: Anatomical (e.g., Mullerian agenesis), genetic (e.g., Turner syndrome), endocrine (e.g., hypothalamic amenorrhea).

Diagnosis: Pregnancy test, FSH, LH, estradiol, karyotype, pelvic ultrasound.

ii) Secondary Amenorrhea: Cessation of menses for ≥3 months in women with prior menstruation.

Causes: Pregnancy, polycystic ovary syndrome (PCOS), hyperprolactinemia, thyroid dysfunction, premature ovarian insufficiency (POI).

Diagnosis: Pregnancy test, prolactin, TSH, FSH, LH, pelvic ultrasound.

Treatment: Address underlying cause (e.g., dopamine agonists for hyperprolactinemia, lifestyle modification for hypothalamic amenorrhea).

b. Dysmenorrhea

Painful menstruation, often due to excessive prostaglandin production.

Treatment: NSAIDs, hormonal contraceptives.

c. Abnormal Uterine Bleeding (AUB)

Causes: Structural (e.g., fibroids, polyps) or non-structural (e.g., ovulatory dysfunction, coagulopathies).

FIGO PALM-COEIN classification: Polyp, Adenomyosis, Leiomyoma, Malignancy; Coagulopathy, Ovulatory dysfunction, Endometrial, Iatrogenic, Not yet classified.

Diagnosis: Ultrasound, hysteroscopy, endometrial biopsy.

Treatment: Hormonal therapy (e.g., levonorgestrel IUD), surgical intervention (e.g., myomectomy).

d. Polycystic Ovarian Syndrome (PCOS)

Definition: A common endocrine disorder characterized by hyperandrogenism, ovulatory dysfunction, and/or polycystic ovarian morphology.

Rotterdam Criteria (2 of 3 required):

1. Oligo- or anovulation.
2. Clinical or biochemical hyperandrogenism (e.g., hirsutism, elevated testosterone).
3. Polycystic ovaries on ultrasound (≥12 follicles or ovarian volume >10 mL).

Pathophysiology: Insulin resistance, hyperandrogenism and disrupted HPG axis feedback.

Clinical Features: Irregular menses, hirsutism, acne, infertility, obesity, metabolic syndrome.

Diagnosis: Rule out other causes (e.g., thyroid dysfunction, hyperprolactinemia).

Treatment:

Lifestyle modification (weight loss, exercise).

Combined oral contraceptives (COCs) for menstrual regulation and hyperandrogenism.

Metformin for insulin resistance.

Clomiphene citrate or letrozole for ovulation induction in infertility.

3. Infertility

Definition: Failure to conceive after 12 months of regular, unprotected intercourse (6 months if age >35).

Endocrine Causes:

Ovulatory dysfunction (e.g., PCOS, hypothalamic amenorrhea).

Hyperprolactinemia (inhibits GnRH).

Thyroid disorders.

Premature ovarian insufficiency.

Diagnosis:

Ovulation assessment (mid-luteal progesterone, ovulation predictor kits).

Semen analysis, hysterosalpingography, ovarian reserve testing (AMH, antral follicle count).

Treatment:

Ovulation induction: Clomiphene, letrozole, gonadotropins.

Assisted reproductive technologies (ART): Intrauterine insemination (IUI), in vitro fertilization (IVF).

Treat underlying endocrine disorders.

4. Hyperprolactinemia

Causes: Prolactinomas, medications (e.g., antipsychotics), hypothyroidism, stress.

Clinical Features: Galactorrhea, amenorrhea, infertility.

Diagnosis: Serum prolactin levels, MRI for pituitary adenomas.

Treatment: Dopamine agonists (cabergoline, bromocriptine), surgery for large adenomas.

5. Premature Ovarian Insufficiency (POI)

Definition: Loss of ovarian function before age 40.

Causes: Genetic (e.g., Turner syndrome), autoimmune, iatrogenic (e.g., chemotherapy).

Clinical Features: Amenorrhea, menopausal symptoms, infertility.

Diagnosis: Elevated FSH (>25 IU/L on two occasions), low estradiol, AMH.

Treatment: HRT for symptom relief, fertility preservation if desired.

6. Menopause

Definition: Permanent cessation of menstruation due to ovarian follicular depletion (average age 51).

Clinical Features: Hot flashes, night sweats, vaginal dryness, mood changes, osteoporosis risk.

Diagnosis: Clinical (12 months of amenorrhea), elevated FSH, low estradiol.

Treatment:

HRT for vasomotor symptoms and bone health (contraindicated in certain conditions, e.g., breast cancer).

Non-hormonal options: SSRIs, gabapentin, lifestyle changes.

Diagnostic Tools in Reproductive Endocrinology

1. Hormonal Assays: FSH, LH, estradiol, progesterone, testosterone, prolactin, TSH, AMH.
2. Imaging: Pelvic ultrasound: Assess ovarian morphology, endometrial thickness.
3. MRI: Evaluate pituitary or hypothalamic lesions.
4. Hysterosalpingography: Assess tubal patency.
5. Ovarian Reserve Testing:

Anti-Mullerian hormone (AMH): Reflects ovarian follicle pool.

Antral follicle count (AFC): Ultrasound-based assessment.

6. Day 3 FSH and estradiol: Elevated FSH indicates diminished reserve.
7. Genetic Testing: Karyotyping for Turner syndrome, FMR1 premutation for POI.
8. Endometrial Biopsy: Evaluate endometrial pathology in AUB.

Therapeutic Approaches

Hormonal Therapies

Combined oral contraceptives (COCs): Regulate menstrual cycles, treat hyperandrogenism.

Progestins: Manage AUB, endometrial hyperplasia.

GnRH agonists/antagonists: Treat endometriosis, precocious puberty.

Dopamine agonists: Treat hyperprolactinemia.

HRT: Manage menopausal symptoms, POI.

Ovulation Induction

Clomiphene citrate: Estrogen receptor antagonist, stimulates FSH/LH.

Letrozole: Aromatase inhibitor, effective in PCOS.

Gonadotropins: Direct stimulation of follicular growth.

Surgical Interventions

Ovarian drilling: For PCOS-related anovulation.

Myomectomy: For fibroids causing AUB or infertility.

Pituitary surgery: For prolactinomas resistant to medical therapy.

Lifestyle Modifications

Weight loss, stress reduction, and exercise for PCOS, hypothalamic amenorrhea.

Clinical Case Examples

Case 1: PCOS

- A 28-year-old woman presents with irregular menses, hirsutism, and infertility.
- Labs: Elevated testosterone, LH:FSH ratio >2, normal prolactin/TSH.
- Ultrasound: Polycystic ovaries.
- Management: Lifestyle modification, COCs for cycle regulation, letrozole for ovulation induction.

Case 2: Secondary Amenorrhea

- A 30-year-old woman with 6 months of amenorrhea, no pregnancy.
- Labs: Low FSH/LH, low estradiol, normal prolactin/TSH.
- Diagnosis: Hypothalamic amenorrhea (due to excessive exercise).
- Management: Reduce exercise, increase caloric intake, consider HRT.

Case 3: Menopause

- A 52-year-old woman reports hot flashes and vaginal dryness.
- Labs: FSH >30 IU/L, low estradiol.
- Management: Low-dose HRT, vaginal estrogen for local symptoms.

Conclusion

Reproductive endocrinology is a dynamic field that bridges gynecology, endocrinology and fertility medicine. Understanding the HPO axis, hormonal interplay and associated disorders is critical for diagnosing and managing reproductive health issues. Advances in diagnostic tools and personalized therapies continue to improve outcomes for patients with menstrual disorders, infertility and menopausal symptoms.

Hormone	Source	Role in Cycle
GnRH	Hypothalamus	Stimulates FSH & LH release
FSH	Anterior Pituitary	Follicle growth, oestrogen production
LH	Anterior Pituitary	Triggers ovulation, corpus luteum formation
Estrogen	Ovarian follicles	Endometrial proliferation, LH surge trigger
Progesterone	Corpus luteum	Endometrial maintenance, suppresses GnRH
Inhibin	Granulosa cells	Negative feedback on FSH
hCG	Placenta (if pregnant)	Maintains corpus luteum

3.2 Physiology of Menstruation

(Dauray-i-Tamth ka mekaniya)

The menstrual cycle is a complex, hormonally regulated process that prepares the female reproductive system for potential pregnancy. It involves cyclic changes in the ovaries, endometrium and hypothalamic-pituitary-ovarian (HPO) axis, resulting in ovulation and in the absence of pregnancy, menstruation.

Introduction to Menstruation

Menstruation is the cyclic shedding of the endometrial lining of the uterus, occurring approximately every 28 days (range: 21–35 days) in reproductive-age women, in the absence of pregnancy. It is a hallmark of female reproductive physiology, driven by the HPO axis, which coordinates ovarian folliculogenesis, ovulation and endometrial preparation for implantation.

The menstrual cycle is divided into three phases: follicular (proliferative), ovulatory and luteal (secretory), culminating in menstruation if implantation does not occur.

Overview of the Menstrual Cycle

The menstrual cycle is orchestrated by the HPO axis, involving the hypothalamus, anterior pituitary and ovaries, with feedback loops regulating hormone production. The cycle is typically 28 days but varies between individuals. It is divided into:

1. Follicular Phase (Days 1–14): Follicular development and endometrial proliferation.
2. Ovulation (Day 14): Release of a mature oocyte.
3. Luteal Phase (Days 15–28): Corpus luteum formation and endometrial preparation for implantation.

Menstruation marks the start of the follicular phase (Day 1) and occurs when progesterone and oestrogen levels decline, triggering endometrial shedding.

Anatomy of the Menstrual Cycle

1. Hypothalamus: Secretes gonadotropin-releasing hormone (GnRH).

2. Anterior Pituitary: Produces follicle-stimulating hormone (FSH) and luteinizing hormone (LH).

3. Ovaries: Contain follicles that produce estrogens, progesterone and androgens; site of folliculogenesis and ovulation.

4. Uterus: The endometrium undergoes cyclic proliferation, differentiation and shedding.

Functional Layer (Stratum Functionalis): Shed during menstruation.

Basal Layer (Stratum Basalis): Regenerates the endometrium post-menstruation.

5. Cervix: Produces cervical mucus, which changes in consistency under hormonal influence.

6. Vagina: Serves as the passage for menstrual flow.

Blood Supply

The endometrium is supplied by spiral (coiled) and straight arteries.

Spiral arteries, sensitive to hormonal changes, constrict during menstruation, leading to ischemia and shedding of the functional layer.

Hormonal Regulation of the Menstrual Cycle

The menstrual cycle is regulated by a dynamic interplay of hormones, with feedback mechanisms ensuring precise control.

Hypothalamic-Pituitary-Gonadal (HPG) Axis

Gonadotropin-Releasing Hormone (GnRH)

Secreted in a pulsatile manner by the hypothalamus.

Pulse frequency and amplitude vary across the cycle:

Follicular phase: High-frequency, low-amplitude pulses favour FSH release.

Luteal phase: Lower-frequency, higher-amplitude pulses favour LH release.

Stimulates the anterior pituitary to release FSH and LH.

Follicle-Stimulating Hormone (FSH)

Promotes follicular growth and granulosa cell proliferation in the ovaries.

Stimulates aromatase activity, leading to oestrogen production.

Luteinizing Hormone (LH)

Triggers ovulation by inducing follicular rupture.

Supports corpus luteum formation and progesterone production.

Feedback Mechanisms

Negative Feedback: Estrogen and progesterone inhibit GnRH, FSH and LH to prevent overstimulation.

Positive Feedback: High estradiol levels in the late follicular phase trigger an LH surge, initiating ovulation.

Ovarian Hormones

1. Estrogens (Estradiol, Estrone)

Produced by growing follicles (granulosa cells).

Promote endometrial proliferation, cervical mucus production and secondary sexual characteristics.

Peak in the late follicular phase, triggering the LH surge.

2. Progesterone

Secreted by the corpus luteum post-ovulation.

Induces endometrial differentiation (secretory phase) and inhibits uterine contractions.

Declines if pregnancy does not occur, triggering menstruation.

3. Inhibin

Secreted by granulosa cells.

Inhibits FSH release, ensuring dominance of a single follicle.

4. Androgens (Testosterone, Androstenedione)

Produced by theca cells; precursors to estrogens.

Modulate libido and follicular development.

Other Hormones

1. Prolactin: Modulates reproductive function; elevated levels can suppress GnRH.
2. Thyroid Hormones: Influence metabolism and reproductive function; hypothyroidism may disrupt ovulation.
3. Adrenal Hormones: Androgens and cortisol can indirectly affect the HPG axis.

Flowchart: Hormonal Interplay in Menstrual Cycle

Hypothalamus
↓ (GnRH pulses)
Anterior Pituitary

↓	↓
FSH	LH
↓	↓
Ovarian Follicles	Theca Cells
↓	↓
Estrogen	Androgens → Estrogen (via granulosa cells)

↓
Endometrial Proliferation
↓
Estrogen Peak → LH Surge → Ovulation
↓
Corpus Luteum Formation
↓
Progesterone Secretion
↓
Endometrial Secretory Phase
↓
No Fertilization → Corpus Luteum Regression
↓
↓ Estrogen & Progesterone
↓
Endometrial Shedding → Menstruation
↓
GnRH Reactivated → New Cycle Begins

Physiology of Menstruation

Controlled by hypothalamic–pituitary–ovarian axis

Cycle length: 21–35 days; average 28 days

Phases

Follicular phase: Estrogen rises, endometrium proliferates

Ovulation: LH surge triggers ovum release

Luteal phase: Progesterone stabilizes endometrium

Menstruation: Hormone withdrawal → endometrial shedding

Phases of the Menstrual Cycle

1. Follicular Phase (Days 1–14)

Ovarian Events

Begins with menstruation (Day 1), marked by low oestrogen and progesterone levels.

FSH stimulates the growth of 5–15 primordial follicles, but only one becomes dominant (Graafian follicle).

The dominant follicle produces increasing amounts of estradiol.

Theca cells produce androgens, which granulosa cells convert to estrogens via aromatase.

Endometrial Events

Menstruation: Shedding of the functional layer due to progesterone and oestrogen withdrawal.

Proliferative Phase: Estradiol stimulates endometrial regeneration and proliferation.

Epithelial cells in the stratum basalis divide, rebuilding the functional layer.

Spiral arteries elongate and endometrial glands proliferate.

Cervical Mucus

Becomes thin, watery and "fertile" (spinnbarkeit) under oestrogen influence, facilitating sperm transport. Duration: Variable (7–21 days); shorter in shorter cycles, longer in longer cycles.

2. Ovulation (Day 14)

Trigger: A surge in LH, induced by a peak in estradiol (positive feedback).

Estradiol levels >200 pg/mL for ~48 hours stimulate the LH surge.

Ovarian Events

The dominant follicle ruptures, releasing the mature oocyte.

Meiosis resumes in the oocyte (arrested at prophase I), completing meiosis I and entering meiosis II (arrested until fertilization).

Endometrial Events Transition from proliferative to secretory phase begins.

Cervical Mucus: Peaks in elasticity and volume, optimizing sperm penetration.

Clinical Signs: Slight rise in basal body temperature (BBT) due to progesterone, Mittelschmerz (ovulation pain).

3. Luteal Phase (Days 15–28)

Ovarian Events

The ruptured follicle transforms into the corpus luteum, which secretes progesterone and less estradiol.

Progesterone peaks ~7 days post-ovulation.

If pregnancy does not occur, the corpus luteum regresses (luteolysis) by day 22–24, reducing progesterone and oestrogen levels.

Endometrial Events

Secretory Phase: Progesterone induces glandular secretion and stromal decidualization.

Endometrial glands produce glycogen-rich secretions.

Spiral arteries coil further, preparing for implantation.

If implantation does not occur, declining progesterone triggers endometrial breakdown.

Cervical Mucus: Thickens under progesterone influence, forming a barrier to sperm.

Duration: Fixed (12–14 days), determined by the lifespan of the corpus luteum.

Menstruation (Days 1–5)

Mechanism

Progesterone and oestrogen withdrawal causes vasoconstriction of spiral arteries, leading to endometrial ischemia.

Ischemia triggers necrosis and shedding of the functional layer.

Matrix metalloproteinases (MMPs) degrade the extracellular matrix, facilitating tissue breakdown.

Prostaglandins (e.g., PGF2α) cause uterine contractions, expelling menstrual blood.

Composition of Menstrual Flow

Blood from spiral arteries (~50%).

Endometrial tissue, mucus and vaginal secretions.

Average blood loss: 30–50 mL (normal range: 10–80 mL).

Hemostasis

Vasoconstriction and platelet aggregation limit bleeding.

The basal layer remains intact, enabling regeneration.

Duration: Typically 3–7 days.

Molecular and Cellular Mechanisms

Endometrial Dynamics

Proliferation: Estrogen upregulates genes for cell division (e.g., cyclin D) and angiogenesis (e.g., VEGF).

Secretory Transformation: Progesterone induces decidualization genes (e.g., prolactin, IGFBP-1) and inhibits proliferation.

Shedding

Progesterone withdrawal upregulates MMPs and inflammatory cytokines (e.g., IL-1, TNF-α).

Prostaglandins (PGF2α, PGE2) mediate vasoconstriction and myometrial contractions.

Ovarian Folliculogenesis

Primordial to Primary Follicles: FSH-independent, driven by local growth factors (e.g., AMH, activin).

Primary to Secondary Follicles: FSH stimulates granulosa cell proliferation and theca cell androgen production.

Antral to Graafian Follicles: The dominant follicle is selected based on FSH receptor density and oestrogen production.

Ovulation: LH induces proteases and prostaglandins, weakening the follicular wall.

Hormonal Signaling

Estrogen Receptors (ERα, ERβ): Mediate endometrial proliferation and gene expression.

Progesterone Receptors (PRA, PRB): Regulate decidualization and inhibit oestrogen-driven proliferation.

Gonadotropin Receptors: FSH and LH receptors on granulosa and theca cells drive follicular development.

Physiological Variations

Cycle Length: Normal range 21–35 days; shorter cycles reflect a shorter follicular phase.

Menarche: Occurs at age 10–15, driven by rising oestrogen levels during puberty.

Perimenopause: Irregular cycles due to declining ovarian reserve and fluctuating hormone levels.

Pregnancy: hCG maintains the corpus luteum, preventing menstruation.

Lactation: Prolactin suppresses GnRH, leading to lactational amenorrhea.

Clinical Relevance

Menstrual Disorders

1. Amenorrhea: Absence of menstruation (e.g., hypothalamic amenorrhea, PCOS).
2. Oligomenorrhea: Infrequent cycles (>35 days).
3. Menorrhagia: Heavy menstrual bleeding (>80 mL).
4. Dysmenorrhea: Painful menstruation, often due to excess prostaglandins.

Diagnostic Tools

Hormone levels: FSH, LH, estradiol, progesterone, prolactin, TSH.

Ultrasound: Assess endometrial thickness, ovarian morphology.

Basal body temperature: Detects ovulation (progesterone-induced rise).

Therapeutic Implications

Hormonal contraceptives: Suppress ovulation and stabilize the endometrium.

NSAIDs: Reduce prostaglandin-mediated pain and bleeding.

Progestins: Treat abnormal uterine bleeding by inducing endometrial atrophy.

Conclusion

The physiology of menstruation reflects a finely tuned interplay of the HPO axis, ovarian hormones and endometrial responses. The follicular phase drives follicular development and endometrial proliferation, ovulation releases a mature oocyte and the luteal phase prepares the endometrium for implantation. In the absence of pregnancy, hormonal withdrawal triggers menstruation, initiating a new cycle.

Key Takeaways

The HPO axis coordinates cyclic hormonal changes, with oestrogen and progesterone as primary mediators.

The endometrium undergoes proliferation, secretion and shedding in response to hormonal changes.

Menstruation results from progesterone withdrawal, leading to spiral artery vasoconstriction and tissue breakdown.

Variations in cycle length and menstrual flow are normal but may indicate pathology when extreme.

Letter	Hormone	Function
F	FSH	Follicle growth
E	Estrogen	Endometrial proliferation
E	LH	Egg release (ovulation)
L	Luteinizing Hormone	Corpus luteum formation
P	Progesterone	Prepares uterus for implantation
G	GnRH	Regulate pituitary hormone release

Mnemonic: "FEEL PG" – Hormones of Menstrual Cycle

3.3 Amenorrhea

(Ihtibas al- tamth)

Definition

Amenorrhea is defined as the absence of menstrual periods in a woman of reproductive age. It is classified into:

Primary Amenorrhea: No menarche by age 15 with normal secondary sexual characteristics or by age 13 without secondary sexual characteristics.

Secondary Amenorrhea: Cessation of menses for ≥3 months in women with previously regular cycles or ≥ 6 months in those with irregular cycles.

Epidemiology

Primary Amenorrhea: Occurs in <1% of women; often linked to genetic or anatomical abnormalities.

Secondary Amenorrhea: More common, affecting 3–5% of women; pregnancy is the most common physiological cause.

Pathophysiology

Amenorrhea results from disruptions at various levels of the reproductive axis or anatomical defects:

1. Hypothalamus: Impaired gonadotropin-releasing hormone (GnRH) secretion affects follicle-stimulating hormone (FSH) and luteinizing hormone (LH) release.
2. Pituitary: Dysfunction reduces FSH/LH production, impairing ovarian stimulation.
3. Ovaries: Failure to produce estrogen or progesterone disrupts endometrial cycling.

4. Uterus/Outflow Tract: Structural abnormalities prevent menstrual flow.
5. Systemic Factors: Thyroid dysfunction, hyperprolactinemia or metabolic disorders alter the HPO axis.

Classification and Etiology

1. Primary Amenorrhea

Causes are categorized by anatomical and hormonal considerations:

a. Outflow Tract Abnormalities

Mullerian Agenesis (Mayer-Rokitansky-Kuster-Hauser Syndrome): Congenital absence of uterus/vagina; normal ovaries and secondary sexual characteristics.

Imperforate Hymen or Transverse Vaginal Septum: Obstructs menstrual flow; presents with cyclic pelvic pain.

b. Gonadal Disorders

Turner Syndrome (45,X): Ovarian dysgenesis, leading to low estrogen, elevated FSH and absent puberty.

Pure Gonadal Dysgenesis (46,XX or 46,XY): Nonfunctional ovaries, normal or ambiguous genitalia.

c. Hypothalamic-Pituitary Dysfunction

Kallmann Syndrome: GnRH deficiency with anosmia; low FSH/LH and estrogen.

Constitutional Delay of Puberty: Delayed but normal pubertal progression.

d. Androgen Excess

Androgen Insensitivity Syndrome (AIS): 46, XY karyotype, female phenotype, absent uterus due to androgen receptor defects.

Congenital Adrenal Hyperplasia (CAH): 21-hydroxylase deficiency causing virilization and amenorrhea.

2. **Secondary Amenorrhea**

Causes are grouped by hormonal and systemic factors:

a. Physiological

Pregnancy: Most common cause; confirmed by β-hCG testing.

Lactation: Prolactin suppresses GnRH.

Menopause: Natural ovarian failure (age >40); premature ovarian insufficiency (POI) if <40.

b. Hypothalamic Causes

Functional Hypothalamic Amenorrhea (FHA): Due to stress, weight loss, excessive exercise or eating disorders (e.g., anorexia nervosa); low GnRH, FSH, LH and estrogen.

c. Pituitary Disorders

Hyperprolactinemia: Prolactinomas or medications (e.g., antipsychotics) suppress GnRH.

Sheehan Syndrome: Postpartum pituitary necrosis causing hypopituitarism.

d. Ovarian Disorders

Polycystic Ovary Syndrome (PCOS): Anovulation due to hyperandrogenism and elevated LH:FSH ratio.

Premature Ovarian Insufficiency (POI): Loss of ovarian function before age 40; elevated FSH, low estrogen.

e. Uterine Causes

Asherman Syndrome: Intrauterine adhesions from curettage or infection, preventing endometrial shedding.

f. Systemic Disorders

Thyroid Dysfunction: Hypothyroidism (menorrhagia or amenorrhea) or hyperthyroidism (oligomenorrhea/amenorrhea).

Cushing Syndrome: Cortisol excess suppresses GnRH.

Chronic Diseases: Renal failure, diabetes or malnutrition disrupt hormonal balance.

Clinical Features

1. Primary Amenorrhea

Symptoms: Absence of menarche; may include cyclic pelvic pain (outflow obstruction) or lack of pubertal development (e.g., Turner syndrome).

Signs

Turner syndrome: Short stature, webbed neck, low hairline.

AIS: Normal breast development, sparse pubic hair.

Kallmann syndrome: Anosmia, delayed puberty.

Outflow obstruction: Pelvic mass, hematocolpos.

2. Secondary Amenorrhea

Symptoms: Cessation of menses, infertility, menopausal symptoms (hot flashes in POI), or galactorrhea (hyperprolactinemia).

Signs

PCOS: Hirsutism, acne, obesity.

FHA: Low BMI, history of stress/exercise.

Hyperprolactinemia: Galactorrhea, visual field defects (macroadenoma).

Thyroid dysfunction: Goiter, weight changes, fatigue.

Diagnostic Approach

A systematic approach is essential to identify the cause of amenorrhea.

History

Menstrual History: Age at menarche (if applicable), cycle regularity, last menstrual period.

Associated Symptoms: Weight changes, stress, exercise, galactorrhea, hirsutism, hot flashes.

Medical History: Chronic diseases, medications (e.g., antipsychotics), obstetric history.

Family History: Delayed puberty, infertility, genetic disorders.

Physical Examination

General: BMI, signs of systemic disease (e.g., Cushing like features, thyroid enlargement).

Pubertal Development: Tanner staging for breast and pubic hair (primary amenorrhea).

Pelvic Exam: Assess for outflow tract abnormalities, uterine size or masses.

Androgen Excess: Hirsutism, acne, virilization.

Laboratory Tests

1. Pregnancy Test: Serum β-hCG to rule out pregnancy in secondary amenorrhea.
2. Hormonal Profile:
   a. FSH and LH:
      - High (>25 IU/L): Ovarian failure (e.g., POI, Turner syndrome).
      - Low/Normal: Hypothalamic or pituitary dysfunction (e.g., FHA, Kallmann syndrome).

   b. Estradiol: Low in hypogonadism; normal/high in PCOS or outflow obstruction.
   c. Prolactin: Elevated in prolactinomas or medication-induced hyperprolactinemia.
   d. Thyroid Function Tests: TSH, free T4 to assess thyroid dysfunction.
   e. Androgens: Testosterone, DHEAS, 17-hydroxyprogesterone for PCOS or CAH.
   f. Anti-Mullerian Hormone (AMH): Low in POI; high in PCOS.
3. Karyotyping: For primary amenorrhea with suspected genetic disorders (e.g., Turner syndrome, AIS).
4. Imaging
   a. Pelvic Ultrasound: Evaluates uterine/ovarian anatomy, polycystic ovaries or hematocolpos.
   b. MRI: Assess pituitary for adenomas or hypothalamic lesions; used in outflow tract anomalies.
   c. Hysterosalpingography (HSG): Detects intrauterine adhesions in Asherman syndrome.

Additional Tests

1. Progesterone Challenge Test: Oral progestin (e.g., medroxyprogesterone 10 mg for 5–10 days) to assess estrogen status; withdrawal bleeding indicates adequate estrogen and a patent outflow tract.
2. Clomiphene Challenge Test: Assess ovarian reserve in suspected POI.
3. ACTH Stimulation Test: For suspected CAH

Management

Management depends on the underlying cause, patient goals (e.g., fertility, symptom relief), and long-term health considerations.

1. Primary Amenorrhea

a. Outflow Tract Abnormalities

Imperforate Hymen/Transverse Septum: Surgical correction (hymenectomy or septum resection).

Mullerian Agenesis: Vaginal dilators or surgical neovagina creation; counseling for infertility (ovaries functional, uterus absent).

b. Gonadal Dysgenesis

Turner Syndrome: Hormone replacement therapy (HRT) with estrogen and progestin to induce puberty and prevent osteoporosis; growth hormone for stature; oocyte donation for fertility.

AIS: Gonadectomy post-puberty (due to malignancy risk in undescended testes); estrogen therapy.

c. Hypothalamic-Pituitary Dysfunction

Kallmann Syndrome: HRT to induce puberty; gonadotropins or pulsatile GnRH for fertility.

Constitutional Delay: Observation or low-dose estrogen to initiate puberty.

2. Secondary Amenorrhea

a. Physiological Causes

Pregnancy/Lactation: Supportive care; breastfeeding cessation may restore cycles.

Menopause/POI: HRT for symptom relief and bone health; oocyte donation for fertility in POI.

b. Hypothalamic Causes

FHA: Address underlying cause (e.g., weight gain, stress reduction); cognitive behavioral therapy for eating disorders; ovulation induction if fertility desired.

c. Pituitary Disorders

Hyperprolactinemia: Dopamine agonists (cabergoline, bromocriptine); surgery for macroadenomas if unresponsive.

Sheehan Syndrome: Replace deficient hormones (e.g., estrogen, thyroid, cortisol).

d. Ovarian Disorders

PCOS: Lifestyle modification (weight loss); combined oral contraceptives (COCs) for cycle regulation and hyperandrogenism; clomiphene or letrozole for ovulation induction.

POI: HRT; fertility counseling (oocyte donation).

e. Uterine Causes

Asherman Syndrome: Hysteroscopic adhesiolysis; estrogen therapy to promote endometrial regrowth.

f. Systemic Disorders

Thyroid Dysfunction: Levothyroxine for hypothyroidism; antithyroid drugs for hyperthyroidism.

Cushing Syndrome: Treat underlying cortisol excess (e.g., adrenalectomy, ketoconazole).

General Principles

a. Hormonal Therapy: COCs or cyclic progestins to regulate cycles and prevent endometrial hyperplasia in estrogenic states (e.g., PCOS).
b. Fertility: Ovulation induction (clomiphene, gonadotropins) or assisted reproductive technologies (ART) like IVF for anovulatory causes.

c. Bone Health: Calcium, vitamin D and HRT in hypoestrogenic states to prevent osteoporosis.
d. Psychosocial Support: Counseling for infertility or genetic diagnoses.

Complications

a. Infertility: Common in PCOS, POI and outflow tract anomalies; requires individualized fertility treatments.
b. Osteoporosis: Risk in hypoestrogenic states (e.g., FHA, POI); mitigated by HRT and lifestyle measures.
c. Endometrial Hyperplasia: Unopposed estrogen in anovulatory states (e.g., PCOS) increases risk; managed with progestins.
d. Psychological Impact: Amenorrhea, especially with infertility or genetic diagnoses, may cause significant distress; referral to mental health professionals may be needed.
e. Cardiovascular/Metabolic Risks: PCOS increases risk of diabetes and cardiovascular disease; regular screening required.

Emerging Research and Advances

a. Genetic Testing: Identifies mutations in POI (e.g., FMR1 premutation) or Kallmann syndrome (e.g., KAL1 gene).
b. AMH as a Biomarker: Guides fertility counseling in POI or PCOS.
c. Neuroendocrine Insights: Role of kisspeptin in regulating GnRH pulsatility; potential therapeutic target in FHA.
d. Fertility Preservation: Oocyte cryopreservation for women at risk of POI (e.g., chemotherapy patients).

Clinical Approach Summary

Step 1: Rule Out Pregnancy: Serum β-hCG in secondary amenorrhea.

Step 2: Assess Estrogen Status:

Progesterone challenge test: Withdrawal bleeding indicates adequate estrogen and patent outflow tract.

Low FSH/LH + low estradiol: Hypothalamic/pituitary dysfunction.

High FSH + low estradiol: Ovarian failure.

Step 3: Targeted investigations:

Prolactin, TSH, androgens for systemic/endocrine causes.

Ultrasound for PCOS or outflow obstruction.

Karyotype/MRI for primary amenorrhea or suspected genetic/anatomical issues.

Step 4: Management:

Treat underlying cause (e.g., dopamine agonists for prolactinomas).

Symptom relief (e.g., HRT for hypoestrogenism).

Fertility optimization if desired (e.g., ART).

Monitor long-term risks (e.g., bone health, metabolic issues).

Ethical and Psychosocial Considerations

a. Informed Consent: Discuss risks of HRT (e.g., thromboembolism) or ART (e.g., ovarian hyperstimulation syndrome).
b. Cultural Sensitivity: Respect patient beliefs about menstruation, fertility or hormonal therapy.
c. Psychological Support: Address emotional impact of infertility, genetic diagnoses or chronic conditions.
d. Fertility Counseling: Offer options like oocyte donation or adoption for non-reversible causes (e.g., Mullerian agenesis, POI).

Conclusion

Amenorrhea is a multifaceted condition requiring a systematic approach to identify its diverse etiologies, ranging from physiological (e.g., pregnancy) to pathological one (e.g., PCOS, Turner syndrome). Understanding the HPO axis and its disruptions is essential for accurate diagnosis and management. Advances in genetic testing, biomarkers and fertility preservation continue to enhance care in reproductive endocrinology.

3.4 Dysmenorrhea

(Usr al- Tamth)

Dysmenorrhea, derived from the Greek words dys (difficult), men (month) and rhea (flow), refers to painful menstruation that interferes with daily activities. It is one of the most common gynecological complaints, affecting school going girls and also women of reproductive age.

Definition

Dysmenorrhea is characterized by crampy, lower abdominal pain that occurs during menstruation, often accompanied by systemic symptoms such as nausea, fatigue, headache or diarrhea. It is classified into two main types:

1. Primary Dysmenorrhea: Painful menstruation without underlying gynecological pathology, typically associated with ovulatory cycles.
2. Secondary Dysmenorrhea: Painful menstruation due to an identifiable gynecological or pelvic condition.

Epidemiology

Prevalence: Dysmenorrhea affects 50–90% of menstruating women, with 10–20% experiencing severe symptoms that impair daily activities.

Age: Primary dysmenorrhea is most common in adolescents and young women, typically starting within 6–12 months of menarche. Secondary dysmenorrhea is more prevalent in older women (20s–30s).

Risk Factors

Early menarche (<12 years)

Heavy or prolonged menstrual flow

Nulliparity

Family history of dysmenorrhea

Smoking, high BMI and stress (for primary dysmenorrhea)

Underlying pelvic pathology (for secondary dysmenorrhea)

Pathophysiology

Primary Dysmenorrhea

Primary dysmenorrhea is primarily driven by prostaglandin-mediated uterine hypercontractility. The key mechanisms include:

1. Prostaglandin Production: During menstruation, endometrial cells release prostaglandins (PGF2α and PGE2) as part of the endometrial shedding process. These prostaglandins:

Stimulate myometrial contractions, leading to uterine ischemia and pain.

Sensitize pain nerve endings, lowering the pain threshold.

2. Uterine Ischemia: Excessive myometrial contractions reduce blood flow to the uterus, causing hypoxia and pain.

3. Other Mediators: Leukotrienes, vasopressin and platelet-activating factors may also contribute to pain and inflammation.

4. Hormonal Influence: Ovulatory cycles are essential for primary dysmenorrhea, as anovulatory cycles (e.g., in early adolescence) typically lack significant pain due to low progesterone levels, which regulate prostaglandin synthesis.

Secondary Dysmenorrhea

Secondary dysmenorrhea results from underlying pelvic or gynecological conditions that exacerbate menstrual pain. Common causes include:

1. Endometriosis: Ectopic endometrial tissue causes inflammation and cyclic pain.
2. Adenomyosis: Endometrial tissue within the myometrium leads to painful uterine contractions.
3. Uterine fibroids: Benign tumors may cause heavy bleeding and pain.
4. Pelvic Inflammatory Disease (PID): Chronic infection or scarring of pelvic organs.
5. Cervical stenosis: Obstruction of menstrual flow, leading to increased intrauterine pressure.
6. Intrauterine Devices (IUDs): Particularly copper IUDs, which may increase prostaglandin release.
7. Congenital anomalies: Such as uterine septum or imperforate hymen, causing outflow obstruction.

Clinical Presentation

Primary Dysmenorrhea

Timing: Pain begins 1–2 days before or with the onset of menstruation and lasts 1–3 days.

Location: Crampy, midline lower abdominal pain, often radiating to the lower back or thighs.

Character: Sharp, spasmodic or dull aching pain.

Associated Symptoms:

Nausea, vomiting or diarrhea

Fatigue, headache or irritability

Dizziness or lightheadedness

Impact: May interfere with school, work or daily activities, but symptoms typically resolve with menstrual flow cessation.

Secondary Dysmenorrhea

Timing: Pain may precede menstruation by several days, persist throughout the cycle or worsen over time.

Location: Pain may be unilateral or diffuse, depending on the underlying pathology.

Associated Symptoms:

Abnormal uterine bleeding (menorrhagia or metrorrhagia)

Dyspareunia (painful intercourse)

Infertility (e.g., in endometriosis or PID)

Systemic symptoms (e.g., fever in PID)

Diagnosis

History

A detailed history is needed to differentiate primary from secondary dysmenorrhea:

Primary Dysmenorrhea:

Onset with menarche or shortly before menses

Pain confined to menstrual period

No history of pelvic pathology or abnormal bleeding

Secondary Dysmenorrhea:

Later onset (after years of painless periods)

Associated symptoms (e.g., dyspareunia, infertility, irregular bleeding)

History of pelvic infections, IUD use or gynecological surgeries

Physical Examination

Primary Dysmenorrhea: Normal pelvic examination, with mild uterine tenderness during menstruation.

Secondary Dysmenorrhea:

Bimanual exam: Uterine or adnexal tenderness, masses or fixed uterus (e.g., in endometriosis).

Speculum exam: Assess for cervical abnormalities or discharge (e.g., in PID).

Signs of systemic illness (e.g., fever in PID).

Investigations

Primary Dysmenorrhea: Diagnosis is clinical and investigations are typically not required unless symptoms are atypical.

Secondary Dysmenorrhea:

Ultrasound (transvaginal or transabdominal): To detect fibroids, ovarian cysts or adenomyosis.

Laparoscopy: Gold standard for diagnosing endometriosis or adhesions.

MRI: For complex cases (e.g., congenital anomalies or adenomyosis).

Cultures/STI testing: If PID is suspected.

Hysteroscopy: To evaluate intrauterine pathology (e.g., polyps, submucosal fibroids).

Endometrial biopsy: If malignancy or endometrial pathology is suspected (rare).

Differential Diagnosis

Endometriosis

Adenomyosis

Uterine fibroids

PID

Ovarian cysts

Ectopic pregnancy

Inflammatory bowel disease

Irritable bowel syndrome

Management

Primary Dysmenorrhea

1. Non-Pharmacological

Heat Therapy: Application of heat to the lower abdomen reduces muscle tension and improves blood flow.

Exercise: Moderate physical activity (e.g., walking) may alleviate symptoms by improving pelvic circulation.

Dietary Modifications: Reducing caffeine, sugar and alcohol intake; increasing omega-3 fatty acids and magnesium.

2. Pharmacological

First-Line: Nonsteroidal anti-inflammatory drugs (NSAIDs) (e.g., ibuprofen 400–800 mg every 6–8 hours, naproxen 500 mg twice daily).

Mechanism: Inhibit prostaglandin synthesis via cyclooxygenase (COX) inhibition.

Timing: Start at the onset of pain or just before menstruation for optimal effect.

Second-Line: Combined oral contraceptives (COCs) or progestin-only pills.

Mechanism: Suppress ovulation, reduce endometrial proliferation and decrease prostaglandin production.

Options: Continuous or cyclic regimens.

3. Other Options

Progestin-releasing IUDs (e.g., levonorgestrel IUD) for long-term management.

Tocolytics (e.g., nifedipine) in refractory cases (rarely used).

Complementary Therapies: Acupuncture, Transcutaneous Electrical Nerve Stimulation (TENS) or herbal drugs (e.g., ginger, fennel).

If symptoms are refractory to NSAIDs or COCs, evaluate for secondary dysmenorrhea.

Secondary Dysmenorrhea

Treat Underlying Cause:

1. Endometriosis: GnRH agonists, aromatase inhibitors or surgical excision of endometriotic lesions.
2. Adenomyosis: Hormonal therapies (e.g., levonorgestrel IUD) or hysterectomy in severe cases.
3. Fibroids: Myomectomy, uterine artery embolization or hormonal therapy.
4. PID: Antibiotics based on culture results or empirical treatment (e.g., ceftriaxone + doxycycline).
5. Cervical Stenosis: Cervical dilation or surgical correction.
6. Symptomatic Relief: NSAIDs or analgesics as adjuncts to specific treatments.

Surgical Management: Reserved for refractory cases (e.g., hysterectomy for adenomyosis or severe endometriosis in women who have completed family).

3.5 Premenstrual syndrome

(Mutalazema sabiq -al-Hayd)

Premenstrual syndrome (PMS) is a condition characterized by a combination of psychological and physical symptoms that begin during the luteal phase of the menstrual cycle (upto 14 days prior to menses), cease by the end of menstruation.

Epidemiology

Prevalence

PMS: Affects 20–40% of women of reproductive age, with varying severity.

Age: Most common in women aged 20–40 years, though symptoms may begin in adolescence and persist till menopause.

Risk Factors

- Family history of PMS
- Personal history of mood disorders (e.g., depression, anxiety)
- Stress, trauma or adverse life events
- High BMI, smoking or poor diet
- Nulliparity or irregular menstrual cycles

Pathophysiology

The exact etiology of PMS remains unclear, but they are thought to result from complex interactions between hormonal fluctuations, neurotransmitter dysregulation and genetic predispositions. Key mechanisms include:

1. Hormonal Fluctuations

PMS occur in ovulatory cycles, suggesting a link to cyclic changes in estrogen and progesterone during the luteal phase.

Progesterone metabolites (e.g., allopregnanolone) interact with the gamma-aminobutyric acid (GABA) receptor system, influencing mood and anxiety.

Abnormal sensitivity to normal hormonal fluctuations, rather than absolute hormone levels, is implicated.

2. Neurotransmitter Dysregulation

Serotonin: Reduced activity in the luteal phase is strongly associated with PMS, contributing to mood symptoms (e.g., irritability, depression).

GABA: Altered GABA receptor sensitivity to progesterone metabolites may exacerbate affective symptoms.

Dopamine and Norepinephrine: Dysregulation may contribute to fatigue, concentration difficulties and mood instability.

3. Genetic Factors

Polymorphisms in serotonin receptor genes and estrogen receptor genes are associated with increased susceptibility to PMS.

4. Psychosocial Factors

Stress, trauma and poor coping mechanisms may amplify symptom severity.

Cultural and societal expectations around menstruation may influence symptom perception.

5. Other Factors

Dysregulated hypothalamic-pituitary-adrenal (HPA) axis activity.

Altered pain perception and inflammatory responses (e.g., prostaglandins) contributing to physical symptoms.

Clinical Presentation

Timing: Symptoms begin in the luteal phase (7–14 days before menstruation) and resolve within a few days of menstrual onset.

Symptoms: Over 150 symptoms are associated with PMS, categorized as:

Physical: Breast tenderness (mastalgia), bloating, weight gain, headache, fatigue, joint or muscle pain, acne.

Emotional: Irritability, mood swings, anxiety, mild depression.

Behavioral: Food cravings (especially for carbohydrates), sleep disturbances, reduced concentration, social withdrawal.

Severity: Symptoms are annoying but typically do not cause significant functional impairment.

Diagnostic Criteria

Clinical diagnosis based on history of cyclic symptoms in the luteal phase that resolve with menses.

Symptoms must be present for at least "two consecutive menstrual cycles" and cause mild to moderate interference with daily life.

No formal diagnostic criteria exist, but the 'American College of Obstetricians and Gynecologists (ACOG)' recommends symptom tracking.

History

Symptom Tracking: Patients should maintain a prospective symptom diary for at least 2 menstrual cycles to confirm the cyclical nature of symptoms and their resolution with menses.

Physical Examination

General Exam: Assess for signs of underlying conditions (e.g., thyroid enlargement, obesity).

Pelvic Exam: Rule out gynecological conditions (e.g., endometriosis, fibroids) if symptoms suggest secondary dysmenorrhea or atypical features.

Investigations

PMS: Typically, no laboratory or imaging tests are required.

Differential Diagnosis

1. Psychiatric Disorders: Major depressive disorder, generalized anxiety disorder, bipolar disorder.
2. Gynecological Conditions: Endometriosis, adenomyosis, uterine fibroids, pelvic inflammatory disease.
3. Endocrine Disorders: Hypothyroidism, hyperprolactinemia.
4. Medical Conditions: Irritable bowel syndrome, migraines, chronic fatigue syndrome.
5. Medication/Substance Effects: Antidepressants, hormonal therapies or substance withdrawal.

Management

General Principles

Management is individualized based on symptom severity, patient preferences and reproductive goals.

Goals: Alleviate symptoms, improve quality of life and minimize side effects.

Treatment involves a combination of lifestyle modifications, non-pharmacological approaches and pharmacological therapies.

Non-Pharmacological Management

1. Lifestyle Modifications

Diet: Reduce caffeine, alcohol and sodium; increase complex carbohydrates, fruits, vegetables and calcium-rich foods (e.g., dairy, leafy greens).

Exercise: Regular aerobic exercise (e.g., 30 minutes most days) improves mood and reduces physical symptoms.

Sleep Hygiene: Maintain consistent sleep patterns to reduce fatigue and irritability.

2. Complementary Therapies

Calcium Supplementation: 1200 mg/day may reduce PMS symptoms (moderate evidence).

Vitamin B6: 50–100 mg/day may alleviate mood symptoms (limited evidence).

Magnesium: 200–400 mg/day may reduce bloating and mood disturbances.

Pharmacological Management

i. Nonsteroidal Anti-Inflammatory Drugs (NSAIDs): For physical symptoms (e.g., breast tenderness, headaches).

Example: Ibuprofen 400–800 mg every 6–8 hours as needed.

ii. Combined Oral Contraceptives (COCs):

Mechanism: Suppress ovulation and stabilize hormonal fluctuations.

Preferred Regimen: Continuous or extended-cycle COCs (e.g., drospirenone-containing pills) to minimize luteal phase symptoms.

iii. Diuretics: For severe bloating or edema.

Example: Spironolactone 25–100 mg/day during the luteal phase.

iv. Analgesics: For headaches or musculoskeletal pain.

Patient Education and Counseling

Educate patients about the cyclical nature of PMS/PMDD and the role of hormonal and neurotransmitter changes.

Encourage symptom tracking to monitor treatment response.

Discuss potential side effects of medications and the importance of adherence.

Complications

Reduced quality of life due to recurrent symptoms.

Absenteeism from work or school.

Strained interpersonal relationships.

Prognosis

Symptoms often improve with lifestyle changes, pharmacological therapy, or spontaneously with age or pregnancy. Symptoms may recur with discontinuation of treatment.

Extra References

American College of Obstetricians and Gynecologists (ACOG) guidelines on PMS.

3.6 Oligomenorrhea

(Qillat-i-Tamth)

Definition

Oligomenorrhea is defined as infrequent menstruation, with menstrual cycles occurring at intervals greater than 35 days but less than 90 days. It typically results in fewer than 4–9 menstrual periods per year, contrasting with the normal cycle length of 21–35 days (average 28 days). Oligomenorrhea often indicates ovulatory dysfunction and is a common presenting symptom in reproductive-age women.

Epidemiology

Prevalence: Affects approximately 10–20% of reproductive-age women.

Common in adolescence and perimenopause due to physiological HPG axis immaturity or decline.

Associated with conditions like polycystic ovary syndrome (PCOS), which accounts for a significant proportion of cases.

Pathophysiology

Oligomenorrhea typically results from disruptions in the hypothalamic-pituitary-ovarian(HPO) axis, leading to irregular ovulation or anovulation. Key mechanisms include:

1. Hypothalamic Dysfunction: Reduced gonadotropin-releasing hormone (GnRH) pulsatility due to stress, excessive exercise, low body weight or chronic illness suppresses follicle-stimulating hormone (FSH) and luteinizing hormone (LH), impairing follicular development.
2. Pituitary Dysfunction: Inadequate FSH or LH secretion disrupts folliculogenesis and ovulation.
3. Ovarian Dysfunction: Conditions like PCOS or premature ovarian insufficiency (POI) reduce ovulatory frequency.
4. Hyperandrogenism: Elevated androgens (e.g., in PCOS) disrupt HPO axis feedback, leading to anovulatory cycles.
5. Endometrial Factors: Less frequent ovulation results in fewer progesterone-driven endometrial cycles, reducing menstrual frequency.

Etiology

Oligomenorrhea can be classified based on the FIGO PALM-COEIN system for abnormal uterine bleeding (AUB), with a focus on non-structural causes:

1. Polycystic Ovarian Syndrome (PCOS): Most common cause; characterized by hyperandrogenism, anovulation and polycystic ovarian morphology.

2. Hypothalamic Amenorrhea: Due to stress, weight loss or excessive exercise, leading to reduced GnRH pulsatility.

3. Hyperprolactinemia: Elevated prolactin (e.g., from prolactinomas or medications) inhibits GnRH, causing anovulation.

4. Thyroid Dysfunction:

Hypothyroidism: Prolongs cycles due to elevated thyrotropin-releasing hormone (TRH), which stimulates prolactin.

Hyperthyroidism: May cause oligomenorrhea or amenorrhea.

5. Premature Ovarian Insufficiency (POI): Early depletion of ovarian follicles reduces ovulatory frequency.

6. Obesity: Insulin resistance and hyperandrogenism disrupt ovulation.

7. Medications: Antipsychotics, antidepressants or anticoagulants

8. Perimenopause: Declining ovarian function leads to irregular cycles.

9. Other: Adrenal disorders (e.g., congenital adrenal hyperplasia), chronic illnesses or eating disorders.

Clinical Features

Infrequent menstrual periods (>35 days apart).

May be associated with:

Hirsutism, acne or obesity (e.g., in PCOS).

Weight loss, fatigue or menopausal symptoms (e.g., in POI).

Galactorrhea (e.g., in hyperprolactinemia).

Potential infertility due to anovulation.

Diagnosis

History and Physical Examination

Assess menstrual history, lifestyle factors (e.g., exercise, weight changes) and symptoms of endocrine disorders (e.g., hirsutism, galactorrhea).

Evaluate body mass index (BMI), thyroid and signs of hyperandrogenism.

Laboratory Tests

Pregnancy test: To rule out pregnancy.

FSH, LH, estradiol: Assess ovarian function (high FSH in POI, high LH:FSH ratio in PCOS).

Prolactin: Elevated in hyperprolactinemia.

Thyroid-stimulating hormone (TSH): To detect thyroid dysfunction.

Testosterone, DHEAS: Assess for hyperandrogenism.

Fasting glucose, insulin: Screen for insulin resistance in PCOS.

Imaging

Pelvic ultrasound: Evaluate for polycystic ovaries or endometrial abnormalities.

MRI: If pituitary pathology (e.g., prolactinoma) is suspected.

Other: Endometrial biopsy if malignancy is suspected (rare).

Management

Management depends on the underlying cause and patient goals (e.g., cycle regulation, fertility).

1. Lifestyle Modifications

Weight loss in obese patients with PCOS (5–10% weight loss can restore ovulation).

Stress reduction and moderate exercise for hypothalamic amenorrhea.

2. Hormonal Therapies

Combined oral contraceptives (COCs): Regulate cycles and reduce hyperandrogenism.

Progestins (e.g., medroxyprogesterone): Induce withdrawal bleeding every 1–3 months to prevent endometrial hyperplasia.

3. Ovulation Induction (for infertility)

Clomiphene citrate or letrozole to stimulate ovulation.

Gonadotropins for resistant cases.

4. Specific Treatments

Dopamine agonists (e.g., cabergoline) for hyperprolactinemia.

Levothyroxine for hypothyroidism.

Metformin for insulin resistance in PCOS.

5. Surgical Options(rare)

Ovarian drilling in PCOS patients unresponsive to medical therapy.

Pituitary surgery for prolactinomas resistant to dopamine agonists.

Complications

Infertility due to anovulation.

Endometrial hyperplasia or cancer due to unopposed oestrogen exposure.

Metabolic syndrome in PCOS (e.g., diabetes, cardiovascular disease).

Psychosocial impact (e.g., anxiety, reduced quality of life).

Clinical Case Examples

1. Oligomenorrhea Case

- A 25-year-old woman presents with menstrual cycles every 60 days and hirsutism.
- Labs: Elevated testosterone, LH:FSH ratio 2.5:1, normal prolactin/TSH.
- Ultrasound: Polycystic ovaries.
- Diagnosis: PCOS.
- Management: Lifestyle modification, COCs for cycle regulation, letrozole for fertility.

Parameters of Menstrual Disorders

Disorder	**Cycle Pattern**	**Bleeding Volume**	**Main Cause**
Amenorrhea	Absent	None	Hormonal, structural
Menorrhagia	Regular but heavy	>80ml	Fibroids, hormonal
Oligomenorrhea	Prolonged intervals	Variable	PCOS, thyroid disorders
Dysmenorrhea	Cyclical pain	Normal	Prostaglandins, endometriosis

3.7 Hypomenorrhea

(*Tahat al Tamt*)

Definition

Hypomenorrhea is defined as abnormally light or scanty menstrual bleeding, with blood loss significantly less than the normal range of 10–80 mL per cycle (typically <10 mL). It is characterized by short menstrual periods (≤2 days) or minimal flow, often described as spotting.

Epidemiology

Less common than oligomenorrhea but often coexists with it.

More prevalent in women using hormonal contraceptives or during perimenopause.

May be normal in some women with no underlying pathology.

Pathophysiology

Hypomenorrhea results from reduced endometrial proliferation or shedding, often due to hormonal or anatomical factors:

1. Low Estrogen Levels: Inadequate oestrogen stimulation leads to thin endometrial lining, reducing menstrual flow.
2. Progesterone Dominance: Hormonal contraceptives or progestin therapy suppress endometrial growth.
3. Endometrial Scarring: Adhesions (e.g., Asherman syndrome) limit functional endometrium.
4. Ovulatory Dysfunction: Anovulatory cycles may produce scanty bleeding due to lack of progesterone-driven endometrial development.
5. Systemic Factors: Malnutrition, chronic illness or stress can reduce hormonal stimulation of the endometrium.

Etiology

1. Hormonal Causes:

Hormonal contraceptives (e.g., COCs, progestin-only pills, levonorgestrel IUD): Suppress endometrial proliferation.

Hypoestrogenic states: Hypothalamic amenorrhea, POI or menopause.

Anovulation: Reduced progesterone leads to minimal endometrial shedding.

2. Anatomical Causes:

Asherman Syndrome: Intrauterine adhesions from curettage, infection or surgery.

Uterine abnormalities: Fibroids or congenital anomalies (e.g., unicornuate uterus).

3. Systemic Causes:

Malnutrition or low body weight: Reduces oestrogen production.

Thyroid dysfunction: Hypothyroidism may cause light menses.

Chronic illnesses: E.g., diabetes, renal disease.

4. Medications: Anticoagulants or antiestrogens (e.g., tamoxifen) may alter menstrual flow.

Physiological Variants: Some women may have scanty menses without pathology.

Clinical Features

Scanty menstrual flow (<10 mL) or spotting.

Short duration of bleeding (≤2 days).

May be associated with:

Infertility or irregular cycles (e.g., in anovulation or POI).

Symptoms of hypoestrogenism (e.g., hot flashes, vaginal dryness).

History of uterine surgery or infection (e.g., in Asherman syndrome).

Often asymptomatic unless associated with infertility or underlying disease.

Diagnosis

History and Physical Examination

Assess menstrual history, contraceptive use, surgical history and symptoms of endocrine disorders.

Pelvic exam to evaluate uterine size, cervical abnormalities or signs of hypoestrogenism.

Laboratory Tests

Pregnancy test: To rule out pregnancy-related spotting.

FSH, LH, estradiol: Low estradiol and high FSH suggest POI or menopause.

Prolactin, TSH: Screen for hyperprolactinemia or thyroid dysfunction.

Complete blood count (CBC): Rule out anaemia or systemic illness.

Imaging

Pelvic ultrasound: Assess endometrial thickness (normal: 8–12 mm in proliferative phase) and uterine anomalies.

Hysterosalpingography or hysteroscopy: Evaluate for intrauterine adhesions or structural abnormalities.

Endometrial Biopsy: To assess endometrial pathology (e.g., atrophy, hyperplasia).

Management

Management focuses on addressing the underlying cause and patient concerns (e.g., fertility, cycle regulation).

Hormonal Therapies

Estrogen therapy: For hypoestrogenic states (e.g., POI, hypothalamic amenorrhea) to promote endometrial growth.

COCs or cyclic progestins: Regulate cycles and increase menstrual flow if desired.

Discontinuation or adjustment of hormonal contraceptives if they are the cause.

Surgical Interventions

Hysteroscopic adhesiolysis: For Asherman syndrome to restore endometrial function.

Myomectomy: For fibroids causing reduced endometrial surface area.

Lifestyle Modifications

Nutritional counselling for malnourished patients.

Stress reduction to restore HPG axis function.

Fertility Treatment

Ovulation induction (e.g., clomiphene, letrozole) for anovulatory patients.

Assisted reproductive technologies (ART) for severe cases.

Observation: If hypomenorrhea is physiological and asymptomatic, no treatment may be needed.

Complications

Infertility due to anovulation or endometrial dysfunction.

Endometrial atrophy, increasing risk of implantation failure.

Psychosocial distress if associated with infertility .

Osteoporosis or cardiovascular risks in hypoestrogenic states (e.g., POI).

Example

Hypomenorrhea Case:

A 30-year-old woman reports spotting for 1–2 days per cycle after a D&C procedure.

Labs: Normal FSH, low estradiol.

Hysteroscopy: Intrauterine adhesions.

Diagnosis: Asherman syndrome.

Management: Hysteroscopic adhesiolysis, oestrogen therapy to promote endometrial regrowth.

Comparative Overview

Feature	Oligomenorrhea	Hypomenorrhea
Definition	Cycles >35 days apart	Scanty menstrual flow (<10 mL)
Primary Cause	Ovulatory dysfunction	Reduced endometrial proliferation
Common Etiologies	PCOS, hypothalamic amenorrhea, hyperprolactinemia	Hormonal contraceptives, Asherman syndrome, hypoestrogenism
Hormonal Abnormalities	Disrupted FSH/LH, hyperandrogenism	Low estradiol, progesterone dominance
Diagnostic test	HPG axis evaluation, ultrasound	Endometrial assessment, oestrogen levels
Treatment Goals	Restore ovulation, regulate cycles	Increase endometrial growth, address anatomical issues

Summary

Oligomenorrhea is primarily an ovulatory disorder, while hypomenorrhea involves inadequate endometrial development.

Both conditions may impact fertility and require careful evaluation of the HPO axis and endometrium.

Treatment is individualized, focusing on restoring normal menstrual function and addressing complications like infertility or endometrial pathology.

3.8 Polymenorrhoea

(*Ta'addud -i-Tamth*)

Polymenorrhea is defined as a menstrual cycle disorder characterized by abnormally frequent menstrual cycles, with cycle lengths typically shorter than 21 days. It is distinguished from other menstrual irregularities such as menorrhagia (heavy menstrual bleeding) or metrorrhagia (irregular bleeding between cycles). Polymenorrhea reflects a disturbance in the hypothalamic-pituitary-ovarian (HPO) axis or local uterine factors that regulate the menstrual cycle.

Epidemiology

Prevalence varies depending on age, reproductive status and underlying conditions.

More common in perimenarcheal (around menarche) and perimenopausal women due to hormonal fluctuations.

Exact incidence is poorly documented, as polymenorrhea is often underreported or misdiagnosed as other menstrual disorders.

Etiology

Polymenorrhea results from shortened follicular or luteal phases of the menstrual cycle, often due to hormonal or structural abnormalities. Common causes include:

1. Hormonal Imbalances

Anovulatory cycles: Lack of ovulation leads to unopposed oestrogen, causing premature endometrial proliferation and shedding.

Luteal phase defects: Shortened luteal phase due to inadequate progesterone production.

Hyperprolactinemia: Elevated prolactin levels disrupt gonadotropin-releasing hormone (GnRH) pulsatility, altering cycle length.

Thyroid dysfunction: Hyperthyroidism accelerates metabolism and GnRH secretion, while hypothyroidism may also disrupt cycle regulation.

Polycystic Ovary Syndrome (PCOS): Though typically associated with oligomenorrhea, some PCOS patients may present with irregular, frequent cycles.

2. Ovarian Causes

Ovarian cysts: Functional cysts (e.g., corpus luteum cysts) may disrupt normal hormonal feedback.

Premature ovarian insufficiency: Declining ovarian reserve can lead to irregular menstrual cycles.

3. Uterine Causes

Endometrial hyperplasia: Excessive endometrial growth due to unopposed oestrogen.

Uterine fibroids or polyps: Structural abnormalities may cause frequent bleeding.

Endometriosis: May contribute to irregular endometrial shedding.

4. Systemic Causes

Stress: Psychological or physical stress disrupts the HPO axis via cortisol and catecholamine release.

Weight fluctuations: Rapid weight loss or gain alters GnRH pulsatility.

Medications: Drugs such as hormonal contraceptives, antipsychotics or antiepileptics may shorten cycles.

Chronic illnesses: Diabetes, liver disease or renal dysfunction can affect hormonal regulation.

5. Iatrogenic Causes

Hormonal contraceptives: Incorrect use or discontinuation of oral contraceptives, intrauterine devices (IUDs) or implants.

Fertility treatments: Ovulation induction agents (e.g., clomiphene) may disrupt cycle length.

Pathophysiology

The menstrual cycle is regulated by the interplay of GnRH, follicle-stimulating hormone (FSH), luteinizing hormone (LH), oestrogen and progesterone. Polymenorrhea typically arises from:

Shortened follicular phase: Accelerated follicular recruitment due to excessive FSH or unopposed oestrogen.

Shortened luteal phase: Inadequate progesterone production or premature corpus luteum regression.

Anovulation: Lack of ovulation leads to irregular endometrial shedding due to unopposed oestrogen.

Endometrial instability: Local uterine factors (e.g., inflammation, fibroids) cause premature endometrial breakdown.

The result is a cycle length shorter than the normal 21–35 days, often with regular but frequent bleeding.

Clinical Features

Menstrual history: Cycles occurring every 14–21 days, with bleeding lasting 3–7 days (normal duration) or shorter.

Associated symptoms

Fatigue, due to frequent blood loss and possible anemia.

Premenstrual syndrome (PMS) symptoms (e.g., bloating, mood changes) may occur with each cycle.

Pelvic pain or dysmenorrhea if associated with endometriosis or fibroids.

Impact on quality of life: Frequent menstruation may cause emotional distress, social inconvenience or reduced productivity.

Diagnosis

Diagnosis is based on a thorough history, physical examination and investigations to identify underlying causes.

1. History

Detailed menstrual history: cycle length, duration and flow characteristics.

Associated symptoms: pain, fatigue or systemic symptoms (e.g., weight loss, galactorrhea).

Medical history: Thyroid disorders, PCOS, stress or medication use.

Lifestyle factors: Diet, exercise, stress or recent weight changes.

2. Physical Examination

General examination: Signs of anemia (pallor), thyroid dysfunction (goitre, tremors), or hyperandrogenism (hirsutism, acne).

Pelvic examination: To assess for uterine enlargement, masses or tenderness suggestive of fibroids, adenomyosis or endometriosis.

3. Investigations

Blood tests

Complete blood count (CBC): To evaluate for anemia due to frequent bleeding.

Thyroid function tests: TSH, free T3, free T4 to rule out thyroid dysfunction.

Serum prolactin: To assess for hyperprolactinemia.

Sex hormones: FSH, LH, oestrogen, progesterone and androgens to evaluate HPO axis function.

Fasting glucose/insulin: To screen for PCOS or metabolic disorders.

Pelvic ultrasound: To identify structural abnormalities (e.g., fibroids, polyps, ovarian cysts).

Endometrial biopsy: Indicated in women >35 years or those with risk factors for endometrial hyperplasia/carcinoma.

Hysteroscopy: To visualize the endometrial cavity for polyps or submucosal fibroids.

MRI/CT: Rarely used, reserved for complex cases (e.g., suspected adenomyosis or malignancy).

4. Menstrual calendar: Patients may be asked to track cycles for 2–3 months

Differential Diagnosis

Metrorrhagia: Irregular bleeding between cycles, not necessarily frequent.

Menorrhagia: Heavy menstrual bleeding with normal cycle length.

Dysfunctional uterine bleeding (DUB): Abnormal bleeding without identifiable organic cause, often anovulatory.

Endometrial hyperplasia/carcinoma: Must be ruled out in older women or those with risk factors (e.g., obesity, unopposed oestrogen).

Bleeding disorders: Von Willebrand disease or thrombocytopenia may mimic polymenorrhea.

Pregnancy complications: Miscarriage or ectopic pregnancy can present with frequent bleeding.

Management

The goal of treatment is to address the underlying cause, normalize cycle length, prevent complications (e.g., anemia) and improve quality of life.

1. General Measures

Lifestyle modification: Stress reduction, weight stabilization and balanced nutrition.

Iron supplementation: For patients with anemia or low ferritin levels.

Menstrual tracking: To monitor treatment response.

2. Medical Management

Hormonal therapies

Combined oral contraceptives (COCs): Regulate cycles by suppressing ovulation and stabilizing the endometrium. Preferred in women without contraindications.

Progestins: Oral (e.g., norethisterone) or intrauterine (e.g., levonorgestrel IUD) to stabilize the endometrium and reduce bleeding frequency.

Gonadotropin-releasing hormone (GnRH) agonists: Used in severe cases (e.g., endometriosis) to suppress ovarian function temporarily.

Non-hormonal therapies

Nonsteroidal anti-inflammatory drugs (NSAIDs): Reduce prostaglandin-mediated bleeding and dysmenorrhea.

Tranexamic acid: To reduce bleeding during menses.

Treatment of underlying conditions

Thyroid dysfunction: Levothyroxine for hypothyroidism or antithyroid drugs for hyperthyroidism.

Hyperprolactinemia: Dopamine agonists (e.g., cabergoline).

PCOS: Metformin or COCs to regulate cycles and address insulin resistance.

3. Surgical Management

Endometrial ablation: For refractory cases with normal uterine anatomy, to reduce or eliminate menstrual bleeding.

Myomectomy or polypectomy: Removal of fibroids or polyps causing frequent bleeding.

Hysterectomy: Last resort for severe, treatment-resistant cases, typically in older women who have completed childbearing.

4. Follow-Up

Regular follow-up to monitor cycle regularity, hemoglobin levels and treatment side effects.

Reassess for underlying conditions if symptoms persist.

Complications

Anemia: Due to frequent blood loss, leading to fatigue, weakness or shortness of breath.

Infertility: Anovulatory cycles or luteal phase defects may impair fertility.

Endometrial hyperplasia/carcinoma: Prolonged unopposed oestrogen exposure increases risk.

Psychosocial impact: Frequent menstruation may lead to anxiety, depression or social withdrawal.

Prognosis

Prognosis depends on the underlying cause and response to treatment.

Most cases are manageable with hormonal therapy or treatment of the underlying condition.

Structural causes (e.g., fibroids) may require surgical intervention but often have good outcomes.

Long-term monitoring is essential in cases with risk of endometrial hyperplasia or malignancy.

Definitions

- Amenorrhea: No menstruation for ≥3 cycles or 6 months
- Dysmenorrhea: Cramping pain during menstruation
- PMS: Cyclic emotional/physical symptoms in luteal phase
- Oligomenorrhea: Cycles >35 days apart
- Polymenorrhea: Cycles <21 days apart
- Metrorrhagia: Irregular bleeding between periods
- Menorrhagia: Bleeding >80 ml or >7 days
- Hirsutism: Male-pattern hair growth in females

Diagnostic Clues

No periods + normal puberty =Primary amenorrhea

Painful menses + nausea = Dysmenorrhea

Mood swings + bloating = PMS

Irregular cycles + acne =PCOS

Heavy bleeding + fatigue = Menorrhagia

Spotting between periods = Metrorrhagia

Excess facial/body hair= Hirsutism

3.9 Menorrhagia

(Kathrat-i-Tamth)

Menorrhagia, also known as heavy menstrual bleeding (HMB), is a common gynecologic condition characterized by excessive menstrual blood loss that interferes with a woman's physical, emotional or social quality of life. It is a subtype of abnormal uterine bleeding (AUB) and requires thorough evaluation to identify underlying causes and implement effective management.

Definition

Menorrhagia is defined as menstrual blood loss exceeding 80 mL per cycle or menstrual bleeding that is abnormally heavy or prolonged (typically lasting >7 days). Clinically, it is often assessed by subjective measures, passing large blood clots (>2.5 cm), or symptoms like fatigue due to anemia. The International Federation of Gynaecology and Obstetrics (FIGO) classifies menorrhagia under the broader category of AUB, using the PALM-COEIN system to categorize causes.

Epidemiology

Prevalence: Affects approximately 10–30% of reproductive-age women, with higher rates in perimenopause.

Impact: Significant burden on quality of life, causing anemia, fatigue and reduced productivity.

Risk Factors: Obesity, nulliparity, age (adolescence and perimenopause) and underlying medical conditions (e.g., bleeding disorders).

Pathophysiology

Menorrhagia results from disruptions in the normal mechanisms regulating menstrual bleeding, including endometrial hemostasis, hormonal balance and uterine structural integrity. Key pathophysiological processes include:

1. Endometrial Hemostasis

Normal menstruation involves vasoconstriction of spiral arteries, mediated by prostaglandins (e.g., PGF2α) and endothelin, to limit blood loss.

In menorrhagia, an imbalance in prostaglandins (increased PGE2 relative to PGF2α) or excessive fibrinolysis (due to elevated plasminogen activators) leads to prolonged or excessive bleeding.

2. Hormonal Imbalance

Unopposed oestrogen (e.g., in anovulatory cycles) causes excessive endometrial proliferation, leading to heavy shedding.

Progesterone deficiency impairs endometrial stabilization, increasing bleeding.

3. Structural Abnormalities

Conditions like fibroids or adenomyosis distort the endometrial cavity, increasing surface area or impairing hemostasis.

4. Systemic Factors

Coagulopathies (e.g., von Willebrand disease) impair clot formation, exacerbating bleeding.

Thyroid dysfunction or chronic illness may disrupt HPG axis regulation.

Etiology

The FIGO PALM-COEIN classification system categorizes causes of AUB, including menorrhagia, into structural (PALM) and non-structural (COEIN) causes:

Structural Causes (PALM)

Polyps (AUB-P): Endometrial or cervical polyps increase bleeding surface area.

Adenomyosis (AUB-A): Endometrial tissue within the myometrium disrupts normal hemostasis.

Leiomyomas (Fibroids, AUB-L):

Submucosal fibroids distort the endometrial cavity, increasing bleeding.

Intramural or subserosal fibroids may cause heavy bleeding via altered vascularity.

Malignancy and Hyperplasia (AUB-M):

Endometrial hyperplasia (often due to unopposed oestrogen) or endometrial cancer can cause heavy bleeding. Cervical or uterine malignancies are rare but serious causes.

Non-Structural Causes (COEIN)

Coagulopathy (AUB-C)

Bleeding disorders (e.g., von Willebrand disease, thrombocytopenia) impair hemostasis.

Anticoagulant therapy (e.g., warfarin, heparin) exacerbates bleeding.

Ovulatory Dysfunction (AUB-O)

Anovulatory cycles (e.g., in PCOS, perimenopause) lead to unopposed oestrogen and excessive endometrial proliferation.

Ovulatory dysfunction is common in adolescence and perimenopause.

Endometrial (AUB-E)

Primary endometrial disorders (e.g., defective hemostasis, excessive fibrinolysis) cause heavy bleeding without structural abnormalities.

Iatrogenic (AUB-I)

Medications (e.g., copper IUD, tamoxifen) or hormonal therapies may cause heavy bleeding.

Not Yet Classified (AUB-N)

Rare or poorly understood causes (e.g., arteriovenous malformations).

Other Contributing Factors

Thyroid Dysfunction: Hypothyroidism may increase bleeding by altering coagulation or HPO axis function.

Obesity: Increases oestrogen production via aromatization in adipose tissue.

Chronic Illness: Liver or renal disease can impair hormone metabolism or coagulation.

Clinical Features

Menstrual Characteristics

Blood loss >80 mL per cycle or subjective heavy bleeding.

Prolonged bleeding (>7 days).

Passage of large clots (>2.5 cm).

Frequent changing of sanitary products (every 1–2 hours).

Associated Symptoms

Fatigue, pallor, or shortness of breath due to anemia.

Pelvic pain or pressure (e.g., with fibroids or adenomyosis).

Irregular cycles if associated with anovulation.

Impact on Quality of Life:

Social embarrassment, reduced productivity or psychological distress.

Interference with daily activities or sexual function.

Diagnosis

Accurate diagnosis requires a systematic approach to identify the underlying cause and assess the severity of bleeding.

History

Menstrual History: Duration, frequency, volume of bleeding and presence of clots.

Associated Symptoms: Pain, infertility or systemic symptoms (e.g., bruising, weight changes).

Medical History: Bleeding disorders, thyroid disease, medications or prior surgeries.

Family History: Coagulopathies or gynaecological conditions.

Quality of Life: Impact on daily activities, work or emotional well-being.

Physical Examination

General: Signs of anemia (pallor, tachycardia), thyroid abnormalities or obesity.

Pelvic Exam: Assess uterine size, tenderness or masses (e.g., fibroids).

Speculum Exam: Evaluate for cervical polyps or lesions.

Laboratory Tests

Complete Blood Count (CBC): Assess for anemia (hemoglobin, hematocrit) and thrombocytopenia.

Coagulation Profile: Prothrombin time (PT), activated partial thromboplastin time (aPTT), and von Willebrand factor testing for coagulopathies.

Hormonal Evaluation

Thyroid-stimulating hormone (TSH): Screen for hypothyroidism.

Prolactin: Rule out hyperprolactinemia.

FSH, LH, estradiol: Assess ovulatory status.

Androgens (testosterone, DHEAS): Evaluate for PCOS.

Pregnancy Test: Rule out pregnancy-related bleeding.

Ferritin: Assess iron stores in anemic patients.

Imaging

Pelvic Ultrasound: First-line imaging to detect fibroids, polyps, adenomyosis or endometrial thickening.

Transvaginal ultrasound is preferred for better resolution.

Saline-Infusion Sonography (SIS): Enhances visualization of endometrial polyps or submucosal fibroids.

MRI: For detailed assessment of adenomyosis or complex fibroids.

Hysterosalpingography: Evaluate tubal patency or uterine cavity abnormalities.

Invasive Procedures

Endometrial Biopsy: Indicated for women >45 years, those with risk factors for endometrial hyperplasia/cancer (e.g., obesity, PCOS) or persistent bleeding.

Hysteroscopy: Visualizes endometrial cavity for polyps, fibroids or adhesions; allows biopsy or resection.

Dilation and Curettage (D&C): Diagnostic and therapeutic for acute heavy bleeding; not routine for diagnosis.

Diagnostic Criteria

Objective: Blood loss >80 mL (measured via alkaline hematin method, rarely used clinically).

Subjective: Patient-reported heavy bleeding impacting quality of life.

Use PALM-COEIN to categorize the cause.

Management

Management of menorrhagia is done according to the underlying cause, severity, patient age, fertility desires and comorbidities. Treatment goals include reducing bleeding, correcting anemia, addressing the underlying cause and improving quality of life.

Medical Management

Non-Hormonal Therapies

1. Non-Steroidal Anti-Inflammatory Drugs (NSAIDs)

E.g., ibuprofen, mefenamic acid.

Reduce prostaglandin production, decreasing bleeding by 20–50%.

Also alleviate dysmenorrhea.

2. Tranexamic Acid:

Antifibrinolytic agent that reduces bleeding by 30–60%.

Taken during menstruation; effective for endometrial causes (AUB-E).

3. Iron Supplementation: Corrects anemia and restores ferritin levels.

Hormonal Therapies

1. Combined Oral Contraceptives (COCs):

Regulate cycles, reduce bleeding by 35–60%, and treat anovulatory bleeding.

Contraindicated in women with thrombotic risk factors.

2. Levonorgestrel-Releasing Intrauterine Device (LNG-IUD):

Reduces bleeding by 70–90%; induces endometrial atrophy.

Preferred for long-term management and contraception.

3. Progestins:

Cyclic (e.g., medroxyprogesterone) or continuous (e.g., norethindrone) to stabilize endometrium.

Effective for anovulatory bleeding or hyperplasia.

4. Gonadotropin-Releasing Hormone (GnRH) Agonists:

E.g., leuprolide; induce a hypoestrogenic state, reducing bleeding.

Used short-term for fibroids or pre-surgery; add-back oestrogen/progestin to minimize side effects.

5. Danazol:

Androgenic steroid that reduces bleeding; limited use due to side effects (e.g., hirsutism).

6. Other:

Desmopressin: For von Willebrand disease to enhance clotting factor release.

Thyroid hormone replacement: For hypothyroidism-related bleeding.

Surgical Management

1. Endometrial Ablation:

Destroys the endometrial lining (e.g., via thermal, radiofrequency, or cryotherapy).

Reduces bleeding by 70–90%; suitable for women not desiring fertility.

Risk of recurrence or need for further intervention.

2. Myomectomy:

Removal of fibroids (hysteroscopic, laparoscopic or abdominal).

Preserves fertility; indicated for submucosal fibroids causing bleeding.

3. Uterine Artery Embolization (UAE):

Occludes uterine arteries to shrink fibroids and reduce bleeding.

Less invasive than hysterectomy; fertility outcomes uncertain.

4. Hysterectomy:

Definitive treatment for refractory menorrhagia or malignancy.

Indicated when fertility is not desired or other treatments fail.

Performed vaginally, laparoscopically, or abdominally.

Polypectomy: Hysteroscopic removal of endometrial or cervical polyps.

D&C: Temporary measure for acute, severe bleeding; not a long-term solution.

Management of Specific Causes

Coagulopathies: Hematologist consultation; desmopressin or clotting factor replacement.

PCOS: COCs, metformin for insulin resistance or ovulation induction for fertility.

Endometrial Hyperplasia: Progestins or LNG-IUD; hysterectomy if atypical hyperplasia or cancer.

Adenomyosis: LNG-IUD, GnRH agonists or hysterectomy for severe cases.

Lifestyle and Supportive Measures

Weight management to reduce unopposed oestrogen in obesity.

Dietary counselling to support iron intake.

Psychosocial support for emotional distress or quality-of-life impact.

Complications

1. Anemia: Iron deficiency anemia due to chronic blood loss; may cause fatigue, pallor or cardiac strain.
2. Endometrial Hyperplasia/Cancer: Risk in unopposed oestrogen states (e.g., PCOS, obesity).
3. Infertility: May occur with structural causes (e.g., fibroids, adenomyosis) or anovulation.
4. Quality of Life: Social, occupational or psychological impact from heavy bleeding or pain.
5. Treatment-Related: Hormonal side effects, surgical complications (e.g., infection, adhesions).

Clinical Case Example

Case: A 42-year-old woman presents with heavy menstrual bleeding for 9 days per cycle, requiring pad changes every hour and fatigue. She has a history of obesity and irregular cycles.

Labs: Hemoglobin 9.5 g/dL, normal TSH, elevated testosterone.

Ultrasound: Thickened endometrium (14 mm), polycystic ovaries.

Diagnosis: AUB-O (anovulatory bleeding due to PCOS).

Management:

LNG-IUD to reduce bleeding.

Iron supplementation for anemia.

Metformin and lifestyle changes for PCOS.

Endometrial biopsy to rule out hyperplasia.

Conclusion

Menorrhagia is a complex condition with diverse etiologies, ranging from structural abnormalities (e.g., fibroids, polyps) to non-structural causes (e.g., coagulopathies, ovulatory dysfunction). Accurate diagnosis using the PALM-COEIN framework, combined with a thorough history, physical examination, laboratory tests and imaging, is essential to identify the underlying cause. Management options include medical therapies (e.g., NSAIDs, LNG-IUD, hormonal treatments) and surgical interventions (e.g., ablation, hysterectomy), individualised to the patient's age, fertility goals, and comorbidities.

Key Takeaways

Menorrhagia is defined as menstrual blood loss >80 mL or bleeding impacting quality of life.

The PALM-COEIN system guides diagnosis by categorizing structural and non-structural causes.

Treatment is individualized, with medical therapies as first-line and surgical options for refractory cases.

Early diagnosis and management prevent complications like anemia and endometrial hyperplasia.

Common Menstrual Disorders – Quick Overview

Amenorrhea	=	Absence of menstruation
Dysmenorrhea	=	Painful menstruation
PMS	=	Physical/emotional symptoms before menses
Oligomenorrhea	=	Infrequent cycles (>35 days apart)
Polymenorrhea	=	Frequent cycles (<21 days apart)
Metrorrhagia	=	Irregular, intermenstrual bleeding
Menorrhagia	=	Excessive/prolonged bleeding
AUB	=	Abnormal uterine bleeding (PALM-COEIN)
Hirsutism	=	Excess hair growth due to androgen excess

Disorder	**Keyword Prompt**	**Recall**
Amenorrhea	No menstruation	"A = Absence"
Menorrhagia	Excessive flow	"M = Massive bleeding"
Oligomenorrhea	Infrequent cycles	"O = Occasional periods"
Dysmenorrhea	Painful menstruation	"D = Discomfort"

3.10 Metrorrhagia

(*Kathrat -i- Tamth*)

Definition

Metrorrhagia is defined as irregular, acyclic uterine bleeding that occurs between menstrual periods or is unrelated to the normal menstrual cycle. It is characterized by unpredictable timing, variable flow and duration, distinguishing it from menorrhagia (heavy menstrual bleeding) or menometrorrhagia (irregular and heavy bleeding).

Epidemiology

Metrorrhagia can occur across all reproductive age groups but is more common in perimenarcheal and perimenopausal women due to hormonal fluctuations.

Prevalence is difficult to quantify precisely, as it is often reported as a symptom rather than a primary diagnosis. It is estimated to affect 10–15% of women seeking gynaecological care.

Associated with conditions like endometrial polyps, leiomyomas, anovulation or malignancy, depending on the age group.

Etiology

Metrorrhagia results from disruptions in the hypothalamic-pituitary-ovarian axis, endometrial abnormalities or systemic conditions. The FIGO (International Federation of Gynaecology and Obstetrics) PALM-COEIN classification system categorizes causes as structural (PALM) or non-structural (COEIN):

Structural Causes (PALM)

1. Polyps (AUB-P): Endometrial or cervical polyps are benign growths that can cause irregular bleeding due to surface erosion or inflammation.
2. Adenomyosis (AUB-A): Endometrial tissue within the myometrium disrupts normal uterine contractility and hemostasis.
3. Leiomyomas (AUB-L): Uterine fibroids, particularly submucosal ones, distort the endometrial cavity, leading to irregular bleeding.
4. Malignancy and Hyperplasia (AUB-M): Endometrial or cervical cancer, or endometrial hyperplasia, especially in postmenopausal women, can present as metrorrhagia.

Non-Structural Causes (COEIN)

1. Coagulopathy (AUB-C): Bleeding disorders (e.g., von Willebrand disease, thrombocytopenia) impair normal hemostasis, leading to irregular bleeding.
2. Ovulatory Dysfunction (AUB-O): Anovulation, common in polycystic ovary syndrome (PCOS), adolescence, or perimenopause, causes unopposed oestrogen exposure, leading to irregular endometrial shedding.
3. Endometrial (AUB-E): Primary endometrial disorders, such as defective local hemostasis or inflammation (endometritis), can cause metrorrhagia.
4. Iatrogenic (AUB-I): Medications (e.g., anticoagulants, hormonal contraceptives, tamoxifen) or intrauterine devices (IUDs) may induce irregular bleeding.
5. Not Yet Classified (AUB-N): Rare or poorly understood causes/ not coming under above categories.

Other Causes

Pregnancy-Related: Ectopic pregnancy, miscarriage or gestational trophoblastic disease.

Infections: Cervicitis, pelvic inflammatory disease (PID) or sexually transmitted infections (e.g., Chlamydia, Gonorrhea).

Systemic Conditions: Thyroid dysfunction, liver disease or renal failure can disrupt hormonal regulation or coagulation.

Trauma: Cervical or vaginal trauma, including postcoital bleeding.

Pathophysiology

Metrorrhagia arises from disruptions in the normal cyclic endometrial proliferation, secretion and shedding regulated by oestrogen and progesterone. Key mechanisms include:

1. Anovulatory Bleeding: Lack of ovulation results in unopposed oestrogen, causing endometrial proliferation without progesterone-induced stabilization, leading to irregular shedding.
2. Structural Abnormalities: Polyps, fibroids or malignancies disrupt the endometrial surface, causing focal bleeding.

3. Coagulation Defects: Impaired clotting mechanisms exacerbate bleeding from the endometrial vasculature.
4. Inflammatory Processes: Endometritis or infections cause vascular fragility and irregular bleeding.
5. Hormonal Imbalance: Dysregulation of the hypothalamic-pituitary-ovarian axis (e.g., in PCOS or stress) leads to dysregulated endometrial stimulation.

Clinical Presentation

Symptoms: Irregular, intermenstrual vaginal bleeding (spotting to heavy flow), often without associated pain. May be accompanied by symptoms of underlying conditions (e.g., pelvic pain in fibroids, systemic symptoms in coagulopathy).

Associated Symptoms

Anovulatory cycles: Symptoms of hyperandrogenism (e.g., hirsutism in PCOS).

Malignancy: Postmenopausal bleeding, weight loss or pelvic pressure.

Pregnancy-related: Positive pregnancy test, abdominal pain or syncope.

Impact: Can lead to anemia (fatigue, pallor), emotional distress or reduced quality of life.

Diagnostic Approach

A systematic approach is critical to identify the underlying cause of metrorrhagia. The following steps are recommended:

1. History

Menstrual History: Timing, frequency, duration and volume of bleeding.

Associated Symptoms: Pain, systemic symptoms or pregnancy symptoms.

Medical History: Thyroid disease, bleeding disorders, liver/renal disease.

Medications: Use of anticoagulants, hormonal therapies or IUDs.

Family History: Bleeding disorders or gynaecological cancers.

Social History: Stress, weight changes or sexual history (e.g., risk of STIs).

2. Physical Examination

General: Signs of anemia (pallor, tachycardia), thyroid dysfunction or systemic disease.

Gynecological: Speculum exam to assess for cervical lesions, polyps or trauma; bimanual exam to evaluate uterine size, adnexal masses or tenderness.

Systemic: Bruising or petechiae suggesting coagulopathy.

3. Laboratory Tests

Pregnancy Test: To rule out pregnancy-related causes.

Complete Blood Count (CBC): Assess for anemia or thrombocytopenia.

Coagulation Profile: PT, aPTT, fibrinogen or von Willebrand factor testing if coagulopathy is suspected.

Thyroid Function Tests: TSH, free T4 to evaluate thyroid dysfunction.

Hormonal Profile: FSH, LH, prolactin or androgens if anovulation or PCOS is suspected.

Infection Screening: Cervical swabs for STIs if infection is suspected.

4. Imaging

Transvaginal Ultrasound (TVUS): First-line imaging to assess endometrial thickness, fibroids, polyps or adnexal masses.

Saline Infusion Sonography (SIS): Enhances visualization of intrauterine pathology (e.g., polyps, submucosal fibroids).

MRI/CT: Reserved for complex cases or suspected malignancy.

5. Invasive Procedures

Endometrial Biopsy: Indicated in women >45 years, postmenopausal bleeding or risk factors for endometrial hyperplasia/cancer (e.g., obesity, PCOS).

Hysteroscopy: Direct visualization of the endometrial cavity to identify and also treat polyps or submucosal fibroids.

Dilation and Curettage (D&C): Diagnostic and therapeutic for acute heavy bleeding or when biopsy is inconclusive.

Management

Management depends on the underlying cause, patient's age, fertility desires and severity of symptoms. The goals are to control bleeding, treat the underlying cause and prevent complications (e.g., anemia).

1. Medical Management

Hormonal Therapy

Combined Oral Contraceptives (COCs): Stabilize endometrial growth in anovulatory bleeding.

Progestins: Oral (e.g., norethindrone) or intrauterine (levonorgestrel IUD) to promote endometrial shedding and prevent hyperplasia.

Gonadotropin-Releasing Hormone (GnRH) Agonists: For severe cases (e.g., fibroids) to induce temporary menopause-like state.

Non-Hormonal Therapy

Tranexamic Acid: Antifibrinolytic to reduce bleeding in acute episodes.

Non-Steroidal Anti-Inflammatory Drugs (NSAIDs): Reduce prostaglandin-mediated bleeding (e.g., ibuprofen).

Treatment of Underlying Conditions

Correct coagulopathies (e.g., desmopressin for von Willebrand disease).

Treat infections with appropriate antibiotics.

Manage systemic conditions (e.g., levothyroxine for hypothyroidism).

2. Surgical Management

Endometrial Ablation: For women with heavy bleeding not responsive to medical therapy, who do not desire future fertility.

Myomectomy: Removal of fibroids while preserving fertility.

Hysterectomy: Definitive treatment for refractory bleeding or malignancy, especially in women who have completed family.

Polypectomy: Removal of endometrial or cervical polyps via hysteroscopy.

3. Supportive Care

Iron Supplementation: For anemia secondary to blood loss.

Counseling: Address psychological impact and educate on treatment options.

4. Special Considerations

Adolescents: Often anovulatory; hormonal regulation with COCs or progestins is first-line.

Perimenopausal Women: Evaluate for malignancy; hormonal therapy or ablation may be considered.

Postmenopausal Women: Any bleeding suggest endometrial biopsy to rule out malignancy.

Pregnancy-Related: Urgent management of ectopic pregnancy or miscarriage.

Complications

Anemia: Chronic blood loss can lead to iron deficiency anemia.

Infertility: Structural causes (e.g., fibroids, adenomyosis) or anovulation may impair fertility.

Malignancy Risk: Persistent metrorrhagia, especially in postmenopausal women, increases suspicion for endometrial or cervical cancer.

Quality of Life: Emotional distress, social embarrassment or disruption of daily activities.

Prognosis

Prognosis depends on the underlying cause. Benign causes (e.g., anovulation, polyps) often respond good to medical or surgical management.

Malignant causes require early detection and treatment for favorable outcomes.

Regular follow-up is essential to monitor response to therapy and detect recurrence.

Prevention

Lifestyle Modifications: Maintain healthy weight, manage stress and avoid unopposed oestrogen exposure (e.g., in obesity or PCOS).

Screening: Regular gynaecological exams to detect structural abnormalities early.

Contraceptive Use: Hormonal contraceptives can regulate cycles and reduce bleeding risk in susceptible individuals.

Key Points

Metrorrhagia is a symptom, not a disease; identifying the underlying cause is crucial.

Use the PALM-COEIN classification to systematically approach diagnosis.

Always rule out pregnancy and malignancy, especially in postmenopausal women.

Individualize management to the patient's age, reproductive goals and severity of bleeding.

Early intervention prevents complications like anemia or progression of undiagnosed malignancy.

3.11 Abnormal Uterine Bleeding

(*Nazf al -Rahim Ghayr Tabi'l*)

Abnormal uterine bleeding (AUB) is a common gynaecological condition encompassing any deviation from normal menstrual bleeding in terms of frequency, duration, volume or regularity. It includes conditions such as menorrhagia, metrorrhagia, oligomenorrhea and hypomenorrhea, among others and significantly impacts quality of life. The International Federation of Gynaecology and Obstetrics (FIGO) introduced the PALM-COEIN classification system to standardize the evaluation and management of AUB.

Definition

AUB is defined as uterine bleeding that is abnormal in volume, frequency, duration or regularity, occurring in non-pregnant women of reproductive age. Normal menstruation occurs every 21–35 days, lasts 3–7 days and involves blood loss of 10–80 mL .

AUB includes:

Heavy menstrual bleeding (HMB): Blood loss >80 mL or subjectively excessive bleeding (previously termed menorrhagia).

Intermenstrual bleeding: Bleeding between menstrual periods (previously termed metrorrhagia).

Infrequent bleeding: Cycles >35 days (oligomenorrhea).

Light bleeding: Blood loss <10 mL (hypomenorrhea).

Prolonged bleeding: Menstruation >7 days.

Irregular bleeding: Cycles with variable intervals.

AUB may occur with or without ovulation and can significantly affect physical, emotional and social well-being, often leading to anemia or infertility.

Epidemiology

Prevalence: Affects 10–35% of women of reproductive age, with higher rates in adolescence and perimenopause.

Impact: Causes anemia, fatigue, reduced quality of life and increased healthcare costs.

Risk Factors: Age (adolescence, perimenopause), obesity, nulliparity, bleeding disorders, hormonal contraceptive use and chronic medical conditions.

Pathophysiology

AUB results from disruptions in the hypothalamic-pituitary-ovarian (HPO) axis, endometrial hemostasis or uterine structural integrity. Key mechanisms include:

1. Hormonal Dysregulation

The HPO axis coordinates gonadotropin-releasing hormone (GnRH), follicle-stimulating hormone (FSH), luteinizing hormone (LH), oestrogen and progesterone to regulate ovulation and endometrial cycle.

Anovulatory cycles (e.g., in polycystic ovary syndrome [PCOS] or perimenopause) lead to unopposed oestrogen, causing excessive endometrial proliferation and irregular shedding.

Progesterone deficiency impairs endometrial stabilization, increasing bleeding volume or duration.

2. Endometrial Hemostasis

Normal menstruation involves spiral artery vasoconstriction (mediated by prostaglandins like PGF2α and endothelin) and controlled fibrinolysis.

AUB may result from increased prostaglandin E2 (PGE2), excessive fibrinolysis (elevated plasminogen activators) or defective angiogenesis.

3. Structural Abnormalities

Lesions like fibroids, polyps or adenomyosis increase endometrial surface area or disrupt hemostasis.

4. Systemic Factors

Coagulopathies (e.g., von Willebrand disease) impair clot formation.

Thyroid dysfunction or chronic illness disrupts HPO axis function or hormone metabolism.

FIGO PALM-COEIN Classification

The FIGO PALM-COEIN system categorizes AUB causes into structural (PALM) and non-structural (COEIN) etiologies, providing a standardized framework for diagnosis:

Structural Causes (PALM)

1. Polyps (AUB-P):

Endometrial or cervical polyps are benign growths that increase bleeding surface area or cause intermenstrual bleeding.

2. Adenomyosis (AUB-A):

Endometrial tissue within the myometrium disrupts hemostasis, causing heavy or painful bleeding.

3. Leiomyomas (Fibroids, AUB-L):

Submucosal fibroids distort the endometrial cavity; intramural/subserosal fibroids alter vascularity.

Classified by FIGO subtype (0–8) based on location.

4. Malignancy and Hyperplasia (AUB-M):

Endometrial hyperplasia (with or without atypia) or endometrial/cervical cancer causes heavy or irregular bleeding. Risk factors include unopposed oestrogen (e.g., obesity, PCOS), tamoxifen use, or Lynch syndrome.

Non-Structural Causes (COEIN)

1. Coagulopathy (AUB-C): Bleeding disorders (e.g., von Willebrand disease, thrombocytopenia) or anticoagulant therapy (e.g., warfarin).
2. Ovulatory Dysfunction (AUB-O): Anovulation (e.g., PCOS, hypothyroidism, perimenopause) leads to unopposed oestrogen and irregular shedding. Ovulatory bleeding may occur with luteal phase defects.
3. Endometrial (AUB-E): Primary endometrial disorders (e.g., defective hemostasis, inflammation or excessive fibrinolysis) in the absence of structural or systemic causes.
4. Iatrogenic (AUB-I): Medications (e.g., hormonal contraceptives, tamoxifen) or devices (e.g., copper IUD) cause irregular bleeding.
5. Not Yet Classified (AUB-N): Rare causes like arteriovenous malformations or cesarean scar defects.

PALM-COEIN Classification of AUB Mnemonic: "PALM COEIN" (According to cause)	
Structural (PALM)	**Non-Structural (COEIN)**
P Polyp	C – Coagulopathy
A Adenomyosis	O – Ovulatory dysfunction
L Leiomyoma (fibroid)	E – Endometrial causes
M Malignancy/hyperplasia	I – Iatrogenic
	N- Not yet classified

Clinical Features

Patterns of AUB

Heavy Menstrual Bleeding (HMB): Excessive volume (>80 mL), large clots (>2.5 cm) or frequent sanitary product changes (every 1–2 hours).

Prolonged Bleeding: Menstruation >7 days.

Intermenstrual Bleeding: Bleeding between periods, often linked to polyps or malignancy.

Irregular Bleeding: Irregular cycle intervals, common in anovulation.

Infrequent/scanty Bleeding: Cycles >35 days or blood loss <10 mL.

Associated Symptoms

Anemia: Fatigue, pallor, shortness of breath.

Pain: Dysmenorrhea (adenomyosis, fibroids) or pelvic pain.

Systemic symptoms: Weight loss (malignancy), galactorrhea (hyperprolactinemia) or hirsutism (PCOS).

Quality of Life: Social embarrassment, reduced productivity, psychological distress or sexual dysfunction.

Diagnosis

Diagnosis of AUB requires a systematic approach to identify the underlying cause, assess bleeding severity and rule out serious conditions like malignancy.

History

Menstrual History: Frequency, duration, volume, regularity and associated symptoms (e.g., clots, pain).

Medical History: Bleeding disorders, thyroid disease, medications (e.g., anticoagulants, hormonal contraceptives) or recent procedures.

Reproductive History: Parity, fertility desires or history of miscarriage.

Family History: Coagulopathies, gynecologic cancers or endocrine disorders.

Quality of Life: Impact on daily activities, work or emotional well-being.

Physical Examination

General: Signs of anemia (pallor, tachycardia), thyroid enlargement, obesity or hirsutism.

Pelvic Exam: Uterine size, tenderness or masses (e.g., fibroids).

Speculum Exam: Cervical lesions, polyps or abnormal discharge.

Laboratory Tests

Complete Blood Count (CBC): Assess hemoglobin, hematocrit and thrombocytopenia.

Coagulation Profile: Prothrombin time (PT), activated partial thromboplastin time (aPTT), von Willebrand factor testing.

Hormonal Evaluation

Thyroid-stimulating hormone (TSH): Screen for hypothyroidism/hyperthyroidism.

Prolactin: Rule out hyperprolactinemia.

FSH, LH, Estradiol: Assess ovulatory status or premature ovarian insufficiency (POI).

Testosterone, DHEAS: Evaluate for PCOS-related hyperandrogenism.

Pregnancy Test: Rule out pregnancy-related bleeding (e.g., miscarriage, ectopic pregnancy).

Ferritin: Assess iron stores in anemic patients.

Imaging

Pelvic Ultrasound: First-line to detect fibroids, polyps, adenomyosis or endometrial thickness.

Transvaginal ultrasound is preferred for better resolution.

Saline-Infusion Sonography (SIS): Enhances visualization of endometrial polyps or submucosal fibroids.

MRI: For detailed assessment of adenomyosis or complex fibroids.

Hysterosalpingography: Evaluates uterine cavity abnormalities or tubal patency.

Invasive Procedures

Endometrial Biopsy: Indicated for women >45 years, those with risk factors for endometrial hyperplasia/cancer (e.g., obesity, PCOS), or persistent/irregular bleeding.

Hysteroscopy: Visualizes endometrial cavity for polyps, fibroids or adhesions; allows biopsy or resection.

Dilation and Curettage (D&C): Diagnostic and therapeutic for acute heavy bleeding; not routine for diagnosis.

Cervical Cytology/Biopsy: Rule out cervical pathology (e.g., cervicitis, cancer).

Diagnostic Criteria

Objective: Blood loss >80 mL (rarely measured; alkaline hematin method).

Subjective: Patient-reported abnormal bleeding impacting quality of life.

PALM-COEIN: Categorize cause to guide management.

Management

Management of AUB is done according to the underlying cause, bleeding severity, patient age, fertility desires and comorbidities. Goals include reducing bleeding, correcting anemia, addressing the etiology and improving quality of life.

Medical Management

Non-Hormonal Therapies

1. Non-Steroidal Anti-Inflammatory Drugs (NSAIDs):

E.g., ibuprofen, mefenamic acid.

Reduce prostaglandin production, decreasing bleeding by 20–50% and alleviating dysmenorrhea.

2. Tranexamic Acid:

Antifibrinolytic; reduces bleeding by 30–60%.

Taken during bleeding episodes; effective for AUB-E or coagulopathies.

3. Iron Supplementation: Corrects anemia and restores ferritin levels.

Hormonal Therapies

1. Combined Oral Contraceptives (COCs):

Regulate cycles, reduce bleeding by 35–60% and treat anovulatory bleeding.

Contraindicated in women with thrombotic risk factors (e.g., smoking, age >35).

2. Levonorgestrel-Releasing Intrauterine Device (LNG-IUD):

Reduces bleeding by 70–90% by inducing endometrial atrophy.

Preferred for long-term management and contraception.

3. Progestins:

Cyclic (e.g., medroxyprogesterone) or continuous (e.g., norethindrone) to stabilize endometrium.

Effective for AUB-O or endometrial hyperplasia.

4. Gonadotropin-Releasing Hormone (GnRH) Agonists:

E.g., leuprolide; induce hypoestrogenic state, reducing bleeding. Used short-term for fibroids or pre-surgery; add-back therapy (oestrogen/progestin) minimizes side effects.

5. Danazol:

Androgenic steroid; reduces bleeding but rarely used due to side effects (e.g., hirsutism).

Specific Treatments

Coagulopathies: Desmopressin (von Willebrand disease), clotting factor replacement.

Hypothyroidism: Levothyroxine to restore normal thyroid function.

Infections: Antibiotics for endometritis or cervicitis.

Surgical Management

1. Endometrial Ablation

Destroys endometrial lining (e.g., thermal, radiofrequency, cryotherapy). Reduces bleeding by 70–90%; suitable for women not desiring fertility. Risk of recurrence or need for further intervention.

2. Myomectomy

Removes fibroids (hysteroscopic, laparoscopic, or abdominal). Preserves fertility; indicated for submucosal fibroids (AUB-L).

3. Uterine Artery Embolization (UAE)

Occludes uterine arteries to shrink fibroids and reduce bleeding. Less invasive than hysterectomy; fertility outcomes uncertain.

4. Hysterectomy

Definitive treatment for refractory AUB or malignancy. Performed vaginally, laparoscopically or abdominally; indicated when fertility is not desired.

5. Polypectomy

Hysteroscopic removal of endometrial or cervical polyps.

6. D&C

Temporary measure for acute, severe bleeding; not a long-term solution.

7. Cervical Procedures

Excision or cautery for cervical lesions (e.g., polyps, cervicitis).

Management of Specific Causes

1. Polyps (AUB-P): Hysteroscopic polypectomy.
2. Adenomyosis (AUB-A): LNG-IUD, GnRH agonists or hysterectomy for severe cases.
3. Fibroids (AUB-L): Myomectomy, UAE or GnRH agonists.
4. Malignancy/Hyperplasia (AUB-M): Progestins or LNG-IUD for hyperplasia; hysterectomy for cancer.
5. Coagulopathy (AUB-C): Hematologic management, tranexamic acid.
6. Ovulatory Dysfunction (AUB-O): COCs, progestins or ovulation induction for fertility.
7. Endometrial (AUB-E): Tranexamic acid, LNG-IUD.
8. Iatrogenic (AUB-I): Adjust or discontinue causative medication/device.

Lifestyle and Supportive Measures

Weight Management: Reduces unopposed oestrogen in obesity-related AUB.

Dietary Counseling: Supports iron intake for anemia.

Psychosocial Support: Addresses emotional distress or quality-of-life impact.

Complications

Anemia: Iron deficiency anemia due to chronic heavy bleeding; causes fatigue, pallor or cardiac strain.

Endometrial Hyperplasia/Cancer: Risk in unopposed oestrogen states (e.g., PCOS, obesity).

Infertility: Associated with anovulation, fibroids or endometrial pathology.

Quality of Life: Social, occupational or psychological impact from heavy or irregular bleeding.

Treatment-Related: Hormonal side effects (e.g., weight gain, mood changes), surgical complications (e.g., infection, adhesions).

Special Populations

1. Adolescents

AUB often due to HPO axis immaturity or coagulopathies (e.g., von Willebrand disease).

Management prioritizes non-invasive options (e.g., COCs, tranexamic acid).

2. Perimenopause

Anovulatory cycles and hyperplasia are common; endometrial biopsy is needed to rule out malignancy.

LNG-IUD or ablation are effective for non-fertility-seeking women.

3. Women Desiring Fertility

Avoid irreversible treatments (e.g., ablation, hysterectomy).

Focus on ovulation induction (e.g., clomiphene) or myomectomy.

4. Postmenopausal Women

Any vaginal bleeding is abnormal and requires urgent evaluation for malignancy.

Endometrial biopsy and imaging are mandatory.

Clinical Case Examples

1. Case 1: Heavy Menstrual Bleeding

A 38-year-old woman presents with heavy periods lasting 9 days, requiring pad changes every hour, and fatigue.

Investigations: Hemoglobin 9.2 g/dL, normal TSH, normal coagulation.

Ultrasound: Submucosal fibroid.

Diagnosis: AUB-L (fibroid-related).

Management: LNG-IUD, iron supplementation, consider myomectomy.

2. Case 2: Irregular Bleeding

A 30-year-old woman reports spotting between periods for 4 months while using a progestin-only pill.

Investigations: Normal hormones, negative pregnancy test.

Hysteroscopy: Endometrial polyp.

Diagnosis: AUB-P (polyp-related) and AUB-I (iatrogenic).

Management: Polypectomy and then combined oral contraceptives.

Conclusion

AUB is a multifaceted condition encompassing heavy, prolonged, irregular or infrequent uterine bleeding, with diverse etiologies classified by the FIGO PALM-COEIN system. Structural causes (e.g., fibroids, polyps) and non-structural causes (e.g., anovulation, coagulopathies) require thorough evaluation through history, physical examination, laboratory tests, imaging and invasive procedures. Management is individualized, balancing medical therapies (e.g., NSAIDs, LNG-IUD) and surgical interventions (e.g., myomectomy, hysterectomy) based on the cause, severity and fertility goals. Early diagnosis and treatment prevent complications like anemia, infertility or malignancy, improving patient outcomes and quality of life.

Key Takeaways

AUB includes deviations from normal menstrual bleeding in volume, frequency or regularity.

The PALM-COEIN system categorizes causes into structural (PALM) and non-structural (COEIN).

Diagnosis requires a systematic approach to identify etiology and rule out malignancy.

Treatment ranges from medical (hormonal, non-hormonal) to surgical, individualize to patient needs.

3.12 Hirsutism

(Shuraniat)

Hirsutism is a common clinical condition characterized by excessive, male-pattern hair growth in women, typically in androgen-sensitive areas such as the face, chest and lower abdomen. It often reflects underlying hormonal imbalances, particularly hyperandrogenism and can significantly impact psychological and social well-being.

Definition

Hirsutism is defined as excessive terminal hair growth in women in areas where hair growth is typically minimal or absent, following a male-pattern distribution (e.g., upper lip, chin, chest, back, abdomen, inner thighs). It is distinct from "hypertrichosis", which involves generalized excessive hair growth in non-androgen-dependent areas and is not necessarily hormonally driven. Hirsutism is often a manifestation of elevated androgen levels or increased sensitivity of hair follicles to androgens.

Epidemiology

Prevalence: Affects 5–15% of reproductive-age women, with higher rates in certain ethnic groups (e.g., Mediterranean, South Asian, Middle Eastern populations).

Risk Factors: Family history of hirsutism, obesity, polycystic ovary syndrome (PCOS) and certain ethnic backgrounds.

Pathophysiology

Hirsutism results from the interaction of androgens with hair follicles in androgen-sensitive skin areas, leading to the transformation of vellus (fine, light) hair into terminal (coarse, dark) hair. Key mechanisms include:

1. Androgen Excess

Androgens (e.g., testosterone, dihydrotestosterone [DHT], androstenedione) stimulate hair follicle growth and prolong the anagen (growth) phase of the hair cycle.

DHT, formed by the enzyme 5α-reductase in hair follicles, is the most potent androgen driving hirsutism.

2. Increased Androgen Sensitivity

Genetic variations in androgen receptor sensitivity or 5α-reductase activity can cause hirsutism even with normal androgen levels (idiopathic hirsutism).

3. Hormonal Regulation

Androgens are produced by the ovaries (testosterone, androstenedione), adrenal glands (dehydroepiandrosterone sulphate [DHEAS]) and peripheral tissues (via conversion).

Sex hormone-binding globulin (SHBG) binds androgens, reducing their bioavailability; low SHBG (e.g., in obesity, PCOS) increases free androgen levels.

4. Endocrine Dysregulation

Conditions like PCOS disrupt the hypothalamic-pituitary-ovarian (HPO) axis, increasing luteinizing hormone (LH) and ovarian androgen production.

Adrenal disorders (e.g., congenital adrenal hyperplasia) elevate adrenal androgens.

Etiology

Hirsutism is classified based on underlying causes, which may involve androgen excess, increased androgen sensitivity or non-androgenic factors.

1. Androgen-Related Causes

Polycystic Ovary Syndrome (PCOS):

Most common cause (70–80% of hirsutism cases).

Characterized by hyperandrogenism, ovulatory dysfunction and polycystic ovarian morphology (Rotterdam criteria).

Elevated LH:FSH ratio stimulates ovarian theca cells to produce androgens.

2. Idiopathic Hirsutism

Hirsutism with normal androgen levels and ovulatory cycles.

Likely due to increased 5α-reductase activity or androgen receptor sensitivity in hair follicles.

Common in women with familial or ethnic predisposition.

3. Congenital Adrenal Hyperplasia (CAH)

Non-classic 21-hydroxylase deficiency is the most common form.

Impaired cortisol synthesis leads to increased adrenocorticotropic hormone (ACTH) and adrenal androgen production (e.g., DHEAS).

4. Ovarian Tumours

Rare androgen-secreting tumours (e.g., Sertoli-Leydig cell tumours, granulosa-theca cell tumours) cause rapid-onset hirsutism and virilization.

5. Adrenal Tumours

Adrenal adenomas or carcinomas secrete androgens (DHEAS, testosterone), causing severe hirsutism.

6. Cushing's Syndrome

Excess cortisol increases adrenal androgen production, contributing to hirsutism.

7. Hyperprolactinemia

Elevated prolactin stimulates adrenal androgen production or disrupts ovarian function, leading to mild hirsutism.

8. Iatrogenic Causes

a. Medications

Androgenic drugs (e.g., danazol, anabolic steroids, progestins).

Non-androgenic drugs (e.g., phenytoin, minoxidil) may cause hypertrichosis rather than true hirsutism.

b. Other Causes

Obesity: Increases insulin resistance, lowering SHBG and raising free androgen levels.

Hypothyroidism: May indirectly increase androgen effects by reducing SHBG.

Acromegaly: Rare; growth hormone excess may enhance androgen activity.

Familial/Ethnic Variation: Normal androgen levels with increased hair growth in certain populations (not pathological).

Severe Hyperandrogenism (Virilization)

Rapid-onset hirsutism with signs of virilization (e.g., clitoromegaly, deepening voice, male-pattern baldness) suggests serious conditions like ovarian/adrenal tumours or severe CAH.

Clinical Features

1. Hair Growth Patterns

Excessive terminal hair in androgen-sensitive areas: upper lip, chin, sideburns, chest, back, lower abdomen, inner thighs. Assessed using the Ferriman-Gallwey score (see Diagnosis).

2. Associated Symptoms

Acne, oily skin, or seborrhoea (common in PCOS).

Irregular menses or amenorrhea (PCOS, hyperprolactinemia).

Obesity, acanthosis nigricans (PCOS, insulin resistance).

Virilization signs (e.g., clitoromegaly, deepening voice) in severe cases.

3. Psychosocial Impact

Anxiety, depression or low self-esteem due to cosmetic concerns.

Social withdrawal or reduced quality of life.

Diagnosis

Diagnosis of hirsutism involves assessing the extent of hair growth, identifying underlying causes, and ruling out serious conditions like tumours or virilization.

History

Hair Growth: Onset (gradual vs. rapid), distribution and progression.

Menstrual History: Regularity, oligomenorrhea or amenorrhea (suggests PCOS or endocrine disorders).

Associated Symptoms: Acne, weight gain, infertility, galactorrhea or virilization signs.

Medical History: Medications, chronic illnesses or recent weight changes.

Family History: Hirsutism, PCOS or endocrine disorders.

Ethnic Background: Influences normal hair growth patterns.

Physical Examination

Ferriman-Gallwey Score: Quantifies hirsutism by scoring hair growth in nine androgen-sensitive areas (e.g., upper lip, chin, chest). Score ≥ 8 indicates hirsutism in most populations; thresholds vary by ethnicity (e.g., ≥ 6 in East Asians).

General: Assess for obesity, acanthosis nigricans, thyroid enlargement or Cushing syndrome like features.

Pelvic Exam: Evaluate for clitoromegaly or ovarian masses (rare).

Skin: Check for acne, seborrhoea, or male-pattern baldness.

Laboratory Tests

1. Androgen Levels:

   a. Total and Free Testosterone: Elevated in PCOS, ovarian/adrenal tumours.
   b. DHEAS: Elevated in adrenal disorders (e.g., CAH, adrenal tumours).
   c. Androstenedione: May be elevated in PCOS or ovarian tumours.
   d. SHBG: Low levels increase free androgen bioavailability (e.g., in obesity, PCOS).

2. 17-Hydroxyprogesterone (17-OHP): Elevated in non-classic CAH; measure in early follicular phase or after ACTH stimulation test.

3. Prolactin: Screen for hyperprolactinemia.

4. TSH: Rule out hypothyroidism.

5. Cortisol: Assess for Cushing's syndrome (e.g., 24-hour urinary free cortisol, dexamethasone suppression test).

6. Fasting Glucose/Insulin: Screen for insulin resistance in PCOS.
7. LH/FSH Ratio: Elevated (>2:1) in PCOS.
8. Pregnancy Test: Rule out pregnancy in amenorrhoeic women.

Imaging

Pelvic Ultrasound: Evaluate for polycystic ovaries (PCOS) or ovarian tumours.

Rotterdam criteria for PCOS: ≥12 follicles (2–9 mm) or ovarian volume >10 mL.

Adrenal Imaging: CT or MRI for suspected adrenal tumours (DHEAS >700 μg/dL or rapid-onset hirsutism).

Pituitary MRI: If hyperprolactinemia or Cushing's syndrome is suspected.

Differential Diagnosis

PCOS: Most common; gradual onset, irregular menses, hyperandrogenism.

Idiopathic Hirsutism: Normal androgens and ovulatory cycles.

Non-Classic CAH: Elevated 17-OHP, often with family history.

Ovarian/Adrenal Tumours: Rapid onset, virilization, markedly elevated androgens.

Hyperprolactinemia: Galactorrhea, amenorrhea, mild hirsutism.

Cushing's Syndrome: Hirsutism with moon facies, striae and central obesity.

Hypertrichosis: Generalized hair growth, often medication-induced or non-androgenic.

Management

Management of hirsutism focuses on reducing hair growth, addressing underlying causes, improving cosmetic outcomes, and managing associated conditions (e.g., infertility, metabolic syndrome). Treatment is based on severity, patient preferences and fertility goals.

Non-Pharmacologic Management

1. Cosmetic Measures

Shaving, Waxing, Plucking: Temporary hair removal; does not affect hair growth rate.

Laser Hair Removal: Targets melanin in hair follicles; effective for long-term reduction in dark hair.

Electrolysis: Destroys hair follicles; permanent but time-consuming.

Depilatory Creams: Chemical hair removal; temporary and may cause skin irritation.

2. Lifestyle Modifications

Weight loss (5–10% body weight) in obese patients with PCOS reduces insulin resistance, increases SHBG and lowers free androgens.

Dietary counselling and exercise to improve metabolic health.

Pharmacologic Management

1. Combined Oral Contraceptives (COCs)

First-line therapy for hirsutism in women not seeking fertility.

Contain ethinyl estradiol and progestin; increase SHBG, reduce free androgens and suppress ovarian androgen production.

Preferred progestins: drospirenone, norgestimate (less androgenic).

Effect on hair growth seen after 6–12 months.

2. Anti-Androgens

Spironolactone (50–200 mg/day):

Androgen receptor antagonist; inhibits 5α-reductase.

Reduces hair growth; side effects include hyperkalaemia, menstrual irregularities.

Requires contraception due to teratogenicity.

Finasteride (2.5–5 mg/day):

Inhibits 5α-reductase, reducing DHT formation.

Less effective than spironolactone; teratogenic.

Flutamide(125–250 mg/day):

Potent androgen receptor blocker; rarely used due to hepatotoxicity.

Cyproterone Acetate (not widely available in the US):

Anti-androgen and progestin; used in some COCs (e.g., ethinyl estradiol/cyproterone).

3. Eflornithine Cream

Topical agent; inhibits ornithine decarboxylase, slowing hair growth.

Used for facial hirsutism; effect seen in 4–8 weeks.

4. Metformin

Improves insulin sensitivity in PCOS, indirectly reducing androgens.

Less effective for hirsutism than COCs or anti-androgens but useful for metabolic management.

5. GnRH Agonists(e.g., leuprolide)

Suppress ovarian androgen production; used in severe cases unresponsive to other therapies.

Requires add-back oestrogen/progestin to prevent hypoestrogenic side effects.

6. Glucocorticoids (e.g., dexamethasone)

Suppress adrenal androgens in non-classic CAH.

Low-dose therapy (0.25–0.5 mg/day); monitor for side effects (e.g., weight gain, osteoporosis).

Management of Specific Causes

PCOS

COCs or anti-androgens for hirsutism.

Metformin and lifestyle changes for insulin resistance.

Ovulation induction (e.g., clomiphene) for fertility.

Non-Classic CAH

Glucocorticoids to suppress adrenal androgens.

COCs or anti-androgens for symptomatic hirsutism.

Ovarian/Adrenal Tumours

Surgical resection (e.g., oophorectomy, adrenalectomy).

Oncology consultation for malignant tumours.

Hyperprolactinemia

Dopamine agonists (e.g., cabergoline, bromocriptine).

Cushing's Syndrome

Treat underlying cause (e.g., pituitary surgery, adrenalectomy).

Iatrogenic

Discontinue or replace causative medication.

Surgical Management

Rarely indicated for hirsutism alone.

Ovarian Drilling: For PCOS patients with resistant anovulation and hirsutism; reduces androgen production.

Tumour Resection: For androgen-secreting ovarian or adrenal tumours.

Monitoring and Follow-Up

Assess Ferriman-Gallwey score every 3–6 months to monitor treatment response.

Monitor for medication side effects (e.g., hyperkalaemia with spironolactone, liver function with flutamide).

Screen for metabolic complications in PCOS (e.g., diabetes, dyslipidaemia).

Repeat imaging or hormonal testing if new symptoms (e.g., virilization) develop.

Complications

Psychosocial: Anxiety, depression or social isolation due to cosmetic concerns.

Metabolic: Increased risk of diabetes, cardiovascular disease in PCOS-related hirsutism.

Infertility: Associated with anovulation in PCOS or hyperprolactinemia.

Malignancy: Rare but serious in cases of androgen-secreting tumours.

Clinical Case Example

Case: A 25-year-old woman presents with excessive facial and chest hair for 2 years, irregular menses and acne. BMI is 30 kg/m^2.

Physical Exam: Ferriman-Gallwey score 12, acanthosis nigricans.

Investigations: Elevated free testosterone, LH:FSH ratio 2.5:1, normal DHEAS, 17-OHP and prolactin.

Ultrasound: Polycystic ovaries.

Diagnosis: Hirsutism due to PCOS.

Management:

COC (ethinyl estradiol/drospirenone) to reduce androgens.

Spironolactone 100 mg/day for hirsutism.

Metformin and lifestyle changes for insulin resistance.

Laser hair removal for cosmetic concerns.

Conclusion

Hirsutism is a common condition driven by androgen excess or increased hair follicle sensitivity, with PCOS being the most frequent cause. Diagnosis involves assessing hair growth severity (Ferriman-Gallwey score), evaluating androgen levels, and ruling out serious conditions like tumours or CAH. Management combines cosmetic measures, hormonal therapies (COCs, anti-androgens) and treatment of underlying disorders.

Key Takeaways

Hirsutism is excessive male-pattern hair growth in women, often due to hyperandrogenism.

PCOS is the leading cause; idiopathic hirsutism and CAH are also common.

Diagnosis requires a thorough history, Ferriman-Gallwey scoring, hormonal testing and imaging.

Treatment includes COCs, anti-androgens, cosmetic measures and management of underlying conditions.

Long Answer Questions

1. Describe the hormonal regulation and endometrial changes during the menstrual cycle. Discuss how dysfunction at any level can lead to menstrual irregularities.
2. Classify amenorrhea into primary and secondary types. Outline the etiologies, diagnostic approach and treatment strategies for each.
3. Explain the PALM-COEIN classification of abnormal uterine bleeding. Provide structural and functional examples with clinical features.
4. Define dysmenorrhea. Differentiate between primary and secondary types and explain the pathophysiology, symptoms and management options for both.
5. Discuss premenstrual syndrome (PMS)—its clinical manifestations, proposed mechanisms, diagnostic criteria and therapeutic strategies.

Short Answer Questions

1. Define oligomenorrhea and polymenorrhea with cycle length parameters.
2. Mention two causes each of primary and secondary amenorrhea.
3. What is the hallmark symptom of menorrhagia and how is it defined clinically?
4. Name two common physical symptoms of premenstrual syndrome.
5. What are two diagnostic tools used to evaluate abnormal uterine bleeding?

Multiple Choice Questions (1 Mark Each)

1. Which hormone triggers ovulation?

a) FSH b) Estrogen c) LH d) Progesterone

Ans: c) LH

2. Normal menstrual cycle length ranges between:

a) 14–24 days b) 21–35 days c) 28–42 days d) 15–30 days

Ans: b) 21–35 days

3. Which condition is characterized by excessive hair growth in females?

a) Amenorrhea b) Menorrhagia c) Hirsutism d) Dysmenorrhea

Ans: c) Hirsutism

4. AUB due to fibroid falls under which PALM-COEIN category?

a) P b) L c) O d) C

Ans: b) L – Leiomyoma

5. Which phase of the cycle is dominated by progesterone?

a) Follicular b) Menstrual c) Luteal d) Ovulatory

Ans: c) Luteal

6. Which hormone regulates the proliferation of endometrial lining?

a) Progesterone b) Estrogen c) FSH d) LH

Ans: b) Estrogen

7. Turner syndrome is associated with:

a) Secondary amenorrhea b) Primary amenorrhea c) Menorrhagia d) PMS

Ans: b) Primary amenorrhea

8. Dysmenorrhea with known uterine pathology is:

a) Primary b) Cyclical c) Secondary d) Pseudomenstrual

Ans: c) Secondary

9. Irregular intermenstrual bleeding is termed:

a) Menorrhagia b) Oligomenorrhea c) Metrorrhagia d) Polymenorrhea

Ans: c) Metrorrhagia

10. Most appropriate initial investigation in heavy menstrual bleeding:

a) Pap smear b) USG pelvis c) HSG d) Laparoscopy

Ans: b) USG pelvis

04

Puberty, Adolescence & its Disorders

(Bulughat, Murahiqa aur Muta'allaqa Amrad)

4.1 *Balughat ka Ta'arrruf* (Introduction of puberty)
4.2 *Badul-ehaza* (Menarche, thelarche, pubarche, adrenarche)
4.3 *Bulughat qabl az waqt* (Precocious puberty)
4.4 *Bulugh-i-Mu'akhkhar* (Delayed puberty)
4.5 *Kathrat-i-tamth Bulughi* (Pubertal Menorrhagia)

Learning Objective (At the end of the session, the students should be able to)

Define *Balughat* (Puberty) & discuss the morphological and hormonal changes in puberty.
Define Menarche, Thelarche, Pubarche & Adrenarche & tanner staging.
Describe & discuss the causes, diagnosis and management of precocious puberty.
Describe & discuss the causes, diagnosis and management of delayed puberty.

4.1 Introduction of puberty

(Balughat ka Ta'arrruf)

Puberty marks a crucial developmental transition from childhood to adulthood, characterized by physical, hormonal and psychological changes that culminate in reproductive maturity. This complex process, driven by the activation of the hypothalamic-pituitary-ovarian (HPO) axis, orchestrates the maturation of secondary sexual characteristics, growth spurts and fertility.

The onset of puberty typically occurs between ages 8 and 13 in females and 9 and 14 in males, influenced by genetic, environmental factors. Asclepius, a Greek physician, aptly described puberty as the "springtime of youth," reflecting the dynamic interplay of hormonal signals that initiate breast development, menarche and other hallmarks of sexual maturation in females. These changes are driven by increased gonadotropin-releasing hormone (GnRH) secretion, stimulating the release of luteinizing hormone (LH) and follicle-stimulating hormone (FSH), which in turn promote ovarian oestrogen production. This cascade also triggers adrenal androgen production, contributing to pubic and axillary hair growth

Definition

Puberty is the developmental period during which a child transits into sexual maturity, marked by the development of secondary sexual characteristics, reproductive capacity and significant physical and psychological changes. It is orchestrated by complex interactions between the hypothalamic-pituitary-ovarian (HPO) axis, adrenal glands and other neuroendocrine systems.

Physiology

Puberty is initiated by the reactivation of the HPO axis, which is dormant during childhood. The hypothalamus begins pulsatile secretion of gonadotropin-releasing hormone (GnRH), stimulating the anterior pituitary to release luteinizing hormone (LH) and follicle-stimulating hormone (FSH).

In females, LH and FSH stimulate ovarian production of estrogens (primarily estradiol), which drive secondary sexual characteristics and reproductive organ development. In males, these hormones stimulate testicular production of testosterone.

Adrenal androgens also contribute to puberty, particularly in the development of pubic and axillary hair (pubarche).

Puberty typically occurs between ages 8–13 in girls and 9–14 in boys, with variations influenced by genetics, nutrition, socioeconomic factors, and environmental exposures.

Stages

Puberty is clinically assessed using the Tanner stages (I–V), which describe the progression of breast development (in females), genital development (in males), and pubic hair growth in both sexes.

In females, key events include thelarche (breast development), pubarche (pubic hair growth) and menarche (onset of menstruation).

Growth spurts occur early in puberty for girls (peak height velocity around Tanner stage II–III) and later for boys (Tanner stage III–IV).

Clinical Relevance

Precocious Puberty: Onset before age 8 in girls or 9 in boys, potentially due to central (GnRH-dependent) or peripheral (GnRH-independent) causes, such as tumours or congenital adrenal hyperplasia.

Delayed Puberty: Absence of secondary sexual characteristics by age 13 in girls or 14 in boys, often due to constitutional delay, hypogonadism or chronic illness.

Key Points

Puberty is a dynamic process driven by neuroendocrine activation.

Timing and progression vary widely but follow predictable patterns.

Abnormal pubertal timing requires thorough evaluation to identify underlying pathologies.

Flowchart: Hormonal Regulation During Puberty

Hypothalamus
↓
GnRH (Gonadotropin-Releasing Hormone)
↓
Anterior Pituitary Gland
↓
FSH & LH (Follicle-Stimulating & Luteinizing Hormones)
↓
Ovaries
↓ ↓
Estrogen Progesterone
↓
Development of Secondary Sexual Characteristics
(Menarche, Thelarche, Pubarche, Growth Spurt)

Hormone	Source	Role in Puberty
GnRH	Hypothalamus	Stimulates FSH & LH release
FSH	Anterior Pituitary	Follicle growth, oestrogen production
LH	Anterior Pituitary	Ovulation, corpus luteum formation
Estrogen	Ovaries	Secondary sexual traits, endometrium
Progesterone	Ovaries	Endometrial maintenance post-ovulation

4.2 Menarche, thelarche, pubarche, adrenarche

(Badul-ehaza)

Menarche

Definition

Menarche is the onset of the first menstrual period, marking a key milestone in female puberty and the beginning of reproductive potential. It typically occurs between ages 10–15, with an average age of 12.4 years in developed countries. (by National Institute of Health)

Physiology

Menarche results from the maturation of the HPO axis, leading to cyclic oestrogen and progesterone production by the ovaries.

Estrogen stimulates endometrial proliferation, while ovulation (if it occurs) leads to progesterone secretion, stabilizing the endometrium. If no pregnancy occurs, hormonal withdrawal causes endometrial shedding, resulting in menstruation.

Early menstrual cycles are often anovulatory (no ovulation), leading to irregular or heavy bleeding, which typically regularizes within 1–2 years.

Factors Influencing Menarche

1. Genetic: Family history strongly influences age at menarche.

2. Nutritional Status: Adequate body fat (approximately 17% body fat) is required to trigger menarche, explaining delayed menarche in underweight girls or those with eating disorders.

3. Environmental: Stress, socioeconomic factors and exposure to endocrine-disrupting drugs can alter timing.

4. Ethnic Variations: Mean age at menarche varies across populations (e.g., earlier in African-American girls compared to Caucasian girls).

Clinical Relevance

Early Menarche (<10 years): Associated with increased risk of obesity, type 2 diabetes, cardiovascular disease and breast cancer due to prolonged oestrogen exposure.

Late Menarche (>15 years): May indicate hypogonadism, Turner syndrome or chronic illness (e.g., celiac disease, hypothyroidism).

One must assess menstrual history to evaluate reproductive health, screen for polycystic ovary syndrome (PCOS) or identify structural abnormalities (e.g., imperforate hymen).

Key Points

Menarche is a hallmark of female puberty, reflecting HPO axis maturity.

Irregular cycles are common in the first 1–2 years post-menarche.

Abnormal timing requires investigation for underlying endocrine or systemic disorders.

Thelarche

Definition

Thelarche is the onset of breast development, typically the first clinical sign of puberty in girls, occurring between ages 8–13 (mean age ~10 years). It is driven by rising oestrogen levels from ovarian activation.

Physiology

Estrogen stimulates proliferation of mammary ductal and stromal tissue, leading to the formation of breast buds (Tanner stage II).

Progressive development includes enlargement of the areola, ductal elongation and adipose tissue deposition (Tanner stages III–V).

Thelarche is primarily mediated by estradiol from the ovaries, though adrenal androgens and local growth factors (e.g., insulin-like growth factor-1) play supportive roles.

Tanner Stages of Breast Development

Stage I: Prepubertal, no glandular tissue.

Stage II: Breast bud formation, small mound under the areola.

Stage III: Further enlargement of breast and areola without separation of contours.

Stage IV: Areola and papilla project above the breast contour.

Stage V: Mature breast, with areola recessed to the breast contour.

Clinical Relevance

Premature Thelarche: Isolated breast development before age 8, often benign and self-limiting but requires evaluation to rule out precocious puberty or oestrogen-secreting tumours.

Asymmetric Development: Common during early thelarche; significant asymmetry warrants investigation for masses or hormonal imbalances.

Absent Thelarche: May indicate primary ovarian failure, androgen excess (e.g., PCOS), or congenital anomalies (e.g., Turner syndrome).

Breast examination is a critical component of gynecologic assessment, as abnormalities may signal endocrine disorders or, rarely, malignancies.

Key Points

Thelarche marks the onset of puberty in most girls.

Estrogen drives breast development through predictable Tanner stages.

Pubarche

Definition

Pubarche is the onset of pubic hair development, typically occurring between ages 8–14 in girls and slightly later in boys. It is primarily driven by adrenal androgens rather than gonadal hormones.

Physiology

Pubarche results from increased adrenal androgen production (dehydroepiandrosterone [DHEA] and androstenedione) during adrenarche, which is converted peripherally to testosterone and dihydrotestosterone (DHT). These androgens stimulate hair follicle growth in androgen-sensitive areas (pubic and axillary regions).

Pubic hair progresses through "Tanner stages"

Stage I: No pubic hair.

Stage II: Sparse, lightly pigmented hair along the labia or base of the penis.

Stage III: Darker, coarser hair spreading over the pubic region.

Stage IV: Adult-type hair, limited to the pubic triangle.

Stage V: Adult distribution, extending to the inner thighs.

Clinical Relevance

Premature Pubarche: Pubic hair development before age 8 in girls or 9 in boys may indicate premature adrenarche, non-classical congenital adrenal hyperplasia (CAH) or androgen-secreting tumours.

Delayed Pubarche: May reflect adrenal insufficiency or hypogonadism. Pubarche is independent of gonadal puberty, so it may occur without thelarche or menarche in certain conditions (e.g., premature adrenarche).

Key Points

Pubarche is driven by adrenal androgens, not gonadal hormones.

It follows a predictable progression through Tanner stages.

Abnormal timing may indicate adrenal or systemic disorders.

Adrenarche

Definition

Adrenarche is the maturation of the adrenal zona reticularis, leading to increased production of adrenal androgens (DHEA, DHEA-sulphate [DHEA-S], and androstenedione) starting around ages 6–8 in both sexes. It is a distinct process from gonadarche (activation of gonadal puberty).

Physiology

Adrenarche is triggered by changes in adrenal enzyme activity (e.g., increased 17,20-lyase activity), independent of the hypothalamo-pituitary gonadal axis.

Adrenal androgens stimulate pubarche (pubic and axillary hair growth) and contribute to sebum production, body odor and mild acne.

Adrenarche precedes gonadarche in most children but is not required for pubertal progression.

Clinical Relevance

Premature Adrenarche: Early adrenal androgen production (before age 6–8) may cause premature pubarche, mild acne or body odor. It is often benign but requires evaluation to exclude CAH, adrenal tumours or precocious puberty.

Exaggerated Adrenarche: Excessive androgen production may lead to hirsutism, acne or insulin resistance, particularly in girls at risk for PCOS.

Adrenal Insufficiency: Failure of adrenarche may occur in conditions like Addison's disease or 21-hydroxylase deficiency, leading to absent pubarche.

Key Points

Adrenarche is the adrenal contribution to puberty, driven by increased androgen production.

It is independent of gonadarche and primarily affects hair growth and skin changes.

Abnormal adrenarche requires investigation for adrenal or metabolic disorders.

Summary

Puberty is a complex, orchestrated process involving the HPO axis and adrenal glands, with menarche, thelarche, pubarche and adrenarche as key milestones in females.

Menarche signifies reproductive maturity but is often preceded by anovulatory cycles.

Thelarche reflects oestrogen-driven breast development and is typically the first sign of puberty in girls.

Pubarche and adrenarche are driven by adrenal androgens, contributing to hair growth and other secondary changes.

4.3 Precocious Puberty

(Bulughat qabl az waqt)

Definition

Precocious puberty is defined as the onset of pubertal changes (secondary sexual characteristics) before age 8 in girls or 9 in boys. It results in early physical and hormonal maturation, which may have significant physical, psychological and social consequences.

Classification

1. Central Precocious Puberty (CPP): Gonadotropin-dependent, caused by premature activation of the hypothalamic-pituitary-ovarian (HPO) axis.
2. Peripheral Precocious Puberty (PPP): Gonadotropin-independent, caused by autonomous sex hormone production or exogenous exposure.
3. Incomplete Precocious Puberty: Isolated development of one pubertal feature (e.g., premature thelarche or premature pubarche) without progression to full puberty.

Etiology

1. Central Precocious Puberty

Idiopathic (most common in girls): No identifiable cause, often familial.

Central Nervous System (CNS) Lesions: Hypothalamic hamartomas, tumours (e.g., gliomas, astrocytomas), hydrocephalus or CNS infections.

Other: Hypothyroidism, neurofibromatosis type 1, or prior cranial irradiation.

2. Peripheral Precocious Puberty

Ovarian Causes: Estrogen-secreting tumours (e.g., granulosa cell tumours), functional ovarian cysts.

Adrenal Causes: Congenital adrenal hyperplasia (CAH), adrenal tumours (e.g., adrenocortical carcinoma).

Exogenous Sources: Exposure to oestrogen-containing creams, medications or environmental endocrine disruptors.

McCune-Albright Syndrome: Triad of precocious puberty, cafe-au-lait spots, and fibrous dysplasia due to GNAS gene mutations.

3. Incomplete Forms

Premature Thelarche: Isolated breast development, often benign and self-limiting.

Premature Pubarche: Early pubic hair growth, often due to premature adrenarche or mild CAH.

Pathophysiology

In CPP, premature pulsatile gonadotropin-releasing hormone (GnRH) secretion stimulates luteinizing hormone (LH) and follicle-stimulating hormone (FSH) release, leading to gonadal activation and sex hormone production.

In PPP, autonomous production of estrogens or androgens (e.g., from tumours) drives pubertal changes without HPG axis activation.

Early puberty accelerates growth and epiphyseal closure, potentially reducing adult height.

Clinical Features

Girls: Early breast development (thelarche), pubic hair (pubarche), menarche, growth spurt, acne or body odor.

Boys: Testicular enlargement, penile growth, pubic hair, voice deepening or growth spurt.

Psychosocial: Mood changes, behavioral issues or social challenges due to physical maturity outpacing emotional development.

Diagnosis

History and Physical Exam: Assess pubertal milestones, Tanner staging, growth velocity and family history.

Laboratory Tests

Basal LH and FSH levels (elevated in CPP).

GnRH stimulation test: Exaggerated LH response confirms CPP.

Estradiol, testosterone or dehydroepiandrosterone sulphate (DHEA-S) levels (elevated in PPP).

Thyroid function tests to rule out hypothyroidism.

Imaging

Bone age X-ray: Advanced in precocious puberty.

Pelvic ultrasound: To detect ovarian cysts or tumours.

Brain MRI: To evaluate CNS lesions in CPP.

Adrenal Evaluation: 17-hydroxyprogesterone or ACTH stimulation test for CAH.

Management

Central Precocious Puberty

GnRH agonists (e.g., leuprolide) to suppress HPO axis activity, delaying puberty progression and preserving height potential.

Treat underlying CNS lesions if present.

Peripheral Precocious Puberty

Treat the underlying cause (e.g., surgical removal of tumours, glucocorticoid therapy for CAH).

Medications to block oestrogen effects (e.g., tamoxifen) in some cases.

Supportive Care: Psychosocial counselling for the child and family to address emotional and social challenges.

Monitoring: Regular follow-up to assess growth, bone age and pubertal progression.

Clinical Relevance

Early puberty increases the risk of short stature, obesity, type 2 diabetes, breast cancer and psychosocial issues.

One must differentiate between benign variants (e.g., premature thelarche) and serious conditions requiring intervention.

Long-term follow-up is essential to monitor reproductive health and adult outcomes.

Key Points

Precocious puberty is classified as central, peripheral, or incomplete, with distinct etiologies.

Diagnosis involves hormonal testing, imaging and bone age assessment.

Treatment aims to halt pubertal progression, preserve height and address underlying causes.

Key Definitions

Menarche ➤ First menstrual bleeding, typically around age 12–13.

Thelarche ➤ Onset of breast development, usually first sign of puberty.

Pubarche ➤ Appearance of pubic hair due to adrenal androgen secretion.

Precocious Puberty ➤ Onset of secondary sexual characteristics before age 8 in girls.

Delayed Puberty ➤ Absence of breast development by age 13 or menarche by age 16.

4.4 Delayed Puberty

(*Bulugh-i-Mu'akhkhar*)

Definition

Delayed puberty is defined as the absence of secondary sexual characteristics by age 13 in girls or 14 in boys, or failure of menarche by age 15 in girls (primary amenorrhea). It reflects a delay in hypothalamo-pituitary ovarian axis activation or gonadal function.

Classification

1. Hypogonadotropic Hypogonadism: Reduced gonadotropin (LH/FSH) secretion due to hypothalamic or pituitary dysfunction.
2. Hypergonadotropic Hypogonadism: Elevated gonadotropins due to primary gonadal failure.
3. Constitutional Delay of Growth and Puberty (CDGP): A benign, self-limiting delay in pubertal onset, often familial.

Etiology

Hypogonadotropic Hypogonadism

Functional: Chronic illness (e.g., celiac disease, inflammatory bowel disease), malnutrition, excessive exercise, eating disorders (e.g., anorexia nervosa) or stress.

Congenital: Kallmann syndrome (anosmia and GnRH deficiency), isolated GnRH deficiency or pituitary disorders.

Acquired: Pituitary tumours, cranial irradiation or trauma.

Hypergonadotropic Hypogonadism

Genetic: Turner syndrome (45,XO), gonadal dysgenesis or Klinefelter syndrome (in males).

Acquired: Chemotherapy, radiation, autoimmune oophoritis or ovarian torsion.

Constitutional Delay: Common in boys, often with a family history of delayed puberty; typically resolves spontaneously by age 18.

Pathophysiology

In hypogonadotropic hypogonadism, impaired GnRH, LH or FSH secretion prevents gonadal stimulation, delaying puberty.

In hypergonadotropic hypogonadism, gonadal failure leads to elevated gonadotropins due to lack of negative feedback.

CDGP reflects a temporary delay in HPO axis activation, with normal eventual progression.

Clinical Features

Girls: Absent breast development (thelarche), pubic hair (pubarche) or menarche by expected ages.

Boys: Absent testicular enlargement (>4 mL) or pubic hair.

Short stature or slow growth velocity may accompany delayed puberty, especially in CDGP or chronic illness.

Psychosocial: Low self-esteem, social isolation or anxiety due to delayed physical development.

Diagnosis

History and Physical Exam: Assess pubertal milestones, growth patterns, family history and signs of chronic illness or genetic syndromes.

Laboratory Tests

Basal LH, FSH and estradiol/testosterone levels (low in hypogonadotropic, high in hypergonadotropic).

GnRH stimulation test to assess pituitary function.

Thyroid function, prolactin and IGF-1 levels to rule out systemic causes.

Karyotyping for suspected Turner syndrome or other genetic conditions.

Imaging

Bone age X-ray: Delayed in CDGP or hypogonadism.

Pelvic ultrasound: To assess ovarian/uterine development.

Brain MRI: To evaluate hypothalamic-pituitary abnormalities.

Screening: Tests for celiac disease, inflammatory markers or adrenal function if systemic illness is suspected.

Management

Constitutional Delay: Reassurance and monitoring; low-dose sex hormone therapy (e.g., estradiol in girls) may be considered for psychosocial reasons.

Hypogonadotropic Hypogonadism

Treat underlying causes (e.g., nutritional rehabilitation, stress management).

Hormone replacement therapy (HRT) with oestrogen (girls) or testosterone (boys) to induce puberty.

GnRH therapy for fertility induction in congenital cases.

Hypergonadotropic Hypogonadism

HRT to induce secondary sexual characteristics and protect bone health.

Address fertility implications (e.g., oocyte donation for Turner syndrome).

Supportive Care: Psychosocial counselling and multidisciplinary care (endocrinology, gynaecology, psychology).

Clinical Relevance

Delayed puberty may indicate serious underlying conditions (e.g., Turner syndrome, pituitary tumours) requiring early intervention.

Long-term management focuses on fertility, bone density and psychosocial well-being.

Key Points

Delayed puberty results from hypogonadotropic or hypergonadotropic hypogonadism or constitutional delay.

Diagnosis requires a systematic evaluation of hormonal, genetic and systemic factors.

4.5 Puberty Menorrhagia

(Kathrat-i-Tamth Bulughi)

Definition

Puberty menorrhagia refers to excessive or prolonged menstrual bleeding (menstrual flow >7 days or blood loss >80 mL per cycle) in adolescent girls within the first 1–2 years post-menarche. It is a common gynaecological complaint during the peripubertal period due to immature hypothalamo-pituitary-ovarian (HPO) axis function.

Etiology

Physiologic (Anovulatory Bleeding): Most common cause; early menstrual cycles are often anovulatory due to incomplete HPO axis maturation, leading to unopposed oestrogen stimulation of the endometrium, irregular shedding and heavy bleeding.

Hematologic Disorders:

Von Willebrand disease (most common coagulopathy, affecting 10–20% of girls with menorrhagia).

Platelet dysfunction, hemophilia or thrombocytopenia.

Endocrine Disorders: Polycystic ovary syndrome (PCOS), hypothyroidism or hyperprolactinemia causing anovulation.

Structural Causes: Rare in adolescents but include uterine fibroids, polyps or adenomyosis.

Medications: Anticoagulants or hormonal contraceptives (if misused).

Infections: Pelvic inflammatory disease or endometritis (rare).

Pathophysiology

Anovulatory cycles lack progesterone, leading to excessive endometrial proliferation and unstable shedding, causing heavy or irregular bleeding.

Coagulopathies exacerbate bleeding by impairing hemostasis at the endometrial level.

Hormonal imbalances (e.g., PCOS) may amplify anovulation, worsening menorrhagia.

Clinical Features

Heavy menstrual bleeding (changing of sanitary pads/tampons every 1–2 hours, passing large clots).

Prolonged menses (>7 days) or irregular cycles.

Symptoms of anemia: Fatigue, pallor, dizziness or shortness of breath.

Psychosocial impact: Embarrassment, school absenteeism or reduced quality of life.

Diagnosis

History: Menstrual history (cycle length, duration, flow volume), family history of bleeding disorders, symptoms of anemia or endocrine issues.

Physical Exam: Signs of anemia, bruising or endocrine disorders (e.g., hirsutism in PCOS).

Laboratory Tests:

Complete blood count (CBC) to assess anemia (hemoglobin <12 g/dL).

Coagulation profile: Prothrombin time (PT), activated partial thromboplastin time (aPTT), von Willebrand factor assay or platelet function tests.

Thyroid function tests, prolactin and androgen levels for endocrine causes.

Pregnancy test to rule out pregnancy-related bleeding.

Imaging: Pelvic ultrasound to exclude structural abnormalities (e.g., fibroids, polyps).

Endometrial Biopsy: Rarely needed in adolescents unless malignancy is suspected.

Management

Supportive Care

Iron supplementation for anemia (oral ferrous sulphate or IV iron for severe cases).

Hydration and nutritional support.

Hormonal Therapy (for anovulatory bleeding)

Combined oral contraceptives (COCs): Stabilize endometrium and regulate cycles.

Progestin-only therapy (e.g., norethindrone, medroxyprogesterone): For acute heavy bleeding or when COCs are contraindicated.

Levonorgestrel-releasing intrauterine device (LNG-IUD): Effective for long-term management in older adolescents.

Non-Hormonal Therapy

Tranexamic acid: Reduces bleeding by stabilizing fibrin clots.

Nonsteroidal anti-inflammatory drugs (NSAIDs): Reduce blood loss and alleviate dysmenorrhea.

Coagulopathy Management

Desmopressin or von Willebrand factor concentrates for von Willebrand disease.

Haematology consultation for other bleeding disorders.

Surgical Intervention: Rarely needed; dilation and curettage (D&C) for intractable bleeding or diagnostic purposes.

Counseling: Educate patients on menstrual hygiene, treatment adherence and psychosocial support.

Clinical Relevance

Puberty menorrhagia is often benign but may reveal serious conditions like coagulopathies or PCOS. Long-term management focuses on cycle regulation, anemia prevention and addressing underlying conditions.

Key Points

Puberty menorrhagia is commonly due to anovulatory cycles but requires evaluation for coagulopathies or endocrine disorders.

Diagnosis involves menstrual history, lab investigations and imaging to exclude structural causes.

Treatment includes hormonal and non-hormonal therapies, with iron supplementation for anemia.

Long Answer Questions

1. Define puberty and adolescence. Describe the physiological changes occurring during this phase.
2. Explain the hormonal regulation of puberty and its impact on reproductive organ development.
3. Discuss the causes, clinical features and management of precocious puberty.
4. Describe delayed puberty and its classification with diagnostic approach.
5. Elaborate on psychosocial changes during adolescence and their influence on reproductive health.

Short Answer Questions

1. What is menarche?
2. Name two secondary sexual characteristics in females.
3. Define precocious puberty.
4. Mention one cause of delayed puberty.
5. What is the role of GnRH in puberty?

Multiple Choice Questions (1 Mark Each)

1. Menarche typically occurs at the age of:

a) 8–9 years b) 10–11 years c) 12–13 years d) 15–16 years

Ans: c) 12–13 years (avg 12.4 years)

2. Thelarche refers to:

a) Onset of menstruation b) Breast development c) Pubic hair growth d) Ovulation

Ans: b) Breast development

3. GnRH is secreted by the:

a) Pituitary gland b) Hypothalamus c) Ovary d) Adrenal gland

Ans: b) Hypothalamus

4. Precocious puberty is defined as onset of secondary sexual characteristics before:

a) 6 years b) 8 years c) 10 years d) 12 years

Ans: b) 8 years

5. Delayed puberty is suspected if menarche has not occurred by age:

a) 12 b) 14 c) 16 d) 18

Ans: c) 16

6. Which hormone initiates follicular development during puberty?

a) LH b) FSH c) Estrogen d) Progesterone

Ans: b) FSH

7. Which of the following is a psychosocial change during adolescence?

a) Menstruation b) Breast development c) Mood swings d) Ovulation

Ans: c) Mood swings

8. Which condition involves early activation of the hypothalamic-pituitary-gonadal axis?

a) Delayed puberty b) Precocious puberty c) Menopause d) Amenorrhea

Ans: b) Precocious puberty

9. Which hormone is responsible for development of secondary sexual characteristics in females?

a) Testosterone b) Estrogen c) Progesterone d) Oxytocin

Ans: b) Estrogen

10. Which of the following is NOT a feature of adolescence?

a) Growth spurt b) Emotional maturity c) Menopause d) Sexual awareness

Ans: c) Menopause

05

Menopause & its Related Problems

(Inqita' al-Tamth aur Muta'allaqa Masael)

5.1 *Marhalah intiqal sinn-i-yas* (Menopausal Transition)
5.2 *Inqita al-Tamth ke taghayyurat/ umar ke sath tabdiliyan* (Menopausal changes/ age related changes)
5.3 *Marhalah Intiql sinn-i-yas ke awarezat* (Perimenopausal abnormalities)
5.4 *Mutalazema sinn-i-yas* (Post Menopausal Syndrome)
5.5 *Nazf-i-Rahim bad sinn-i-yas* (Post Menopausal Bleeding)

Learning Objective (At the end of the session, the students should be able to):

Describe menopausal transition.
Enumerate the Menopausal Changes/ Age-related changes.
Describe in *Layyan ul Izaam* & *Nakhrul (Hashsatul) Izaam* (Osteomalacia & Osteoporosis).
Enumerate the Perimenopausal abnormalities.
Describe & discuss the Post-Menopausal Syndrome and its management.
Enumerate the causes of Post-Menopausal Bleeding and describe its management.

5.1 Menopausal Transition

(*Marhalah intiqal Sinn-i-yas*)

Menopause marks a significant milestone in a woman's reproductive life, signaling the permanent cessation of menstruation due to the loss of ovarian follicular activity. It is a natural biological process, not a disease, but its associated physiological and psychological changes can profoundly impact health and quality of life. The menopausal transition, also known as perimenopause, is the period of gradual endocrine and reproductive changes leading to menopause.

Definitions

Menopause: Defined by the World Health Organization (WHO) as the permanent cessation of menstruation resulting from the loss of ovarian follicular function, diagnosed retrospectively after 12 consecutive months of amenorrhea without other pathological or physiological causes. The average age of natural menopause in developed countries is approximately 51 years, though this varies across populations and is influenced by genetic, environmental and lifestyle factors.

Menopausal Transition (Perimenopause): The period of transition from reproductive to non-reproductive status, characterized by irregular menstrual cycles and fluctuating hormone levels. It typically begins in a woman's 40s and ends with the final menstrual period (FMP). The Stages of Reproductive Aging Workshop (STRAW+10) criteria provide a standardized framework for classifying reproductive aging, dividing the menopausal transition into early and late stages based on menstrual cycle variability and hormonal changes.

Postmenopause: The phase following the FMP, encompassing the remainder of a woman's life. It is subdivided into early (first 8 years after FMP) and late postmenopause, reflecting ongoing physiological adjustments

Epidemiology

Menopause is a universal phenomenon for women who reach midlife, with the global median age ranging from 45 to 55 years. In developed countries, the average age is around 51–52 years, while in developing countries, it may occur earlier (e.g., 48–50 years) due to factors such as nutritional status, socioeconomic conditions and smoking. Approximately 10% of women experience premature menopause (before age 40), and 1% experience primary ovarian insufficiency (POI), defined as menopause before age 40 due to ovarian failure. Ethnicity, genetics and lifestyle factors, such as smoking or low body mass index, can influence the timing of menopause.

Physiology of Menopause and Menopausal Transition

The menopausal transition and menopause result from the progressive depletion of ovarian follicles, leading to a decline in ovarian hormone production, primarily oestrogen and progesterone. Key physiological changes include:

1. Follicular Depletion: Women are born with a finite number of ovarian follicles (approximately 1–2 million at birth), which decline to fewer than 1,000 by menopause. This depletion accelerates in the late 30s and 40s, reducing the pool of responsive follicles.
2. Hormonal Changes: During the menopausal transition, follicle-stimulating hormone (FSH) levels rise due to decreased ovarian feedback from inhibin B and estradiol. Estrogen levels

fluctuate, often leading to anovulatory cycles and irregular menstruation. Luteinizing hormone (LH) levels also increase, though less in comparison to FSH. In postmenopause, estradiol and progesterone levels stabilize at low levels, while FSH and LH remain elevated.

3. Endocrine Impact: The decline in oestrogen affects multiple systems, including the hypothalamic-pituitary-ovarian axis, cardiovascular system, bone metabolism and thermoregulatory centres in the brain, contributing to menopausal symptoms and long-term health risks.

Clinical Features

The menopausal transition and menopause are associated with a spectrum of symptoms and health changes.

1. Menstrual Irregularity: The hallmark of perimenopause is cycle variability, with shorter or longer cycles or unpredictable bleeding patterns.
2. Vasomotor Symptoms (VMS): Hot flashes and night sweats affect up to 80% of women, peaking in late perimenopause and early postmenopause. These are caused by hypothalamic sensitivity to declining oestrogen levels, triggering thermoregulatory dysfunction.
3. Urogenital Symptoms: Vaginal dryness, dyspareunia and urinary symptoms (e.g., urgency, recurrent infections) result from genitourinary syndrome of menopause (GSM), driven by oestrogen deficiency affecting urogenital tissues.
4. Psychological and Cognitive Symptoms: Mood changes, irritability, anxiety and cognitive complaints, though their direct link to hormonal changes versus psychosocial factors remains under study.
5. Other Symptoms: Sleep disturbances, fatigue, joint pain and weight gain are common, often multifactorial in origin.
6. Long-Term Health Risks: Estrogen deficiency increases risks of osteoporosis, cardiovascular disease and metabolic syndrome. Bone loss accelerates in the first 5–7 years postmenopause, while cardiovascular risk rises due to changes in lipid profiles and endothelial function.

Clinical Significance

Symptom Management: Hormone therapy (HT) remains the most effective treatment for vasomotor and urogenital symptoms, though its use requires individualized risk-benefit assessment. Non-hormonal therapies, lifestyle modifications and complementary approaches are also widely utilized.

Health Screening and Prevention: Menopause is a critical window for assessing cardiovascular risk, bone health and mental well-being. Screening for osteoporosis, lipid disorders and breast cancer is essential, alongside counselling on lifestyle factors such as diet, exercise and smoking cessation.

Cultural and Psychosocial Context: Menopausal experiences vary widely across cultures, influenced by societal attitudes, access to healthcare and individual expectations. Addressing these factors ensures culturally sensitive care.

Conclusion

Menopause and the menopausal transition represent a dynamic period of physiological, psychological and social change.

5.2 Menopausal changes/ age related changes

(*Inqita al-Tamth ke taghayyurat/ umar ke sath tabdiliyan*)

Menopause represents the permanent cessation of menstruation due to the depletion of ovarian follicular activity, typically occurring around the age of 51 in most populations. The physiological and systemic changes associated with menopause, compounded by age-related processes, affect multiple organ systems and have significant clinical implications. These changes are driven primarily by the decline in ovarian hormone production, particularly oestrogen and progesterone, but are also influenced by aging processes independent of hormonal shifts.

Physiological Basis of Menopausal Changes

1. Ovarian Follicular Depletion

Women are born with approximately 1–2 million ovarian follicles, which decline to fewer than 1,000 by menopause. This depletion accelerates in the late 30s and 40s, reducing the number of functional follicles capable of ovulation.

The loss of granulosa cells leads to decreased production of inhibin B, resulting in elevated follicle-stimulating hormone (FSH) levels as the hypothalamic-pituitary-ovarian axis attempts to stimulate folliculogenesis.

Estradiol levels decline significantly postmenopause, stabilizing at low levels (<20 pg/mL), while progesterone production ceases due to anovulation.

2. Hormonal Changes

Estrogen Decline: Estradiol, the primary ovarian oestrogen, decreases, affecting tissues with oestrogen receptors, including the brain, cardiovascular system, bones and urogenital tract.

Gonadotropin Elevation: FSH and luteinizing hormone (LH) levels rise due to reduced negative feedback from ovarian hormones.

Androgen Shifts: Ovarian androgen production (e.g., testosterone, androstenedione) decreases, though adrenal androgens partially compensate. Peripheral aromatization of androgens to estrogens becomes a significant source of oestrogen postmenopause.

3. Systemic Effects

a. Thermoregulatory Dysfunction: Estrogen withdrawal affects the hypothalamic thermoregulatory centre, leading to vasomotor symptoms (VMS) such as hot flashes and night sweats.
b. Tissue Changes: Estrogen deficiency causes atrophy of oestrogen-dependent tissues, notably the vaginal and urethral epithelium, contributing to genitourinary syndrome of menopause (GSM).
c. Metabolic Shifts: Reduced oestrogen alters lipid metabolism (increased LDL, decreased HDL) and insulin sensitivity, increasing cardiovascular and metabolic syndrome risks.

Clinical Manifestations of Menopausal Changes

1. Vasomotor Symptoms (VMS)

Hot flashes and night sweats affect 60–80% of women, peaking in early postmenopause. Hot flashes are characterized by sudden warmth, flushing and sweating, lasting 1–5 minutes, often triggered by stress, heat or caffeine.

Pathophysiology involves hypothalamic sensitivity to oestrogen fluctuations, disrupting the thermoregulatory set point.

2. Genitourinary Syndrome of Menopause (GSM)

Vaginal dryness, dyspareunia and urinary symptoms (e.g., urgency, recurrent infections) result from atrophy of the vaginal, vulvar and urethral epithelium due to oestrogen deficiency.

Symptoms may persist or worsen postmenopause, affecting sexual function and quality of life.

3. Musculoskeletal Changes

Bone Loss: Estrogen deficiency accelerates bone resorption by osteoclasts, leading to a 2–3% annual bone loss in the first 5–7 years postmenopause. This increases the risk of osteoporosis and fractures (e.g., hip, vertebral).

Joint and Muscle Symptoms: Arthralgia and myalgia are reported, potentially linked to oestrogen's anti-inflammatory effects.

4. Cardiovascular Changes

Estrogen withdrawal increases cardiovascular risk through adverse changes in lipid profiles (elevated LDL, triglycerides), endothelial dysfunction and increased vascular stiffness.

Postmenopausal women face a 2–3-fold higher risk of coronary artery disease compared to premenopausal women of similar age.

5. Psychological and Cognitive Changes

Mood changes, anxiety and irritability are common, potentially exacerbated by sleep disruption from night sweats.

Cognitive complaints (e.g., memory lapses, "brain fog") are reported, though evidence linking these directly to menopause versus aging or psychosocial factors is mixed.

6. Skin and Connective Tissue Changes

Decreased collagen and elastin due to oestrogen deficiency lead to skin thinning, dryness and reduced elasticity.

Hair thinning and changes in hair distribution (e.g., increased facial hair due to relative androgen excess) are common.

7. Age-Related Changes

While menopause-specific changes are driven by hormonal decline, aging itself contributes to overlapping physiological changes:

a. Cardiovascular Aging: Independent of menopause, aging increases arterial stiffness, hypertension risk and oxidative stress, compounding menopausal cardiovascular risks.
b. Neurodegenerative Changes: Age-related declines in neuronal elasticity and neurotransmitter function may contribute to cognitive changes, distinct from menopausal effects.
c. Metabolic Decline: Aging reduces basal metabolic rate and muscle mass, contributing to weight gain and insulin resistance, which are exacerbated by menopausal hormonal shifts.
d. Immune Function: Immunosenescence reduces immune responsiveness, increasing susceptibility to infections and chronic diseases, which may interact with menopausal changes.

Clinical Implications

Screening and Prevention: Screening is necessary for osteoporosis (e.g., DEXA scans), cardiovascular risk (lipid profiles, blood pressure) and metabolic disorders (glucose levels). Counselling on lifestyle modifications (e.g., weight-bearing exercise, calcium/vitamin D intake) is essential.

Symptom Management: Hormone therapy (HT) is effective for VMS and GSM but requires individualized risk-benefit assessment. Non-hormonal options (e.g., SSRIs, gabapentin) and lifestyle interventions are alternatives.

Long-Term Health: Menopause is a critical window for addressing long-term risks, including cardiovascular disease, osteoporosis and cognitive decline, through preventive strategies and early intervention.

Hormonal Changes During Menopause

Ovarian Aging Begins

↓

↓ Estrogen & Progesterone Production

↓

↓ Negative Feedback to Hypothalamus

↓

↑ GnRH Secretion

↓

↑ FSH & LH Levels (Pituitary Response)

↓

No Ovulation → Menstrual Cessation

↓

Menopause Confirmed (12 Months Amenorrhea)

Key Definitions

Menopause ➤ Permanent cessation of menstruation after 12 months of amenorrhea.

Perimenopause ➤ Transition phase with fluctuating hormones and irregular cycles.

Postmenopause ➤ Life stage after menopause; increased risk of chronic conditions.

5.3 Perimenopausal abnormalities

(Marhalah Intiql sinn-i-Yas ke awarezat)

The menopausal transition, or perimenopause, is the period of reproductive aging leading to menopause, characterized by irregular menstrual cycles and fluctuating hormone levels. Perimenopause typically begins in the mid-40s and ends with the final menstrual period. Abnormalities during this phase arise from the hormonal fluctuations and ovarian dysfunction, leading to clinical challenges in diagnosis and management. These abnormalities can significantly impact quality of life and require careful evaluation to distinguish physiological changes from pathological conditions.

Physiological Basis of Perimenopausal Abnormalities

1. Hormonal Fluctuations

During perimenopause, ovarian follicular reserve diminishes, leading to irregular ovulation and disturbed oestrogen and progesterone levels. FSH levels rise intermittently, reflecting reduced inhibin B feedback.

Anovulatory cycles increases, resulting in unopposed oestrogen exposure in some cycles, which can cause endometrial hyperplasia.

Progesterone deficiency due to anovulation contributes to irregular bleeding patterns.

2. Ovarian Dysfunction

The declining number of functional follicles leads to disturbed follicular development, with some cycles producing high oestrogen peaks (luteal out-of-phase surges) and others resulting in low oestrogen levels.

Corpus luteum function becomes inconsistent, reducing progesterone production and altering menstrual cycle dynamics.

3. Hypothalamic-Pituitary Sensitivity

The hypothalamic-pituitary-ovarian axis becomes less responsive to feedback signals, contributing to irregular ovulation and menstrual cycle variability.

Clinical Manifestations of Perimenopausal Abnormalities

1. Menstrual Irregularities

Cycle Variability: Perimenopause is marked by shortened cycles (due to early follicular recruitment), prolonged cycles or skipped periods. The Stages of Reproductive Aging Workshop (STRAW+10) classifies early perimenopause as cycles varying by ≥7 days and late perimenopause as ≥60 days of amenorrhea.

Abnormal Uterine Bleeding (AUB): Heavy menstrual bleeding (menorrhagia), irregular bleeding or spotting is common due to anovulatory cycles and unopposed oestrogen stimulating endometrial proliferation. AUB requires evaluation to rule out pathology (e.g., endometrial hyperplasia, polyps, fibroids).

2. Vasomotor Symptoms (VMS)

Hot flashes and night sweats often emerge in perimenopause, particularly in the late transition, due to fluctuating oestrogen levels disrupting hypothalamic thermoregulation.

Symptoms may be more severe during periods of rapid oestrogen decline.

3. Urogenital Symptoms

Early signs of GSM, such as vaginal dryness or discomfort during intercourse, may appear due to intermittent oestrogen declines affecting urogenital tissues.

Urinary symptoms (e.g., urgency, frequency) may also emerge, though less severe than in postmenopause.

4. Psychological and Cognitive Symptoms

Mood swings, anxiety and irritability are common, potentially exacerbated by hormonal fluctuations, sleep disruption or psychosocial stressors (e.g., midlife transitions, caregiving responsibilities).

Cognitive complaints, such as difficulty in concentrating, are reported but may reflect sleep disturbance or stress, rather than direct hormonal effects.

5. Endometrial Abnormalities

Endometrial Hyperplasia: Unopposed oestrogen in anovulatory cycles can lead to endometrial proliferation, increasing the risk of simple or complex hyperplasia, with or without atypia. Atypical hyperplasia is a precursor to endometrial cancer.

Polyps and Fibroids: Estrogen fluctuations may exacerbate pre-existing benign growths, contributing to AUB.

6. Ovarian Cysts

Functional ovarian cysts (e.g., follicular or luteal cysts) may occur due to disturbed follicular development. Most are benign and resolve spontaneously, but require monitoring to exclude malignancy.

7. Fertility Challenges

Despite declining fertility, ovulation can occur anytime, leading to a risk of unintended pregnancy. Contraception is recommended until 12 months of amenorrhea (menopause).

Pathological considerations

Perimenopausal abnormalities must be distinguished from pathological conditions mimicking physiological changes:

1. Endometrial Cancer: Heavy or irregular bleeding suggests endometrial evaluation (e.g., ultrasound, biopsy) to exclude malignancy, particularly in women over 45 or with risk factors (e.g., obesity, PCOS).
2. Thyroid Dysfunction: Hypothyroidism or hyperthyroidism can mimic perimenopausal symptoms (e.g., irregular cycles, mood changes) and should be ruled out with thyroid function tests.
3. Anemia: Heavy menstrual bleeding can lead to iron-deficiency anemia, requiring evaluation of hemoglobin and ferritin levels.

4. Ovarian Pathology: Persistent ovarian cysts or masses require imaging (e.g., transvaginal ultrasound) and tumour markers (e.g., CA-125) to exclude ovarian cancer.

Diagnostic Evaluation

History and Physical Exam: Assess menstrual patterns, symptom severity and risk factors (e.g., obesity, smoking). Do pelvic examination to evaluate for structural abnormalities.

Laboratory Tests: FSH levels (>25 IU/L in the early follicular phase) and estradiol may support perimenopause but are not diagnostic due to variability. Thyroid function tests and complete blood count are indicated for atypical symptoms.

Imaging and Procedures: Transvaginal ultrasound assesses endometrial thickness (normal <5 mm in postmenopausal women; perimenopausal thresholds vary). Endometrial biopsy is indicated for AUB in women over 45 or with risk factors.

STRAW+10 Criteria: Provides a standardized framework for staging reproductive aging based on menstrual cycle changes and hormonal markers.

Management of Perimenopausal Abnormalities

1. Menstrual Irregularities

Hormonal Therapies: Low-dose combined oral contraceptives or progestin therapy (e.g., levonorgestrel IUD) can regulate cycles and reduce bleeding in non-smokers without contraindications.

Non-Hormonal Options: Tranexamic acid or NSAIDs can reduce heavy bleeding.

2. Vasomotor Symptoms

Low-dose hormone therapy (e.g., estradiol with progestin in women with a uterus) is effective for VMS but requires risk assessment (e.g., for thromboembolism, breast cancer).

Non-hormonal options include SSRIs (e.g., paroxetine), SNRIs, or gabapentin.

3. Endometrial Protection

Progestin therapy or endometrial monitoring is essential for women with unopposed oestrogen exposure to prevent hyperplasia.

Surgical options (e.g., endometrial ablation, hysterectomy) are considered for refractory AUB or hyperplasia.

4. Contraception

Low-dose combined hormonal contraceptives or progestin-only methods are suitable until menopause is confirmed. Barrier methods or copper IUDs are alternatives for women with contraindications to hormonal therapy.

5. Lifestyle Interventions

Weight management, stress reduction and smoking cessation can mitigate symptoms and reduce health risks.

Conclusion

Menopausal changes and age-related changes reflect the interplay of hormonal decline and aging processes, affecting multiple systems and necessitating comprehensive care. Perimenopausal abnormalities, driven by hormonal fluctuations and ovarian dysfunction, present diagnostic and management challenges due to their overlap with pathological conditions.

5.4 Post Menopausal Syndrome

(Mutalazema sinn-i-yas)

Postmenopausal syndrome refers to the group of symptoms and physiological changes experienced by women following menopause, defined as the permanent cessation of menstruation due to the loss of ovarian follicular activity, typically diagnosed after 12 consecutive months of amenorrhea. Occurring in the postmenopausal phase—spanning early postmenopause (first 8 years after the final menstrual period [FMP]) and late postmenopause—this syndrome encompasses vasomotor, urogenital, psychological and systemic symptoms driven primarily by oestrogen deficiency, with contributions from aging and psychosocial factors. Postmenopausal syndrome significantly impacts quality of life and increases long-term health risks.

Definition and Epidemiology

Definition: Postmenopausal syndrome includes symptoms and health changes resulting from the permanent decline in ovarian hormone production, particularly estradiol and progesterone, following menopause. It is distinct from menopausal transition (perimenopause) symptoms due to its persistence in the absence of menstrual cycles and stabilized low hormone levels.

Epidemiology: Menopause occurs at a median age of 51 years in developed countries, with variations (48–50 years in lower-income regions) influenced by genetics, nutrition, smoking and socioeconomic factors. Approximately 80% of postmenopausal women experience symptoms, with 20–30% reporting severe symptoms impacting daily life. Vasomotor symptoms (VMS) and genitourinary syndrome of menopause (GSM) are the most prevalent features, while long-term risks like osteoporosis and cardiovascular disease affect a significant proportion of women.

Pathophysiology

The hallmark of postmenopausal syndrome is the profound reduction in ovarian oestrogen and progesterone production due to follicular depletion, leading to systemic effects across oestrogen-dependent tissues. Key pathophysiological mechanisms include:

1. Hormonal Changes

a. Estrogen Deficiency: Postmenopause, estradiol levels stabilize at <20 pg/mL, with estrone (from peripheral aromatization of adrenal androgens) becoming the dominant oestrogen. This decline affects tissues with oestrogen receptors, including the brain, cardiovascular system, bones and urogenital tract.
b. Progesterone Absence: Cessation of ovulation eliminates progesterone production, altering endometrial and systemic homeostasis.

c. Gonadotropin Elevation: Follicle-stimulating hormone (FSH) levels remain elevated (>25 IU/L), and luteinizing hormone (LH) levels increase due to loss of ovarian feedback.
d. Androgen Decline: Ovarian testosterone and androstenedione production decreases, though adrenal androgens provide some compensation, contributing to relative androgen excess in some women.

2. Thermoregulatory Dysregulation

Estrogen deficiency disrupts the hypothalamic thermoregulatory centre, narrowing the thermoneutral zone and triggering vasomotor symptoms like hot flashes and night sweats. This is mediated by altered serotonin and norepinephrine signaling in the hypothalamus.

3. Tissue Atrophy

Estrogen-dependent tissues, such as the vaginal and urethral epithelium, undergo atrophy, leading to GSM. Reduced collagen and elastin in connective tissues contribute to skin and musculoskeletal changes. Bone resorption accelerates due to increased osteoclast activity, driven by the loss of oestrogen's protective effects on bone remodelling.

4. Metabolic and Cardiovascular Effects

Estrogen deficiency alters lipid metabolism (increased LDL, decreased HDL, elevated triglycerides) and impairs endothelial function, increasing cardiovascular risk.

Reduced insulin sensitivity and changes in fat distribution (increased visceral adiposity) contribute to metabolic syndrome.

5. Neurological Effects

Estrogen's neuroprotective effects diminish, potentially exacerbating age-related cognitive changes and mood dysregulation, though direct causation remains under study.

Clinical Manifestations

Postmenopausal syndrome presents with a spectrum of symptoms and long-term health changes, varying in severity and duration among individuals:

1. Vasomotor Symptoms (VMS)

Hot Flashes and Night Sweats: Affect 60–80% of postmenopausal women, characterized by sudden warmth, flushing and sweating, often lasting 1–5 minutes. Night sweats disrupt sleep, contributing to fatigue. Symptoms peak in early postmenopause and may persist for 7–10 years or longer in some women (up to 20% experience VMS into their 60s).

Risk factors include smoking, obesity and African descent, while Asian women report lower rates.

2. Genitourinary Syndrome of Menopause (GSM)

Vaginal Symptoms: Vaginal dryness, itching, and dyspareunia result from atrophy of the vaginal epithelium, reduced lubrication and loss of elasticity. These affect 50–70% of postmenopausal women and worsen over time without treatment.

Urinary Symptoms: Urinary urgency, frequency, nocturia and recurrent urinary tract infections (UTIs) arise from urethral and bladder mucosal thinning.

GSM impacts sexual function, quality of life and relationship dynamics, yet many women do not seek treatment due to stigma or lack of awareness.

3. Psychological and Cognitive Symptoms

Mood changes (e.g., irritability, anxiety, depression) affect 20–40% of women, often exacerbated by sleep disruption, VMS or psychosocial stressors (e.g., career transitions).

Cognitive complaints, such as memory lapses or difficulty concentrating ("brain fog"), are reported, though evidence linking these directly to oestrogen deficiency versus aging or stress is inconclusive.

4. Musculoskeletal Changes

Osteoporosis: Bone loss accelerates at 2–3% per year in early postmenopause, increasing fracture risk (e.g., hip, vertebral, wrist). By age 70, 30–40% of women have osteoporosis.

Joint Pain: Arthralgia is common, potentially due to oestrogen's anti-inflammatory effects or age-related osteoarthritis.

5. Cardiovascular and Metabolic Changes

Postmenopausal women face a 2–3-fold increased risk of coronary artery disease due to adverse lipid profiles, endothelial dysfunction and increased arterial stiffness.

Weight gain and visceral fat accumulation are common, contributing to metabolic syndrome, type 2 diabetes and hypertension.

6. Skin and Hair Changes

Reduced collagen leads to skin thinning, dryness and wrinkling. Hair thinning and increased facial hair (due to relative androgen excess) are also reported.

7. Sexual Dysfunction

Decreased libido, reduced sexual arousal and dyspareunia (due to GSM) affect sexual health, compounded by psychological and relational factors.

Diagnosis

Diagnosis of postmenopausal syndrome is primarily clinical, based on a history of amenorrhea for ≥12 months and associated symptoms, with exclusion of other causes. Key diagnostic points include:

1. History: Assess timing of FMP, symptoms and their impact on quality of life. Inquire about risk factors (e.g., smoking, family history of osteoporosis or cardiovascular disease).

2. Physical Examination: Evaluate for signs of oestrogen deficiency (e.g., vaginal atrophy, skin changes) and systemic health (e.g., blood pressure, BMI).

3. Laboratory Tests:

FSH levels (>25 IU/L) and low estradiol (<20 pg/mL) confirm postmenopausal status but are rarely necessary unless age or symptoms are atypical (e.g., premature menopause).

Thyroid function tests rule out hypothyroidism, which mimics some symptoms.

Lipid profile, fasting glucose and hemoglobin A1c assess cardiovascular and metabolic risk.

4. Imaging:

Dual-energy X-ray absorptiometry (DEXA) screens for osteoporosis in women ≥65 or younger with risk factors (e.g., early menopause, low BMI).

Transvaginal ultrasound evaluates endometrial thickness if abnormal bleeding is reported (postmenopausal bleeding requires investigation to exclude endometrial cancer).

Differential Diagnosis

Rule out thyroid disorders, depression, anemia or malignancy (e.g., endometrial or ovarian cancer) for atypical symptoms.

Management

Management of postmenopausal syndrome aims to alleviate symptoms, improve quality of life and mitigate long-term health risks. Treatment is individualized based on symptom severity, patient preferences and risk profiles.

1. Hormone Therapy (HT)

Indications: Most effective for VMS and GSM in women <60 years or within 10 years of menopause, with minimal contraindications (e.g., history of breast cancer, thromboembolism or cardiovascular disease).

Regimens

a. Estrogen Therapy: Oral, transdermal or vaginal estradiol for women without a uterus.

b. Combined Estrogen-Progestin Therapy: For women with a uterus to prevent endometrial hyperplasia.

c. Vaginal Estrogen: Low-dose vaginal oestrogen (e.g., creams, tablets, rings) effectively treats GSM with minimal systemic absorption.

Risks and Benefit: HT reduces VMS, GSM and fracture risk but carries risks (e.g., thromboembolism, breast cancer with combined therapy). The "timing hypothesis" suggests lower risks when initiated early in postmenopause.

Duration: Shortest duration and lowest dose needed, typically reassessed annually.

2. Non-Hormonal Therapies

Vasomotor Symptoms:

Selective serotonin reuptake inhibitors (SSRIs, e.g., paroxetine 7.5 mg) and serotonin-norepinephrine reuptake inhibitors (SNRIs, e.g., venlafaxine) reduce hot flashes by 50–60%.

Gabapentin or clonidine are alternatives but less effective.

GSM: Non-hormonal vaginal moisturizers and lubricants provide symptomatic relief, though less effective than vaginal oestrogen.

Cognitive and mood Symptoms: Cognitive-behavioral therapy (CBT), antidepressants or counselling address psychological symptoms.

3. Lifestyle Interventions

Diet and Exercise: Weight-bearing exercise, calcium (1200 mg/day) and vitamin D (800–1000 IU/day) support bone health. A heart-healthy diet (e.g., Mediterranean diet) reduces cardiovascular risk.

Sleep Hygiene: Addressing night sweats through cooling techniques and sleep routines improves sleep quality.

Smoking Cessation and Weight Management: Critical for reducing VMS and long-term health risks.

4. Bone Health

Pharmacotherapy: Bisphosphonates, denosumab or selective oestrogen receptor modulators (SERMs, e.g., raloxifene) prevent or treat osteoporosis in high-risk women.

Screening: DEXA every 1–2 years for women with osteopenia or osteoporosis.

5. Cardiovascular and Metabolic Health

Statins, antihypertensives or metformin may be indicated based on risk profiles.

Regular screening for lipids, blood pressure and glucose is essential.

6. Complementary Therapies

Limited evidence supports phytoestrogens, black cohosh, or acupuncture for VMS. Patients should be counselled on variable efficacy and potential risks.

Long-Term Health Implications

Postmenopausal syndrome is associated with increased risks of chronic conditions, necessitating proactive management:

a. Osteoporosis: Accelerated bone loss increases fracture risk, contributing to morbidity and mortality. Early screening and treatment are critical.
b. Cardiovascular Disease: The leading cause of death in postmenopausal women, driven by oestrogen deficiency and age-related vascular changes.
c. Metabolic Syndrome: Increased visceral fat and insulin resistance elevate risks of diabetes and hypertension.
d. Cognitive Decline: While controversial, some studies suggest oestrogen deficiency may accelerate age-related cognitive decline, particularly in women with early or surgical menopause.
e. Cancer Risk: Postmenopausal bleeding or unopposed oestrogen exposure (e.g., in obesity) increases endometrial cancer risk, requiring urgent monitoring.

Clinical and Psychosocial Considerations

Individualized Care: Treatment decisions must consider patient preferences, cultural attitudes and access to care. Many women underreport symptoms due to stigma or lack of awareness.

Psychosocial Impact: Menopause often coincides with midlife transitions, amplifying psychological symptoms. Supportive counselling and education empower women to manage this phase.

Health Equity: Access to menopause care varies globally, with disparities in low-resource settings.

Menopause-Related Disorders

> Menopause may cause HAVOCS in the body:

Letter	Disorder/Symptom	Description
H	Hot Flashes	Sudden warmth, flushing, sweating
A	Atrophy of Vagina	Dryness, thinning, dyspareunia
V	Vaginal Dryness	↓ Lubrication, ↑ pH
O	Osteoporosis	↓ Bone density, ↑ fracture risk
C	Coronary Artery Disease	↑ Risk due to ↓ oestrogen
S	Sleep Disturbances	Insomnia, night sweats

Common Symptoms

- Hot flashes
- Night sweats
- Mood swings
- Vaginal dryness
- Sleep disturbances
- Weight gain
- Osteoporosis
- Urinary incontinence

Symptom	Management Approach
Hot flashes	Lifestyle changes, HRT, SSRIs
Vaginal dryness	Lubricants, topical oestrogen
Osteoporosis	Calcium, Vitamin D, bisphosphonates
Mood changes	Counseling, SSRIs, exercise
Sleep issues	Sleep hygiene, melatonin, HRT

5.5 Post Menopausal Bleeding

(Nazf-i-Rahim bad Sinn-i-Yas)

Postmenopausal bleeding (PMB) is defined as any vaginal bleeding occurring in a woman at least 12 months after her final menstrual period (FMP), marking the onset of menopause. PMB is a clinical symptom, as it may indicate benign conditions, such as atrophic changes or serious pathology, including endometrial cancer. Given its association with malignancy in a significant proportion of cases, PMB warrants prompt and thorough evaluation.

Definition and Epidemiology

Definition: PMB is vaginal bleeding occurring after 12 consecutive months of amenorrhea in a postmenopausal woman, typically after the age of 50. It excludes bleeding due to hormone therapy (HT) or other iatrogenic causes, which should be evaluated separately.

Epidemiology: PMB affects approximately 5–10% of postmenopausal women. The incidence varies with age, risk factors and underlying pathology. While 90% of cases are due to benign causes, 10–15% are associated with endometrial cancer or hyperplasia, making PMB a red-flag symptom requiring urgent investigation. Risk factors for malignancy include advanced age (>60 years), obesity, unopposed oestrogen exposure, diabetes, hypertension and a history of irregular perimenopausal bleeding.

Etiology

PMB arises from a spectrum of benign and malignant causes, primarily affecting the genital tract but occasionally involving non-gynecologic sources. The most common etiologies include:

1. Benign Causes

a. Atrophic Endometrium/Vaginitis: The most common cause (50–60% of cases), resulting from oestrogen deficiency leading to thinning of the endometrial and vaginal mucosa, destructive testing, causing fragility and bleeding.

b. Endometrial Polyps: Benign growths in the endometrium (10–15% of cases) that may bleed due to irritation or necrosis.

c. Uterine Fibroids: Submucosal fibroids may cause bleeding, though less common postmenopause.

d. Genitourinary Syndrome of Menopause (GSM): Atrophic changes in the vaginal or cervical epithelium can lead to bleeding from minor trauma.

e. Cervical or Vaginal Lesions: Erosions, ulcers or trauma from intercourse or foreign bodies (e.g., pessaries) may cause bleeding.

f. Hormone Therapy: Unscheduled bleeding may occur in women on HT, particularly with inadequate progestin opposition in combined regimens.

2. Malignant Causes

a. Endometrial Cancer: Accounts for 7–15% of PMB cases. Type 1 endometrial cancers (oestrogen-dependent) are more common in postmenopausal women, often presenting with bleeding due to endometrial proliferation.
b. Endometrial Hyperplasia: A precursor to cancer, often caused by unopposed oestrogen (e.g., obesity, tamoxifen use), presenting as simple, complex or atypical hyperplasia.
c. Cervical Cancer: Less common but may cause PMB, particularly in advanced stages.
d. Ovarian or Fallopian Tube Cancer: Rare causes of PMB, typically associated with advanced disease.
e. Other Malignancies: Sarcomas (e.g., leiomyosarcoma) or metastatic cancers to the genital tract are rare.

3. Other Causes

a. Coagulopathy: Anticoagulant therapy (e.g., warfarin) or bleeding disorders (e.g., von Willebrand disease) may contribute to PMB.
b. Foreign Bodies: Pessaries or retained tampons can cause irritation and bleeding.
c. Non-Gynecological causes: Hematuria or rectal bleeding may be mistaken for vaginal bleeding, requiring differentiation.

Pathophysiology

The pathophysiology of PMB depends on the underlying cause:

a. Atrophic Changes: Estrogen deficiency postmenopause leads to thinning of the endometrial lining (<4 mm) and vaginal epithelium, increasing susceptibility to microtrauma and bleeding.
b. Endometrial Proliferation: Unopposed oestrogen (e.g., from obesity, HT or oestrogen-producing tumours) stimulates endometrial growth, leading to hyperplasia or cancer, which disrupts vascular integrity and causes bleeding.
c. Neoplastic Processes: Malignant tumours disrupt normal tissue architecture, leading to abnormal vasculature and bleeding.
d. Vascular Fragility: Aging and oestrogen deficiency weaken pelvic vasculature, increasing the risk of spontaneous bleeding from atrophic tissues.

Clinical Evaluation

A systematic approach to PMB is critical to identify the underlying cause and rule out malignancy.

1. History

Bleeding Characteristics: Assess the amount, frequency, duration and pattern of bleeding (e.g., spotting, heavy bleeding, postcoital).

Associated Symptoms: Pelvic pain, weight loss or systemic symptoms may suggest malignancy. GSM symptoms (e.g., vaginal dryness, dyspareunia) suggest atrophy.

Risk Factors: Obesity, diabetes, hypertension, tamoxifen use, late menopause (>55 years), nulliparity, or family history of endometrial or breast cancer increase malignancy risk.

Medical History: Review HT use, anticoagulants, or bleeding disorders.

Menopausal Status: Confirm ≥12 months of amenorrhea to distinguish PMB from perimenopausal bleeding.

2. Physical Examination

General Exam: Assess for signs of systemic disease (e.g., cachexia, lymphadenopathy) or coagulopathy (e.g., bruising).

Pelvic Exam: Inspect the vulva, vagina and cervix for lesions, atrophy or trauma. Bimanual exam evaluates uterine size, shape and adnexal masses.

Speculum Exam: Visualize the cervix and vagina for sources of bleeding (e.g., polyps, erosions).

3. Diagnostic Tests

Transvaginal Ultrasound (TVUS): Measures endometrial thickness. An endometrial stripe ≤4 mm in a postmenopausal woman has a high negative predictive value (99%) for endometrial cancer. Thickness >4 mm indicates further investigation.

Endometrial Biopsy: Gold standard for evaluating endometrial pathology. Performed via opd-based pipelle biopsy or hysteroscopy with directed biopsy for abnormal TVUS findings or persistent bleeding.

Hysteroscopy: Visualizes the endometrial cavity for focal lesions (e.g., polyps, submucosal fibroids) and allows targeted biopsy.

Laboratory Tests: Complete blood count (CBC) to assess anemia, coagulation studies for bleeding disorders and thyroid function tests to rule out systemic causes.

Additional Imaging: Pelvic MRI or CT may be indicated for suspected malignancy or adnexal masses. CA-125 levels may be considered for suspected ovarian cancer.

Differential Diagnosis

Distinguish PMB from perimenopausal bleeding (incomplete amenorrhea), hematuria, or rectal bleeding.

Rule out iatrogenic causes (e.g., HT, anticoagulants) and non-gynaecological sources (e.g., bladder or colorectal pathology).

Management

Management of PMB depends on the underlying cause, with a focus on treating the condition, alleviating symptoms and preventing recurrence.

1. Benign Causes

Atrophic Endometrium/Vaginitis

Vaginal Estrogen: Low-dose vaginal oestrogen (e.g., estradiol cream, tablets, or rings) restores mucosal integrity, reducing bleeding. Systemic absorption is minimal, making it safe for most women.

Moisturizers and Lubricants: Non-hormonal options for women with contraindications to oestrogen.

Endometrial Polyps

Hysteroscopic Polypectomy: Surgical removal of polyps under direct visualization.

Uterine Fibroids

Observation: Small, asymptomatic fibroids may not require treatment.

Surgical Options: Myomectomy or hysterectomy for symptomatic or large fibroids.

GSM

Topical treatments as above, combined with pelvic floor therapy for urinary symptoms.

2. Malignant Causes

Endometrial Cancer

Surgical Management: Total hysterectomy with bilateral salpingo-oophorectomy (BSO) is the primary treatment for early-stage disease. Lymph node assessment may be required.

Adjuvant Therapy: Radiation, chemotherapy, or hormonal therapy (e.g., progestins) for advanced or high-risk disease.

Endometrial Hyperplasia

Progestin Therapy: Oral progestins (e.g., medroxyprogesterone) or levonorgestrel IUD for non-atypical hyperplasia.

Hysterectomy: Recommended for atypical hyperplasia due to high risk of progression to cancer.

Cervical Cancer

Treatment depends on stage, ranging from local excision (e.g., cone biopsy) to hysterectomy, radiation or chemoradiation.

Ovarian/Fallopian Tube Cancer

Surgical debulking followed by chemotherapy (e.g., carboplatin/paclitaxel) is standard.

3. Other Causes

Coagulopathy: Adjust anticoagulant therapy or treat underlying bleeding disorder.

Foreign Bodies: Removal of pessaries or other objects, with treatment of secondary infections if present.

4. Supportive Care

Anemia Management: Iron supplementation or transfusion for severe anemia due to heavy bleeding.

Counseling: Educate patients about the cause, prognosis and need for follow-up to alleviate anxiety and ensure compliance.

Prognosis

Benign Causes: Atrophic changes, polyps and fibroids generally have an excellent prognosis with appropriate treatment. Recurrence is possible if underlying factors (e.g., oestrogen imbalance) persist.

Malignant Causes: Endometrial cancer has a 5-year survival rate of 80–90% for early-stage disease but poorer outcomes for advanced stages. Atypical hyperplasia carries a 20–50% risk of progression to cancer if untreated. Cervical and ovarian cancers have variable prognoses based on stage and histology.

Recurrent PMB: Persistent or recurrent bleeding after negative evaluation requires repeat investigation, as malignancy may develop over time.

Clinical and Preventive Considerations

Urgent Evaluation: PMB is considered a potential sign of malignancy until proven otherwise. Prompt investigation (within 2–4 weeks) is critical to avoid delays in diagnosing cancer.

Risk Factor Modification: Address obesity, diabetes and unopposed oestrogen exposure (e.g., via progestin therapy in HT users) to reduce the risk of endometrial hyperplasia and cancer.

Patient Education: Inform patients about the importance of reporting PMB and the low but significant risk of malignancy to encourage timely presentation.

Screening and Follow-Up: Women with a history of PMB, particularly those with hyperplasia, require regular follow-up (e.g., annual TVUS or biopsy) to monitor for recurrence or progression.

Conclusion

Postmenopausal bleeding is a common yet potentially serious symptom that requires systematic evaluation to distinguish benign from malignant causes. Atrophic changes are the most frequent etiology, but the 10–15% risk of endometrial cancer necessitates thorough investigation, including transvaginal ultrasound and endometrial biopsy. Management is tailored to the underlying cause, ranging from vaginal oestrogen for atrophy to surgical intervention for malignancy.

Long Answer Questions

1. Define menopause and describe its physiological changes and hormonal alterations.
2. Discuss the symptoms, diagnosis and management of postmenopausal syndrome.
3. Explain the pathophysiology and treatment of osteoporosis in postmenopausal women.
4. Describe the role and risks of hormone replacement therapy (HRT) in menopause.
5. Elaborate on genitourinary changes during menopause and their clinical implications.

Short Answer Questions

1. What is the average age of menopause in Indian women?
2. Name two common vasomotor symptoms of menopause.
3. Define postmenopausal bleeding.
4. Mention one non-hormonal therapy for menopausal symptoms.
5. What is the role of oestrogen in bone health?

Multiple Choice Questions (1 Mark Each)

1. Menopause is confirmed after:

a) 3 months of amenorrhea b) 6 months c) 12 months d) 18 months

Ans: c) 12 months

2. Most common symptom of menopause:

a) Vaginal bleeding b) Hot flashes c) Pelvic pain d) Weight loss

Ans: b) Hot flashes

3. Osteoporosis in menopause is due to deficiency of:

a) Progesterone b) Estrogen c) Testosterone d) FSH

Ans: b) Estrogen

4. Postmenopausal bleeding may indicate:

a) Fibroid b) Endometrial carcinoma c) PCOS d) Cervical polyp

Ans: b) Endometrial carcinoma

5. Which hormone rises significantly after menopause?

a) Estrogen b) Progesterone c) FSH d) GnRH

Ans: c) FSH

6. Common genitourinary symptom in menopause:

a) Dysuria b) Dyspareunia c) Amenorrhea d) Menorrhagia

Ans: b) Dyspareunia

7. HRT is contraindicated in:

a) Osteoporosis b) Hot flashes c) Breast cancer history d) Vaginal dryness

Ans: c) Breast cancer history

8. Menopausal uterus shows:

a) Hypertrophy b) Atrophy c) Fibrosis d) Hyperplasia

Ans: b) Atrophy

9. Which vitamin is essential in postmenopausal bone health?

a) Vitamin A b) Vitamin B12 c) Vitamin D d) Vitamin K

Ans: c) Vitamin D

10. Senile vaginitis is caused by:

a) Infection b) Estrogen deficiency c) Trauma d) Allergy

Ans: b) Estrogen deficiency

06

Hormone & Phytohormone Therapy in Gynecological Disorders

(Amrad-i-Niswan mein hormone aur Nabati hormone)

6.1 *Istebdal-e-hormone Muaaleja* (Hormone Replacement Therapy)
6.2 *Nabati* Hormones (Phytohormones)

Learning Objective (At the end of the session, the students should be able to):

Describe in brief Hormone Replacement Therapy (HRT)
Enlist the Phytohormones & describe their mechanism of action

6. Hormone & Phytohormone therapy in gynecological Disorders

(*Amrad-i-Niswan mein hormone aur Nabati hormone*)

Hormones play a pivotal role in regulating female reproductive physiology, influencing menstrual cycles, fertility, pregnancy and menopausal transitions. In gynaecology, hormone replacement therapy (HRT), also known as menopausal hormone therapy (MHT), is a cornerstone for managing conditions associated with hormonal deficiencies, particularly during menopause and perimenopause.

Hormones in Gynecological physiology

Hormones orchestrate the complex interplay of reproductive and systemic functions in women. The primary hormones relevant to gynaecology include estrogens, progesterone, androgens and gonadotropins, each with distinct roles and interactions.

1. Estrogens

Types: Estradiol (E2, predominant in reproductive years), estrone (E1, dominant postmenopause), and estriol (E3, prominent in pregnancy).

Sources: Primarily produced by ovarian follicles (estradiol), with peripheral conversion of androgens to estrone in adipose tissue and adrenal glands.

Physiological Roles

Reproductive System: Stimulates endometrial proliferation, cervical mucus production and vaginal epithelial maturation. Supports follicular development and ovulation.

Systemic Effects: Maintains bone density by inhibiting osteoclast activity, modulates lipid profiles (increases HDL, decreases LDL), supports cardiovascular health and regulates thermoregulatory centres in the hypothalamus.

Menopause: Declining estradiol levels postmenopause lead to vasomotor symptoms (VMS), genitourinary syndrome of menopause (GSM), bone loss and increased cardiovascular risk.

2. Progesterone

Source: Produced by the corpus luteum post-ovulation and by the placenta during pregnancy.

Physiological Roles

Reproductive System: Promotes endometrial secretory transformation, prevents endometrial hyperplasia and maintains pregnancy by inhibiting uterine contractions.

Systemic Effects: Modulates mood and sleep via neurosteroid metabolites (e.g., allopregnanolone) and counteracts oestrogen's proliferative effects.

Menopause: Absence of progesterone contributes to irregular bleeding in perimenopause and increases endometrial cancer risk if unopposed oestrogen is present.

3. Androgens

Types: Testosterone, dehydroepiandrosterone (DHEA) and androstenedione.

Sources: Produced by ovaries and adrenal glands, with peripheral conversion to estrogens via aromatization.

Physiological Roles

Reproductive System: Supports libido, sexual arousal and ovarian follicular health.

Systemic Effects: Contributes to muscle mass, bone density and energy levels. Relative androgen excess postmenopause may lead to hirsutism or hair thinning.

Menopause: Ovarian androgen production declines, impacting sexual function and vitality.

4. Gonadotropins

Types: Follicle-stimulating hormone (FSH) and luteinizing hormone (LH).

Source: Secreted by the anterior pituitary, regulated by gonadotropin-releasing hormone (GnRH) from the hypothalamus.

Physiological Roles

Reproductive System: FSH stimulates follicular growth, while LH triggers ovulation and corpus luteum formation.

Menopause: Elevated FSH (>25 IU/L) and LH levels result from reduced ovarian feedback, serving as diagnostic markers of menopause.

5. Other Hormones

Inhibin: Produced by granulosa cells, inhibits FSH secretion. Declines in perimenopause, contributing to rising FSH levels.

Anti-Mullerian Hormone (AMH): Reflects ovarian reserve, declining with age and nearing zero at menopause.

Thyroid Hormones: Influence menstrual regularity and metabolism, with dysfunction mimicking menopausal symptoms.

Cortisol and Adrenal Hormones: Adrenal androgens (e.g., DHEA) contribute to postmenopausal oestrogen production via peripheral conversion.

Hormonal Changes in Menopause

Menopause, defined as 12 consecutive months of amenorrhea due to ovarian follicular depletion, results in profound hormonal changes:

1. Estrogen Decline: Estradiol levels drop to <20 pg/mL, with estrone becoming the primary circulating oestrogen.
2. Progesterone Absence: Cessation of ovulation eliminates progesterone production.
3. Gonadotropin Elevation: FSH and LH levels rise due to loss of ovarian feedback from inhibin and estradiol.
4. Androgen Reduction: Ovarian testosterone production decreases, though adrenal androgens partially compensate.

These changes drive the symptoms of postmenopausal syndrome (e.g., VMS, GSM, bone loss) and increase risks of osteoporosis, cardiovascular disease and metabolic syndrome, forming the basis for HRT.

6.1 Hormone Replacement Therapy

(*Istebdal-e-hormone Muaaleja*)

HRT involves the administration of exogenous hormones (primarily estrogens and progestogens) to alleviate symptoms of hormonal deficiency and mitigate long-term health risks. It is most commonly used to manage menopausal symptoms but also has applications in other gynaecological conditions, such as premature ovarian insufficiency (POI) and hypogonadism.

Indications for HRT

1. Menopausal Symptoms

Vasomotor Symptoms (VMS): Hot flashes and night sweats, affecting 60–80% of women, are the primary indication for systemic HRT.

Genitourinary Syndrome of Menopause (GSM): Vaginal dryness, dyspareunia and urinary symptoms (e.g., urgency, recurrent UTIs) respond well to local (vaginal) oestrogen therapy.

Psychological Symptoms: Mood swings, irritability, or sleep disturbances may improve with HRT.

2. Bone Health

HRT reduces bone resorption and fracture risk in postmenopausal women, particularly in the first 5–7 years postmenopause.

3. Premature Ovarian Insufficiency (POI)

Women with menopause before age 40 require HRT to manage symptoms and prevent long-term complications (e.g., osteoporosis, cardiovascular disease) until the average age of natural menopause (~51 years).

4. Other Indications

Hypogonadism (e.g., due to surgical menopause or pituitary dysfunction).

Adjunct therapy in specific conditions (e.g., endometrial preparation in assisted reproductive technology).

HRT Regimens

HRT regimens are prescribed according to the patient's menopausal status, symptoms and uterine status (intact vs. post-hysterectomy). Key regimens include:

1. Estrogen-Only Therapy

Indications: Women without a uterus (post-hysterectomy).

Forms:

Oral: Conjugated equine estrogens (CEE, 0.3–0.625 mg/day) or estradiol (1–2 mg/day).

Transdermal: Estradiol patches (25–100 µg/day) or gels (0.5–1.5 mg/day), which bypass first-pass hepatic metabolism, reducing thromboembolism risk.

Vaginal: Low-dose estradiol (e.g., 10 µg tablets, 0.01% cream) for GSM, with minimal systemic absorption.

Advantages: Effective for VMS and GSM; preserves bone density.

Risks: Increases endometrial cancer risk in women with a uterus, requiring progestogen opposition.

2. Combined Estrogen-Progestogen Therapy

Indications: Women with an intact uterus to prevent endometrial hyperplasia.

Progestogens: Micronized progesterone (100–200 mg/day), medroxyprogesterone acetate (MPA, 2.5–10 mg/day), or levonorgestrel intrauterine device (IUD).

Regimens:

Continuous Combined: Daily oestrogen and progestogen to avoid withdrawal bleeding (e.g., CEE 0.625 mg + MPA 2.5 mg).

Sequential/Cyclic: Estrogen daily with progestogen for 10–14 days/month, mimicking menstrual cycles and causing scheduled bleeding.

Advantages: Reduces endometrial cancer risk; effective for VMS and GSM.

Risks: Progestogens may attenuate oestrogen's cardiovascular benefits and increase breast cancer risk with long-term use.

3. Vaginal Estrogen Therapy

Indications: GSM symptoms (vaginal dryness, dyspareunia, urinary issues).

Forms: Estradiol tablets (10 µg), creams (0.01%) or rings (7.5 µg/day).

Advantages: Localized effect with minimal systemic absorption; safe for most women, including those with contraindications to systemic HRT.

Risks: Minimal, though endometrial monitoring is recommended with prolonged use.

4. Tibolone

A synthetic steroid with estrogenic, progestogenic and androgenic properties, used for VMS and bone health. Dose: 2.5 mg/day.

Advantages: Reduces VMS and fracture risk; may improve libido.

Risks: Similar to combined HRT, with potential increased stroke risk in older women.

5. Androgen Therapy

Indications: Rarely used, primarily for hypoactive sexual desire disorder (HSDD) in postmenopausal women.

Forms: Transdermal testosterone (off-label in many regions).

Risks: Virilization, lipid profile changes and limited long-term safety data.

Benefits of HRT

1. Symptom Relief

Vasomotor symptom: Reduces hot flash frequency and severity by 75–90%.

Genitourinary syndrome of menopause: Improves vaginal lubrication, elasticity and urinary symptoms.

Psychological: May improve mood and sleep indirectly via VMS relief.

2. Bone Health

Reduces bone loss by 2–3% annually and lowers fracture risk by 20–40% (hip, vertebral, non-vertebral fractures).

3. Cardiovascular Effects (Controversial)

The "timing hypothesis" suggests cardiovascular benefit when HRT is initiated <10 years postmenopause or before age 60, improving endothelial function and lipid profiles.

Benefits are less clear in older women or those with established cardiovascular disease.

4. Other Benefits

May reduce colorectal cancer risk with combined HRT. Improves skin elasticity and connective tissue health.

Risks of HRT

1. Cardiovascular Risks

Thromboembolism: Oral oestrogen increases venous thromboembolism (VTE) risk 2–3-fold, particularly in the first year. Transdermal oestrogen has lower risk.

Stroke: Slight increase in stroke risk with oral HRT, especially in women >60 years.

2. Breast Cancer

Combined oestrogen-progestogen therapy increases breast cancer risk after 5 years of use (relative risk ~1.3). Estrogen-only therapy has minimal or no increased risk.

Risk diminishes after discontinuation.

3. Endometrial Cancer

Estrogen-only therapy in women with a uterus increases endometrial cancer risk 5–10-fold. Combined therapy mitigates this risk.

4. Gallbladder Disease

Oral HRT increases risk of cholelithiasis and cholecystitis.

5. Other Risks

Minor side effects include breast tenderness, bloating and mood changes. Long-term use requires ongoing risk-benefit assessment.

Contraindications to HRT

Absolute

History of breast cancer, endometrial cancer or oestrogen-dependent malignancies.

Active VTE or history of unprovoked VTE.

Uncontrolled hypertension, active liver disease or undiagnosed vaginal bleeding.

Relative

Cardiovascular disease, high VTE risk (e.g., obesity, smoking), or strong family history of breast cancer.

Non-Hormonal Alternatives

For women with contraindications to HRT or who prefer non-hormonal options:

VMS: SSRIs (e.g., paroxetine 7.5 mg), SNRIs (e.g., venlafaxine), gabapentin or clonidine reduce hot flashes by 50–60%.

GSM: Vaginal moisturizers, lubricants (a selective oestrogen receptor modulator [SERM]).

Bone Health: Bisphosphonates, denosumab or raloxifene.

Psychological Symptoms: Cognitive-behavioral therapy (CBT) or antidepressants.

Clinical Considerations

1. Individualized Therapy

Individualise HRT based on age, time since menopause, symptoms, risk factors and patient preferences. The "lowest dose for the shortest duration" principle guides therapy.

Women <60 years or within 10 years of menopause derive the greatest benefit with the lowest risk.

2. Monitoring

Regular follow-up (every 6–12 months) to assess symptom control, side effects and risks.

Endometrial surveillance (e.g., transvaginal ultrasound, biopsy) for women with abnormal bleeding.

Breast cancer screening (mammography) and cardiovascular risk assessment (lipid profile, blood pressure) are essential.

3. Discontinuation

Gradual tapering reduces symptom recurrence compared to abrupt cessation.

Reassess need for HRT annually, balancing benefits and risks.

4. Special Populations

Premature Ovarian Insufficiency: Requires higher-dose HRT (e.g., 2 mg estradiol or equivalent) until age 51 to mimic physiological levels.

Surgical Menopause: Immediate HRT initiation post-oophorectomy to prevent severe symptoms and long-term risks, unless contraindicated.

Breast Cancer Survivors: Non-hormonal therapies are preferred; vaginal oestrogen may be considered in some cases with oncology consultation.

5. Psychosocial Factors

Education and counselling address stigma and misconceptions. Psychosocial stressors may exacerbate symptoms, requiring individualized holistic care.

Long-Term Health Implications

HRT reduces several long-term risks associated with menopause:

1. Osteoporosis: Reduces fracture risk, though symptoms gradually re-appear after discontinuation.
2. Cardiovascular Disease: Potential benefit in early postmenopause, but risks increase in older women or with prolonged use.

3. Cognitive Health: Limited evidence suggests early HRT may reduce dementia risk, but data are inconclusive.
4. Cancer Risk: Combined HRT increases breast cancer risk, while oestrogen-only therapy reduces colorectal cancer risk.

6.2 Phytohormones

(Nabati Hormones)

Phytohormones, commonly referred to as phytoestrogens, are naturally occurring plant-derived compounds that structurally or functionally mimic mammalian estrogens, offering potential therapeutic benefits in gynaecology. These compounds are increasingly utilized as alternatives or adjuncts to hormone replacement therapy (HRT) for managing menopausal symptoms, particularly in women seeking non-hormonal options or those with contraindications to conventional HRT.

Definition and Classification

Phytohormones are plant-derived compounds with oestrogen-like activity due to their structural similarity to 17β-estradiol, enabling them to bind to oestrogen receptors (ERs). They are classified into several groups based on chemical structure:

1. Isoflavones: The most studied phytoestrogens, found in soybeans and legumes, including genistein, daidzein and glycitein.

2. Lignans: Present in flaxseeds, whole grains and vegetables, with enterolactone and enterodiol formed via gut microbiota metabolism.

3. Coumestans: Found in clover and alfalfa, with coumestrol as the primary estrogenic compound.

4. Stilbenes: Present in grapes and red wine, with resveratrol exhibiting weak estrogenic activity.

Phytohormones act as selective oestrogen receptor modulators (SERMs), exerting estrogenic or anti-estrogenic effects depending on the tissue, receptor subtype and endogenous oestrogen levels . Their weaker binding affinity compared to estradiol results in milder effects, making them appealing for managing mild menopausal symptoms .

Sources of Phytohormones

Phytohormones are abundant in plant-based foods and herbal supplements:

Soy Products: Tofu, soy milk contain isoflavones (40–100 mg/100 g) [3].

Flaxseeds: Rich in lignans (300–1000 mg/100 g), particularly secoisolariciresinol diglucoside (SDG) [4].

Legumes: Red clover, chickpeas and lentils provide isoflavones and coumestans [1].

Whole Grains: Oats, barley, and rye contain lignans [4].

Fruits and Vegetables: Berries, apples and cruciferous vegetables supply lignans and stilbenes [1].

Herbs: Red clover (Trifolium pratense) and black cohosh (Actaea racemosa) are used in supplements for menopausal symptoms, though black cohosh's mechanism may involve serotonergic rather than phytoestrogenic pathways [5].

Mechanisms of Action

Phytohormones exert their effects through multiple pathways:

1. Estrogen Receptor Binding

Phytohormones bind to ERα and ERβ, with a preference for ERβ, which is prevalent in bone, brain and urogenital tissues but less so in the breast and endometrium [2].

Their binding affinity is 100–1000 times weaker than estradiol, resulting in partial agonist or antagonist effects [1].

In low-oestrogen states (e.g., postmenopause), phytohormones act as weak agonists; in high-oestrogen environments (e.g., premenopause), they may act as antagonists by competing with endogenous estrogens [6].

2. Non-Receptor Effects

Phytohormones modulate signaling pathways, including tyrosine kinase, nuclear factor-kappa B (NF-κB) and antioxidant pathways, contributing to anti-inflammatory and antiproliferative effects [7].

They influence gene transcription via interaction with co-activators or co-repressors in oestrogen-responsive tissues [2].

3. Metabolism by Gut Microbiota

Isoflavones like daidzein are metabolized by gut bacteria into equol, a compound with stronger estrogenic activity. Only 30–50% of individuals produce equol, impacting clinical efficacy [8].

Lignans are converted to enterolactone and enterodiol, which exert estrogenic and antioxidant effects [4].

4. Other Hormonal Effects

Phytohormones may reduce FSH and LH levels by providing partial estrogenic feedback to the hypothalamic-pituitary-ovarian axis [9].

Some isoflavones (e.g., genistein) inhibit aromatase, reducing endogenous oestrogen synthesis, which may be relevant in oestrogen-dependent conditions [10].

Clinical Applications in Gynaecology

Phytohormones are primarily used to manage menopausal symptoms but have potential applications in other hormonal conditions:

1. Menopausal Symptoms

Vasomotor Symptoms (VMS): Soy isoflavones and red clover extracts are studied for reducing hot flashes and night sweats [11].

Genitourinary Syndrome of Menopause (GSM): Limited evidence supports phytohormones for vaginal dryness and urinary symptoms [12].

Psychological Symptoms: Mood and sleep improvements may occur indirectly via VMS relief [13].

2. Bone Health

Isoflavones and lignans may reduce bone resorption by acting on ERβ in osteoblasts, potentially lowering osteoporosis risk [14].

3. Cardiovascular Health

Phytohormones improve lipid profiles (e.g., reducing LDL cholesterol) and endothelial function, potentially decreasing cardiovascular risk [15].

4. Other Conditions

Endometriosis and Fibroids: Preliminary studies suggest anti-estrogenic effects may reduce proliferation in these conditions [16].

Polycystic Ovary Syndrome (PCOS): Isoflavones may improve insulin sensitivity and androgen profiles [17].

Breast Cancer Prevention: Observational studies suggest dietary phytohormones may reduce breast cancer risk, particularly in Asian populations [18].

Efficacy of Phytohormones

Clinical efficacy varies due to differences in compound type, dose, formulation and individual factors:

Vasomotor Symptoms

Meta-analyses indicate soy isoflavones (40–80 mg/day) reduce hot flash frequency by 20–30% compared to placebo, with greater effects in equol producers [11].

Red clover isoflavones show inconsistent results, with some trials reporting no significant benefit [19].

Black cohosh (20–40 mg/day) may reduce VMS, but its mechanism is likely non-phytoestrogenic [5].

Bone Health

Isoflavones (50–100 mg/day) increase lumbar spine BMD by 1–2% after 1–2 years, less effective than HRT or bisphosphonates [14].

Flaxseed lignans show minimal BMD effects [4].

Cardiovascular Health

Soy isoflavones reduce LDL cholesterol by 5–10% and improve endothelial function, but long-term cardiovascular outcomes are unclear [15].

Genitourinary Symptoms

Oral phytohormones show limited improvement in vaginal dryness; topical preparations are understudied [12].

Psychological Symptoms

Mixed results, with some studies showing mood and sleep benefits secondary to VMS relief [13].

Factors influencing efficacy include dose, duration (effects may take 8–12 weeks), and equol production [8].

Safety and Risks

Phytohormones are generally safe at dietary doses, but high-dose supplements raise concerns:

1. Endometrial Safety

Short-term use (<2 years) of isoflavones or lignans shows no increased risk of endometrial hyperplasia or cancer [20].

Long-term data are limited and high doses may stimulate endometrial proliferation in susceptible women [21].

2. Breast Cancer Risk

Epidemiological studies suggest dietary soy reduces breast cancer risk, particularly in Asian populations with lifelong exposure [18].

High-dose supplements in breast cancer survivors are controversial due to potential estrogenic effects, though no consistent evidence shows harm [22].

3. Cardiovascular and Thromboembolic Risk

Phytohormones do not increase venous thromboembolism risk, unlike oral HRT [15].

4. Gastrointestinal and Allergic Reactions

High doses of soy or flaxseed may cause bloating, nausea, or allergic reactions [23].

5. Drug Interactions

Phytohormones may interfere with tamoxifen or aromatase inhibitors due to SERM-like effects [24].

Soy may inhibit thyroid hormone absorption in hypothyroidism [25].

6. Regulation and Quality

Supplements lack stringent regulation, leading to variability in potency and purity. Standardized products are recommended [26].

Clinical Considerations

1. Patient Selection

Phytohormones are suitable for women with mild to moderate menopausal symptoms, those preferring natural therapies, or those with HRT contraindications (e.g., breast cancer, VTE risk) [27].

Severe symptoms may require HRT for better efficacy [11].

2. Dosing and Administration

Soy Isoflavones: 40–80 mg/day, preferably from diet or standardized supplements [11].

Flaxseed: 40 g/day ground flaxseed or 10–20 mg/day lignan extracts [4].

Red Clover: 40–80 mg/day isoflavones [19].

Black Cohosh: 20–40 mg/day, though not a true phytohormone [5].

3. Counseling and Monitoring

Educate patients on variable efficacy and the need for 8–12 weeks to assess benefits [11].

Monitor for side effects (e.g., gastrointestinal, allergic reactions) and endometrial health in long-term users [20].

Regular gynaecological exams and transvaginal ultrasound are recommended for women on high-dose supplements [21].

4. Cultural and Dietary Context

Asian populations with high lifelong phytoestrogen intake may experience greater benefits due to gut microbiota adaptations [8].

Cultural preferences for natural remedies influence use, requiring patient-centered counselling [27].

5. Combination with Other Therapies

Phytohormones can be combined with lifestyle interventions or non-hormonal therapies (e.g., SSRIs for VMS) [13].

Avoid combining with HRT or tamoxifen without specialist consultation [24].

Conclusion

Phytohormones offer a promising, though less potent, alternative to HRT for managing menopausal symptoms and supporting bone and cardiovascular health. Their SERM-like properties provide tissue-specific benefits, particularly for women with mild symptoms or HRT contraindications. However, variable efficacy, limited long-term safety data and regulatory challenges necessitate cautious use and patient education.

References

1. Patisaul HB, Jefferson W. The pros and cons of phytoestrogens. *Front Neuroendocrinol*. 2010;31(4):400-419. doi:10.1016/j.yfrne.2010.03.003
2. Kuiper GG, Lemmen JG, Carlsson B, et al. Interaction of estrogenic chemicals and phytoestrogens with oestrogen receptor β. *Endocrinology*. 1998;139(10):4252-4263. doi:10.1210/endo.139.10.6216
3. Messina M. Soy and health update: evaluation of the clinical and epidemiologic literature. *Nutrients*. 2016;8(12):754. doi:10.3390/nu8120754
4. Adolphe JL, Whiting SJ, Juurlink BH, et al. Health effects with consumption of the flax lignan secoisolariciresinol diglucoside. *Br J Nutr*. 2010;103(7):929-938. doi:10.1017/S0007114509992753
5. Leach MJ, Moore V. Black cohosh (Cimicifuga spp.) for menopausal symptoms. *Cochrane Database Syst Rev*. 2012;2012(9):CD007244. doi:10.1002/14651858.CD007244.pub2
6. Turner JV, Agatonovic-Kustrin S, Singh J. In vitro screening of phytoestrogens for estrogenic and antiestrogenic activity. *Drug Dev Ind Pharm*. 2007;33(10):1051-1061. doi:10.1080/03639040701377367
7. Sirotkin AV, Harrath AH. Phytoestrogens and their effects. *Eur J Pharmacol*. 2014;741:230-236. doi:10.1016/j.ejphar.2014.07.057
8. Setchell KD, Brown NM, Lydeking-Olsen E. The clinical importance of the metabolite equol—a clue to the effectiveness of soy and its isoflavones. *J Nutr*. 2002;132(12):3577-3584. doi:10.1093/jn/132.12.3577
9. Eden JA. Managing menopause: a review of the role of phytoestrogens. *Climacteric*. 2012;15(3):204-209. doi:10.3109/13697137.2011.620193
10. Rice S, Whitehead SA. Phytoestrogens and breast cancer—promoters or protectors? *Endocr Relat Cancer*. 2006;13(4):995-1015. doi:10.1677/erc.1.01159

11. Chen MN, Lin CC, Liu CF. Efficacy of phytoestrogens for menopausal symptoms: a meta-analysis and systematic review. *Climacteric*. 2015;18(2):260-269. doi:10.3109/13697137.2014.950662
12. Franco OH, Chowdhury R, Troup J, et al. Use of plant-based therapies and menopausal symptoms: a systematic review and meta-analysis. *JAMA*. 2016;315(23):2554-2563. doi:10.1001/jama.2016.8012
13. Gartoulla P, Hickey M. Menopause management: how you can do better. *Curr Obstet Gynecol Rep*. 2014;3(2):105-111. doi:10.1007/s13669-014-0079-8
14. Marini H, Minutoli L, Polito F, et al. Effects of the phytoestrogen genistein on bone metabolism in osteopenic postmenopausal women: a randomized trial. *Ann Intern Med*. 2007;146(12):839-847. doi:10.7326/0003-4819-146-12-200706190-00005
15. Sacks FM, Lichtenstein A, Van Horn L, et al. Soy protein, isoflavones, and cardiovascular health: an American Heart Association Science Advisory. *Circulation*. 2006;113(7):1034-1044. doi:10.1161/CIRCULATIONAHA.106.171052
16. Clowes JA, Peel NF, Eastell R. The effect of phytoestrogens on bone. *Curr Osteoporos Rep*. 2004;2(2):62-68. doi:10.1007/s11914-004-0013-7
17. Khani B, Mehrabian F, Khalesi E, Eshraghi A. Effect of soy phytoestrogen on metabolic and hormonal parameters of women with polycystic ovary syndrome. *J Obstet Gynaecol Res*. 2011;37(10):1373-1378. doi:10.1111/j.1447-0756.2011.01537.x
18. Wu AH, Yu MC, Tseng CC, Pike MC. Epidemiology of soy exposures and breast cancer risk. *Br J Cancer*. 2008;98(1):9-14. doi:10.1038/sj.bjc.6604145
19. Lethaby A, Marjoribanks J, Kronenberg F, et al. Phytoestrogens for menopausal vasomotor symptoms. *Cochrane Database Syst Rev*. 2013;2013(12):CD001395. doi:10.1002/14651858.CD001395.pub4
20. Tempfer CB, Bentz EK, Leodolter S, et al. Phytoestrogens in clinical practice: a review of the literature. *Fertil Steril*. 2007;87(6):1243-1249. doi:10.1016/j.fertnstert.2007.01.120
21. Unfer V, Casini ML, Costabile L, et al. Endometrial effects of long-term treatment with phytoestrogens: a randomized, double-blind, placebo-controlled study. *Fertil Steril*. 2004;82(1):145-148. doi:10.1016/j.fertnstert.2003.11.041
22. Messina M, McCaskill-Stevens W, Lampe JW. Addressing the soy and breast cancer relationship: review, commentary, and workshop proceedings. *J Natl Cancer Inst*. 2006;98(18):1275-1284. doi:10.1093/jnci/djj356
23. Bedell S, Nachtigall M, Naftolin F. The pros and cons of plant estrogens for menopause. *J Steroid Biochem Mol Biol*. 2014;139:225-236. doi:10.1016/j.jsbmb.2012.12.004
24. Ju YH, Doerge DR, Allred KF, et al. Dietary genistein negates the inhibitory effect of tamoxifen on growth of oestrogen-dependent human breast cancer (MCF-7) cells implanted in athymic mice. *Cancer Res*. 2002;62(9):2474-2477.
25. Messina M, Redmond G. Effects of soy protein and soybean isoflavones on thyroid function in healthy adults and hypothyroid patients: a review of the relevant literature. *Thyroid*. 2006;16(3):249-258. doi:10.1089/thy.2006.16.249
26. Fitzpatrick LA. Phytoestrogens—mechanism of action and effect on bone. *Climacteric*. 2003;6(3):178-184. doi:10.1080/cmt.6.3.178.184
27. North American Menopause Society. Nonhormonal management of menopause-associated vasomotor symptoms: 2015 position statement of The North American Menopause Society. *Menopause*. 2015;22(11):1155-1172. doi:10.1097/GME.0000000000000546

Hormonal Therapy Decision Tree

Patient Presentation

↓

Menstrual Irregularity?

↓

Yes → Evaluate Cycle Pattern

↓

Anovulatory? → Clomiphene / Letrozole

Ovulatory but irregular? → Progesterone therapy

↓

No → Consider Other Endocrine Causes

↓

Refer for Endocrine Workup

Hormonal Therapy in Gynecological Disorders

Gynecological Disorder Identified

↓

Evaluate Hormonal Imbalance

↓

Select Therapy Type:

↓	↓	↓
Estrogen	Progesterone	Combination
↓	↓	↓
Menopause Osteoporosis	Amenorrhea Dysmenorrhea	Contraception PCOS

↓

Monitor Response & Side Effects

↓

Adjust Dosage or Switch Therapy

Long Answer Questions

1. Describe the role of oestrogen and progesterone in female reproductive physiology and their therapeutic applications.
2. Discuss hormonal therapy in menopause, including indications, contraindications and side effects.
3. Explain the use of phytoestrogens in gynaecological disorders with examples and mechanisms.

4. Elaborate on hormonal management of menstrual irregularities and infertility.
5. Describe the classification and clinical use of synthetic and natural hormones in gynaecology.

Short Answer Questions

1. Define phytoestrogens.
2. Name two synthetic estrogens used in gynaecology.
3. Mention one indication for progesterone therapy.
4. What is the role of GnRH analogues in gynaecology?
5. List two sources of plant-based hormones.

Multiple Choice Questions (1 Mark Each)

1. Which hormone is primarily responsible for endometrial proliferation?

a) Progesterone b) Estrogen c) FSH d) LH

Ans: b) Estrogen

2. Phytoestrogens are commonly derived from:

a) Dairy products b) Soybeans c) Meat d) Fish

Ans: b) Soybeans

3. GnRH analogues are used in the treatment of:

a) Menorrhagia b) Endometriosis c) Vaginitis d) Fibroids

Ans: b) Endometriosis

4. Which of the following is a selective oestrogen receptor modulator (SERM)?

a) Mifepristone b) Tamoxifen c) Clomiphene d) Danazol

Ans: b) Tamoxifen

5. Which hormone is used to trigger ovulation in infertility treatment?

a) Estrogen b) Progesterone c) LH d) hCG

Ans: d) hCG

6. Common side effect of long-term oestrogen therapy:

a) Osteoporosis b) Breast tenderness c) Weight loss d) Hypotension

Ans: b) Breast tenderness

7. Which plant is a rich source of phytoestrogens?

a) Aloe vera b) Fenugreek c) Soy d) Neem

Ans: c) Soy

8. Progesterone therapy is contraindicated in:

a) Menorrhagia b) Pregnancy c) Liver disease d) Amenorrhea

Ans: c) Liver disease

9. Which hormone is used in emergency contraception?

a) Estrogen   b) Progesterone   c) Levonorgestrel   d) FSH

Ans: c) Levonorgestrel

10. Phytohormones act by binding to:

a) Enzymes   b) DNA   c) Hormone receptors   d) Blood proteins

Ans: c) Hormone receptors

07

Diseases of Vulva

(Amrad-i-farj)

7.1 *Hikkat-ul-farj* (Pruritus Vulvae)
7.2 *Quruh al-farj* (Ulcers of Vulva)
7.3 *Iltihab-i-farj* (Vulvitis)
7.4 *Huzal* (Atrophy)
7.5 *Kyas wa Sal'at* (Cysts & Neopalsm)
7.6 *Alam-i-farj* (Vulvodynia)
7.7 *Mutalazemai Iltihab-i-Dehliz-i-farj* (Vulval vestibulitis Syndrome)

Learning Objectives (At the end of the session, the students should be able to):

Describe the causes of *Hikkat-ul-Farj* (Pruritus Vulvae) and describe its diagnosis, management & complications .

Describe the causes, types, diagnosis, management and complications of *Quruh-al-Farj* (Ulcers of Vulva)

Describe the causes, diagnosis, management and complications of *Iltihab–e-Farj* (Vulvitis) .

Describe the causes, diagnosis, management & complications of *Huzaal* (Atrophy) of the vagina.

Explain in brief the causes, classification, diagnosis, stages, management and complications of *Kyas & Sal'at* (Cysts & Neoplasm)

Enumerate the causes of Vulvodynia and describe its management.

Explain Vulval vestibulitis syndrome in brief.

7. Diseases of Vulva

(*Amrad-i-farj*)

The vulva, comprising the external genitalia including the labia majora, labia minora, clitoris, vestibule and perineum, is susceptible to various dermatological, inflammatory, infectious and neoplastic conditions.

7.1 Pruritus Vulvae

(*Hikka al-farj*)

Definition

Pruritus vulvae is persistent itching of the vulvar skin, often a symptom rather than a primary condition, caused by various underlying dermatological, infectious or systemic disorders.

Etiology

Infections: Candidiasis, bacterial vaginosis, trichomoniasis, herpes simplex virus (HSV).

Dermatological Conditions: Lichen simplex chronicus, lichen sclerosus, lichen planus, contact dermatitis, eczema, psoriasis.

Systemic Causes: Diabetes mellitus, liver disease, renal failure, thyroid disorders.

Allergic/Irritant Factors: Soaps, detergents, perfumes, synthetic clothing, sanitary products.

Neoplastic: Vulvar intraepithelial neoplasia (VIN), squamous cell carcinoma.

Others: Poor hygiene, psychogenic factors or idiopathic causes.

Clinical Features

Intense itching, worse at night, leading to scratching and excoriation.

Erythema, edema or lichenification (thickened skin) in chronic cases.

Associated symptoms like discharge or pain, depending on the underlying cause.

Diagnosis

History: Duration, triggers, hygiene practices, systemic symptoms and allergies.

Physical Examination: Inspect for skin changes (erythema, lichenification, excoriations or lesions).

Investigations

Swabs for microscopy and culture (bacterial, fungal or viral).

Skin biopsy for suspected dermatoses or neoplasia.

Blood tests for systemic causes (e.g., fasting glucose, thyroid function, liver/renal function tests).

Patch Testing: For suspected allergic contact dermatitis.

Management

General Measures:

Avoid irritants (scented products, tight clothing).

Maintain hygiene with mild, fragrance-free cleansers.

Use cotton underwear and avoid overwashing.

Specific Treatment

Treat underlying infections (e.g., antifungals for candidiasis, antivirals for HSV).

Topical corticosteroids (e.g., hydrocortisone 1% for mild cases, clobetasol for lichen sclerosus).

Antihistamines (e.g., hydroxyzine) for night time itching.

Treat systemic conditions (e.g., optimize glycemic control in diabetes).

Counseling: Address psychogenic factors and educate on avoiding scratching.

Prognosis

Depends on the underlying cause. Infections and contact dermatitis resolve with treatment, while chronic dermatoses like lichen sclerosus require long-term management.

Diseases of the Vulva (Classify by etiology)

Infectious	Inflammatory	Neoplastic	Functional
Candidiasis	Lichen sclerosus	VIN, SCC	Vulvodynia
Trichomoniasis	Lichen planus	Melanoma	Bartholin cyst
Herpes	Contact dermatitis	Paget's disease	Pruritus
HPV	Psoriasis	Basal cell carcinoma	Dyspareunia

Symptom		**Likely Condition**
Itching + white plaques	=	Lichen sclerosus
Painful ulcer	=	Herpes simplex
Painless lump	=	Bartholin cyst
Pigmented lesion	=	Melanoma
Chronic pain	=	Vulvodynia.

Patient Presents with Vulvar Symptoms
↓
History Taking
(Discharge, Itching, Pain, Lesion Type)
↓
Physical Examination
(Speculum + Vulvar Inspection)
↓
Identify Lesion Type:
↓ ↓ ↓ ↓
Papule Plaque Ulcer Nodule
↓ ↓ ↓ ↓
Color, Margin, Surface, Location
↓
Differential Diagnosis
↓
Lab Tests (Swab, Biopsy, pH, Culture)
↓
Final Diagnosis → Treatment Plan

7.2 Ulcers of Vulva

(*Quruh al-farj*)

Definition

Vulvar ulcers are breaches in the epithelial surface of the vulva, often painful, caused by infectious, inflammatory, neoplastic or traumatic etiologies.

Etiology

Infectious

Herpes simplex virus (most common).

Syphilis (primary chancre).

Chancroid (*Haemophilus ducreyi*).

Lymphogranuloma venereum (*Chlamydia trachomatis*).

Granuloma inguinale (*Klebsiella granulomatis*).

Non-Infectious

Aphthous ulcers (autoimmune or idiopathic).

Behcet's disease (recurrent oral and genital ulcers).

Crohn's disease (perianal and vulvar involvement).

Trauma (e.g., sexual trauma, chemical burns).

Neoplastic (e.g., squamous cell carcinoma, basal cell carcinoma).

Iatrogenic

Post-surgical or radiation-induced ulcers.

Clinical Features

Painful or painless ulcers, depending on etiology (e.g., painful in HSV, painless in syphilis).

Single or multiple ulcers, with associated erythema, edema or discharge.

Systemic symptoms like fever, lymphadenopathy or malaise in infectious causes.

Chronic ulcers may suggest malignancy or autoimmune disease.

Diagnosis

History: Sexual history, trauma, systemic symptoms, recurrence.

Physical Examination: Note ulcer characteristics (size, number, edges, base, tenderness).

Investigations

Viral PCR for HSV.

Serology for syphilis (VDRL, TPHA).

Swabs or tissue biopsy for bacterial culture or histopathology.

Autoimmune workup (e.g., ANA for suspected Behcet's).

Biopsy for chronic or suspicious ulcers to rule out malignancy.

Management

Infectious Causes

HSV: Acyclovir, valacyclovir or famciclovir (oral or topical).

Syphilis: Penicillin G (single-dose intramuscular for primary syphilis).

Chancroid: Azithromycin or ceftriaxone.

Lymphogranuloma venereum: Doxycycline or erythromycin.

Granuloma inguinale: Azithromycin or doxycycline.

Non-Infectious Causes

Aphthous ulcers: Topical steroids, analgesics.

Behcet's: Systemic steroids, colchicine or immunosuppressants.

Crohn's: Anti-TNF agents, steroids or surgical consultation.

Supportive Care: Pain management, wound care and hygiene.

Malignancy: Refer for surgical excision, radiotherapy or chemotherapy.

Prognosis: Infectious ulcers resolve with appropriate antimicrobial therapy. Chronic or neoplastic ulcers may require prolonged treatment and have a guarded prognosis.

7.3 Vulvitis

(*Iltihab-e-farj*)

Definition

Vulvitis is inflammation of the vulvar skin and mucosa, often secondary to infections, allergies or irritants.

Etiology

Infectious: Candida albicans (most common), bacterial vaginosis, herpes simplex virus.

Allergic/Irritant: Contact dermatitis from soaps, perfumes or latex.

Dermatological: Psoriasis, eczema, lichen planus.

Systemic: Estrogen deficiency (postmenopausal), diabetes mellitus.

Clinical Features

Erythema, swelling and tenderness of the vulva.

Itching, burning or pain.

Discharge (e.g., thick white discharge in candidiasis).

Fissures or excoriations in severe cases.

Diagnosis

History: Onset, triggers, associated vaginal discharge or systemic symptoms.

Physical Examination: Inspect for erythema, edema or specific lesions (e.g., satellite lesions in candidiasis).

Investigations

Vaginal/vulvar swabs for microscopy and culture.

Skin biopsy for chronic or atypical cases.

Patch testing for allergic causes.

Management

General Measures: Avoid irritants and maintain hygiene. Use emollients to soothe skin.

Specific Treatment: Antifungals (e.g., clotrimazole cream or oral fluconazole) for candidiasis. Antibiotics for bacterial infections. Topical steroids for allergic or dermatological causes.

Education: Advise on loose clothing and avoiding douching.

Prognosis

Acute vulvitis resolves with treatment of the underlying cause.

Chronic cases may recur if triggers persist.

Key Definitions

Lichen Sclerosus ➤ Chronic inflammatory condition with white, thin, parchment-like vulvar skin.

Bartholin's Cyst ➤ Obstruction of Bartholin gland duct causing painless swelling.

Vulvodynia ➤ Chronic vulvar pain without identifiable cause, lasting ≥3 months.

VIN ➤ Premalignant lesion of vulvar epithelium, often HPV-related.

Squamous Cell Carcinoma ➤ Most common vulvar cancer, often arising from VIN or lichen sclerosus.

7.4 Atrophy

(*Huzal*)

Definition

Vulval atrophy (also known as genitourinary syndrome of menopause) is thinning and drying of the vulvar and vaginal tissues due to oestrogen deficiency, commonly seen in postmenopausal women.

Etiology

Primary Cause: Decreased oestrogen levels (menopause, postpartum or iatrogenic, e.g., oophorectomy).

Contributing Factors: Aging, smoking or chemotherapy.

Clinical Features

Dryness, itching and burning of the vulva.

Thin, pale or shiny vulvar skin.

Dyspareunia (painful intercourse).

Recurrent urinary tract infections or urinary symptoms (e.g., urgency).

Diagnosis

History: Menopausal status, symptoms of dryness or dyspareunia.

Physical Examination: Thin, pale mucosa, loss of rugae or fissures.

Investigations

Usually clinical diagnosis.

Vaginal pH testing (>5 in atrophy).

Rule out infections or dermatoses with swabs or biopsy if needed.

Management

Hormonal Therapy

Topical oestrogen (e.g., estradiol cream or vaginal ring) is first-line.

Systemic hormone replacement therapy (HRT) for women with systemic menopausal symptoms.

Non-Hormonal Therapy

Moisturizers and lubricants for symptom relief.

Ospemifene (oral selective oestrogen receptor modulator) for dyspareunia.

General Measures: Avoid irritants, maintain hygiene and counsel on sexual health.

Prognosis

Symptoms improve significantly with oestrogen therapy.

Long-term management may be needed in postmenopausal women.

7.5 Cysts & Neopalsm

(*Kyas wa Sal'at*)

A. Vulvar Cysts

Definition

Benign, fluid-filled sacs in the vulvar region, often asymptomatic unless large or infected.

Types and Etiology

1. Bartholin's Cyst/Abscess: Obstruction of Bartholin's gland duct, often due to infection (e.g., Escherichia coli, Neisseria gonorrhoeae).
2. Skene's Gland Cyst: Obstruction of paraurethral glands.
3. Sebaceous/Epidermal Cysts: Blocked sebaceous glands or hair follicles.
4. Mucous Cysts: Arise from minor vestibular glands.

Clinical Features

Painless lump (unless infected).

Pain, swelling, or dyspareunia if large or abscessed.

Bartholin's abscess: Tender, erythematous mass with systemic symptoms (fever, malaise).

Diagnosis

Clinical Examination: Palpation of a cystic mass, noting size, location, and tenderness.

Investigations

Ultrasound to confirm cystic nature.

Culture of abscess fluid to guide antibiotic therapy.

Biopsy if malignancy is suspected (rare).

Management

1. Asymptomatic Cysts: Observation.

2. Symptomatic Cysts:

Bartholin's cyst/abscess: Incision and drainage, marsupialization, or Word catheter placement.

Antibiotics for infected cysts (e.g., amoxicillin-clavulanate).

3. Recurrent Cysts: Consider Bartholin's gland excision.

Prognosis

Most resolve with treatment; recurrence is possible with incomplete drainage.

B. Vulvar Neoplasms

Definition

Vulvar neoplasms encompass a spectrum of benign, premalignant and malignant tumours arising from the tissues of the vulva, which includes the labia majora, labia minora, clitoris, vestibule and perineum. These neoplasms range from benign growths, such as fibromas and condylomas, to premalignant conditions like vulvar intraepithelial neoplasia (VIN) and malignant tumours, predominantly squamous cell carcinoma.

Classification

Vulvar neoplasms are classified based on their malignant potential and histological origin:

1. Benign Neoplasms

a. Epithelial: Epidermal cysts, seborrheic keratosis, hidradenoma papilliferum.
b. Mesenchymal: Fibroma, lipoma, leiomyoma, hemangioma.
c. Infectious/HPV-related: Condyloma acuminata (genital warts).

2. Premalignant Neoplasms

a. Vulvar Intraepithelial Neoplasia (VIN):
b. Usual-type VIN (uVIN): Associated with human papillomavirus (HPV).
c. Differentiated VIN (dVIN): Associated with chronic dermatoses like lichen sclerosus.

3. Malignant Neoplasms

Primary:

a. Squamous cell carcinoma (SCC): Most common, ~85–90% of vulvar cancers.
b. Melanoma (~5%).
c. Basal cell carcinoma (~1–2%).
d. Extramammary Paget's disease (rare).
e. Adenocarcinoma (e.g., Bartholin's gland carcinoma, rare).
f. Sarcomas (e.g., leiomyosarcoma, extremely rare).

Secondary: Metastatic tumours (e.g., from cervix, endometrium, or breast).

Etiology and Risk Factors

The etiology of vulvar neoplasms varies by type:

Benign Neoplasms

1. Often idiopathic or related to chronic irritation (e.g., epidermal cysts from blocked sebaceous glands).
2. Condyloma acuminata: Caused by low-risk HPV types (e.g., HPV 6, 11).

Premalignant Neoplasms (VIN)

1. Usual-type VIN: High-risk HPV infection (e.g., HPV 16, 18), smoking, immunosuppression (e.g., HIV, organ transplant).
2. Differentiated VIN: Chronic inflammatory dermatoses (e.g., lichen sclerosus, lichen planus), often in older women.

Malignant Neoplasms

1. Squamous Cell Carcinoma

a. HPV-related SCC (40–50%): Linked to high-risk HPV, younger women, multifocal lesions.
b. Non-HPV-related SCC: Associated with lichen sclerosus or lichen planus, older women, unifocal lesions.

2. Melanoma: UV exposure (less relevant), genetic predisposition (e.g., BRAF mutations).

3. Basal Cell Carcinoma: Chronic sun exposure (rare on vulva), genetic syndromes (e.g., Gorlin syndrome).

4. Paget's Disease: Often idiopathic; may be associated with underlying adenocarcinoma (10–20% of cases).

Risk Factors

HPV infection.

Smoking.

Immunosuppression (e.g., HIV, chronic steroid use).

Chronic vulvar dermatoses.

Age (>65 years for non-HPV-related SCC).

Prior history of cervical or vaginal neoplasia.

Epidemiology

Benign Neoplasms: Common, especially condyloma acuminata in sexually active women.

VIN: Incidence increasing due to higher HPV prevalence; more common in younger women (20–50 years).

Malignant Neoplasms: Vulvar cancer accounts for ~5% of gynecologic cancers.

Incidence

~2–7 per 100,000 women annually, rising with age.

SCC is the most common, with peak incidence in women >65 years.

Melanoma and Paget's disease are rare, with incidence <0.5 per 100,000.

Clinical Features

Benign Neoplasms

Condyloma Acuminata: Soft, warty, pedunculated or sessile growths; often asymptomatic but may cause itching or discomfort.

Fibroma/Lipoma: Painless, slow-growing, subcutaneous masses.

Hidradenoma: Small, firm nodules, occasionally painful if ulcerated.

Premalignant Neoplasms (VIN)

Asymptomatic or present with pruritus, burning or pain.

Lesions: Multifocal, warty, or plaque-like (uVIN); unifocal, scaly or ulcerated (dVIN).

Pigmentation changes (hyper- or hypopigmentation).

Malignant Neoplasms

a. Squamous Cell Carcinoma

Persistent ulcer, mass or plaque.

Pruritus, pain, bleeding or discharge.

Inguinal lymphadenopathy in advanced cases.

b. Melanoma

Asymmetrical, pigmented lesions with irregular borders.

Rapid growth, bleeding or ulceration.

c. Basal Cell Carcinoma

Pearly, rolled-edge nodule or ulcer.

Slow-growing, rarely metastatic.

d. Paget's Disease

Erythematous, eczematous or scaly patches.

Intense pruritus or burning.

Often mistaken for dermatitis.

General Symptoms (advanced malignancy)

Weight loss, fatigue or symptoms of metastasis (e.g., bone pain).

Diagnosis

Accurate diagnosis is critical for appropriate management and requires a systematic approach:

1. History

Duration, symptoms (pruritus, pain, bleeding).

Sexual history (for HPV-related lesions).

Risk factors (smoking, immunosuppression, prior HPV-related cancers).

History of vulvar dermatoses or prior treatments.

2. Physical Examination

Inspect the vulva for lesion characteristics (size, number, color, texture, ulceration).

Palpate for depth of invasion and inguinal lymphadenopathy.

Examine vagina and cervix to rule out synchronous malignancies.

3. Investigations

a. Biopsy: Gold standard for diagnosis.

Punch or excisional biopsy for histopathological evaluation.

b. Immunohistochemistry (e.g., p16 for HPV-related VIN/SCC, HMB-45 for melanoma).

c. HPV Testing: PCR for high-risk HPV in suspected uVIN or SCC.

Imaging:

d. Ultrasound, CT or MRI for staging malignant tumours (assess depth of invasion, lymph node involvement or metastasis).

e. PET-CT for advanced cases or suspected metastasis.

f. Lymph Node Evaluation: Fine needle aspiration (FNA) or sentinel lymph node biopsy for suspicious nodes.

g. Colposcopy: To evaluate multifocal VIN or synchronous cervical/vaginal lesions.

4. Staging (for Malignant Neoplasms)

FIGO staging for vulvar cancer (2021 update)

Stage I: Tumour confined to vulva or perineum (IA: ≤2 cm, ≤1 mm invasion; IB: >2 cm or >1 mm invasion).

Stage II: Tumour extends to adjacent structures (e.g., urethra, vagina, anus).

Stage III: Regional lymph node involvement.

Stage IV: Distant metastasis or fixed/ulcerated lymph nodes.

Management

Management depends on the type, stage and extent of the neoplasm, with a multidisciplinary approach involving gynecologic oncologists, dermatologists and pathologists.

1. Benign Neoplasms

Asymptomatic: Observation with regular follow-up.

Symptomatic: Surgical excision (e.g., for fibromas, lipomas).

Condyloma Acuminata:

Topical therapies: Imiquimod (immune modulator), podophyllotoxin or trichloroacetic acid.

Cryotherapy, laser ablation or surgical excision for resistant lesions.

HPV vaccination (preventive for uninfected patients).

2. Premalignant Neoplasms (VIN)

Usual-type VIN:

Topical Therapy: Imiquimod 5% cream (3 times weekly for 12–16 weeks).

Ablative Therapy: CO2 laser ablation for multifocal lesions.

Surgical Excision: Wide local excision for unifocal or high-grade lesions.

Follow-Up: Regular monitoring due to high recurrence risk (20–40%).

Differentiated VIN:

Surgical excision preferred due to higher malignant potential.

Monitor for progression to SCC.

3. Malignant Neoplasms

a. Squamous Cell Carcinoma

Early-Stage (I–II):

Wide local excision with 1–2 cm margins.

Sentinel lymph node biopsy for tumours >1 mm invasion or >2 cm.

Advanced-Stage (III–IV):

Radical vulvectomy with inguinofemoral lymphadenectomy.

Adjuvant radiotherapy for positive margins or lymph node involvement.

Chemotherapy (e.g., cisplatin-based) for metastatic disease.

Recurrent Disease: Re-excision, radiotherapy or palliative care.

b. Melanoma

Wide local excision with 1–2 cm margins.

Sentinel lymph node biopsy for staging.

Immunotherapy (e.g., checkpoint inhibitors) or targeted therapy (e.g., BRAF inhibitors) for advanced cases.

c. Basal Cell Carcinoma

Local excision with clear margins.

Mohs micrographic surgery for cosmetically sensitive areas.

d. Paget's Disease

Wide local excision; recurrence is common (30–50%).

Investigate for underlying adenocarcinoma (e.g., colorectal or urogenital).

Topical imiquimod for non-invasive disease (off-label).

Supportive Care

Pain management, wound care and psychological support.

Lymphedema management post-lymphadenectomy.

Prevention

HPV vaccination (quadrivalent or nonavalent) to prevent HPV-related VIN and SCC.

Smoking cessation and management of chronic dermatoses.

Regular screening in high-risk populations (e.g., immunosuppressed patients).

Prognosis

Benign Neoplasms: Excellent prognosis; recurrence rare unless incomplete excision.

VIN: Recurrence rates high (20–40% for uVIN, 10–15% for dVIN); progression to SCC in 5–10% of untreated cases.

Malignant Neoplasms:

Squamous Cell Carcinoma

Stage I: 5-year survival >80%.

Stage III–IV: 5-year survival 20–50%, depending on lymph node status.

Melanoma: Poorer prognosis; 5-year survival ~50% for localized disease, <20% for metastatic.

Basal Cell Carcinoma: Excellent prognosis (>95% cure rate with excision).

Paget's Disease: High recurrence rate; prognosis depends on underlying malignancy.

Complications

Surgical: Wound infection, dehiscence, lymphedema, sexual dysfunction.

Radiotherapy: Skin fibrosis, ulceration or chronic pain.

Psychosocial: Body image issues, sexual dysfunction or anxiety.

Metastatic Disease: Poor quality of life, systemic symptoms.

Follow-Up

Benign Neoplasms: Annual examination if observed; post-excision follow-up to monitor recurrence.

VIN: Every 3–6 months for 2 years, then annually to monitor for recurrence or progression.

Malignant Neoplasms: Every 3 months for 2 years, then every 6 months for 3 years, then annually.

Physical examination, imaging and symptom review to detect recurrence or metastasis.

7.6 Vulvodynia

(*Alam-i-farj*)

Definition

Vulvodynia is chronic vulvar pain or discomfort, lasting ≥3 months, without a clear identifiable cause.

Etiology

Multifactorial: Neurogenic (altered pain processing), muscular (pelvic floor dysfunction), inflammatory or psychogenic factors.

Associations: History of recurrent infections, hormonal changes or psychological stress.

Types

Generalized vulvodynia: Pain throughout the vulva.

Localized vulvodynia (e.g., vestibulodynia): Pain confined to the vestibule.

Clinical Features

Burning, stinging or rawness of the vulva.

Pain with intercourse (dyspareunia) or touch (allodynia).

Normal-appearing vulva in most cases.

Diagnosis

History: Chronic pain, triggers (e.g., intercourse, tampons) and impact on quality of life.

Physical Examination: Cotton swab test to map painful areas; rule out infections or dermatoses.

Investigations: Swabs to exclude infections, biopsy if dermatological cause suspected.

Diagnosis of Exclusion: Rule out other causes of vulvar pain.

Management

Multidisciplinary Approach

1. Topical Therapy: Lidocaine gel for symptom relief; avoid prolonged use to prevent irritation.
2. Systemic Therapy: Tricyclic antidepressants (e.g., amitriptyline), gabapentin, or SSRIs for neuropathic pain.
3. Pelvic Floor Therapy: Physiotherapy to address muscle hypertonicity.
4. Psychological Support: Cognitive-behavioral therapy for associated anxiety or depression.
5. Lifestyle Modifications: Avoid irritants, use lubricants during intercourse.
6. Surgical Option: Vestibulectomy for refractory localized vulvodynia.

Prognosis

Variable; some improve with multimodal therapy, while others have persistent symptoms.

7.7 Vulval vestibulitis Syndrome

(*Mutalazemai Iltihab-i-Dehliz-i-farj*)

Definition

Vulvar vestibulitis syndrome, now termed provoked vestibulodynia, is a subtype of vulvodynia characterized by pain localized to the vaginal vestibule, typically provoked by touch or pressure.

Etiology

Hypothesized Causes: Chronic inflammation, nerve hypersensitivity, pelvic floor dysfunction, or hormonal influences (e.g., oral contraceptive use).

Associations: History of recurrent candidiasis, HPV or psychological stress.

Clinical Features

Severe pain on vestibular contact (e.g., during intercourse, tampon insertion or examination).

Erythema of the vestibule in some cases.

Normal vulvar appearance in others.

Diagnosis

History: Pain with penetration, duration ≥3 months.

Physical Examination: Cotton swab test reveals tenderness at vestibular sites (e.g., 4 and 8 o'clock positions).

Investigations: Rule out infections (swabs) or dermatoses (biopsy if indicated).

Management

1. Conservative

Topical lidocaine or compounded oestrogen/testosterone creams.

Pelvic floor physiotherapy to relax hypertonic muscles.

Psychological counselling for sexual dysfunction or stress.

2. Medical

Gabapentin or amitriptyline for neuropathic pain.

Botulinum toxin injections for refractory cases.

3. Surgical

Vestibulectomy (removal of painful vestibular tissue) for severe, refractory cases.

4. Education

Avoid irritants and use lubricants.

Prognosis

Many patients improve with conservative measures.

Surgical outcomes are favorable in refractory cases (success rates ~60–80%).

Summary Table

Condition	**Key Etiology**	**Clinical Features**	**Diagnosis**	**Management**	**Prognosis**
Pruritus Vulvae	Infections, dermatoses, systemic diseases	Itching, erythema, excoriation	Swabs, biopsy, blood tests	Treat cause, topical steroids, hygiene	Good with treatment
Vulvar Ulcers	HSV, syphilis, Behcet's, malignancy	Painful/painless ulcers, systemic symptoms	PCR, serology, biopsy	Antimicrobials, steroids, excision	Variable, depends on cause
Vulvitis	Candida, contact dermatitis, dermatoses	Erythema, itching, discharge	Swabs, biopsy	Antifungals, steroids, avoid irritants	Good with treatment
Vulval Atrophy	Estrogen deficiency	Dryness, dyspareunia, thin mucosa	Clinical, pH testing	Topical oestrogen, lubricants	Excellent with therapy
Vulval Cysts	Bartholin's gland obstruction, sebaceous cysts	Painless lump, pain if infected	Ultrasound, culture	Drainage, antibiotics, excision	Good, recurrence possible
Vulval Neoplasms	HPV, lichen sclerosus, melanoma	Ulcer, mass, bleeding	Biopsy, imaging	Excision, radiotherapy, chemotherapy	Variable, stage-dependent

| **Vulvodynia**| Neuropathic, muscular, psychogenic | Chronic burning, dyspareunia | Cotton swab test, exclusion | Multimodal (topical, systemic, therapy) | Variable, often chronic |

|**Vestibulodynia** | Inflammation, nerve hypersensitivity | Vestibular pain on contact | Cotton swab test, exclusion | Topical therapy, physiotherapy, surgery | Good with multimodal approach |

Long Answer Questions

1. Classify vulvar diseases and describe the clinical features and treatment of vulvar infections.
2. Discuss lichen sclerosus of the vulva—etiology, diagnosis and management.
3. Explain the types, symptoms and treatment of vulvar neoplasms.
4. Describe Bartholin's gland disorders and their clinical implications.
5. Elaborate on vulvodynia—classification, diagnosis and therapeutic options.

Short Answer Questions

1. What is lichen sclerosus?
2. Name two common causes of vulvar itching.
3. Define vulvodynia.
4. Mention one symptom of vulvar carcinoma.
5. What is the function of Bartholin's glands?

Multiple Choice Questions (1 Mark Each)

1. Lichen sclerosus commonly affects:

a) Cervix b) Vulva c) Vagina d) Uterus

Ans: b) Vulva

2. Bartholin's cyst is caused by:

a) Hormonal imbalance b) Gland obstruction c) STI d) Trauma

Ans: b) Gland obstruction

3. Most common symptom of vulvar carcinoma:

a) Amenorrhea b) Dyspareunia c) Pruritus d) Menorrhagia

Ans: c) Pruritus

4. Vulvodynia is defined as:

a) Vulvar infection b) Vulvar pain without identifiable cause c) Vulvar swelling d) Vulvar discharge

Ans: b) Vulvar pain without identifiable cause

5. Which of the following is a premalignant vulvar lesion?

a) Bartholin's abscess b) Vulvar intraepithelial neoplasia (VIN) c) Lichen simplex d) Vulvar candidiasis

Ans: b) Vulvar intraepithelial neoplasia (VIN)

6. Common fungal infection of the vulva:

a) Trichomoniasis b) Gonorrhea c) Candidiasis d) Chlamydia

Ans: c) Candidiasis

7. Vulvar carcinoma is most commonly:

a) Adenocarcinoma b) Squamous cell carcinoma c) Melanoma d) Sarcoma

Ans: b) Squamous cell carcinoma

8. Whiff test is used to diagnose:

a) Vulvar carcinoma b) Bacterial vaginosis c) Vulvodynia d) Bartholin's cyst

Ans: b) Bacterial vaginosis

9. Which condition presents with white, thin, parchment-like vulvar skin?

a) Lichen sclerosus b) Psoriasis c) Herpes d) VIN

Ans: a) Lichen sclerosus

10. Treatment of uncomplicated Bartholin's cyst includes:

a) Hysterectomy b) Marsupialization c) Chemotherapy d) Cryotherapy

Ans: b) Marsupialization

08

Diseases of Vagina

(Amrad al-mahbil)

8.1 *Sayalan-al-Rahim wa Ghayr Tabi-I mahbil Ilfrazat* (Excessive & Abnormal Vaginal Discharge)
8.2 *Iltihab-i-mahbil aur Iltihab-i-mahbil jursoomi* (Vaginitis & Bacterial vaginosis)
8.3 *Quruh-i-mahbil* (Ulcers of vagina)
8.4 *Khuraj-i-mahbil aur Istirkha-i-mahbil* (Prolapse of vagina)
8.5 *Tashannuj-i-mahbil* (Vaginismus)
8.6 *Jemay-i-molim* (Dyspareunia)
8.7 *Akyas wa Sal'at* (Cysts & Neopalsm)

Learning Objective (At the end of the session, the students should be able to)

Evaluate the etiopathogenesis, diagnosis, management & complications of *Sailan-al-Rahim wa Ghair Tabaiee Mahbili Afrazaat* (Excessive & Abnormal Vaginal Discharge).
Discuss the etiology, types, diagnosis, management and complications of *Iltihab-e-Mahbil* (Vaginitis & Bacterial Vaginosis).
Describe the causes, diagnosis, management and complications of *Qurooh-e-Mahbil* (Ulcers of Vagina).
Elaborate the causes, types, diagnosis, management and complications of *Khurooj-e-Mahbil* & *Isterkhai Mahbil* (Prolapse of Vagina).
Describe the causes, types, diagnosis, and management of *Tashannuj-e-Mahbil* (Vaginismus) & *Moallam-e-jima* (Dyspareunia).
Explain briefly the causes, stages, diagnosis, management and complications of *Daweera* & *Sulaat* (Cysts & Neoplasm) of the Vagina.

8.1 Excessive & Abnormal Vaginal Discharge

(*Sayalan-al-Rahim wa Ghayr Tabi-I mahbil Ilfrazat*)

Vaginal discharge is a normal physiological phenomenon in women of reproductive age, consisting of a mixture of cervical mucus, vaginal epithelial cells, transudate and resident microbial flora. "Excessive vaginal discharge" is defined as an increase in the volume of discharge beyond what is typical for an individual, often perceived as bothersome or requiring frequent changes of undergarments or sanitary protection. "Abnormal vaginal discharge" refers to discharge that deviates from normal in terms of color, consistency, odor or associated symptoms such as itching, irritation or pain.

Normal vaginal discharge is typically clear to white, odorless or mildly odorous and varies in quantity and consistency with the menstrual cycle, influenced by hormonal changes. Abnormal discharge may indicate an underlying pathological condition, including infections, inflammatory processes or neoplastic changes.

Physiology of Normal Vaginal Discharge

Vaginal discharge is primarily produced by:

a. Cervical glands: Secrete mucus under the influence of oestrogen and progesterone, which fluctuates during the menstrual cycle.

b. Vaginal epithelium: Contributes desquamated cells and transudate.

c. Microbial flora: Predominantly "Lactobacillus" species, which maintain an acidic vaginal pH (3.8–4.5) through lactic acid production, protecting against pathogens.

The volume and characteristics of normal discharge vary:

a. Menstrual cycle: Discharge is scanty post-menstruation, increases and becomes clear and stretchy (spinnbarkeit) at ovulation and thickens in the luteal phase.

b. Pregnancy: Increased discharge due to elevated oestrogen levels.

c. Postmenopause: Scanty discharge due to decreased oestrogen and vaginal atrophy.

Etiology of Excessive and Abnormal Vaginal Discharge

Abnormal vaginal discharge may result from infectious, non-infectious or neoplastic causes. The following are common etiologies:

1. Infectious Causes

a. Bacterial Vaginosis (BV)

Cause: Overgrowth of anaerobic bacteria (e.g., Gardnerella vaginalis, Prevotella, Mobiluncus) with a reduction in Lactobacillus species.

Characteristics: Thin, greyish-white discharge with a characteristic "fishy" odor, worse after intercourse or menses. pH > 4.5.

Symptoms: Often asymptomatic; may cause mild itching or irritation.

Risk factors: Douching, multiple sexual partners, antibiotic use.

b. Vulvovaginal Candidiasis

Cause: Overgrowth of 'Candida' species, primarily 'Candida albicans' (80–90%) or non-albicans species (e.g., 'C. glabrata').

Characteristics: Thick, white, "cottage cheese-like" discharge, minimal to no odor. pH normal (4.0–4.5).

Symptoms: Intense vulvar itching, erythema and dysuria.

Risk factors: Diabetes, antibiotic use, pregnancy, immunosuppression, high-oestrogen states (e.g., oral contraceptives).

c. Trichomoniasis

Cause: Trichomonas vaginalis, a flagellated protozoan.

Characteristics: Frothy, yellow-green discharge with a foul odor. pH > 4.5.

Symptoms: Vaginal irritation, dysuria, dyspareunia; may be asymptomatic in up to 50% of cases.

Risk factors: Multiple sexual partners, unprotected intercourse.

d. Cervicitis

Cause: Commonly Chlamydia trachomatis or Neisseria gonorrhoeae; less commonly Herpes simplex virus (HSV) or Mycoplasma genitalium .

Characteristics: Purulent or mucopurulent cervical discharge, often with postcoital bleeding.

Symptoms: May be asymptomatic or associated with pelvic pain, dyspareunia or abnormal uterine bleeding.

e. Other Infections

Aerobic vaginitis: Caused by Escherichia coli, Streptococcus spp., or Staphylococcus spp., presenting with sticky, yellow discharge and inflammation.

Foreign body: Retained tampons or condoms may cause foul-smelling, purulent discharge.

2. Non-Infectious Causes

a. Physiological Excess

Increased discharge during ovulation, pregnancy or sexual arousal.

Use of hormonal contraceptives or hormone replacement therapy.

b. Allergic/Irritant Reactions

Cause: Contact dermatitis from soaps, perfumes, lubricants or latex condoms.

Characteristics: Clear or serous discharge with vulvar erythema and itching.

c. Atrophic Vaginitis

Cause: Estrogen deficiency in postmenopausal women or breastfeeding mothers.

Characteristics: Thin, watery or serosanguinous discharge; vaginal dryness.

Symptoms: Burning, dyspareunia and spotting.

d. Cervical Ectropion

Cause: Eversion of endocervical columnar epithelium, often in young women or those on oral contraceptives.

Characteristics: Clear or mucoid discharge, sometimes blood-tinged.

3. Neoplastic Causes

a. Cervical or Endometrial Cancer:

Characteristics: Watery, blood-stained or foul-smelling discharge.

Symptoms: Postcoital bleeding, pelvic pain or abnormal uterine bleeding.

b. Vaginal or Vulvar Cancer:

Rare, often presenting with persistent discharge and ulceration.

4. Other Causes

Fistulae: Vesicovaginal or rectovaginal fistulae may cause continuous watery or faecal-smelling discharge.

Desquamative Inflammatory Vaginitis: Rare, characterized by purulent discharge and vaginal erythema.

Clinical Evaluation

A systematic approach to evaluating excessive or abnormal vaginal discharge is essential for accurate diagnosis and management.

1. History

Characteristics of Discharge: Onset, duration, color, consistency, odor and volume.

Associated Symptoms: Itching, irritation, dysuria, dyspareunia, pelvic pain or abnormal bleeding.

Menstrual History: Cycle regularity, menarche, menopause or pregnancy status.

Sexual History: Number of partners, unprotected intercourse, history of sexually transmitted infections (STIs).

Risk Factors: Recent antibiotic use, douching, diabetes, immunosuppression or foreign body use.

Other: Recent travel, hygiene practices or exposure to allergens/irritants.

2. Physical Examination

External Genitalia: Inspect for erythema, edema, lesions or excoriations.

Vaginal Examination: Note discharge characteristics, vaginal wall appearance and presence of foreign bodies.

Cervical Examination: Assess for mucopurulent discharge, friability or ectropion.

Bimanual Examination: Evaluate for pelvic tenderness or masses.

3. Diagnostic Tests

a. Vaginal pH Testing

Normal: 3.8–4.5.

Elevated (>4.5): Suggests BV or trichomoniasis.

b. Wet Mount Microscopy

Clue cells: Epithelial cells studded with bacteria (BV).

Motile trichomonad: Diagnostic for trichomoniasis.

Pseudohyphae or budding yeast: Suggests candidiasis.

c. Whiff Test

Add 10% potassium hydroxide (KOH) to discharge; a fishy odor indicates BV.

d. Gram Stain or Culture

For confirming BV, candidiasis or aerobic vaginitis.

e. Nucleic Acid Amplification Tests (NAATs)

Detect Chlamydia trachomatis, Neisseria gonorrhoeae or Trichomonas vaginalis.

f. Pap Smear/Cervical Cytology

Screen for cervical pathology if indicated.

g. Colposcopy or Biopsy

For suspected neoplastic causes.

h. Other

Pregnancy test if indicated.

Imaging (e.g., ultrasound) for pelvic masses or fistulae.

Diagnostic Criteria

Bacterial Vaginosis (Amsel's Criteria): At least three of the following:

1. Homogeneous, greyish-white discharge.
2. Vaginal pH > 4.5.
3. Positive whiff test.
4. Clue cells on wet mount.

Vulvovaginal Candidiasis: Clinical symptoms plus microscopy or culture confirming Candida spp.

Trichomoniasis: Motile trichomonads on wet mount or positive NAAT.

Cervicitis Mucopurulent discharge and positive NAAT for Chlamydia or Gonococcus.

Management

Management depends on the underlying cause and should address both symptoms and the etiology.

1. Infectious Causes

a. Bacterial Vaginosis

Treatment: Metronidazole 500 mg orally twice daily for 7 days or clindamycin 2% vaginal cream for 7 days.

Partner treatment: Not routinely recommended.

Recurrence: Consider maintenance therapy with metronidazole gel.

b. Vulvovaginal Candidiasis

Treatment: Fluconazole 150 mg single dose orally or topical azoles (e.g., clotrimazole 1% cream for 7 days).

Recurrent candidiasis: Weekly fluconazole for 6 months.

Non-albicans species: May require boric acid intravaginal suppositories.

c. Trichomoniasis

Treatment: Metronidazole 2 g single dose or tinidazole 2 g single dose.

Partner treatment: Essential to prevent reinfection.

d. Cervicitis

Chlamydia: Azithromycin 1 g single dose or doxycycline 100 mg twice daily for 7 days.

Gonorrhea: Ceftriaxone 500 mg intramuscularly single dose (add azithromycin if co-infection suspected).

Partner treatment: Recommended for STIs.

2. Non-Infectious Causes

a. Atrophic Vaginitis

Treatment: Topical oestrogen (e.g., estradiol vaginal cream or ring).

Non-hormonal options: Moisturizers or lubricants.

b. Allergic/Irritant Reactions

Treatment: Remove offending agent; consider short-term topical corticosteroids for severe inflammation.

c. Cervical Ectropion

Often self-limiting; may require cryotherapy or cauterization if persistent.

3. Neoplastic Causes

Colposcopy, biopsy and management of suspected malignancies.

4. General Measures

Hygiene: Avoid douching and irritants (e.g., scented soaps, tight clothing).

Education: Counsel on safe sexual practices and STI prevention.

Follow-up: Ensure resolution of symptoms and re-evaluate for persistent or recurrent discharge.

Complications

Bacterial Vaginosis: Associated with preterm birth, pelvic inflammatory disease (PID) and increased STI susceptibility.

Trichomoniasis: Increased risk of HIV transmission and preterm delivery.

Cervicitis: May progress to PID, infertility or ectopic pregnancy if untreated.

Neoplastic Causes: Delayed diagnosis may lead to advanced malignancy.

Prevention

Promote safe sexual practices, including condom use.

Discourage douching and overuse of vaginal hygiene products.

Regular gynecologic screening for early detection of cervical abnormalities.

Manage underlying conditions (e.g., diabetes, immunosuppression).

Conclusion

Excessive and abnormal vaginal discharge is a common clinical presentation with a wide range of etiologies, from benign physiological changes to serious infections or malignancies. A thorough history, physical examination and targeted diagnostic testing are critical for accurate diagnosis. Treatment should be tailored to the underlying cause, with attention to patient education and prevention of recurrence. Prompt recognition and management of abnormal discharge can prevent complications and improve patient outcomes.

8.2 Vaginitis & Bacterial Vaginosis

(*Iltihab-e-Mahbil*)

Introduction

Vaginitis is a common gynecologic condition characterized by inflammation or irritation of the vaginal mucosa, often presenting with abnormal vaginal discharge, itching, irritation or odor. It encompasses a spectrum of disorders, including infectious and non-infectious causes, with bacterial vaginosis (BV), vulvovaginal candidiasis and trichomoniasis being the most prevalent. Bacterial vaginosis, the most common cause of vaginitis, is a polymicrobial syndrome resulting from an imbalance in the vaginal microbiome.

Vaginitis

Definition

Vaginitis refers to inflammation or irritation of the vaginal mucosa, typically presenting with symptoms such as abnormal vaginal discharge, pruritus, burning, irritation or malodor. It may be caused by infectious agents (bacteria, fungi, or protozoa), non-infectious factors (e.g., allergies, chemical irritants), or hormonal changes (e.g., atrophic vaginitis).

Epidemiology

Vaginitis is one of the most common reasons for gynecologic consultations, affecting women of all ages, particularly during reproductive years.

Prevalence

Bacterial vaginosis: 20–60% of women with vaginitis, higher in sexually active women and certain populations (e.g., those with multiple partners).

Vulvovaginal candidiasis: 20–25% of vaginitis cases, with 75% of women experiencing at least one episode in their lifetime.

Trichomoniasis: 5–15% of vaginitis cases, more common in areas with high STI prevalence.

Risk factors include sexual activity, douching, antibiotic use, hormonal changes and immunosuppression.

Etiology

Vaginitis can be broadly categorized into infectious and non-infectious causes:

1. Infectious Causes

Bacterial Vaginosis (BV): Polymicrobial dysbiosis with overgrowth of anaerobic bacteria.

Vulvovaginal Candidiasis: Primarily caused by Candida albicans or non-albicans Candida species.

Trichomoniasis: Caused by Trichomonas vaginalis, a flagellated protozoan.

Aerobic Vaginitis: Caused by aerobic bacteria such as Escherichia coli, Streptococcus spp., or Staphylococcus spp.

Cervicitis: Often due to Chlamydia trachomatis or Neisseria gonorrhoeae, presenting with vaginal discharge.

2. Non-Infectious Causes

Atrophic Vaginitis: Estrogen deficiency in postmenopausal or breastfeeding women.

Allergic/Irritant Vaginitis: Contact dermatitis from soaps, perfumes or hygiene products.

Desquamative Inflammatory Vaginitis: Rare, idiopathic condition with purulent discharge and mucosal inflammation.

3. Other Causes

Foreign bodies (e.g., retained tampons or condoms).

Cervical ectropion or neoplastic conditions (rare).

Pathophysiology

The vaginal ecosystem is maintained by a balance of resident microbial flora, predominantly Lactobacillus species, which produce lactic acid to maintain an acidic vaginal pH (3.8–4.5). This acidic environment inhibits the growth of pathogenic organisms. Disruption of this balance due to hormonal changes, antibiotics, douching or sexual activity can lead to overgrowth of pathogenic microbes or inflammation, resulting in vaginitis.

Vaginitis: Broader Management Considerations

Clinical Evaluation

A systematic approach is critical for diagnosing vaginitis:

1. History

Discharge characteristics (color, consistency, odor, volume).

Associated symptoms (itching, burning, dysuria, dyspareunia).

Menstrual, sexual and medical history (e.g., recent antibiotics, diabetes, immunosuppression).

Hygiene practices and exposure to irritants.

2. Physical Examination

External genitalia: Inspect for erythema, edema or lesions.

Vaginal examination: Assess discharge, mucosal appearance and foreign bodies.

Cervical examination: Check for mucopurulent discharge or friability.

Bimanual examination: Evaluate for pelvic tenderness or masses.

3. Diagnostic Testing

Vaginal pH: Normal (3.8-4.5) in candidiasis; elevated (>4.5) in BV or trichomoniasis.

Wet mount microscopy: Clue cells (BV), pseudohyphae (candidiasis) or motile trichomonads.

Whiff test: Positive in BV.

NAATs: For Chlamydia, Gonococcus or Trichomonas.

Culture: For recurrent or atypical infections.

Cervical cytology or colposcopy: If neoplastic causes are suspected.

Management of Other Vaginitis Causes

1. Vulvovaginal Candidiasis

Treatment- Single-dose fluconazole 150 mg orally or topical azoles (e.g., clotrimazole 1% cream for 7 days). Recurrent cases: Weekly fluconazole for 6 months.

Non-albicans species: Boric acid 600 mg vaginal suppositories for 14 days.

Patient counselling: Manage predisposing factors (e.g., diabetes control, avoid antibiotics when possible).

2. Trichomoniasis

Treatment: Metronidazole 2 g single dose or tinidazole 2 g single dose.

Partner treatment: Essential to prevent reinfection.

Follow-up: Retest after 3 months due to high reinfection rates.

3. Atrophic Vaginitis

Treatment: Topical oestrogen (e.g., estradiol cream or vaginal ring).

Non-hormonal options: Vaginal moisturizers or lubricants for symptom relief.

4. Allergic/Irritant Vaginitis

Treatment: Remove irritants; short-term topical corticosteroids for severe cases.

Prevention: Avoid scented products and tight clothing.

5. Aerobic Vaginitis

Treatment: Topical clindamycin or metronidazole; antibiotics based on culture results.

Management: Address underlying inflammation and restore vaginal flora.

Complications

Infectious vaginitis: Increased STI susceptibility, PID or obstetric complications.

Atrophic vaginitis: Vaginal dryness, dyspareunia and recurrent urinary tract infections.

Chronic vaginitis: Psychosocial impact, including reduced quality of life and sexual dysfunction.

Prevention

Promote vaginal health through good hygiene practices (e.g., unscented soaps, cotton underwear).

Encourage safe sexual practices and regular STI screening.

Advise against douching and overuse of antibiotics.

Routine gynecologic care, including Pap smears and pelvic exams, for early detection of abnormalities.

Conclusion

Vaginitis, including bacterial vaginosis, is a common clinical entity of women's health. Bacterial vaginosis, characterized by a shift in vaginal microbiota, is the leading cause of abnormal vaginal discharge and requires careful diagnosis using Amsel's criteria or Nugent scoring. Management involves targeted antimicrobial therapy, with attention to recurrence and complications, particularly in pregnancy. A comprehensive approach to vaginitis, including thorough history-taking, physical examination and diagnostic testing, ensures accurate identification of the underlying cause and appropriate treatment. Preventive strategies and patient education are essential to reduce the burden of vaginitis and its associated complications.

Key References

Centres for Disease Control and Prevention (CDC). (2021). Sexually Transmitted Infections Treatment Guidelines.

American College of Obstetricians and Gynecologists (ACOG). Vaginitis in Nonpregnant Patients. Practice Bulletin No. 215.

Sobel, J. D. (2019). Vulvovaginal candidiasis and bacterial vaginosis. In Infectious Diseases of the Female Genital Tract.

Bacterial Vaginosis

Definition

Bacterial vaginosis (BV) is a polymicrobial syndrome characterized by a shift in the vaginal microbiota from Lactobacillus dominant flora to an overgrowth of anaerobic and facultative bacteria, such as Gardnerella vaginalis, Prevotella spp., Mobiluncus spp., and Atopobium vaginae . It is the most common cause of abnormal vaginal discharge in women of reproductive age.

Epidemiology

Prevalence

BV affects 20–60% of women presenting with vaginal discharge, with higher rates in sexually active women, African American populations and those with multiple sexual partners.

Recurrence: Up to 30–50% of women experience recurrence within 3–6 months of treatment.

Risk Factors

Sexual activity (multiple partners, new partner, unprotected intercourse).

Douching or use of vaginal hygiene products.

Antibiotic use, which disrupts vaginal flora.

Smoking and low socioeconomic status.

Intrauterine device (IUD) use (controversial).

Pathophysiology

BV results from a disruption of the vaginal microbiome, leading to:

1. Reduction in Lactobacillus species: Loss of lactic acid production increases vaginal pH (>4.5), creating a favorable environment for anaerobic bacteria.
2. Overgrowth of anaerobes: Gardnerella vaginalis and other anaerobes produce enzymes (e.g., sialidases) and volatile amines, contributing to discharge and odor.
3. Biofilm formation: Gardnerella forms a biofilm on vaginal epithelial cells, promoting adherence of other anaerobes and resistance to treatment.
4. Immune response: Minimal inflammation in BV, explaining the absence of significant erythema or pain in most cases.

Clinical Features

Symptoms

Thin, greyish-white or yellowish vaginal discharge.

Characteristic "fishy" odor, often more pronounced after intercourse or menses due to amine release in alkaline environments.

Mild or no vaginal irritation; many women are asymptomatic (up to 50%).

Associated Symptoms: Rarely, mild itching or burning; no significant pelvic pain unless complicated by co-infections.

Complications

Increased risk of sexually transmitted infections (e.g., HIV, herpes simplex virus).

Obstetric complications: Preterm birth, low birth weight, premature rupture of membranes and postpartum endometritis.

Gynecologic complications: Pelvic inflammatory disease (PID), post-surgical infections.

Diagnosis

Diagnosis of BV is based on clinical and laboratory criteria. The two primary diagnostic approaches are Amsel's criteria (clinical) and Nugent score (microbiological).

1. Amsel's Criteria (requires at least three of four)

Homogeneous, thin, greyish-white discharge.

Vaginal pH > 4.5 (measured using pH paper).

Positive whiff test: Fishy odor upon adding 10% potassium hydroxide (KOH) to vaginal discharge.

Clue cells on wet mount microscopy (vaginal epithelial cells coated with bacteria, obscuring cell borders).

2. Nugent Score

Gram stain of vaginal discharge is scored (0–10) based on the relative proportions of Lactobacillus (large Gram-positive rods), Gardnerella /anaerobes (small Gram-variable rods) and Mobiluncus (curved Gram-negative rods).

Score interpretation:

0–3 Normal flora (Lactobacillus-dominant).

4–6 Intermediate flora.

7–10 Bacterial vaginosis.

3. Other Diagnostic Tools

Tests: DNA probes or nucleic acid amplification tests (NAATs) for Gardnerella or other BV-associated bacteria.

Culture: Not routinely recommended due to the polymicrobial nature of BV.

Differential Diagnosis

1. Vulvovaginal candidiasis: Thick, white, curd-like discharge, normal pH; pseudohyphae on microscopy.
2. Trichomoniasis: Frothy, yellow-green discharge; motile trichomonads on wet mount.
3. Aerobic vaginitis Purulent discharge, significant inflammation and aerobic bacteria on culture.
4. Cervicitis: Purulent cervical discharge, often with bleeding or pelvic pain.

Management

Treatment of bacterial vaginosis aims to restore the vaginal microbiome, alleviate symptoms and reduce complications. Both symptomatic and asymptomatic cases (e.g., in pregnancy or before gynecologic procedures) may require treatment.

1. First-Line Treatments (CDC Guidelines)

Metronidazole

Oral: 500 mg twice daily for 7 days (preferred for efficacy).

Vaginal gel (0.75%): Once daily for 5 days.

Clindamycin

Vaginal cream (2%): Once daily for 7 days.

Oral: 300 mg twice daily for 7 days.

Tinidazole: 2 g orally once daily for 2 days or 1 g daily for 5 days.

2. Alternative Regimens

Secnidazole: 2 g single-dose oral therapy (convenient but less commonly used).

Metronidazole: Vaginal suppositories for patients intolerant to oral therapy.

3. Management of Recurrent Bacterial Vaginosis

Maintenance therapy: Metronidazole gel 0.75% twice weekly for 4–6 months.

Probiotics: Oral or vaginal Lactobacillus supplementation to restore flora. (Limited evidence)

Biofilm disruption: Investigational therapies targeting Gardnerella biofilms (e.g., boric acid).

4. Partner Treatment

Not routinely recommended, as BV is not considered a sexually transmitted infection, though sexual activity is a risk factor. Consider treating partners in cases of recurrent BV or if the partner is female (due to shared vaginal flora).

5. Special Populations

Pregnancy

Treat symptomatic BV to reduce preterm birth risk.

Prefer Metronidazole 500 mg orally twice daily for 7 days (safe in all trimesters).

Avoid clindamycin cream in late pregnancy due to risk of preterm labor.

Breastfeeding

Metronidazole is excreted in breast milk; consider single-dose regimens to minimize exposure.

Immunocompromised patients

May require prolonged or combination therapy due to higher recurrence rates.

Complications

Obstetric

Preterm birth, premature rupture of membranes, low birth weight and chorioamnionitis.

Postpartum endometritis or post-abortion infections.

Gynecologic

Increased susceptibility to STIs (HIV, HSV, Chlamydia, Gonorrhea).

Pelvic inflammatory disease or post-surgical infections (e.g., after hysterectomy).

Recurrent BV: Chronic symptoms impact quality of life and may require long-term management.

Prevention

Patient Education

Avoid douching and vaginal irritants (e.g., scented soaps, tight clothing).

Promote safe sexual practices, including condom use.

Lifestyle Modifications

Smoking cessation and management of underlying conditions (e.g., diabetes).

Limit sexual partners to reduce microbiome disruption.

Screening

Routine screening is not recommended for asymptomatic women, except in pregnancy or before gynecologic procedures (e.g., IUD insertion).

Diagnostic Approach to Vaginal Infections

Patient Presents with Vaginal Discharge
↓
History Taking
(Color, Odor, Duration, Associated Symptoms)
↓
Physical Examination
(Speculum + Vaginal Inspection)
↓
Initial Tests:
↓ ↓ ↓
Vaginal pH — Whiff Test — Wet Mount Microscopy
↓
Identify Likely Cause:
↓ ↓ ↓
BV → pH > 4.5 + Clue Cells
Candida → pH < 4.5 + Pseudohyphae
Trichomonas → pH > 5 + Motile Protozoa
↓
Confirm Diagnosis → Begin Targeted Treatment

Key Definitions

Bacterial Vaginosis (BV) ➤ Overgrowth of anaerobic bacteria; fishy odor, clue cells, ↑ pH.

Candidiasis ➤ Fungal infection; curdy white discharge, itching, pseudohyphae.

Trichomoniasis ➤ Protozoal STI; frothy green discharge, strawberry cervix.

Atrophic Vaginitis ➤ Estrogen deficiency; dryness, thinning, postmenopausal.

Cytolytic Vaginosis ➤ Excess lactobacilli; acidic pH, white discharge, irritation.

Diagnostic Clues

Symptom	Likely Diagnosis
Fishy odor + clue cells	Bacterial Vaginosis
Curdy discharge + itching	Candidiasis
Frothy green discharge	Trichomoniasis
Dryness + thin mucosa	Atrophic Vaginitis
Acidic pH + cytolysis	Cytolytic Vaginosis

8.3 Ulcers of vagina

(*Quruh-i-mahbil*)

Introduction

Vaginal ulcers are localized defects or erosions in the vaginal mucosa, often accompanied by inflammation, pain or discomfort. They may result from infectious, inflammatory, autoimmune, traumatic or neoplastic processes. Vaginal ulcers are relatively uncommon but significant clinical finding, as they may indicate serious underlying conditions, including sexually transmitted infections (STIs), autoimmune diseases or malignancies.

Definition

A vaginal ulcer is defined as a disruption of the vaginal mucosal epithelium, exposing the underlying submucosal tissue. Ulcers may be single or multiple, superficial or deep, and are often associated with symptoms such as pain, burning, discharge or dyspareunia. They differ from erosions, which are superficial and do not penetrate the basement membrane, and from excoriations, which are caused by scratching or trauma.

Epidemiology

Prevalence: Vaginal ulcers are less common than vulvar ulcers but are frequently underdiagnosed due to their internal location and variable presentation. Exact prevalence varies depending on the underlying cause (e.g., STIs, autoimmune diseases).

Population: Most common in sexually active women of reproductive age, though postmenopausal women (due to atrophic changes) and immunocompromised individuals are also at risk.

Geographic variation: Higher incidence of infectious causes (e.g., herpes simplex virus, syphilis) in regions with high STI prevalence.

Risk factors: Sexual activity, immunosuppression (e.g., HIV, chemotherapy), trauma, autoimmune diseases and poor hygiene.

Etiology

Vaginal ulcers may arise from a variety of causes, which can be broadly classified as infectious, non-infectious (inflammatory, autoimmune, traumatic), or neoplastic.

1. Infectious Causes

a. Herpes Simplex Virus (HSV)

Pathogen HSV-2 (most common) or HSV-1.

Characteristics: Painful, shallow ulcers or vesicles on the vaginal mucosa, often preceded by prodromal symptoms (tingling, burning).

Epidemiology: Most common cause of genital ulcers globally recurrent episodes are common.

b. Syphilis (Treponema pallidum)

Primary syphilis: Single, painless chancre (ulcer) with indurated borders, typically appearing 2–6 weeks post-exposure.

Secondary syphilis: Mucocutaneous lesions, including mucous patches or condylomata lata, may involve the vagina.

c. Chancroid (Haemophilus ducreyi)

Characteristics: Painful, soft ulcers with ragged edges, often accompanied by suppurative lymphadenopathy.

d. Lymphogranuloma Venereum (LGV)

Pathogen: Chlamydia trachomatis serotypes L1–L3.

Characteristics: Transient, painless genital ulcers followed by painful lymphadenopathy (buboes).

e. Other Infections

Cytomegalovirus (CMV): Ulcers in immunocompromised patients.

Epstein-Barr Virus (EBV): Rare, associated with systemic illness.

Tuberculosis: Chronic, indolent ulcers in endemic areas.

Fungal infections: Rare, typically in immunocompromised patients (e.g., candidiasis causing deep erosions).

2. Non-Infectious Causes

a. Autoimmune/Inflammatory Diseases

Behcet's Disease: Recurrent, painful genital and oral ulcers, often with uveitis or skin lesions.

Lichen Planus: Erosive lesions with lacy, white patches (Wickham's striae).

Lichen Sclerosus: Atrophic, white patches that may ulcerate, more common on the vulva but can extend to the vagina.

Crohn's Disease: Perineal or vaginal fistulae and ulcers, often with gastrointestinal symptoms.

Pemphigus Vulgaris: Painful, flaccid bullae and ulcers due to autoantibodies against desmogleins.

b. Trauma

Causes: Mechanical injury (e.g., intercourse, foreign bodies, tampons), chemical irritation (e.g., douches, spermicides), or iatrogenic (e.g., post-surgical).

Characteristics: Variable, often painful, with a clear history of trauma.

c. Atrophic Vaginitis

Cause: Estrogen deficiency (postmenopause, breastfeeding, or anti-oestrogen therapy).

Characteristics: Thin, friable mucosa prone to erosions or ulcers, often with vaginal dryness and dyspareunia.

3. Neoplastic Causes

Vaginal Cancer: Squamous cell carcinoma or adenocarcinoma may present as ulcerated lesions.

Vulvar Cancer: May extend to the vaginal mucosa, presenting as persistent, non-healing ulcers.

Metastatic Disease: Rare, from cervical, endometrial or other primaries.

4. Other Causes

Drug Reactions: Fixed drug eruptions or Stevens-Johnson syndrome/toxic epidermal necrolysis (SJS/TEN) may cause mucosal ulceration.

Idiopathic Aphthous Ulcers: Painful, recurrent ulcers with no identifiable cause, often associated with systemic conditions (e.g., stress, nutritional deficiencies).

Pathophysiology

The development of vaginal ulcers depends on the underlying etiology:

1. Infectious ulcers

Pathogens (e.g., HSV, Treponema pallidum) invade the mucosal epithelium, causing cell lysis, inflammation and ulceration. Immune responses (e.g., T-cell mediated in HSV) contribute to tissue damage.

2. Autoimmune ulcers

Autoantibodies or immune complexes (e.g., in Behcet's or pemphigus) target mucosal components, leading to epithelial breakdown.

3. Traumatic ulcers

Direct mechanical or chemical injury disrupts the mucosal barrier, exposing submucosal tissue.

4. Atrophic ulcers

Estrogen deficiency reduces mucosal thickness and vascularity, making the vagina prone to friction-induced ulceration.

5. Neoplastic ulcers

Malignant transformation leads to tissue necrosis and ulceration due to tumour invasion or ischemia.

The vaginal mucosa's response to injury involves inflammation, recruitment of immune cells, and attempts at repair. Chronic or recurrent ulcers may result from persistent infection, immune dysregulation, or failure of mucosal healing.

Clinical Features

Symptoms

Pain: Common in infectious (e.g., HSV, chancroid) and autoimmune ulcers; absent in primary syphilis.

Discharge: May accompany ulcers, especially in infections (e.g., purulent in chancroid, serous in HSV).

Itching or burning: Common in HSV, candidiasis or lichen planus.

Dyspareunia: Frequent due to mucosal sensitivity.

Systemic symptoms: Fever, malaise or lymphadenopathy in HSV, LGV or secondary syphilis.

Physical Findings

Ulcer characteristics: Size, number, depth, borders (indurated in syphilis, ragged in chancroid), and base (clean, necrotic or purulent).

Location: Vaginal mucosa, vestibule or extending to the vulva.

Associated findings: Vesicles (HSV), white patches (lichen planus), or lymphadenopathy (LGV, chancroid).

Chronicity: Recurrent ulcers suggest HSV, Behcet's, or aphthous ulcers; persistent, non-healing ulcers raise suspicion for malignancy.

Diagnosis

Accurate diagnosis of vaginal ulcers requires a systematic approach, integrating history, physical examination and diagnostic testing.

1. History

Symptom onset and duration: Acute (e.g., HSV) vs. chronic (e.g., malignancy).

Pain: Painful (HSV, chancroid) vs. painless (syphilis).

Sexual history: Number of partners, unprotected intercourse, history of STIs.

Associated symptoms: Oral ulcers, skin lesions, or systemic symptoms (e.g., in Behcet's or Crohn's).

Medical history: Autoimmune diseases, immunosuppression, recent trauma or medication use.

Hygiene practices: Use of irritants, douches or foreign bodies.

2. Physical Examination

External genitalia: Inspect for vesicles, erythema or lymphadenopathy.

Vaginal examination: Use a speculum to visualize ulcers, noting size, number and characteristics.

Bimanual examination: Assess for pelvic tenderness or masses.

Systemic examination: Check for oral ulcers, skin lesions or joint involvement (e.g., in Behcet's).

3. Diagnostic Testing

a. Microbiological Tests

HSV: Polymerase chain reaction (PCR) from ulcer swab is gold standard, viral culture less sensitive.

Syphilis: Dark-field microscopy (if available) or serology (RPR/VDRL, confirmed by treponemal tests like TPPA or FTA-ABS).

Chancroid: Culture or PCR for Haemophilus ducreyi (often unavailable; diagnosis often clinical).

LGV: NAAT for Chlamydia trachomatis serotypes L1–L3.

Other Cultures or PCR: For CMV, tuberculosis or fungi in immunocompromised patients.

b. Histopathology and Biopsy

Indicated for persistent, non-healing ulcers or suspected malignancy.

Autoimmune conditions (e.g., pemphigus, lichen planus) may show characteristic findings (e.g., acantholysis in pemphigus).

c. Other Tests

Vaginal pH and wet mount: To rule out coexisting vaginitis (e.g., BV, candidiasis).

Blood tests: HIV testing, autoimmune serologies (e.g., ANA, anti-desmoglein antibodies).

Colposcopy: For detailed visualization of vaginal or cervical ulcers.

Imaging: Pelvic ultrasound or MRI if fistulae or malignancy are suspected.

4. Differential Diagnosis

Infectious: HSV, syphilis, chancroid, LGV, tuberculosis.

Autoimmune: Behcet's, Lichen planus, pemphigus, Crohn's.

Neoplastic: Squamous cell carcinoma, adenocarcinoma.

Traumatic: Mechanical or chemical injury.

Other: Aphthous ulcers, drug reactions, atrophic vaginitis.

Management

Management of vaginal ulcers depends on the underlying cause, with a focus on treating the etiology, alleviating symptoms and preventing complications.

1. Infectious Causes

a. Herpes Simplex Virus

Treatment

First episode: Acyclovir 400 mg three times daily for 7–10 days, valacyclovir 1 g twice daily for 7–10 days, or famciclovir 250 mg three times daily for 7–10 days.

Recurrent episodes: Shorter regimens (e.g., acyclovir 800 mg three times daily for 2 days).

Suppressive therapy: Acyclovir 400 mg twice daily or valacyclovir 500 mg daily for frequent recurrences.

Symptom relief: Analgesics, topical lidocaine or sitz baths.

Partner counselling: Advise on transmission risk and condom use.

b. Syphilis

Treatment: Benzathine penicillin G 2.4 million units intramuscularly (single dose for primary/ secondary syphilis; three weekly doses for late latent syphilis).

Alternatives: Doxycycline 100 mg twice daily for 14 days (non-pregnant patients with penicillin allergy).

Partner treatment: Essential for sexual contacts within 90 days.

c. Chancroid

Treatment: Azithromycin 1 g single dose, ceftriaxone 250 mg intramuscularly single dose, or erythromycin 500 mg three times daily for 7 days.

Follow-up: Monitor for resolution and lymphadenopathy.

d. Lymphogranuloma Venereum

Treatment: Doxycycline 100 mg twice daily for 21 days or erythromycin 500 mg four times daily for 21 days.

Management of buboes: Aspiration if fluctuant; avoid incision to prevent fistulae.

e. Other Infections

Tuberculosis: Standard anti-tubercular therapy (e.g., isoniazid, rifampin, pyrazinamide, ethambutol for 6–9 months).

CMV or fungal infections: Antiviral (e.g., ganciclovir) or antifungal therapy (e.g., fluconazole) based on culture results.

2. Non-Infectious Causes

a. Autoimmune/Inflammatory Diseases

Behcet's Disease: Topical or systemic corticosteroids; colchicine or immunosuppressive agents (e.g., azathioprine) for severe cases.

Lichen Planus: Topical corticosteroids (e.g., clobetasol); systemic steroids or methotrexate for erosive disease.

Pemphigus Vulgaris: High-dose systemic corticosteroids and immunosuppressants (e.g., rituximab, azathioprine).

Crohn's Disease: Systemic therapy (e.g., anti-TNF agents like infliximab) and surgical management of fistulae.

b. Atrophic Vaginitis

Treatment: Topical oestrogen (e.g., estradiol cream 0.01% or vaginal ring); non-hormonal moisturizers for mild cases.

Contraindications: Avoid oestrogen in patients with hormone-sensitive cancers.

c. Traumatic Ulcers

Treatment: Remove offending agent (e.g., foreign body); promote healing with sitz baths or barrier creams. Prevention Counsel on safe sexual practices and hygiene.

3. Neoplastic Causes

Management: Biopsy, staging and treatment (e.g., surgery, radiation, or chemotherapy for vaginal cancer). Follow-up: Long-term monitoring for recurrence.

4. General Measures

Symptom relief: Analgesics, topical anesthetics or sitz baths for pain.

Hygiene: Advise gentle cleansing with unscented soaps and avoidance of irritants.

Sexual abstinence: Until ulcers heal, especially in infectious cases.

Counseling: Address psychosocial impact, including sexual dysfunction or stigma.

Complications

Infectious ulcers

Secondary bacterial infections.

Increased HIV transmission risk (e.g., in HSV or chancroid).

Scarring or adhesions in chronic infections.

Autoimmune ulcers

Chronic pain, sexual dysfunction or vaginal stenosis.

Systemic complications (e.g., uveitis in Behcet's, gastrointestinal involvement in Crohn's).

Neoplastic ulcers

Local invasion, metastasis or obstruction.

Psychosocial

Anxiety, depression or reduced quality of life due to chronic symptoms or recurrence.

Prevention

STI prevention: Promote condom use, regular STI screening and partner treatment.

Hygiene: Avoid douching, chemical irritants or traumatic practices.

Vaccination: HPV vaccination to reduce risk of vaginal/vulvar cancers.

Management of chronic conditions: Control autoimmune diseases or diabetes to minimize mucosal vulnerability.

Screening: Regular gynecologic exams for early detection of neoplastic or inflammatory conditions.

Conclusion

Vaginal ulcers represent a complex clinical entity with diverse etiologies, ranging from infectious causes like HSV and syphilis to autoimmune conditions like Behcet's disease and rare neoplastic processes. Accurate diagnosis requires a thorough history, physical examination, and targeted diagnostic testing, including PCR, serology, or biopsy. Management is etiology-specific, with an emphasis on treating the underlying cause, alleviating symptoms and preventing complications. Preventive strategies, including safe sexual practices and regular gynecologic care, are critical to reducing the incidence and impact of vaginal ulcers.

Key References

Centers for Disease Control and Prevention (CDC) (2021). Sexually Transmitted Infections Treatment Guidelines.

American College of Obstetricians and Gynecologists (ACOG). Vulvovaginal Health. Practice Bulletin No. 224.

Sobel, J. D. (2019). Genital Ulcer Disease . In Infectious Diseases of the Female Genital Tract.

James, W. D., et al. (2020). Andrews' Diseases of the Skin Clinical Dermatology.

Common Causes of Vaginitis "BaCT SOAP"

Letter	Cause	Description
Ba	Bacterial Vaginosis	Fishy odor, clue cells, ↑ pH
C	Candida albicans	Curdy white discharge, itching
T	Trichomonas vaginalis	Frothy green discharge, motile protozoa
S	Senile Vaginitis	Postmenopausal, dryness, irritation
O	Overgrowth (Cytolytic)	Excess lactobacilli, acidic pH
A	Allergic/Irritant	Reaction to soaps, chemicals
P	Physiological	Normal discharge in pregnancy/puberty

8.4 Prolapse of Vagina

(Khurooj-e-Mahbil & Isterkhai)

Introduction

Vaginal prolapse, a subset of pelvic organ prolapse (POP), is a condition characterized by the descent of the vaginal walls or apex due to weakened pelvic floor support structures. It is a common gynecologic condition that significantly impacts quality of life, causing symptoms such as pelvic pressure, urinary dysfunction and sexual difficulties. Vaginal prolapse is often associated with other pelvic organ prolapses, including uterine prolapse or enterocele.

Definition

Vaginal prolapse refers to the downward displacement of the vaginal walls (anterior, posterior or apical) due to weakened pelvic floor muscles, ligaments and connective tissues. It is classified based on the vaginal compartment affected:

a. Anterior vaginal prolapse (cystocele): Descent of the anterior vaginal wall, often involving the bladder.

b. Posterior vaginal prolapse (rectocele): Descent of the posterior vaginal wall, often involving the rectum.

c. Apical vaginal prolapse: Descent of the vaginal apex (post-hysterectomy) or cervix (with uterus intact), sometimes accompanied by enterocele (small bowel herniation).

Vaginal prolapse is a component of pelvic organ prolapse, quantified using standardized systems such as the Pelvic Organ Prolapse Quantification (POP-Q) system.

Epidemiology

Prevalence: Pelvic organ prolapse, including vaginal prolapse, affects approximately 30–50% of women, with symptomatic prolapse reported in 3–6% of women. Prevalence increases with age and parity.

Age: Most common in postmenopausal women due to oestrogen deficiency and age-related tissue weakening.

Risk factors

Parity (especially vaginal deliveries).

Aging and menopause.

Obesity, chronic constipation or chronic cough (increased intra-abdominal pressure).

Connective tissue disorders (e.g., Ehlers-Danlos syndrome).

Previous pelvic surgery (e.g., hysterectomy).

Geographic variation: Higher prevalence in populations with limited access to obstetric care or high rates of multiparity.

Etiology and Risk Factors

Vaginal prolapse results from the failure of pelvic support structures, including muscles, ligaments and fascia. Key etiological factors include.

1. Obstetric Factors

Vaginal delivery, particularly prolonged labor, forceps delivery or large fetal size, causes stretching or tearing of pelvic floor muscles (e.g., levator ani) and ligaments (e.g., uterosacral, cardinal).

Multiparity increases cumulative trauma to pelvic tissues.

2. Aging and Hormonal Changes

Estrogen deficiency in menopause reduces collagen strength and vaginal tissue elasticity, weakening support structures. Age-related degeneration of pelvic floor muscles and connective tissues.

3. Increased Intra-Abdominal Pressure

Chronic conditions such as obesity, chronic constipation, chronic cough (e.g., from COPD) or heavy lifting elevate intra-abdominal pressure, stressing pelvic supports.

4. Connective Tissue Disorders

Genetic conditions (e.g., Marfan syndrome, Ehlers-Danlos syndrome) impair collagen integrity, predisposing to prolapse. Weakened endopelvic fascia and ligaments contribute to prolapse.

5. Pelvic Surgery

Hysterectomy or other pelvic surgeries may disrupt uterosacral or cardinal ligaments, leading to apical prolapse.

Surgical trauma to pelvic floor muscles increases risk.

6. Other Factors

Pelvic trauma or radiation therapy.

Neurological conditions (e.g., spina bifida, spinal cord injury) impairing pelvic floor muscle function.

Lifestyle factors, such as smoking, which may degrade connective tissue.

Pathophysiology

The pelvic floor comprises muscles (levator ani, coccygeus), ligaments (uterosacral, cardinal) and endopelvic fascia, which support the vagina, uterus, bladder, and rectum. Vaginal prolapse occurs when these structures are weakened or damaged, leading to descent of vaginal compartments. Key mechanisms include:

a. Muscle damage: Levator ani injury during childbirth reduces pelvic floor strength, allowing organ descent.
b. Ligament attenuation: Stretching or tearing of uterosacral or cardinal ligaments compromises apical support.
c. Fascial defects: Tears in the pubocervical fascia (anterior) or rectovaginal fascia (posterior) lead to cystocele or rectocele, respectively.
d. Intra-abdominal pressure: Chronic elevation exacerbates prolapse by pushing pelvic organs downward.
e. Estrogen deficiency: Reduces collagen synthesis and mucosal thickness, weakening vaginal support.

The degree of prolapse varies from mild (descent within the vagina) to severe (protrusion beyond the vaginal introitus). Apical prolapse often exacerbates anterior or posterior prolapse due to loss of central support.

Clinical Features

Symptoms

Pelvic pressure or heaviness: Sensation of a “bulge” or “something falling out,” worse with standing or straining.

Vaginal bulge: Visible or palpable protrusion, particularly in advanced prolapse.

Urinary symptoms

Cystocele: Stress urinary incontinence, incomplete bladder emptying or recurrent urinary tract infections (UTIs).

Urethral kinking: Urinary retention or obstructive voiding.

Bowel symptoms

Rectocele: Difficulty with defecation, need for manual splinting (pressing perineum to evacuate stool), or faecal incontinence.

Sexual dysfunction: Dyspareunia, reduced sexual satisfaction or partner discomfort.

Vaginal symptoms: Discharge, irritation or ulceration of exposed mucosa in severe prolapse.

Back or pelvic pain: Less common, associated with advanced prolapse or coexisting conditions.

Physical Findings

Inspection Visible vaginal bulge or protrusion beyond the introitus in advanced cases.

Speculum examination: Descent of anterior (cystocele), posterior (rectocele), or apical (vault/cervix) vaginal walls, assessed at rest and with Valsalva manoeuvre.

Bimanual examination: Evaluate for coexisting uterine prolapse or pelvic masses.

Associated findings: Atrophic vaginal mucosa in postmenopausal women, stress incontinence, or rectal prolapse.

Classification (Pelvic Organ Prolapse Quantification, POP-Q)

A standardized system measuring vaginal descent at nine points relative to the hymen.

Stage 0: No prolapse.

Stage I: Descent >1 cm above hymen.

Stage II: Descent between 1 cm above and 1 cm below hymen.

Stage III: Descent >1 cm below hymen but not complete eversion.

Stage IV: Complete vaginal eversion.

Diagnosis

Diagnosis of vaginal prolapse is primarily clinical, based on history and physical examination, with adjunctive tests to assess severity and complications.

1. History

Symptoms: Pelvic pressure, bulge sensation, urinary or bowel dysfunction, sexual difficulties.

Obstetric history: Number of vaginal deliveries, complications (e.g., forceps, prolonged labor).

Medical history: Menopause, chronic cough, constipation, connective tissue disorders or prior pelvic surgery.

Lifestyle factors: Obesity, heavy lifting or smoking.

2. Physical Examination

External genitalia: Inspect for protrusion or mucosal changes.

Speculum examination: Assess anterior, posterior and apical compartments at rest and during Valsalva.

POP-Q measurement: Quantify prolapse severity using standardized points (e.g., Aa, Ba, C, Ap, Bp).

Pelvic floor muscle assessment: Evaluate levator ani strength (e.g., Oxford scale 0–5).

Rectal examination: Confirm rectocele or assess anal sphincter tone.

3. Diagnostic Testing

Urodynamic testing: For complex urinary symptoms (e.g., mixed incontinence, voiding dysfunction).

Pelvic ultrasound or MRI: To evaluate for enterocele, pelvic masses or complex prolapse.

Cystoscopy or proctoscopy: If bladder or rectal involvement is suspected (e.g., hematuria, rectal bleeding).

Urinalysis: To rule out UTI in patients with urinary symptoms.

Differential Diagnosis

1. Uterine prolapse: Descent of the cervix/uterus, often coexisting with vaginal prolapse.
2. Pelvic mass tumours (e.g., fibroids, ovarian cysts) mimicking prolapse symptoms.
3. Vaginal wall cysts: Gartner's duct or Bartholin's gland cysts.
4. Rectal prolapse: Protrusion of rectal mucosa, distinguished by rectal examination.

Management

Management of vaginal prolapse is individualized based on symptom severity, prolapse stage, patient preferences and comorbidities. Options include conservative, non-surgical and surgical approaches.

1. Conservative Management

Indications: Mild symptoms (Stage I–II), asymptomatic prolapse or patients unfit for surgery.

1. Pelvic floor muscle training (PFMT): Supervised Kegel exercises to strengthen levator ani muscles. Effective for mild prolapse and stress urinary incontinence.

2. Lifestyle modifications: Weight loss in obese patients.

3. Management of chronic cough or constipation (e.g., smoking cessation, laxatives).

4. Avoidance of heavy lifting.

5. Vaginal oestrogen therapy: For postmenopausal women with atrophic mucosa.

Improves tissue integrity and may reduce symptoms (e.g., estradiol cream 0.01% or vaginal ring).

2. Non-Surgical Management

Pessaries

Silicone or plastic devices inserted into the vagina to support prolapsed organs.

Types: Ring (most common), Gellhorn, donut or cube pessaries.

Indications: Symptomatic prolapse, patient preference for non-surgical treatment or temporary management (e.g., during pregnancy).

Fitting: Requires trial and follow-up to ensure comfort and prevent complications (e.g., erosion, discharge).

Maintenance: Regular removal, cleaning and vaginal oestrogen to prevent ulceration.

3. Surgical Management

Indications Severe symptoms (Stage III–IV), failure of conservative measures or significant impact on quality of life.

Anterior vaginal prolapse (cystocele)

Anterior colporrhaphy: Plication of pubocervical fascia to repair anterior wall defects.

Paravaginal repair: Reattachment of fascia to pelvic sidewall for lateral defects.

Mesh augmentation: Controversial due to complications (e.g., erosion, pain); reserved for recurrent cases.

Posterior vaginal prolapse (rectocele)

Posterior colporrhaphy: Repair of rectovaginal fascia to support posterior wall.

Perineorrhaphy: Reinforcement of perineal body for associated perineal laxity.

Apical prolapse

Sacrocolpopexy: Gold standard for vaginal vault prolapse (post-hysterectomy); mesh attaches vaginal apex to sacrum.

Uterosacral ligament suspension: Reattachment of vaginal apex to uterosacral ligaments.

Sacrospinous ligament fixation: Suturing vaginal apex to sacrospinous ligament.

Colpocleisis: Obliterative procedure for elderly patients unfit for reconstructive surgery (closes vaginal canal).

Concomitant procedures

Hysterectomy for coexisting uterine prolapse.

Anti-incontinence surgery (e.g., mid-urethral sling) for stress urinary incontinence.

Minimally invasive approaches: Laparoscopic or robotic-assisted sacrocolpopexy for reduced recovery time.

4. General Measures

Symptom management: Analgesics or sitz baths for discomfort; topical treatments for mucosal irritation.

Patient counselling: Discuss treatment options, risks (e.g., recurrence, mesh complications), and postoperative care.

Follow-up: Regular assessment for symptom resolution, pessary maintenance or surgical complications.

Complications

Untreated prolapse

Ulceration or infection of exposed vaginal mucosa.

Urinary retention, recurrent UTIs, or hydronephrosis (severe cystocele).

Bowel obstruction or faecal incontinence (severe rectocele).

Pessary complications

Vaginal erosion, discharge or fistula formation.

Discomfort or expulsion, if poorly fitted.

Surgical complications

Recurrence (10–30% depending on procedure).

Mesh complications (erosion, pain, dyspareunia).

Urinary or bowel injury, bleeding or infection.

De novo urinary incontinence or sexual dysfunction.

Prevention

1. Obstetric care: Minimize pelvic floor trauma during vaginal delivery (e.g., avoid prolonged second stage, judicious use of forceps). Encourage cesarean delivery in high-risk cases (controversial).
2. Lifestyle modifications: Maintain healthy weight, treat chronic cough or constipation and avoid heavy lifting.

3. Pelvic floor exercises: Routine PFMT in postpartum women to strengthen pelvic muscles.
4. Hormonal therapy: Vaginal oestrogen in postmenopausal women to maintain tissue integrity.

Screening

Regular gynaecological exams to detect early prolapse in high-risk populations (e.g., multiparous women, post-hysterectomy).

Conclusion

Vaginal prolapse is a prevalent condition resulting from weakened pelvic support structures, leading to descent of the vaginal walls or apex. It is associated with significant morbidity, including pelvic pressure, urinary and bowel dysfunction and impaired quality of life. Management options range from conservative measures (PFMT, pessaries) to surgical repair (e.g., colporrhaphy, sacrocolpopexy), individualised to patient needs and prolapse severity. Preventive strategies, including obstetric care and lifestyle modifications, are critical to reducing incidence.

Diseases of the Vagina (Classify by Etiology)

Infectious	Inflammatory	Atrophic	Congenital
Candidiasis	Contact Dermatitis	Postmenopausal Vaginitis	Vaginal Agenesis
Bacterial Vaginosis	Allergic Vaginitis	Senile Vaginitis	Transverse Septum
Trichomoniasis	Irritant Vaginitis	Estrogen Deficiency	Imperforate Hymen
Herpes Simplex	Cytolytic Vaginosis		

8.5 Vaginismus

(*Tashannuj-i-mahbil*)

Introduction

Vaginismus is a sexual pain disorder characterized by involuntary, recurrent or persistent contraction of the pelvic floor muscles, particularly the pubococcygeus muscle, surrounding the vaginal introitus. This involuntary muscle spasm prevents vaginal penetration, causing significant distress and impacting sexual function, gynecologic examinations and quality of life. Vaginismus is classified as a genito-pelvic pain/penetration disorder (GPPPD) in the Diagnostic and Statistical Manual of Mental Disorders (DSM-5).

Definition

Vaginismus is defined as the involuntary, recurrent or persistent contraction of the perivaginal pelvic floor muscles in response to attempted vaginal penetration, including sexual intercourse, tampon insertion or gynecologic examination. The condition may be lifelong (primary, present from the first attempt at penetration) or acquired (secondary, developing after a period of normal function). Severity ranges from mild (allowing partial penetration with discomfort) to severe (preventing all penetration).

Epidemiology

Prevalence: Estimated to affect 1–17% of women globally, with variability due to underreporting and cultural differences in sexual health disclosure.

Age: Most common in reproductive-age women, particularly those initiating sexual activity or undergoing gynecologic procedures.

Risk factors

Psychological factors: Anxiety, fear of pain or history of sexual trauma.

Cultural or religious beliefs emphasizing sexual purity.

History of pelvic pain or gynecologic conditions.

Geographic variation: Higher prevalence in cultures with restrictive attitudes toward sexuality or limited sexual education.

Etiology

Vaginismus is multifactorial, often resulting from a combination of physical, psychological and relational factors. It is classified as primary or secondary, based on onset and may be situational or generalized.

1. Psychological and Emotional Causes

Fear of pain: Anticipation of pain during penetration, often based on prior experiences or misinformation.

Sexual trauma: History of sexual abuse, assault or negative sexual experiences.

Anxiety or stress: General anxiety disorders, performance anxiety or fear of intimacy.

Cultural or religious factors: Upbringing emphasizing shame, guilt or prohibition of sexual activity.

Relationship issues: Lack of trust, poor communication or partner dynamics contributing to anxiety.

2. Physical Causes

Pelvic floor dysfunction: Hypertonic pelvic floor muscles due to chronic tension or injury.

Gynecologic conditions: Endometriosis, vulvodynia or vaginal infections causing pain that triggers muscle spasms.

Postpartum changes: Perineal trauma or episiotomy scars from childbirth.

Atrophic vaginitis: Estrogen deficiency in postmenopausal or breastfeeding women, leading to vaginal dryness and pain.

Congenital anomalies: Rare, such as vaginal septum or imperforate hymen, causing mechanical obstruction.

3. Relational and Sociocultural Factors

Partner-related issues, such as aggressive or coercive behavior.

Lack of sexual education or negative societal attitudes toward sexuality.

Stressful life events (e.g., infertility, relationship conflicts).

Pathophysiology

Vaginismus involves a reflex contraction of the pelvic floor muscles, particularly the pubococcygeus and bulbocavernosus muscles, in response to attempted vaginal penetration. This reflex is mediated by the autonomic nervous system and influenced by psychological and physical triggers:

1. Neuromuscular mechanism: Hypertonicity of pelvic floor muscles creates a vicious cycle of pain, fear and further muscle contraction. The reflex may be conditioned by prior painful experiences.

2. Psychological reinforcement: Fear of pain or penetration activates the sympathetic nervous system, heightening muscle tension and reinforcing avoidance behaviors.

3. Pain perception: Central sensitization in chronic cases amplifies pain perception, even with minimal stimuli.

4. Hormonal influence: Estrogen deficiency may reduce vaginal lubrication and elasticity, exacerbating discomfort and triggering spasms.

The interplay of psychological distress and physical pain creates a feedback loop, where fear of penetration leads to muscle contraction, which causes pain and reinforces fear.

Clinical Features

Symptoms

1. Inability to achieve vaginal penetration (e.g., during intercourse, tampon insertion or gynaecological exams).
2. Pain or burning sensation during attempted penetration, ranging from mild discomfort to severe pain.
3. Anticipatory anxiety or fear before sexual activity or pelvic exams.
4. Avoidance of sexual activity or gynaecological care due to fear of pain.
5. Emotional distress, including frustration, embarrassment or low self-esteem.

Associated Symptoms

1. Dyspareunia (painful intercourse), if partial penetration is possible.
2. Vaginal tightness or “hitting a wall” sensation reported by patients or partners.
3. Urinary symptoms (e.g., hesitancy, incomplete voiding) due to pelvic floor dysfunction.
4. Relationship strain or sexual dysfunction in partners.

Physical Findings

Involuntary contraction of vaginal introitus during attempted speculum or digital examination.

Hypertonic pelvic floor muscles on palpation, often with tenderness.

Normal vaginal anatomy in primary vaginismus; possible scarring or atrophy in secondary cases.

Absence of organic lesions in most cases, though coexisting conditions (e.g., vulvodynia, endometriosis) may be present.

Diagnosis

Diagnosis of vaginismus is primarily clinical, based on history and physical examination, with a focus on ruling out organic causes and assessing psychological factors.

1. History

Symptom characteristics: Onset (lifelong vs. acquired), context (situational vs. generalized), and severity of pain or penetration difficulty.

Sexual history: Previous sexual experiences, trauma or cultural/religious influences.

Gynecologic history: Menstrual history, obstetric history or prior pelvic pain conditions.

Psychosocial history: Anxiety, depression, relationship dynamics or history of abuse.

Medical history: Chronic pain syndromes, neurologic disorders or hormonal status.

2. Physical Examination

Approach: Conduct in a sensitive, patient-centered manner to minimize anxiety. Explain procedures and obtain consent.

External genitalia: Inspect for signs of vulvodynia, lichen sclerosus or trauma.

Pelvic examination

Attempt gentle single-digit examination to assess pelvic floor muscle tone and trigger points.

Avoid forceful speculum insertion, if severe spasm is present.

Note any anatomic abnormalities (e.g., vaginal septum, scarring).

Pelvic floor assessment: Evaluate muscle strength and hypertonicity using digital palpation.

3. Diagnostic Testing

Vaginal swabs or cultures: To rule out infections (e.g., candidiasis, bacterial vaginosis).

Hormonal evaluation: Assess for oestrogen deficiency in postmenopausal or breastfeeding women.

Imaging: Pelvic ultrasound or MRI if structural abnormalities (e.g., vaginal septum, pelvic mass) are suspected.

Psychological assessment: Screening for anxiety, depression or trauma using validated tools (e.g., GAD-7, PHQ-9).

Urodynamic testing: If urinary symptoms suggest pelvic floor dysfunction.

4. Differential Diagnosis

Vulvodynia: Localized vulvar pain without muscle spasm.

Dyspareunia: Painful intercourse due to endometriosis, pelvic inflammatory disease or atrophic vaginitis.

Vaginal atrophy: Pain and dryness in postmenopausal women, without involuntary spasms.

Congenital anomalies: Vaginal septum or imperforate hymen causing mechanical obstruction. Neurologic disorders: Conditions like multiple sclerosis affecting pelvic floor innervation.

5. DSM-5 Criteria for Genito-Pelvic Pain/Penetration Disorder

Persistent or recurrent difficulties with one or more of:

Vaginal penetration during intercourse.

Marked vulvovaginal or pelvic pain during penetration.

Fear or anxiety about pain in anticipation of penetration.

Marked tensing or tightening of pelvic floor muscles during attempted penetration.

Symptoms cause significant distress and are not better explained by another condition.

Management

Management of vaginismus is multidisciplinary, addressing physical, psychological and relational factors. Treatment is done according to the patient's needs, severity and underlying causes.

1. Non-Surgical Management

a. Pelvic Floor Physical Therapy

Goal: Desensitize pelvic floor muscles and reduce hypertonicity.

Techniques

Pelvic floor muscle training to improve relaxation and control.

Biofeedback to monitor muscle tension.

Manual therapy to release trigger points.

Dilator therapy: Gradual use of vaginal dilators to desensitize the vagina to penetration, starting with the smallest size and progressing under guidance.

b. Psychotherapy

Cognitive Behavioral Therapy (CBT): Addresses fear, anxiety and negative beliefs about penetration.

Sex therapy: Improves sexual communication, reduces performance anxiety and enhances intimacy.

Trauma-focused therapy: For patients with a history of sexual abuse (e.g., Eye Movement Desensitization and Reprocessing, EMDR).

c. Education and Counseling

Provide accurate information about vaginal anatomy, sexual function and vaginismus.

Involve partners to foster understanding and support.

Address cultural or religious barriers through sensitive counselling.

d. Medical Therapy

Topical lidocaine: Reduces pain during dilator use or intercourse.

Vaginal oestrogen: For postmenopausal women with atrophic vaginitis.

Anxiolytics or antidepressants: For severe anxiety or depression, prescribed cautiously.

Botulinum toxin (Botox): Rarely used for refractory cases; injected into pelvic floor muscles to reduce spasms (investigational).

2. Surgical Management

Indications: Rare, reserved for anatomic abnormalities (e.g., vaginal septum, imperforate hymen) or refractory cases.

Procedures: Hymenectomy for imperforate hymen. Vaginoplasty for congenital anomalies. Perineal or pelvic floor surgery for severe scarring or trauma.

Surgery does not address psychological components and should be combined with therapy.

3. General Measures

Pain management: Analgesics or topical anesthetics for discomfort during therapy.

Lubricants: Water-based lubricants to reduce friction during dilator use or intercourse.

Partner involvement: Encourage open communication and joint therapy sessions.

Follow-up: Regular monitoring to assess progress, adjust therapy and address setbacks.

4. Multidisciplinary Approach

Collaboration among gynaecologists, pelvic floor physical therapists, psychologists and sex therapists.

Plan treatment to address both physical (muscle spasms) and psychological (fear, anxiety) components.

Complications

Sexual dysfunction: Persistent avoidance of intercourse, reduced libido or partner dissatisfaction.

Relationship strain: Frustration, communication breakdown or infidelity.

Psychological impact: Anxiety, depression, low self-esteem or body image issues.

Infertility: Difficulty with intercourse may prevent conception.

Delayed gynaecological care: Avoidance of pelvic exams may delay diagnosis of other conditions (e.g., cervical cancer).

Prevention

Sexual education: Provide comprehensive education on sexual health and anatomy to reduce fear and misinformation.

Trauma prevention: Early intervention for sexual abuse or trauma to prevent conditioned responses.

Pelvic floor health: Encourage pelvic floor exercises postpartum to maintain muscle tone.

Gynecological care: Use gentle, patient-centered techniques during pelvic exams to minimize trauma.

Cultural sensitivity: Address societal or religious barriers to sexual health through community education.

Conclusion

Vaginismus is a complex genito-pelvic pain/penetration disorder characterized by involuntary pelvic floor muscle contractions that prevent vaginal penetration. It arises from a combination of psychological, physical and relational factors, requiring a multidisciplinary approach to diagnosis and management. Clinical evaluation involves a detailed history, sensitive physical examination and exclusion of organic causes. Treatment focuses on pelvic floor physical therapy, psychotherapy and patient education, with surgical intervention reserved for rare cases. Preventive strategies, including sexual education and trauma-informed care, are essential to reduce incidence.

Key References

American College of Obstetricians and Gynecologists (ACOG). (2020). Female Sexual Dysfunction. Practice Bulletin No. 213.

American Psychiatric Association. (2013). Diagnostic and Statistical Manual of Mental Disorders (DSM-5).

Pacik, P. T., & Geletta, S. (2017). Vaginismus: A Review of the Literature on the Classification/Diagnosis, Etiology, and Treatment. Sexual Medicine Reviews.

Rosenbaum, T. Y. (2018). Pelvic Floor Involvement in Sexual Dysfunction. In Urogynaecology and Reconstructive Pelvic Surgery.

8.6 Dyspareunia

(*Jemay-i-molim*)

Definition

Dyspareunia is defined as persistent or recurrent genital pain that occurs just before, during or after sexual intercourse, causing distress or interpersonal difficulty. It is a common gynaecological complaint that can affect individuals of any gender but is more frequently reported in women. Dyspareunia is not a diagnosis in itself but a symptom that warrants thorough evaluation to identify underlying causes.

Epidemiology

Prevalence: Estimates vary widely, ranging from 8% to 22% in women, with higher rates in postmenopausal women (up to 45%) and lower rates in men (1–5%). The prevalence may be underestimated due to underreporting caused by stigma or embarrassment.

Age and Demographics: Dyspareunia can occur across all age groups, with specific causes varying by life stage (e.g., postpartum, menopause). It is more commonly reported in women with lower socioeconomic status, history of sexual trauma or chronic medical conditions.

Classification

Dyspareunia is classified based on its timing, location and etiology:

1. Temporal Classification

Entry Dyspareunia: Pain at the vaginal introitus or during initial penetration.

Deep Dyspareunia: Pain with deep vaginal penetration, often associated with pelvic structures.

2. Etiologic Classification

Superficial: Pain localized to the vulva, vestibule or vaginal opening.

Deep: Pain involving deeper pelvic structures (e.g., cervix, uterus, adnexa).

3. Primary vs. Secondary

Primary: Present since the onset of sexual activity.

Secondary: Develops after a period of pain-free intercourse.

4. Situational vs. Generalized

Situational: Occurs in specific contexts (e.g., with certain partners or positions).

Generalized: Occurs consistently across all sexual encounters.

Pathophysiology

Dyspareunia results from a complex interplay of physical, psychological and social factors. The underlying mechanisms may involve

1. Local Tissue Factors: Inflammation, infection or trauma to the vulva, vagina or pelvic organs can cause pain. For example, vaginal dryness due to hypoestrogenism or vulvar dermatoses can lead to superficial pain, while endometriosis or pelvic adhesions may cause deep pain.
2. Neuromuscular Factors: Hypertonic pelvic floor muscles (vaginismus) or nerve hypersensitivity (e.g., vulvodynia) can contribute to pain.
3. Psychological Factors: Anxiety, depression or a history of sexual trauma may amplify pain perception or lead to involuntary pelvic floor muscle contraction.
4. Vascular and Hormonal Factors: Reduced blood flow or oestrogen deficiency (e.g., menopause, postpartum) can lead to vaginal atrophy and discomfort.

Etiology

The causes of dyspareunia are multifactorial and can be broadly categorized into organic, psychogenic and mixed etiologies. Common causes include:

1. Superficial Dyspareunia

Vulvar Conditions

Vulvodynia or provoked vestibulodynia (pain with contact to the vaginal vestibule).

Vulvar dermatoses (e.g., lichen sclerosus, lichen planus).

Infections (e.g., candidiasis, herpes simplex virus).

Vaginal Conditions

Vaginal atrophy (due to menopause, breastfeeding or hormonal contraceptive use).

Vaginismus (involuntary pelvic floor muscle contraction).

Trauma or scarring (e.g., episiotomy, vaginal surgery).

Infectious Causes

Bacterial vaginosis, trichomoniasis or sexually transmitted infections.

Congenital Anomalies

Vaginal septum or imperforate hymen.

2. Deep Dyspareunia

a. Pelvic Inflammatory Disease (PID): Chronic pelvic pain from prior infections.
b. Endometriosis: Ectopic endometrial tissue causing cyclic or constant pelvic pain.
c. Adenomyosis: Endometrial tissue within the myometrium, leading to deep pain.
d. Pelvic Adhesions: Post-surgical or post-inflammatory scarring.
e. Uterine or Ovarian Pathology: Fibroids, ovarian cysts or malignancy.
f. Gastrointestinal Causes: Irritable bowel syndrome, constipation or inflammatory bowel disease.
g. Urological Causes: Interstitial cystitis, urethritis or bladder pain syndrome.

3. Psychological and Relational Factors

Anxiety, depression or stress.

History of sexual trauma or abuse.

Relationship conflict or lack of arousal/lubrication.

4. Iatrogenic Causes

Post-surgical scarring (e.g., hysterectomy, pelvic surgery).

Radiation therapy causing vaginal stenosis or fibrosis.

Medications (e.g., aromatase inhibitors, selective serotonin reuptake inhibitors).

Clinical Presentation

Patients with dyspareunia may present with:

Burning, stinging, sharp or aching pain.

Pain localized to the vulva, vaginal introitus or deep pelvis.

Associated symptoms such as vaginal dryness, itching or abnormal discharge.

Psychological distress, reduced sexual desire or relationship strain.

Symptoms may be exacerbated during specific activities (e.g., intercourse, tampon insertion) or in certain positions.

Diagnosis

A thorough history and physical examination are critical for identifying the underlying cause of dyspareunia. The diagnostic approach includes:

1. History

Pain Characteristics: Onset, duration, location, intensity and quality (e.g., burning, sharp).

Sexual History: Timing (entry or deep), situational or generalized and impact on sexual function.

Gynecological History: Menstrual history, obstetric history, prior infections or surgeries.

Psychosocial History: History of trauma, stress or relationship status.

Medical History: Chronic conditions (e.g., diabetes, autoimmune disorders), medications or allergies.

2. Physical Examination

External Genital Examination: Inspect for erythema, lesions or atrophy. Perform a cotton swab test for vulvodynia (to assess vestibular tenderness).

Pelvic Examination: Assess for vaginal dryness, atrophy, or masses. Evaluate pelvic floor muscle tone for vaginismus.

Bimanual Examination: Palpate for uterine or adnexal tenderness, masses or adhesions.

Speculum Examination: Check for vaginal or cervical abnormalities, discharge or lesions.

3. Diagnostic Tests

Infection Screening: Vaginal swabs for microscopy, culture or PCR to rule out candidiasis, bacterial vaginosis or STIs.

Imaging: Pelvic ultrasound, MRI or CT to evaluate for masses, endometriosis or adhesions.

Laparoscopy: Considered for suspected endometriosis or pelvic pathology, if imaging is inconclusive.

Biopsy: For vulvar lesions or suspected dermatoses.

Psychological Assessment: Referral to a psychologist or counsellor, if psychogenic factors are suspected.

Differential Diagnosis

Vulvodynia

Vaginismus

Endometriosis

Pelvic inflammatory disease

Interstitial cystitis

Uterine fibroids

Ovarian cysts

Psychosexual disorders

Management

Management of dyspareunia is multidisciplinary and done according to the underlying cause. A stepwise approach includes:

1. General Measures

Patient Education: Discuss the condition, its causes and treatment options to reduce anxiety and improve compliance.

Lubricants and Moisturizers: Water-based or silicone-based lubricants for vaginal dryness; vaginal moisturizers for long-term hydration.

Sexual Counseling: Address relationship status or psychosexual issues with a therapist.

2. Medical Management

Hormonal Therapy: Topical or systemic oestrogen for vaginal atrophy in postmenopausal or postpartum women.

Antibiotics/Antifungals: Treat underlying infections (e.g., fluconazole for candidiasis, metronidazole for bacterial vaginosis).

Analgesics: Topical lidocaine or analgesics for vulvodynia.

Botulinum Toxin: For severe vaginismus to relax pelvic floor muscles.

Antidepressants or Anticonvulsants: Low-dose tricyclic antidepressants (e.g., amitriptyline) or gabapentin for neuropathic pain.

3. Surgical Management

Laparoscopy: For excision of endometriotic lesions or adhesiolysis.

Vestibulectomy: Rarely used for refractory provoked vestibulodynia.

Hysterectomy: Considered in severe cases of adenomyosis or fibroids, if conservative measures fail.

4. Physical Therapy

Pelvic floor physical therapy to address hypertonic muscles or vaginismus.

Dilator therapy to improve pelvic floor relaxation.

5. Psychological Therapy

Cognitive-behavioral therapy (CBT) for pain management or trauma-related dyspareunia.

Couples therapy to address relational factors.

6. Lifestyle Modifications

Avoid irritants (e.g., scented products, tight clothing).

Optimize sexual practices (e.g., adequate foreplay, position changes).

Prognosis

The prognosis depends on the underlying cause and the patient's response to treatment. Organic causes like infections or atrophy often resolve with targeted therapy, while chronic conditions like endometriosis or vulvodynia may require long-term management. Psychological factors can complicate recovery but respond well to multidisciplinary care.

Complications

Sexual dysfunction (e.g., low libido, arousal difficulties).

Relationship strain or marital discordance.

Chronic pelvic pain syndrome.

Psychological distress, including anxiety or depression.

Prevention

Regular gynecologic care to address infections or hormonal changes early.

Education on sexual health and safe practices.

Psychological support for individuals with a history of trauma.

8.7 Cysts & Neoplasm

(*Akyas wa salat*)

A vaginal cyst is a fluid-filled or semi-solid sac that forms on or within the vaginal wall. They are usually benign (non-cancerous) and often asymptomatic, but can sometimes cause discomfort or complications depending on their size, location or underlying cause.

Types of Vaginal Cysts

Vaginal cysts can vary based on their origin and location. The most common types include:

1. Bartholin's Gland Cysts

Location: Occur near the vaginal opening, within the Bartholin's glands, which are located on either side of the vaginal opening and produce lubricating fluid.

Cause: Develop when the gland's duct becomes blocked, causing fluid to accumulate.

Characteristics: Typically soft, painless and unilateral, but can become painful if infected (forming a Bartholin's abscess).

2. Gartner's Duct Cysts

Location: Found along the vaginal wall, often deeper within the tissue.

Cause: Arise from remnants of the Wolffian (mesonephric) ducts, which are embryonic structures that typically regress in females.

Characteristics: Usually asymptomatic and discovered incidentally during pelvic examinations.

3. Mullerian Cysts

Location: Can occur anywhere along the vaginal wall.

Cause: Develop from remnants of the Mullerian ducts, which form parts of the female reproductive system during fetal development.

Characteristics: Often filled with mucus and may vary in size.

4. Inclusion Cysts (Epidermal/Epithelial Inclusion Cysts).

Location: Typically on the vaginal surface or near the vaginal opening.

Cause: Result from trauma, such as childbirth or surgery, where epithelial tissue becomes trapped under the vaginal lining.

Characteristics: Small, firm and usually painless, unless irritated.

5. Sebaceous Cysts

Location: Found on the skin of the vulva or outer vaginal area.

Cause: Occur when sebaceous glands (oil-producing glands) become blocked.

Characteristics: Small, round and may contain cheesy or oily material.

6. Endometriotic Cysts (rare).

Location: Can form in the vaginal wall in cases of endometriosis.

Cause: Endometrial tissue grows abnormally outside the uterus, forming cysts.

Characteristics: May cause pain, especially during menstruation.

Causes and Risk Factors

Vaginal cysts typically develop due to:

1. Blockage of Glands or Ducts: Common in Bartholin's gland cysts, where fluid retention occurs due to obstruction.
2. Congenital Factors: Gartner's duct and Mullerian cysts arise from embryonic remnants.
3. Trauma or Injury: Childbirth, episiotomy or surgery can lead to inclusion cysts.
4. Infections: Infections in the Bartholin's gland (e.g., from bacteria like Escherichia coli or sexually transmitted infections like Gonorrhea or Chlamydia) can cause cyst formation or abscesses.
5. Endometriosis: Abnormal growth of endometrial tissue can lead to cysts.
6. Hormonal Changes: May influence gland activity, potentially contributing to cyst formation.

Risk Factors

History of vaginal trauma or surgery.

Sexually transmitted infections.

Endometriosis or pelvic inflammatory disease.

Pregnancy or childbirth.

Symptoms

Many vaginal cysts are asymptomatic and discovered during routine gynaecological examinations. When symptoms occur, they may include:

1. A palpable lump or mass in the vaginal area.
2. Discomfort or pain during sexual intercourse, walking or sitting.
3. Swelling or redness near the vaginal opening (especially with Bartholin's gland cysts).
4. Pain, if the cyst becomes infected or forms an abscess: Pressure or a feeling of fullness in the vaginal area.
5. In rare cases, difficulty in urinating or defecating, if the cyst is large.

Diagnosis

Diagnosing a vaginal cyst typically involves:

1. Medical History and Symptoms: Enquire symptoms, medical history and any recent trauma or infections.

2. Pelvic Examination: A physical examination to locate and assess the cyst's size, texture and tenderness.

3. Imaging

Ultrasound: Used to visualize the cyst's size, location and contents (fluid-filled vs. solid).

MRI/CT Scan: Rarely needed, but used for complex or deep cysts to rule out other conditions.

4. Biopsy or Aspiration: If there's suspicion of malignancy (rare), a sample of the cyst's contents or tissue may be examined.

5. Culture Testing: If infection is suspected, a swab of the cyst fluid may be tested to identify the causative organism.

Treatment

Treatment depends on the cyst's type, size, symptoms and whether it's infected. Options include:

1. Observation

Asymptomatic, small cysts (especially Gartner's duct or inclusion cysts) may not require treatment and are monitored for changes.

2. Small, non-infected cysts

Warm Compresses or Sitz Baths: Soaking the area in warm water several times a day can promote drainage and reduce discomfort, especially for Bartholin's gland cysts.

Pain Relief: Analgesics (e.g., ibuprofen) for mild discomfort.

3. Medical Interventions

Antibiotics: Prescribed if the cyst is infected or an abscess is present.

Drainage: For large or painful Bartholin's gland cysts, perform a minor procedure to drain the cyst, often under local anaesthesia.

Marsupialization: A surgical technique where the cyst is opened and stitched to create a permanent drainage pathway, commonly used for recurrent Bartholin's gland cysts.

Catheter Insertion: A small catheter (e.g., Word catheter) may be inserted into a Bartholin's gland cyst for several weeks to allow continuous drainage and prevent recurrence.

4. Surgical Removal

Indicated for large, persistent or symptomatic cysts (e.g., Gartner's duct or Mullerian cysts).

Complete removal of the Bartholin's gland (rare) may be considered for recurrent infections or cysts.

5. Specific Treatment

Endometriotic cysts may require hormonal therapy or management of endometriosis.

Infections caused by STIs require specific antibiotic or antiviral treatment.

Complications

While most vaginal cysts are benign, potential complications include:

1. Infection: Leading to abscess formation, which is painful and may require urgent treatment.
2. Recurrence: Common with Bartholin's gland cysts, if the underlying duct obstruction isn't resolved.
3. Pain or Discomfort: Large cysts can interfere with daily activities or sexual intercourse.
4. Rare Malignant Transformation: Extremely rare, but cysts with unusual features (e.g., solid components) may need evaluation for cancer.

Prevention

While not all vaginal cysts can be prevented, some strategies may reduce the risk:

1. Practice good hygiene to prevent infections.
2. Use protection during sexual activity to reduce the risk of STIs.
3. Seek prompt treatment for vaginal infections or trauma.
4. Regular check-ups to detect asymptomatic cysts early.

Prognosis

Most vaginal cysts are benign and resolve with minimal intervention or no treatment. Symptomatic or infected cysts often respond well to drainage, antibiotics or surgery. Recurrence is possible, particularly with Bartholin's gland cysts, but proper management reduces this risk.

Vaginal Neoplasms

Definition

Vaginal neoplasms refer to abnormal growths or tumours arising from the vaginal tissue, which may be benign, premalignant or malignant. Primary vaginal neoplasms are rare, accounting for approximately 1–2% of all gynecologic malignancies, while secondary (metastatic) tumours are more common. These tumours can originate from the vaginal epithelium, connective tissue or other structures and may present significant diagnostic and therapeutic challenges.

Epidemiology

Primary vaginal neoplasm: Constitutes 1–3% of gynecologic cancers, with an incidence of approximately 0.7 per 100,000 women annually.

Age distribution: Most common in postmenopausal women (peak incidence: 60–70 years), though certain subtypes (e.g., rhabdomyosarcoma) occur in paediatric populations.

Risk factors

Human papillomavirus (HPV) infection (particularly high-risk strains 16 and 18) for squamous cell carcinoma.

History of cervical or vulvar intraepithelial neoplasia or cancer.

In utero exposure to diethylstilbesterol (DES) for clear cell adenocarcinoma.

Chronic vaginal irritation or immunosuppression (e.g., HIV, organ transplantation).

Smoking and low socioeconomic status increase risk for squamous cell carcinoma.

Classification

Vaginal neoplasms are classified based on their origin (primary vs. secondary) and histological type.

1. Benign Neoplasms

Vaginal cysts: Gartner's duct cysts, Mullerian cysts or inclusion cysts.

Fibroepithelial polyps: Benign growths of connective tissue and epithelium.

Leiomyomas: Rare, benign smooth muscle tumours.

Haemangiomas: Vascular tumours, typically congenital.

Endometriosis: Ectopic endometrial tissue causing cystic or nodular lesions.

2. Vaginal intraepithelial neoplasia (VAIN)

Dysplastic changes in the vaginal epithelium, graded as VAIN 1 (mild), VAIN 2 (moderate), or VAIN 3 (severe/carcinoma in situ). Strongly associated with HPV infection.

3. Malignant Neoplasms

Primary vaginal cancers

1. Squamous cell carcinoma (SCC): Most common (80–90% of cases), linked to HPV and chronic irritation.
2. Adenocarcinoma: Rare (5–10%), includes clear cell adenocarcinoma (DES-related) and endometrioid types.
3. Melanoma: Extremely rare (2–5%), arising from vaginal melanocytes.
4. Sarcomas: Leiomyosarcoma or embryonal rhabdomyosarcoma (sarcoma botryoides, common in children).
5. Small cell carcinoma: Rare, aggressive neuroendocrine tumour.

Secondary (metastatic) cancers: More common than primary cancers, originating from:

Cervix, endometrium or ovary (via direct extension or lymphatic spread).

Distant sites (e.g., breast, colon or lung) via hematogenous spread.

Etiology and Risk Factors

1. HPV infection: High-risk HPV strains (16, 18) are implicated in squamous cell carcinoma and VAIN.
2. DES exposure: Historical use of DES in pregnancy (1940s–1970s) is linked to clear cell adenocarcinoma in exposed offspring.
3. Prior gynecologic malignancy: History of cervical or vulvar cancer increases risk due to field cancerization or HPV-related multicentric disease.
4. Chronic irritation: Pessaries, prolapse or chronic vaginitis may predispose to squamous cell carcinoma.
5. Immunosuppression: HIV, immunosuppressive therapy or organ transplantation increases risk of HPV-related neoplasms.
6. Radiation history: Prior pelvic radiation for other cancers may induce secondary vaginal malignancies.
7. Genetic factors: Rare associations with Lynch syndrome (for adenocarcinoma) or Li-Fraumeni syndrome (for sarcomas).

Pathophysiology

Squamous cell carcinoma: Arises from the vaginal epithelium, often preceded by VAIN. HPV-driven oncogenesis involves E6 and E7 viral proteins, which inactivate p53 and Rb tumour suppressor genes, leading to uncontrolled cell proliferation.

Adenocarcinoma: Clear cell subtype is linked to DES-induced Mullerian anomalies, while endometrioid adenocarcinoma may arise from endometriosis or direct extension from the uterus.

Sarcomas: Embryonal rhabdomyosarcoma results from malignant transformation of mesenchymal cells, presenting as grape-like masses in young girls.

Metastatic tumours: Spread via direct extension (cervix, uterus), lymphatic channels or hematogenous routes, with the vagina acting as a common site for metastases due to its rich vascular and lymphatic supply.

Clinical Features

Symptoms

1. Vaginal bleeding: Postmenopausal bleeding, postcoital bleeding or irregular bleeding (most common presentation).
2. Vaginal discharge: Watery, bloody or foul-smelling discharge.
3. Pelvic pain: Due to local invasion or mass effect.
4. Dyspareunia: Painful intercourse, particularly with superficial lesions.
5. Urinary or bowel symptoms: Advanced tumours may cause urinary retention, frequency or constipation due to invasion of adjacent structures.
6. Asymptomatic: Early lesions or VAIN may be detected incidentally during routine gynaecological examinations.

Signs

1. Visible or palpable mass, ulcer or plaque on vaginal examination.
2. Friable, bleeding lesions in squamous cell carcinoma.
3. Grape-like masses in paediatric rhabdomyosarcoma.
4. Speculum exam may reveal abnormal vaginal mucosa or nodularity.

Diagnosis

Diagnosis requires a combination of clinical evaluation, imaging and histopathologic confirmation.

1. History

Detailed gynaecological history: Menstrual irregularities, prior HPV-related disease, DES exposure or radiation.

Risk factor assessment: Smoking, immunosuppression or prior gynecologic cancers.

Symptom review: Bleeding, discharge, pain or systemic symptoms (e.g., weight loss in advanced malignancy).

2. Physical Examination

Speculum examination: To visualize vaginal lesions, ulcers or masses.

Bimanual and rectovaginal examination: To assess tumour size, mobility and invasion into parametria or rectum.

Lymph node assessment: Inguinal and pelvic nodes for metastasis.

3. Investigations

Biopsy: Essential for histological diagnosis. Colposcopy-directed biopsy for VAIN or early lesions; excisional biopsy for larger tumours.

Colposcopy: To identify VAIN or early squamous cell carcinoma, often using acetic acid or Lugol's iodine to highlight abnormal areas.

Cytology: Vaginal or cervical Pap smear may detect VAIN or early malignancy but is less sensitive for advanced tumours.

Imaging

Pelvic MRI: Preferred for assessing tumour size, local invasion and lymph node involvement.

CT scan: To evaluate distant metastases (lungs, liver or bones).

PET-CT: For staging and detecting metastatic disease.

Cystoscopy/proctoscopy: To assess bladder or rectal involvement in advanced cases.

Tumour markers: Limited utility; CA-125 may be elevated in adenocarcinoma, SCC antigen in squamous cell carcinoma.

4. Staging

Vaginal cancer is staged using the FIGO (International Federation of Gynaecology and Obstetrics) system or TNM classification .

Stage I: Tumour confined to the vagina.

Stage II: Tumour invades paravaginal tissues but not pelvic sidewall.

Stage III: Tumour extends to pelvic sidewall or involves regional lymph nodes.

Stage IV: IVA (invasion of bladder/rectum) or IVB (distant metastases).

VAIN is graded as 1, 2 or 3 based on the depth of epithelial involvement.

Differential Diagnosis

Benign lesions: Vaginal cysts, polyps or condylomas.

Cervical cancer: May extend to the vagina, mimicking primary vaginal cancer.

Endometrial cancer: Direct extension or metastasis to the vagina.

Vulvar cancer: May involve the lower vagina.

Infections: Chronic vaginitis or herpes simplex virus lesions.

Endometriosis: May present as vaginal nodules or bleeding.

Metastatic tumours: From cervix, uterus, ovary or distant sites.

Management

Management depends on the tumour type, stage, patient age, fertility desires and comorbidities. Multidisciplinary care involving gynecologic oncologists, radiation oncologists and medical oncologists is essential.

1. Benign Neoplasms

Observation: For asymptomatic cysts or polyps.

Surgical excision: For symptomatic or enlarging lesions (e.g., fibroepithelial polyps, leiomyomas).

Laser or cryotherapy: For small, superficial benign lesions.

2. Vaginal Intraepithelial Neoplasia (VAIN)

VAIN 1/2: Observation with regular follow-up, as spontaneous regression is common.

VAIN 2/3

Topical therapies: 5-fluorouracil (5-FU) cream or imiquimod to induce local immune response.

Laser ablation: For localized lesions.

Surgical excision: Wide local excision for multifocal or recurrent VAIN.

Intravaginal radiation: Rarely used for refractory cases.

HPV vaccination may reduce recurrence risk in HPV-related VAIN.

3. Primary Vaginal Cancer

Early-stage (Stage I-II)

Radiation therapy: Primary treatment modality, combining external beam radiotherapy (EBRT) and brachytherapy to achieve local control.

Surgery: Limited role due to anatomical constraints. Wide local excision or partial vaginectomy for small, superficial tumours. Radical vaginectomy with pelvic lymphadenectomy is rarely performed.

Advanced-stage (Stage III–IV)

Chemoradiation: Concurrent cisplatin-based chemotherapy with EBRT and brachytherapy for improved outcomes.

Palliative therapy: For stage IVB, including systemic chemotherapy (e.g., cisplatin, 5-FU) or supportive care.

Special Cases

Clear cell adenocarcinoma: Surgery (radical hysterectomy/vaginectomy) may be considered in young patients, followed by adjuvant radiation.

Rhabdomyosarcoma: Multimodal therapy with chemotherapy (vincristine, actinomycin-D, cyclophosphamide), surgery and radiation for paediatric cases.

4. Metastatic Vaginal Tumours

Treatment focuses on the primary cancer (e.g., cervical, endometrial).

Palliative radiation or chemotherapy for symptomatic vaginal metastases.

5. Follow-Up

Regular pelvic exams, imaging and Pap smears every 3–6 months for 2 years, then annually.

Monitor for recurrence, particularly in the vagina, pelvis or distant sites.

Address long-term side effects of radiation (e.g., vaginal stenosis, sexual dysfunction).

Complications

Treatment-related

Radiation: Vaginal stenosis, fistulae (vesicovaginal, rectovaginal), or chronic pelvic pain.

Surgery: Sexual dysfunction, urinary incontinence or lymphedema.

Chemotherapy: Myelosuppression, neuropathy or renal toxicity.

Disease-related

Local invasion: Bladder, rectal or pelvic sidewall involvement.

Metastasis: Lungs, liver or bones in advanced stages.

Psychosocial impact: Sexual dysfunction, body image issues or emotional distress.

Prognosis

Benign tumours: Excellent prognosis with surgical removal or observation.

VAIN: High cure rates with early intervention; recurrence risk is 10–20% with HPV-related lesions.

Primary vaginal cancer

Stage I: 5-year survival rate ~70–85%.

Stage II: ~50–60%.

Stage III-IV: < 30%, with poor prognosis in metastatic disease.

Histology-specific: Clear cell adenocarcinoma and rhabdomyosarcoma have better outcomes with multimodal therapy in young patients.

Metastatic tumours: Prognosis depends on the primary cancer and extent of spread.

Prevention

HPV vaccination: Reduces risk of HPV-related squamous cell carcinoma and VAIN.

Screening: Routine Pap smears and HPV testing to detect VAIN or early cancers.

DES exposure counselling: For women with in utero exposure, regular gynaecological examinations.

Smoking cessation: Reduces risk of squamous cell carcinoma.

Management of chronic irritation: Prompt treatment of vaginitis or prolapse.

Long Answer Questions

1. Classify vaginal diseases, describe the clinical features and treatment of vaginitis.
2. Discuss the etiology, diagnosis and management of vaginal infections including candidiasis and trichomoniasis.
3. Explain the causes and treatment of atrophic vaginitis in postmenopausal women.
4. Describe congenital anomalies of the vagina and their clinical implications.
5. Elaborate on the diagnostic approach to abnormal vaginal discharge.

Short Answer Questions

1. What is bacterial vaginosis?
2. Name two symptoms of vaginal candidiasis.
3. Define atrophic vaginitis.
4. Mention one cause of vaginal ulceration.
5. What is the normal vaginal pH in reproductive-age women?

Multiple Choice Questions (1 Mark Each)

1. Common fungal cause of vaginitis:

a) Trichomonas b) Candida albicans c) Gonococcus d) Chlamydia

Ans: b) Candida albicans

2. Vaginal pH in healthy reproductive-age women is:

a) 3.5–4.5 b) 5.5–6.5 c) 6.5–7.5 d) 7.5–8.5

Ans: a) 3.5–4.5

3. Fishy odor in vaginal discharge suggests:

a) Candidiasis b) Bacterial vaginosis c) Trichomoniasis d) Herpes

Ans: b) Bacterial vaginosis

4. Curdy white discharge with itching is characteristic of:

a) Trichomoniasis b) Gonorrhea c) Candidiasis d) Chlamydia

Ans: c) Candidiasis

5. Which test is used to detect clue cells?

a) Wet mount b) Gram stain c) KOH prep d) Pap smear

Ans: a) Wet mount

6. Atrophic vaginitis is commonly seen in:

a) Adolescents b) Pregnancy c) Postmenopausal women d) Menstruating women

Ans: c) Postmenopausal women

7. Trichomoniasis presents with:

a) Frothy green discharge b) Curdy white discharge c) Bloody discharge d) No discharge

Ans: a) Frothy green discharge

8. Which of the following is NOT a cause of vaginitis?

a) Candida b) Trichomonas c) HPV d) Gardnerella

Ans: c) HPV

9. Congenital absence of vagina is called:

a) Vaginal atresia b) Vaginal stenosis c) Vaginal agenesis d) Imperforate hymen

Ans: c) Vaginal agenesis

10. Which condition may present with vaginal ulceration?

a) Herpes simplex b) Candidiasis c) Bacterial vaginosis d) Fibroid

Ans: a) Herpes simplex

09

Diseases of Uterus

(Amrad al-Rahim)

9.1 *Su Mizaj-i-Rahim* (Abnormal Temperament of Uterus)
9.2 *Iltihab-I' Unuq-i-Rahim* (Cervicitis)
9.3 *Ta'akkul unuq-i-Rahim* (Cervical Erosion)
9.4 *Iltihabe-i-Rahim* (Inflammation of Uterus)
9.5 *Maylan-al-Rahim/Eujaj-al-Rahim* (Displacement of Uterus)
9.6 *Inzilaq-i-Rahim/ Khuruj-i-Rahim* (Prolapse of Uterus)
9.7 *Inqilab-i-Raahim* (Inversion of Uterus)
9.8 *Rahmi daroon-i-rahmiyat/Uzal-i-Guddi* (Adenomyosis)
9.9 *Bawasir-al-Rahim* (Polyps of Uterus)
9.10 *Akyas wa Sal'at* (Cysts & Neopalsm)

Learning Objective (At the end of the session, the students should be able to)

Interpret *Su-e-Mizaj-e-Rahim* (Abnormal Temperament of Uterus) & explore its management.
Describe the causes, types, diagnosis, management and complications of *Iltihab-e-Unaq-Ur-Rahim* (Cervicitis).
Discuss the causes, diagnosis and management of *Taakkul- Unaq-Ur-Rahim* (Cervical Erosion / Ectopy).
Explain the causes, types, diagnosis, management and complications of *Iltihab-e-Rahim* (Inflammation of the Uterus).
Describe the causes, diagnosis, management and complications of *Mailan wa Aujaj-Ur-Rahim* (Displacement of Uterus) & *Inzalaq-e-Rahim/ Khurooj-e-Rahim* (Prolapse of Uterus).
Demonstrate gradation of Uterine Prolapse.
Describe the causes, diagnosis & complications of *Inqilab-e- Rahim* (Inversion of Uterus).
Describe & demonstrate pelvic floor exercises to patients.
Perform & demonstrate the technique of Pessary Insertion.
Describe & discuss the causes, diagnosis, management and complications of *Daroon–e-Rehmiyat* (Adenomyosis).
Describe the causes, types, diagnosis, management and complications of *Bawaseer ur Rahim* (Polyp of Uterus).
Observe and describe Polypectomy.
Explain briefly the causes, stages, diagnosis and complications of *Daweera & Sulaat* (Cysts & Neoplasm).

9.1 Abnormal Temperament of Uterus

(*Su Mizaj-i-Rahim*)

The Unani system of medicine, also known as Greco-Arabic medicine, is a holistic healing tradition rooted in the teachings of Greek physicians like Hippocrates (460–370 BC) and Galen (129–200 CE), further developed by Arab and Persian scholars such as Avicenna (Ibn Sina, 980–1037 CE) and Rhazes (Al-Razi, 854–925 CE). It is widely practiced in South Asia, particularly in India, and emphasizes the balance of four humors (*Akhlat*)-blood (*Dam*), phlegm (*Balgham*), yellow bile (*Safra*), and black bile (*Sauda*)-and their corresponding temperaments (*Mizaj*) to maintain health. The uterus, as a vital organ, is subject to temperamental imbalances that contribute to various gynaecological disorders.

Concept of Temperament (*Mizaj*) in Unani Medicine

Temperament (*Mizaj*) is a foundational concept in Unani medicine, describing the unique physical, psychological and physiological characteristics of an individual or organ, determined by the balance of four elements (*Arkan*)—fire (hot and dry), air (hot and moist), water (cold and moist) and earth (cold and dry). These elements combine to produce four temperaments:

Sanguine (*Damavi*): Hot and moist, associated with blood.

Phlegmatic (*Balghami*): Cold and moist, associated with phlegm.

Choleric (*Safravi*): Hot and dry, associated with yellow bile.

Melancholic (*Saudavi*): Cold and dry, associated with black bile.

Each organ, including the uterus, has its own temperament, which is typically balanced (*Mizaj-e-Mu'tadil*) for optimal function. The uterus is considered to have a cold and moist temperament in its normal state, conducive to its reproductive functions, such as menstruation, gestation and parturition. An imbalance in this temperament, termed *Su'-i-Mizaj Rahim* (abnormal uterine temperament), leads to gynaecological disorders.

Abnormal Uterine Temperament (*Su'-i-Mizaj Rahim*)

Abnormal uterine temperament occurs when the uterus deviates from its balanced state due to qualitative or quantitative changes in humors or external factors. These imbalances are classified into:

1. Simple Imbalance (*Su'-i-Mizaj Sada*): Alteration in the quality of the uterine temperament without accumulation of abnormal humors (e.g., excessive heat, coldness, dryness or moisture).
2. Material Imbalance (*Su'-i-Mizaj Maddi*): Accumulation of pathological humors (e.g., phlegm, bile) in the uterus, altering its function.
3. Compound Imbalance: Combination of simple and material imbalances, leading to complex disorders.

The four types of abnormal uterine temperament are:

1. Hot and Dry (*Har Yabis)*: Excessive heat and dryness, often linked to dominance of yellow bile (Safra).
2. Hot and Moist (*Har Ratab*): Excessive heat and moisture, associated with blood (*Dam*).
3. Cold and Dry (*Barid Yabis*): Excessive coldness and dryness, linked to black bile (*Sauda*).

4. Cold and Moist (*Barid Ratab*): Excessive coldness and moisture, associated with phlegm (*Balgham*).

Etiology of Abnormal Uterine Temperament

According to Unani scholars, abnormal uterine temperament results from:

1. Dominance of Humors (*Ghalaba-i-Akhlat*): Excessive production or retention of one humor (e.g., phlegm in cold and moist temperament) disrupts uterine function. For example, dominance of phlegm (*Balgham*) may cause viscosity of menstrual blood, leading to amenorrhea. (https://www.academia.edu/40887421/Gynaecological_Disorders_in_the_light_of_Unani_System_of_Medicine)
2. Weakness of Uterine Faculties (*Du'fe Quwwat-i-Rahim*): Impairment in the uterus's digestive (*Hadima*), retentive (Masika), or expulsive (*Dafi'a*) faculties, leading to conditions like leucorrhoea or infertility. (https://onlinelibrary.wiley.com/doi/10.1155/2022/5718501)
3. External Factors (*Asbab-e-Sittah Zaruriyyah)*: Imbalances in the six essential factors of health:
    a. Air (*Hawa*): Poor environmental conditions.
    b. Food and Drink (*Makool-wo-Mashroob*): Inappropriate diet (e.g., cold, heavy foods promoting phlegm).
    c. Bodily Movement and Repose (*Harkat-wo-Sukoon-e-Jismiah*): Sedentary lifestyle or excessive exertion.
    d. Mental Work and Rest (*Harkat-wo-Sukoon Nafsaniah*): Stress, anxiety, or emotional disturbances.
    e. Sleep and Wakefulness: Insomnia or excessive sleep.
    f. Retention and Excretion (*Ehtabaas wa Istafraagh*): Retention of waste (e.g., constipation) or excessive purging. (https://www.britannica.com/science/Unanimedicine) (https://ayush.delhi.gov.in/ayush/unani)
    g. Psychological Factors: Anger, stress or sudden shocks, which may exacerbate uterine disorders like hysteria (*Ikhtinaq-ur-Rahim*). (https://www.ncbi.nlm.nih.gov/pmc/articles/PMC5217817/)
    h. Uterine Structural Abnormalities: Displacement, inflammation (*Waram-e-Rahim*) or congenital deformities.
    i. Infections: Reproductive tract infections, such as metritis (*Waram-e-Rahim*) or vaginitis (*Waram-e-Mahbil*), which alter temperament. (https://onlinelibrary.wiley.com/doi/10.1155/2022/5718501)
    j. Lifestyle Factors: Obesity, which is associated with cold and wet temperament, or excessive fatigue. (https://pubmed.ncbi.nlm.nih.gov/33977688/)

Associated Gynecological Disorders

Abnormal uterine temperament is implicated in various gynaecological conditions described in Unani literature:

1. Amenorrhea (*Ihtibas-e-Tamth*): Often linked to cold and wet temperament due to phlegm dominance, causing viscous menstrual blood and obstruction (*Sudda*). (https://pubmed.ncbi.nlm.nih.gov/33977688/)(https://www.academia.edu/40887421/Gynaecological_Disorders_in_the_light_of_Unani_System_of_Medicine)

2. Dysmenorrhea (*Usr-e-Tamth*): Associated with temperamental changes (e.g., cold or dry temperament) leading to painful menstruation due to cervical obstruction or humor imbalance. (https://www.researchgate.net/publication/302588238_Diagnostic_and_Management_of_Dysmenorrhea_in_Unani_GreekoArab_System_of_Medicine)

3. Leucorrhoea (*Sailan-ur-Rahim*): Caused by weakness of uterine faculties or abnormal humor accumulation (e.g., phlegm or blood), leading to excessive vaginal discharge (white, yellow, red, or black). (https://www.academia.edu/40887421/Gynaecological_Disorders_in_the_light_of_Unani_System_of_Medicine)

4. Menorrhagia (*Kasrat-e-Haiz*): Linked to hot and moist temperament, causing excessive menstrual bleeding due to blood humor dominance. (https://www.academia.edu/40887421/Gynaecological_Disorders_in_the_light_of_Unani_System_of_Medicine)

5. Infertility (*Uqr*): Resulting from temperamental imbalances (e.g., cold and dry or hot and dry) affecting uterine receptivity or ovum quality. (https://www.researchgate.net/publication/336969493_Gynaecological_Disorders_in_the_light_of_Unani_System_of_Medicine)

6. Polycystic Ovarian Disease (PCOD): Associated with phlegmatic temperament and obesity, leading to anovulation and menstrual irregularities due to phlegm-induced viscosity. (https://www.academia.edu/40887421/Gynaecological_Disorders_in_the_light_of_Unani_System_of_Medicine)

7. Hysteria (*Ikhtinaq-ur-Rahim*): Historically attributed to uterine dysfunction, involving the heart and brain, often linked to cold temperament or retained humors (e.g., seminal fluid, putrefied matter). Symptoms include a sensation of an "air ball" rising from the pelvis (*Bao-Gola*). (https://www.ncbi.nlm.nih.gov/pmc/articles/PMC5217817/)

8. Uterine Tumours (*Sul'ah-ur-Rahim*): May arise from chronic humor imbalances, particularly melancholic (cold and dry) temperament. (https://www.researchgate.net/publication/336969493_Gynaecological_Disorders_in_the_light_of_Unani_System_of_Medicine)

9. Hydrometra (*Isthasqa-ur-Rahim*): Fluid accumulation in the uterus due to cold and moist temperament. (https://www.researchgate.net/publication/336969493_Gynaecological_Disorders_in_the_light_of_Unani_System_of_Medicine)

Pathophysiology

In Unani medicine, the uterus's normal cold and moist temperament supports its functions of menstruation, conception and gestation. Abnormal temperament disrupts these functions:

1. Hot and Dry Temperament: Excessive yellow bile (*Safra*) causes inflammation (*Waram-e-Rahim),* irritation, or excessive menstrual flow (menorrhagia). It may lead to conditions like vaginitis or metritis.
2. Hot and Moist Temperament: Blood humor (*Dam*) dominance results in hyperemia, leading to menorrhagia or prolonged bleeding.
3. Cold and Dry Temperament: Black bile (*Sauda*) accumulation causes uterine atrophy, dryness or infertility due to reduced receptivity.
4. Cold and Moist Temperament: Phlegm (*Balgham*) dominance increases viscosity of uterine secretions or menstrual blood, leading to amenorrhea, leucorrhoea or PCOD. (https://onlinelibrary.wiley.com/doi/10.1155/2022/5718501)[](https://pubmed.ncbi.nlm.nih.gov/33977688/)

The uterus's faculties (*Quwa*) are also affected:

Digestive Faculty (*Quwwat-i-Hadima*): Impaired digestion of nutrients in the uterus leads to abnormal discharge or humor accumulation.

Retentive Faculty (*Quwwat-i-Masika*): Weak retention causes miscarriage or infertility.

Expulsive Faculty (*Quwwat-i-Dafi'a*): Impaired expulsion results in retained menstrual blood or products of conception, contributing to amenorrhea or dysmenorrhea. (https://onlinelibrary.wiley.com/doi/10.1155/2022/5718501)

Clinical Features

Symptoms of abnormal uterine temperament vary depending on the type of imbalance and associated disorder:

Hot and Dry

Painful menstruation (dysmenorrhea).

Scanty, dark menstrual blood.

Vaginal irritation or pruritus (*Hikkat-ul-Farj*).

Pelvic pain or inflammation signs (e.g., warmth, redness).

Hot and Moist

Heavy or prolonged menstrual bleeding (menorrhagia).

Bright red vaginal discharge.

Systemic symptoms like fever or flushing.

Cold and Dry

Amenorrhea or oligomenorrhea.

Infertility or recurrent miscarriage.

Dryness of vaginal mucosa.

Cold and Moist

Excessive vaginal discharge (leucorrhoea, white or yellow).

Amenorrhea or irregular cycles.

Pelvic heaviness or bloating.

Associated obesity or sluggish metabolism. (https://onlinelibrary.wiley.com/doi/10.1155/2022/5718501)[](https://pubmed.ncbi.nlm.nih.gov/33977688/)

Hysteria (*Ikhtinaq-ur-Rahim*)

Sensation of an "air ball" rising from the pelvis (*Bao-Gola*).

Choking sensation (*Ikhtinaq-ur-Rahim*).

Anxiety, fainting, or seizures resembling epilepsy. (https://www.ncbi.nlm.nih.gov/pmc/articles/PMC5217817/)

General Symptoms

Fatigue, emotional disturbances (e.g., anxiety, depression).

Digestive issues (e.g., constipation, flatulence).

Systemic effects of humor imbalance (e.g., pallor in phlegmatic temperament, jaundice in bilious temperament).

Diagnosis

Diagnosis in Unani medicine relies on assessing the patient's general and uterine temperament, humor balance and clinical symptoms. Key diagnostic methods include:

1. History and Clinical Assessment

Menstrual history (e.g., regularity, volume, pain).

Associated symptoms (e.g., vaginal discharge, infertility, psychological symptoms).

Evaluation of lifestyle factors (*Asbab-e-Sittah Zaruriyyah*).

Risk factors: Obesity, stress or poor diet.

2. Pulse Examination (*Nabz)*

Pulse characteristics reflect humor dominance (e.g., rapid pulse in hot temperament, slow in cold temperament).

3. Urine and Stool Analysis (Baul and *Baraz*)

Urine: Color, consistency and sediments indicate humor imbalance (e.g., thick, white urine in phlegmatic temperament).

Stool: Constipation or abnormal consistency suggests humor retention.

4. Physical Examination

Assess complexion, body habitus and emotional state to determine general temperament.

Pelvic examination for uterine size, position or discharge.

5. Temperament Assessment

Qualitative and quantitative evaluation of uterine temperament using standardized questionnaires or clinical signs (e.g., hotness/coldness, wetness/dryness).

Correlation with general body temperament (e.g., cold and wet temperament linked to amenorrhea). (https://pubmed.ncbi.nlm.nih.gov/33977688/) (https://www.ncbi.nlm.nih.gov/pmc/articles/PMC7187550/)

6. Modern Adjuncts

Transvaginal ultrasound to assess uterine size, endometrial thickness or ovarian pathology (e.g., PCOD).

Laboratory tests to rule out infections or hormonal imbalances, though not traditionally part of Unani diagnostics.

Management

Unani treatment aims to restore the uterus's normal temperament (cold and moist) by correcting humor imbalances and addressing underlying causes. The principle of treatment is *Ilaj-bil-Zid*, where drugs or interventions with opposite temperament are used to counteract the abnormality. Treatment modalities include: (https://onlinelibrary.wiley.com/doi/10.1155/2022/5718501)

1. Dietotherapy (*Ilaj-bil-Ghiza*)

According to the patient's temperament and condition:

Hot and Dry Temperament: Cool and moist foods (e.g., cucumber, watermelon, barley water).

Hot and Moist Temperament: Dry and cool foods (e.g., lentils, pomegranate).

Cold and Dry Temperament: Hot and moist foods (e.g., dates, almonds, warm milk).

Cold and Moist Temperament: Hot and dry foods (e.g., ginger, cinnamon, honey). (https://www.researchgate.net/publication/321386220_FUNDAMENTALS_OF_UNANI_SYSTEM_OF_MEDICINE-A_REVIEW)

Avoid foods that exacerbate humor imbalance (e.g., heavy, cold foods in phlegmatic conditions).

2. Pharmacotherapy (*Ilaj-bil-Dawa*)

Single Drugs

Myrrh (Commiphora myrrha): Used for amenorrhea, leucorrhoea and uterine tumours due to its hot and dry properties. (https://www.researchgate.net/publication/336969493_Gynaecological_Disorders_in_the_light_of_Unani_System_of_Medicine)

Miswak (Salvadora persica): Anti-inflammatory, used for vaginal infections.

Clove (Syzygium aromaticum): Hot, used for cold temperament disorders.

Amla (Emblica officinalis): Cold, used for hot temperament conditions.

Compound Formulations

1. *Sufoof-e-Sailan:* Polyherbal powder for leucorrhoea, containing dry and astringent herbs. (https://www.academia.edu/40887421/Gynaecological_Disorders_in_the_light_of_Unani_System_of_Medicine)
2. *Majoon-e-Falasafa*: Hot and dry temperament, used for phlegmatic disorders like amenorrhea. (https://www.researchgate.net/publication/322655260_Introduction_and_Principles_of_Unani_Medicine)
3. *Khamira*: General tonic for vital organs, used in hysteria or weakness-related disorders. (https://www.researchgate.net/publication/340444054_Determination_of_Human_Temperament_Mizaj-e-Insani_An_Overview_of_the_Theory_and_Practice_of_Unani_Medicine)

Dosage forms: Decoctions, powders (*Sufoof),* pastes (*Majoon*) or oils for local application.

3. Regimental Therapy (*Ilaj-bil-Tadbeer*)

a. *Nutool* (Irrigation): Pouring herbal decoctions (e.g., chamomile, myrrh) over the pelvic region to correct temperament or disperse toxic humors. (https://www.researchgate.net/

publication/340444054_Determination_of_Human_Temperament_Mizaj-e-Insani_An_Overview_of_the_Theory_and_Practice_of_Unani_Medicine)

b. *Hijama* (Cupping): Used to remove excess humors, particularly in hot or bilious temperaments.
c. *Fasd* (Venesection): Rarely used, for excess humor accumulation (e.g., blood in menorrhagia).
d. Massage (*Dalk*): With hot oils (e.g., sesame oil) for cold temperament disorders.
e. Exercise: Moderate physical activity to improve circulation and expel excess humors.

4. Surgery (*Ilaj-bil-Yad*)

Reserved for structural abnormalities (e.g., uterine tumours, severe prolapse) when other treatments fail. (https://www.researchgate.net/publication/321386220_FUNDAMENTALS_OF_UNANI_SYSTEM_OF_MEDICINE-A_REVIEW)

5. Lifestyle Modifications

Address *Asbab-e-Sittah Zaruriyyah*: Ensure clean air, balanced sleep, stress management and regular excretion (e.g., treat constipation). (https://www.britannica.com/science/Unani-medicine)

Psychological support for hysteria or stress-related disorders.

6. Management of Specific Conditions

a. Amenorrhea: Hot and dry drugs (e.g., saffron, cinnamon) to expel viscous phlegm. (https://pubmed.ncbi.nlm.nih.gov/33977688/)
b. Dysmenorrhea: Analgesic herbs (e.g., fennel, chamomile) and heat/ diathermy therapies to relieve obstruction. (https://www.researchgate.net/publication/302588238_Diagnostic_and_Management_of_Dysmenorrhea_in_Unani_GreekoArab_System_of_Medicine)
c. Leucorrhoea: Astringent and dry drugs (e.g., Acacia nilotica, *Sufoof-e-Sailan*). (https://www.academia.edu/40887421/Gynaecological_Disorders_in_the_light_of_Unani_System_of_Medicine)
d. Infertility: Drugs to correct uterine temperament (e.g., hot and moist for cold and dry uterus) and improve ovulation. (https://www.ncbi.nlm.nih.gov/pmc/articles/PMC7187550/)
e. Hysteria: Sedative drugs (e.g., valerian) and psychological counselling to address emotional triggers. (https://www.ncbi.nlm.nih.gov/pmc/articles/PMC5217817/)

Complications

Chronic Gynecological Disorders: Untreated temperament imbalances may lead to persistent amenorrhea, infertility or recurrent infections.

Malignant Transformation: Chronic humor imbalances, particularly melancholic (cold and dry), may contribute to uterine tumours or endometrial hyperplasia, increasing cancer risk. (https://www.ncbi.nlm.nih.gov/books/NBK470297/)

Systemic Effects: Humor imbalances may affect other organs (e.g., heart, brain in hysteria), causing symptoms like seizures or depression. (https://www.ncbi.nlm.nih.gov/pmc/articles/PMC5217817/)

Infertility and Pregnancy Complications: Abnormal temperament may lead to anovulation, miscarriage or obstetric issues. (https://www.ncbi.nlm.nih.gov/pmc/articles/PMC7187550/)

Prognosis

Favorable: Early correction of temperament through diet, lifestyle and pharmacotherapy often resolves symptoms, especially in simple imbalances.

Recurrent: Humoral imbalances or chronic conditions (e.g., PCOD, uterine tumours) require prolonged treatment and may recur.

Poor: Advanced structural abnormalities or malignant transformation have a worse prognosis, requiring surgical intervention.

Prevention

Maintain *Asbab-e-Sittah Zaruriyyah*: Balanced diet, exercise, sleep and emotional well-being to prevent humor imbalances. (https://www.britannica.com/science/Unani-medicine)

Dietary Management: Advise diet according to individual temperament (e.g., avoid cold, heavy foods in phlegmatic individuals).

Regular Excretion: Treat constipation or urinary retention to prevent humor accumulation.

Screening in High-Risk Groups: Women with obesity, PCOS or stress-related disorders should be monitored for temperamental changes. (https://pubmed.ncbi.nlm.nih.gov/33977688/)

Drugs Prophylaxis: Use tonics (e.g., Khamira) to strengthen uterine faculties and maintain temperament balance. (https://www.researchgate.net/publication/340444054_Determination_of_Human_Temperament_Mizaj-e-Insani_An_Overview_of_the_Theory_and_Practice_of_Unani_Medicine)

Key Points

1. The organ uterus in a female has cold and moist temperament; abnormal temperament (*Su'-i-Mizaj Rahim*) results from humor imbalances or external factors.
2. Common types of abnormal temperament include hot and dry, hot and moist, cold and dry and cold and moist, each linked to specific gynaecological disorders.
3. Common disorders include amenorrhea, dysmenorrhea, leucorrhoea, menorrhagia, infertility, PCOD and hysteria, with cold and moist temperament prevalent in conditions like amenorrhea and PCOD.
4. Diagnosis involves assessing general and uterine temperament through history, pulse, urine/stool analysis and clinical signs, supplemented by modern tools like ultrasound.
5. Treatment follows the *Ilaj-bil-Zid* principle, using dietotherapy, pharmacotherapy (single and compound drugs), regimental therapies (e.g., *Nutool*, *Hijama*), and lifestyle modifications.
6. Prevention emphasizes balancing the six essential factors (*Asbab-e-Sittah Zaruriyyah*) and interventions according to the patient's temperament.
7. Unani medicine offers a holistic approach, integrating physical, psychological and environmental factors, but requires further research to standardize temperament assessment and validate treatments.

Patient Presents with Uterine Symptoms

↓

History Taking

(Menstrual pattern, pain, fertility, discharge)

↓

Physical Examination

(Bimanual palpation, speculum exam)

↓

Initial Investigations:

↓ ↓ ↓

USG Pelvis CBC & Hormones Endometrial Biopsy

↓

Identify Likely Condition:

↓

Fibroid → Enlarged, firm uterus

Endometriosis → Dysmenorrhea, infertility

AUB → Irregular bleeding, hormonal imbalance

Endometrial CA → Postmenopausal bleeding

↓

Confirm Diagnosis → Begin Targeted Treatment

9.2 Cervicitis

(Iltihab-i[1]Unuq-i-Rahim)

Definition

Cervicitis is the inflammation of columnar epithelium of the uterine endocervix, sometimes termed endocervicitis, can be acute, often caused by infections, or chronic, defined as cervicitis lasting 3 months or longer, which is typically linked to non-infectious sources. Cervicitis is a significant gynaecological entity due to its potential to cause discomfort, complications and its association with sexually transmitted infections (STIs).

Etiology

Cervicitis can result from infectious or non-infectious causes:

1. Infectious Causes

Bacterial

Chlamydia trachomatis: The most common cause, often asymptomatic but can lead to mucopurulent cervicitis.

Neisseria gonorrhoeae: Causes purulent or mucopurulent cervical discharge.

Mycoplasma genitalium: Emerging as a significant cause of non-gonococcal, non-chlamydial cervicitis.

Bacterial vaginosis: Associated organisms (e.g., Gardnerella vaginalis): May contribute to cervicitis in some cases.

Viral

Herpes simplex virus (HSV): Typically presents with painful cervical ulcerations or vesicles.

Human papillomavirus (HPV): May cause chronic inflammation, though more commonly associated with cervical dysplasia.

Other Pathogens

Trichomonas vaginalis

Rarely, Treponema pallidum (syphilis) or Candida species.

2. Non-Infectious Causes

Chemical irritants (e.g., douches, spermicides, or latex condoms).

Mechanical irritation (e.g., tampons, cervical caps or pessaries).

Allergic reactions to contraceptives or hygiene products.

Systemic inflammatory conditions (e.g., autoimmune disorders).

Cervical trauma or foreign bodies.

Epidemiology

The exact prevalence of cervicitis is difficult to determine due to the lack of a standard definition, underdiagnosis due to lack of symptoms. Cervicitis is prevalent among sexually active women, particularly those aged 15–25 years, due to higher rates of STIs.

Risk factors include:

Multiple sexual partners or a partner with an STI.

Unprotected sexual intercourse.

History of STIs.

Use of intrauterine devices (IUDs) or other cervical interventions.

Poor hygiene practices or use of irritating vaginal products.

Chronic cervicitis is more common in multiparous women or those with a history of cervical procedures.

Pathophysiology

The cervix, composed of squamous epithelium (ectocervix) and columnar epithelium (endocervix), is susceptible to infection and irritation.

Infectious agents invade the cervical mucosa, triggering an inflammatory response characterized by the infiltration of neutrophils, lymphocytes and plasma cells.

In acute cervicitis, there is often mucopurulent or purulent discharge due to infection of the endocervical glands.

Chronic cervicitis may result in persistent inflammation, leading to epithelial changes, metaplasia or even predisposing to cervical intraepithelial neoplasia (CIN) in cases of HPV-related inflammation.

Non-infectious causes lead to localized irritation, edema and potential micro-abrasions, increasing susceptibility to secondary infections.

Clinical Features

1. Symptoms

Often asymptomatic, especially in chlamydial infections.

Abnormal vaginal discharge (mucopurulent, purulent or serous).

Postcoital bleeding or intermenstrual bleeding.

Vaginal or pelvic discomfort, dyspareunia (painful intercourse).

In severe cases (e.g., HSV), painful cervical ulcerations or systemic symptoms like fever.

2. Signs on Examination

Cervical erythema or friability (easily induced bleeding).

Mucopurulent or purulent discharge from the cervical os.

Cervical edema or tenderness on palpation.

Presence of ulcers or vesicles in HSV-related cervicitis.

In chronic cases, Nabothian cysts or cervical erosions may be visible.

Diagnosis

Diagnosis is based on clinical evaluation, laboratory testing and exclusion of other conditions.

1. History and Physical Examination

Detailed sexual history, including STI exposure and contraceptive use.

Speculum examination to assess cervix and discharge.

Bimanual examination to rule out pelvic inflammatory disease (PID).

2. Laboratory Tests

Nucleic Acid Amplification Tests (NAATs): Gold standard for detecting Chlamydia trachomatis and Neisseria gonorrhoeae from cervical swabs.

Wet Mount Microscopy: To identify Trichomonas vaginalis or clue cells (bacterial vaginosis).

Viral Testing: PCR for HSV or HPV if clinically indicated.

Culture or Serology: For Mycoplasma genitalium or rare pathogens.

pH Testing and Whiff Test: To evaluate for bacterial vaginosis.

3. Additional Tests

Colposcopy: If chronic cervicitis or suspicion of cervical dysplasia.

Cervical biopsy: In cases of persistent inflammation or suspicion of malignancy.

Screening for other STIs (e.g., HIV, syphilis) is recommended due to co-infection risk.

4. Differential Diagnosis

Cervical ectropion

Cervical polyps.

Cervical intraepithelial neoplasia (CIN) or cervical cancer.

Endometritis or pelvic inflammatory disease.

Vaginitis (e.g., candidiasis, bacterial vaginosis).

Management

Management depends on the underlying cause, severity and patient factors.

1. Infectious Cervicitis

Chlamydia trachomatis: Azithromycin 1 g orally (single dose) or doxycycline 100 mg orally twice daily for 7 days.

Neisseria gonorrhoeae: Ceftriaxone 500 mg intramuscularly (single dose) plus azithromycin 1 g orally (to cover potential co-infection with chlamydia).

Mycoplasma genitalium: Azithromycin or moxifloxacin (due to increasing resistance to azithromycin).

Herpes Simplex Virus: Acyclovir 400 mg orally three times daily for 7–10 days or valacyclovir 1 g orally twice daily for 7–10 days.

Trichomonas vaginalis: Metronidazole 2 g orally (single dose) or 500 mg twice daily for 7 days.

Partner treatment is essential for STIs to prevent reinfection.

Abstinence from sexual intercourse until treatment completion and symptom resolution.

2. Non-Infectious Cervicitis

Remove or avoid irritants (e.g., discontinue irritating douches or spermicides).

Short-term topical corticosteroids for severe inflammation (rarely needed).

Treat underlying systemic conditions if present.

3. Chronic Cervicitis

Address underlying infections or irritants.

Cryotherapy, electrocautery or loop electrosurgical excision procedure (LEEP) for persistent cases with cervical erosions or metaplasia (rare).

Regular follow-up to monitor for complications like CIN.

4. General Measures

Patient education on safe sexual practices and STI prevention.

Screening and treatment of sexual partners.

Follow-up testing to confirm resolution of infection (e.g., test of cure for chlamydia or gonorrhoea in pregnant women or persistent symptoms).

Complications

Pelvic Inflammatory Disease (PID): Ascending infection from untreated cervicitis can lead to endometritis, salpingitis or tubo-ovarian abscess.

Infertility: Chronic inflammation or scarring from PID.

Ectopic Pregnancy: Due to tubal damage from untreated infections.

Chronic Pelvic Pain: Persistent inflammation may cause long-term discomfort.

Increased HIV Transmission: Cervical inflammation increases susceptibility to HIV.

Cervical Dysplasia or Cancer: Chronic HPV-related cervicitis may progress to CIN or cervical cancer.

Prevention

Consistent use of condoms to reduce STI transmission.

Regular STI screening in high-risk populations.

HPV vaccination to prevent HPV-related cervicitis and cervical cancer.

Avoidance of vaginal irritants or allergens.

Routine gynaecological examinations and Pap smears for early detection of cervical abnormalities.

Prognosis

Acute cervicitis typically resolves with appropriate treatment of the underlying cause.

Chronic cervicitis may require prolonged management and monitoring for complications.

Early detection and treatment of STIs significantly reduce the risk of sequelae like PID or infertility.

Special Conditions

Pregnancy: Cervicitis in pregnancy increases the risk of preterm labor, chorioamnionitis and neonatal infections. Safe antibiotics (e.g., azithromycin, erythromycin) should be used.

Adolescents: Higher risk of STIs; sensitive counselling and confidentiality are critical.

Immunocompromised Patients: May present with atypical or severe symptoms, requiring aggressive management.

9.3 Cervical Erosion

(*Ta'akkul unuq-i-Rahim*)

Definition

Cervical erosion, also known as cervical ectropion, is a benign condition characterized by the presence of columnar epithelium (normally found in the endocervical canal) on the ectocervix, replacing the usual squamous epithelium. Despite its name, it is not a true erosion (loss of tissue) but rather a normal anatomical variation or a response to hormonal or inflammatory changes.

Etiology

Cervical erosion results from the eversion of the endocervical columnar epithelium onto the ectocervix, often due to:

1. Hormonal Influences

Puberty: Increased oestrogen levels stimulate columnar epithelium growth.

Pregnancy: Elevated oestrogen and progesterone levels promote ectropion.

Oral Contraceptive Pills (OCPs): Estrogen-containing contraceptives can induce or exacerbate ectropion.

Menstrual Cycle Variations: More prominent during the proliferative phase due to oestrogen surges.

2. Congenital Factors

Common in adolescents and young women due to an immature squamocolumnar junction.

3. Inflammatory or Traumatic Causes

Chronic cervicitis (e.g., due to Chlamydia trachomatis or Neisseria gonorrhoeae).

Cervical trauma from procedures (e.g., biopsy, cryotherapy or IUD insertion).

Repeated vaginal infections or irritants (e.g., douches, tampons).

4. Other Factors

Multiparity: Repeated cervical stretching during childbirth may contribute.

Rarely associated with systemic conditions affecting cervical tissue (e.g., connective tissue disorders).

Epidemiology

Cervical ectropion is highly prevalent in:

Adolescents and young women (15–30 years).

Pregnant women (up to 80% may show some degree of ectropion).

Women using oestrogen-containing contraceptives.

It is less common in postmenopausal women due to lower oestrogen levels, which cause retraction of the squamocolumnar junction.

No ethnic or geographic predisposition is noted, though prevalence may be higher in populations with limited access to gynaecological care due to underdiagnosis.

Pathophysiology

The cervix consists of two epithelial types:

i) Ectocervix: Covered by stratified squamous epithelium, which is protective.

ii) Endocervix: Lined by single-layered columnar epithelium, which is glandular and secretes mucus.

The junction between these two epithelia, known as the squamocolumnar junction (SCJ), is dynamic and influenced by hormonal and environmental factors.

In cervical ectropion, the columnar epithelium extends onto the ectocervix, often due to oestrogen-primed proliferation. This epithelium appears red, velvety and friable because it is thinner and more vascular than squamous epithelium.

The exposed columnar epithelium is prone to irritation, inflammation or bleeding upon contact (e.g., during intercourse or speculum examination).

Over time, chronic irritation or hormonal changes may lead to “squamous metaplasia”, where columnar epithelium is replaced by squamous epithelium, restoring the normal ectocervical appearance.

Clinical Features

1. Symptoms

Often asymptomatic and discovered incidentally during pelvic examination.

Abnormal vaginal discharge: Mucoid, clear or occasionally blood-tinged due to friable tissue.

Postcoital bleeding: Due to the fragility of columnar epithelium.

Intermenstrual spotting or irregular bleeding.

Mild pelvic discomfort or vaginal irritation in some cases, especially if associated with cervicitis.

2. Signs

Speculum examination reveals a red, velvety or granular appearance around the cervical os, contrasting with the pale pink squamous epithelium.

Friability: The area may bleed easily upon contact (e.g., with a swab or speculum).

No ulceration or erosion is present, distinguishing it from true cervical pathology.

The cervix may appear enlarged or everted, especially in pregnancy.

Diagnosis

Diagnosis is primarily clinical, supported by investigations to rule out other conditions.

1. History and Physical Examination

Assess for risk factors (e.g., pregnancy, OCP use, sexual history or recent cervical procedures).

Speculum examination to visualize the characteristic red, velvety ectocervical area.

Bimanual examination to exclude pelvic tenderness or masses suggestive of other pathology.

2. Laboratory Tests

a. Cervical Swabs: To rule out infectious causes like Chlamydia trachomatis, Neisseria gonorrhoeae or Trichomonas vaginalis using Nucleic acid amplification tests (NAATs) or wet mount microscopy.
b. Pap Smear: To screen for cervical dysplasia or malignancy, as ectropion may coexist with human papillomavirus (HPV)-related changes.
c. Colposcopy: Indicated if atypical cells are found on Pap smear, persistent bleeding occurs, or malignancy is suspected.
d. Cervical Biopsy: Rarely needed but performed if colposcopy shows suspicious lesions or to rule out cervical intraepithelial neoplasia (CIN) or cancer.

Differential Diagnosis

a. Cervicitis: Inflammatory condition often associated with infection; may coexist with ectropion.
b. Cervical Polyps: Benign growths that may bleed or cause discharge.
c. Cervical Intraepithelial Neoplasia (CIN): Precancerous changes requiring colposcopy and biopsy for confirmation.

d. Cervical Cancer: Rare but must be excluded, especially in women with risk factors (e.g., HPV infection, smoking).
e. Endometriosis: Endometrial tissue on the cervix may mimic ectropion.
f. Trauma or Foreign Bodies: May cause localized irritation resembling ectropion.

Management

Cervical ectropion is often a physiological condition and may not require treatment unless symptomatic or associated with complications.

1. Asymptomatic Cases

Observation and reassurance, as ectropion often resolves spontaneously (e.g., after pregnancy, discontinuation of OCPs, or menopause).

Regular follow-up with Pap smears as per cervical cancer screening guidelines.

2. Symptomatic Cases

Address Underlying Causes:

Treat coexisting infections (e.g., antibiotics for chlamydia or gonorrhoea, metronidazole for trichomoniasis).

Discontinue or modify irritants (e.g., switch from oestrogen-containing OCPs to progesterone-only methods).

Minimally Invasive Treatments (for persistent symptoms like postcoital bleeding or excessive discharge):

Cryotherapy: Freezing the affected area to promote squamous metaplasia; effective for small areas.

Electrocautery: Thermal ablation to destroy columnar epithelium and encourage squamous regrowth.

Laser Therapy: Less commonly used but effective for precise treatment.

Loop Electrosurgical Excision Procedure (LEEP): Reserved for cases with coexisting dysplasia or severe symptoms.

Post-Treatment Care: Advise abstinence from sexual intercourse for 4–6 weeks to allow healing and reduce infection risk.

3. Patient Education

Counsel on the benign nature of ectropion and its association with hormonal changes.

Promote safe sexual practices and STI screening to prevent complications.

Encourage cervical cancer screening protocols.

Complications

Chronic Cervicitis: Persistent irritation or coexisting infections may lead to inflammation.

Increased STI Susceptibility: The exposed columnar epithelium is more vulnerable to pathogens like HIV, HPV or Chlamydia.

Cervical Dysplasia: Chronic irritation or HPV infection may predispose to CIN, especially in high-risk individuals.

Infertility or Pregnancy complications: Rarely, untreated infections associated with ectropion may ascend, causing pelvic inflammatory disease (PID) or preterm labor.

Prevention

Regular gynaecological examinations and Pap smears for early detection of abnormalities.

HPV vaccination to reduce the risk of HPV-related cervical changes.

Consistent condom use to prevent STIs that may exacerbate ectropion.

Avoidance of vaginal irritants (e.g., harsh douches, spermicides).

Consideration of alternative contraception (e.g., progesterone-only methods) in women prone to symptomatic ectropion.

Prognosis

Cervical ectropion is a benign condition with an excellent prognosis.

Asymptomatic cases often resolve spontaneously with hormonal changes (e.g., post-pregnancy or menopause).

Symptomatic cases respond well to treatment, with low recurrence rates if underlying causes are addressed.

Regular monitoring is essential to detect any progression to dysplasia or malignancy, particularly in women with HPV infection.

Special Conditions

Pregnancy: Ectropion is common and usually resolves postpartum. Invasive treatments are avoided unless absolutely necessary (e.g., suspicion of malignancy).

Adolescents: Reassurance is key, as ectropion is often physiological and resolves with maturation of the cervix.

Postmenopausal Women: Ectropion is rare due to low oestrogen levels; its presence suggest investigation for other pathology (e.g., malignancy). Women with STI Risk: Routine STI screening is critical, as ectropion may mask or coexist with cervicitis.

9.4 Inflammation of the Uterus (Endometritis)

(*Iltihab-i-Rahim)*

Definition

Endometritis is defined as an infection or inflammation of the endometrium. It may occur as an acute or chronic condition and is often associated with infection, though non-infectious causes also exist. Endometritis is a significant gynaecological entity due to its potential to cause pelvic pain, infertility and complications in pregnancy.

Etiology

Endometritis can be caused by infectious or non-infectious factors:

1. Infectious Causes

Bacterial

Polymicrobial: Common after childbirth or gynaecological procedures, involving organisms such as Escherichia coli, Streptococcus (e.g., Group B Streptococcus), Staphylococcus and anaerobes (e.g., Bacteroides, Peptostreptococcus).

Sexually Transmitted Infections (STIs): Chlamydia trachomatis and Neisseria gonorrhoeae are frequent causes, particularly in non-puerperal cases.

Mycoplasma genitalium: Increasingly recognized as a cause of endometritis.

Mycobacterium tuberculosis: Rare but significant in endemic areas, causing chronic granulomatous endometritis.

Viral: Rare, but herpes simplex virus (HSV) or cytomegalovirus (CMV) may be implicated in immunocompromised patients.

Fungal: Extremely rare, typically in immunocompromised individuals (e.g., Candida species).

2. Non-Infectious Causes

Retained products of conception (e.g., after miscarriage, abortion or delivery).

Intrauterine devices (IUDs), especially in the early post-insertion period.

Foreign bodies (e.g., retained tampons or surgical material).

Chemical irritants (e.g., from intrauterine instillations or douches).

Autoimmune or idiopathic chronic inflammation (rare).

3. Predisposing Factors

Puerperal Endometritis: Most common after cesarean delivery, prolonged labor, premature rupture of membranes, or multiple vaginal examinations during labor.

Non-Puerperal Endometritis: Associated with STIs, gynaecological procedures (e.g., dilation and curettage, hysteroscopy), or IUD use.

Other Risk Factors: Poor hygiene, immunosuppression, diabetes or multiple sexual partners.

Epidemiology

Puerperal Endometritis: Occurs in 1–3% of vaginal deliveries and 5–15% of cesarean deliveries, with higher rates in low-resource settings.

Non-Puerperal Endometritis: More common in sexually active women aged 15–35 years, particularly those with STI risk factors.

Tuberculous Endometritis: Rare in developed countries but prevalent in tuberculosis-endemic regions.

Risk factors include low socioeconomic status, lack of access to healthcare and high-risk sexual behavior.

Pathophysiology

The endometrium is normally protected by cervical mucus and immune defences, but breaches (e.g., childbirth, procedures, or STIs) allow pathogens to ascend into the uterine cavity.

Acute endometritis involves an inflammatory response with neutrophil infiltration, edema and possible microabscess formation.

Chronic endometritis is characterized by plasma cell infiltration, lymphoid aggregates and stromal changes. It may be subclinical, contributing to infertility or recurrent pregnancy loss.

In puerperal endometritis, polymicrobial infections from vaginal flora or skin contaminants invade the endometrium, often facilitated by retained placental tissue or blood clots.

Tuberculous endometritis results in granulomatous inflammation with caseation, potentially causing scarring and synechiae (Asherman's syndrome).

Chronic inflammation may disrupt endometrial receptivity, affecting implantation and increasing miscarriage risk.

Clinical Features

1. Acute Endometritis

Symptoms

Pelvic or lower abdominal pain.

Fever (often >38°C), chills or malaise (common in puerperal cases).

Abnormal uterine bleeding (e.g., heavy or prolonged lochia in postpartum cases).

Foul-smelling vaginal discharge (purulent or serosanguinous).

Dyspareunia or general discomfort.

Signs

Uterine tenderness on bimanual examination.

Cervical motion tenderness (if associated with pelvic inflammatory disease [PID]).

Purulent or malodorous lochia in postpartum cases.

Systemic signs (e.g., tachycardia, fever) in severe cases.

2. Chronic Endometritis

Symptoms

Often asymptomatic or subtle.

Chronic pelvic pain or discomfort.

Irregular menstrual bleeding or spotting.

Infertility or recurrent pregnancy loss.

Signs

Subtle uterine tenderness or normal pelvic examination.

Endometrial irregularities on imaging or hysteroscopy.

3. Tuberculous Endometritis

Symptoms include infertility, amenorrhea or chronic pelvic pain.

Systemic symptoms (e.g., weight loss, night sweats) may be present.

Diagnosis

Diagnosis combines clinical evaluation, laboratory tests and imaging, with a focus on identifying the underlying cause.

1. History and Physical Examination

Assess for risk factors (e.g., recent delivery, gynaecological procedures, STI exposure).

Speculum examination to evaluate discharge or cervical abnormalities.

Bimanual examination for uterine tenderness, cervical motion tenderness or adnexal masses.

2. Laboratory Tests

Cervical Swabs: Nucleic acid amplification tests (NAATs) for Chlamydia trachomatis, Neisseria gonorrhoeae or Mycoplasma genitalium.

Endometrial Sampling: Biopsy or curettage for histopathology (e.g., plasma cells in chronic endometritis, granulomas in tuberculosis).

Blood Tests: Complete blood count (leukocytosis in acute cases), erythrocyte sedimentation rate (ESR), or C-reactive protein (CRP) for inflammation.

Microbiology: Endometrial or lochia cultures (though often contaminated in puerperal cases).

Tuberculosis Testing: PCR, culture or interferon-gamma release assays for suspected tuberculous endometritis.

3. Imaging

Ultrasound: To detect retained products of conception, endometrial thickening or fluid collections.

Hysteroscopy: Visualizes endometrial irregularities, adhesions or chronic inflammation.

MRI/CT: Rarely used but may identify abscesses or structural abnormalities in severe cases.

Differential Diagnosis

Pelvic Inflammatory Disease (PID): Involves broader pelvic structures (e.g., fallopian tubes, ovaries).

Cervicitis: Limited to the cervix but may coexist.

Retained products of conception: Common postpartum or post-abortion.

Endometriosis: Causes cyclic pelvic pain and may mimic chronic endometritis.

Uterine fibroids or adenomyosis: May present with abnormal bleeding or pain.

Endometrial Cancer: Must be ruled out in chronic cases, especially in older women.

Management

Treatment depends on the cause, severity and clinical scenario.

Acute Endometritis

Antibiotics (targeting polymicrobial or specific pathogens):

Puerperal Endometritis

Broad-spectrum regimens: Clindamycin 900 mg IV every 8 hours + gentamicin 5 mg/kg IV daily (gold standard for postpartum cases).

Alternative: Ampicillin-sulbactam or piperacillin-tazobactam for severe cases.

Transition to oral antibiotics (e.g., doxycycline or metronidazole) once afebrile for 24–48 hours.

STI-Related Endometritis

Ceftriaxone 500 mg IM (single dose) + doxycycline 100 mg orally twice daily for 14 days for N. gonorrhoeae and C. trachomatis.

Azithromycin or moxifloxacin for Mycoplasma genitalium.

Supportive Care

Analgesics (e.g., ibuprofen) for pain and fever.

Hydration and rest.

Surgical Intervention

Dilation and curettage (D&C) for retained products of conception.

Drainage of abscesses in rare cases of severe infection.

Chronic Endometritis

Antibiotic

Doxycycline 100 mg orally twice daily for 14 days or metronidazole 500 mg orally twice daily for 14 days (empiric treatment).

Repeat endometrial biopsy to confirm resolution if symptoms persist.

Hormonal Therapy: Considered in idiopathic cases to stabilize the endometrium.

Hysteroscopy: To evaluate and treat adhesions or structural abnormalities.

Tuberculous Endometritis

Standard anti-tuberculosis therapy (e.g., isoniazid, rifampicin, ethambutol, pyrazinamide) for 6–9 months. Multidisciplinary care involving infectious disease management.

Non-Infectious Causes

Remove IUDs or foreign bodies, if implicated.

Treat underlying autoimmune conditions or discontinue irritants.

General Measures

Partner treatment for STIs to prevent reinfection.

Patient education on safe sexual practices and hygiene.

Follow-up to ensure symptom resolution and rule out complications.

Complications

1. Pelvic Inflammatory Disease (PID): Ascending infection can lead to salpingitis, tubo-ovarian abscess or peritonitis.
2. Infertility: Chronic endometritis disrupts endometrial receptivity, contributing to implantation failure.
3. Recurrent Pregnancy Loss: Due to endometrial scarring or inflammation.
4. Asherman's Syndrome: Intrauterine adhesions from chronic inflammation or repeated curettage.
5. Sepsis: In severe puerperal endometritis, particularly after cesarean delivery.
6. Chronic Pelvic Pain: Persistent inflammation may cause long-term discomfort.

Prevention

Aseptic techniques during childbirth, cesarean delivery or gynaecological procedures.

Routine STI screening and treatment in high-risk populations.

Early removal of retained products of conception or foreign bodies.

Use of prophylactic antibiotics during cesarean delivery (e.g., cefazolin).

HPV vaccination and safe sexual practices to reduce STI-related endometritis.

Regular gynaecological follow-up for women with IUDs or risk factors.

Prognosis

Acute endometritis typically resolves with prompt antibiotic therapy, with low morbidity if treated early. Chronic endometritis may persist or recur, requiring prolonged treatment and monitoring, especially in infertility cases. Tuberculous endometritis has not a favourable prognosis for fertility due to scarring, but systemic outcomes are favorable with appropriate therapy. Early diagnosis and management are necessary to prevent complications like PID or infertility.

Special Considerations

1. Postpartum Period: Puerperal endometritis requires aggressive treatment to prevent sepsis, especially after cesarean delivery.
2. Pregnancy: Antibiotics safe for pregnancy (e.g., ampicillin, clindamycin) are used, and D&C is avoided unless absolutely necessary.
3. Infertility Patients: Chronic endometritis is increasingly recognized as a cause of recurrent implantation failure; endometrial biopsy is key for diagnosis.
4. Immunocompromised Patients: May present with atypical pathogens or severe disease, requiring individualised therapy.
5. Tuberculosis-Endemic Areas: Consider tuberculous endometritis in women with infertility or chronic pelvic pain.

Diseases of the Uterus

↓

.Classify by Etiology

↓	↓	↓	↓
Structural	**Infectious**	**Functional**	**Neoplastic**
↓	↓	↓	↓
Fibroids Adenomyosis Congenital Anomalies	Endometritis Pyometra Tuberculosis PID	AUB Dysmenorrhea Infertility Prolapse	Endometrial Hyperplasia Endometrial Carcinoma Uterine Sarcoma Polyps

9.5 Displacement of Uterus

(*Maylan-al-Rahim* / Eujaj-*al- Rahim*)

Definition

Uterine displacement refers to an abnormal position or orientation of the uterus within the pelvic cavity. The most common forms include retroversion, retroflexion, anteversion, anteflexion and uterine prolapse . While often asymptomatic, uterine displacement can contribute to gynaecological symptoms or complications, particularly in severe cases or when associated with other pelvic pathology.

Anatomy and Normal Position

The uterus is a pear-shaped, muscular organ located in the pelvis between the bladder and rectum.

Normal Position: The uterus is typically anteverted (tilted forward at the cervix relative to the vagina) and anteflexed (the uterine body is flexed forward over the cervix). The angle between the cervix and vagina is approximately 90°, and the uterine body forms an angle of about 120° with the cervix.

The uterus is supported by ligaments (e.g., uterosacral, cardinal, round ligaments) and the pelvic floor muscles. Displacement occurs when these supports are compromised or when congenital or acquired factors alter uterine positioning.

Types of Uterine Displacement

1. Retroversion

The uterus is tilted backward so that the cervix points toward the anterior vaginal wall, and the fundus is directed toward the sacrum.

May be congenital (common, often asymptomatic) or acquired (e.g., due to pelvic adhesions or endometriosis).

2. Retroflexion

The uterine body is flexed backward relative to the cervix, while the cervix remains in its normal position. Often associated with retroversion.

3. Anteversion (if excessive)

The uterus is tilted excessively forward, beyond the normal anteverted position.

Rare and usually asymptomatic unless extreme.

4. Anteflexion (if excessive)

The uterine body is sharply flexed forward over the cervix, forming a more acute angle than normal. It may cause symptoms if associated with obstruction of menstrual flow.

5. Uterine Prolapse

Descent of the uterus into or through the vaginal canal due to weakened pelvic support structures.

Graded by severity

First-degree: Cervix descends into the upper vagina.

Second-degree: Cervix reaches the vaginal introitus.

Third-degree: Cervix and uterus protrude outside the vaginal introitus .

Complete prolapse: Entire uterus and cervix is outside .

6. Uterine Inversion (Rare)

The uterus turns inside out, often during or after childbirth, due to excessive traction on the umbilical cord or fundal pressure.

Can be acute (postpartum) or chronic (rare, associated with tumours or weakening of uterine walls).

Etiology

Uterine displacement may be congenital or acquired, with the following causes:

1. Congenital

Developmental anomalies leading to retroversion or retroflexion (common in 20–30% of women).

Weak pelvic ligaments or abnormal uterine shape (e.g., bicornuate uterus).

2. Acquired

Pelvic Floor Weakness

Multiparity, vaginal deliveries or prolonged labor.

Aging or menopause (decreased oestrogen weakens pelvic tissues).

Obesity or chronic increased intra-abdominal pressure (e.g., chronic cough, constipation).

Pelvic Adhesions

Endometriosis or pelvic inflammatory disease (PID) causing retroversion.

Previous pelvic surgery (e.g., cesarean section, myomectomy).

Trauma or Procedures

Childbirth trauma or postpartum inversion.

Mishandling of uterus during gynaecological procedures.

Tumours or Masses

Fibroids, ovarian cysts or pelvic tumours pushing the uterus out of position.

Other Factors

Chronic constipation or straining.

Connective tissue disorders (e.g., Ehlers-Danlos syndrome).

Epidemiology

Retroversion/Retroflexion: Found in 20–30% of women, often asymptomatic and considered a normal variant.

Uterine Prolapse: More common in postmenopausal women and multiparous women, with prevalence increasing with age (up to 40% in women over 50 in some studies).

Uterine Inversion: Rare, occurring in approximately 1 in 2,000–20,000 deliveries.

Risk factors include multiparity, menopause, obesity and a history of pelvic surgery or infections.

Pathophysiology

Retroversion/Retroflexion: Results from laxity of supporting ligaments (e.g., uterosacral or round ligaments) or adhesions pulling the uterus backward. This may impair uterine mobility, potentially contributing to symptoms like dysmenorrhea or infertility in rare cases.

Uterine Prolapse: Weakening of pelvic floor muscles (e.g., levator ani) and ligaments (e.g., cardinal, uterosacral) allows descent of the uterus. Risk is exacerbated by vaginal deliveries, chronic straining, or oestrogen deficiency.

Uterine Inversion: Occurs when the uterine fundus collapses into the endometrial cavity, often due to excessive traction during delivery or a weakened uterine wall (e.g., from myometrial thinning or tumours). This can lead to severe haemorrhage or shock in acute cases.

Displaced uteri may cause mechanical issues (e.g., pressure on adjacent organs like the bladder or rectum) or impair fertility by altering endometrial or tubal function.

Clinical Features

1. Retroversion/Retroflexion

Symptoms: Often asymptomatic. May include:

Dysmenorrhea or pelvic pain (if associated with endometriosis or adhesions).

Dyspareunia (deep pelvic pain during intercourse).

Infertility or recurrent miscarriage (rare).

Signs: Uterus palpated posteriorly on bimanual examination; fundus not felt anteriorly.

2. Uterine Prolapse

Symptoms

Sensation of pelvic heaviness or “something falling out.”

Vaginal bulging or protrusion.

Urinary symptoms (incontinence, urgency, or difficulty voiding).

Bowel symptoms (constipation or incomplete evacuation).

Dyspareunia or sexual dysfunction.

Signs

Descent of the cervix or uterus on speculum examination, exacerbated by Valsalva manoeuvre.

Cervical elongation or vaginal wall prolapse (cystocele, rectocele) may coexist.

Ulceration or bleeding of the exposed cervix in severe cases.

3. Uterine Inversion

Symptoms (Acute)

Severe pelvic pain and vaginal bleeding postpartum.

Shock (hypovolemic or neurogenic) due to haemorrhage or vagal stimulation.

Signs

Absence of palpable uterine fundus abdominally.

Palpable or visible mass in the vagina or at the introitus.

Chronic inversion may present with irregular bleeding or pelvic pain.

Diagnosis

Diagnosis is primarily clinical, supported by imaging or procedures when needed.

1. History and Physical Examination

Assess for risk factors (e.g., parity, menopause, recent vaginal delivery, pelvic surgery).

Speculum Examination: Visualizes cervical position or prolapse; Valsalva manoeuvre accentuates prolapse.

Bimanual Examination: Determines uterine position (retroverted vs. anteverted) and mobility (fixed vs. mobile).

Pelvic Organ Prolapse Quantification (POP-Q): Standardized system to grade prolapse severity.

2. Imaging

Ultrasound: Transvaginal or transabdominal to confirm uterine position, detect masses or evaluate for retained products in inversion.

MRI: Useful for complex cases (e.g., suspected adhesions, tumours or chronic inversion).

CT: Rarely used, but may identify associated pelvic pathology.

3. Additional Tests

Hysteroscopy: To evaluate the endometrial cavity in chronic inversion or infertility cases.

Urodynamic Testing: For prolapse with urinary symptoms to assess bladder function.

Endometrial Biopsy: If abnormal uterine bleeding suggests coexisting pathology (e.g., endometrial cancer).

4. Differential Diagnosis

Endometriosis or PID: May cause retroversion or pelvic pain.

Uterine Fibroids or Tumours: Can mimic prolapse or cause displacement.

Cervical/Vaginal Pathology: Polyps or malignancy may resemble prolapse.

Pelvic Congestion Syndrome: Can cause pelvic pain similar to retroversion.

Submucous Fibroid or Endometrial Polyp: May mimic inversion in rare cases.

Management

Management depends on the type of displacement, symptoms and patient factors.

1. Retroversion/Retroflexion

Asymptomatic: No treatment needed; considered a normal variant.

Symptomatic

Treat underlying causes (e.g., antibiotics for PID, surgery for endometriosis).

Pessary: Temporary device to reposition the uterus in severe cases (rarely used).

Surgical Correction: Rarely indicated, but procedures like uterosacral ligament suspension or round ligament plication may be considered for persistent symptoms or infertility (controversial efficacy).

2. Uterine Prolapse

Conservative Management

Pelvic Floor Exercises (Kegels): Strengthen pelvic muscles, effective for mild cases.

Pessary: Vaginal device to support the uterus; ideal for women unfit for surgery or during pregnancy.

Lifestyle Modifications: Weight loss, treatment of chronic cough or constipation.

Surgical Management

Vaginal Hysterectomy: For severe prolapse in women who have completed childbearing.

Uterine-Sparing Procedures: Sacrospinous hysteropexy or sacrocolpopexy to preserve fertility.

Colporrhaphy: Repair of associated cystocele or rectocele.

Obliterative Procedures (e.g., LeFort colpocleisis): For elderly patients unfit for major surgery.

Hormonal Therapy: Estrogen replacement (topical or systemic) in postmenopausal women to improve tissue strength before surgery.

3. Uterine Inversion

Acute Inversion (Medical Emergency)

Immediate manual repositioning under anaesthesia, often with tocolytics (e.g., terbutaline) to relax the uterus.

Fluid resuscitation and blood transfusion for shock or haemorrhage.

Surgical intervention (e.g., Huntington or Haultain procedure) if manual repositioning fails.

Chronic Inversion

Surgical correction via abdominal or vaginal approach (e.g., Spinelli or Kustner procedure).

Hysterectomy if fertility is not desired, or if the uterus is non-viable.

4. General Measures

Patient education on symptoms, risk factors and prevention.

STI screening and treatment if PID is suspected.

Regular follow-up for prolapse or symptomatic retroversion to monitor progression.

Complications

Retroversion/Retroflexion

Chronic pelvic pain or dyspareunia (if associated with adhesions or endometriosis).

Infertility (controversial, rare).

Uterine Prolapse

Urinary incontinence or retention.

Recurrent urinary tract infections.

Bowel dysfunction (e.g., constipation).

Cervical ulceration or infection in severe prolapse.

Uterine Inversion

Severe haemorrhage or hypovolemic shock.

Infection or sepsis.

Infertility or Asherman's syndrome in chronic cases.

Increased STI Risk: Displaced uterus may predispose to ascending infections.

Prevention

Pelvic Floor Strengthening: Kegel exercises post-delivery or in high-risk women.

Proper Obstetric Care: Avoid excessive traction during delivery to prevent inversion.

Management of Risk Factors: Treat chronic cough, constipation, or obesity.

Prophylactic Measures: Estrogen therapy in postmenopausal women to maintain pelvic tissue integrity.

STI Prevention: Condom use and regular screening to reduce PID-related adhesions.

Prognosis

Retroversion/Retroflexion: Excellent prognosis, as most cases are asymptomatic and require no intervention.

Uterine Prolapse: Good outcomes with conservative or surgical management, though recurrence is possible if risk factors persist.

Uterine Inversion: Acute cases have a good prognosis with prompt treatment; chronic cases may lead to fertility issues or require hysterectomy.

Regular follow-up is essential to monitor for complications or recurrence.

Special Conditions

Pregnancy

Retroversion may cause urinary retention in early pregnancy (resolves as uterus grows).

Prolapse often improves during pregnancy but may worsen postpartum.

Inversion is a postpartum emergency requiring immediate intervention.

Postmenopausal Women: Prolapse is more common; oestrogen therapy and pessaries are often first-line treatments.

Infertility: Retroversion is rarely a sole cause but may require evaluation for coexisting conditions (e.g., endometriosis).

Adolescents: Congenital retroversion is common and usually asymptomatic; reassurance is key.

Definitions

Fibroid (Leiomyoma) ➤ Benign tumor of uterine smooth muscle; causes menorrhagia, pressure symptoms.

Adenomyosis ➤ Endometrial tissue invades myometrium; leads to dysmenorrhea, bulky uterus.

Endometritis ➤ Infection of endometrial lining; presents with fever, pelvic pain, discharge.

Endometrial Hyperplasia ➤ Excessive proliferation of endometrium due to unopposed estrogen.

Endometrial Carcinoma ➤ Most common uterine cancer; postmenopausal bleeding is hallmark symptom.

Uterine Prolapse ➤ Descent of uterus due to pelvic floor weakness; graded by severity.

Clinical Clues

Symptom	Likely Diagnosis
Heavy bleeding + firm uterus	Fibroid
Dysmenorrhea + infertility	Endometriosis
Postmenopausal bleeding	Endometrial carcinoma
Fever + foul discharge	Endometritis
Bulky uterus + pain	Adenomyosis
Pelvic pressure + descent	Uterine prolapse

9.6 *Inzalaq-e-Rahim/ Khurooj-e-Rahim*

(Prolapse of Uterus)

Definition

Uterine prolapse is a form of pelvic organ prolapse characterized by the descent of the uterus into or through the vaginal canal due to weakened pelvic support structures. It is a common gynaecological condition, particularly in older or multiparous women, and can significantly impact quality of life due to associated symptoms affecting urinary, bowel and sexual function.

Anatomy and Pathophysiology

The uterus is supported by a complex network of ligaments (uterosacral, cardinal, round ligaments) and pelvic floor muscles (primarily the levator ani, including pubococcygeus and iliococcygeus muscles). The endopelvic fascia and perineal body also contribute to stability.

Pathophysiology

Weakening of pelvic support structures allows the uterus to descend, often accompanied by prolapse of adjacent structures (e.g., bladder [cystocele], rectum [rectocele], or vaginal vault).

Contributing factors include:

Loss of Muscle Tone: Due to aging, childbirth trauma, or chronic strain (e.g., obesity, constipation).

Ligamentous Laxity: Estrogen deficiency (post-menopause) or connective tissue disorders (e.g., Ehlers-Danlos syndrome).

Increased Intra-abdominal Pressure: From chronic cough, heavy lifting, or obesity.

The descent stretches vaginal walls, leading to protrusion of the cervix or uterus into the vagina or beyond the introitus.

Grading of Uterine Prolapse

(Pelvic Organ Prolapse Quantification [POP-Q] system or Baden-Walker system):

First-degree: Cervix descends into the upper vagina but remains above the introitus.

Second-degree: Cervix reaches the vaginal introitus.

Third-degree: Cervix and part of the uterus protrude outside the introitus.

Procidentia (Complete Prolapse): Entire uterus protrudes outside the vagina, often with eversion of vaginal walls.

Etiology

Uterine prolapse results from a combination of predisposing, inciting, and promoting factors:

1. Predisposing Factors

Childbirth: Vaginal deliveries, especially multiple or traumatic (e.g., prolonged labor, large fetus, or instrumental delivery), damage pelvic floor muscles and ligaments.

Aging: Postmenopausal oestrogen decline reduces tissue elasticity and strength.

Congenital Factors: Inherent weakness in connective tissue (e.g., Marfan syndrome, Ehlers-Danlos syndrome).

2. Inciting Factors

Obstetric Trauma: Lacerations, overstretching, or nerve damage during delivery.

Pelvic Surgery: Hysterectomy or other procedures may weaken supporting structures.

Pelvic Masses: Fibroids or tumours increasing pelvic pressure.

3. Promoting Factors

Chronic Intra-abdominal Pressure: Obesity, chronic cough (e.g., COPD), constipation, or heavy lifting.

Menopause: Estrogen deficiency accelerates tissue atrophy.

Lifestyle Factors: Sedentary behavior or inadequate pelvic floor rehabilitation post-delivery.

Epidemiology

Prevalence Up to 40% of women over 50 years show some degree of pelvic organ prolapse, with uterine prolapse being a subset. Severe prolapse (third-degree or procidentia) is less common, affecting ~2–10% of women.

Risk factors

Multiparity (especially >3 vaginal deliveries).

Postmenopausal status.

Obesity (BMI >30).

Chronic respiratory conditions or constipation.

Occupational heavy lifting.

More prevalent in populations with limited access to obstetric care or higher rates of vaginal deliveries.

Clinical Features

1. Symptoms

Pelvic Pressure or Heaviness: A sensation of “something falling out,” worse with standing or straining.

Vaginal Bulging: Visible or palpable protrusion at the introitus (in severe cases).

Urinary Symptoms

Stress urinary incontinence (leakage with coughing/sneezing).

Urgency or incomplete bladder emptying (due to kinking of the urethra).

Recurrent urinary tract infections (UTIs) from urinary stasis.

Bowel Symptoms

Constipation or difficulty with defecation (due to rectocele or pressure).

Faecal incontinence (rare, in severe cases).

Sexual Dysfunction

Dyspareunia (painful intercourse) or reduced sexual satisfaction.

Low Back or Pelvic Pain: Particularly with prolonged standing.

Abnormal Bleeding: From cervical ulceration or irritation in severe prolapse (procidentia).

2. Signs

Speculum Examination: Descent of the cervix or uterus into the vaginal canal, accentuated by Valsalva manoeuvre.

Cervical Changes: Elongation, erosion, or ulceration in exposed prolapse.

Associated Prolapse: Cystocele (anterior vaginal wall), rectocele (posterior vaginal wall), or enterocele (small bowel prolapse).

POP-Q Staging: Quantifies prolapse severity by measuring descent relative to the hymen.

Diagnosis

Diagnosis is primarily clinical, with imaging or tests to rule out complications or associated conditions.

1. History

Assess obstetric history (number of deliveries, complications), menopausal status, and risk factors (e.g., obesity, chronic cough).

Evaluate symptoms (pelvic pressure, urinary/bowel dysfunction, sexual issues).

Screen for systemic conditions (e.g., connective tissue disorders).

2. Physical Examination

Speculum Examination: Visualize cervical descent; Valsalva manoeuvre or standing examination may reveal prolapse.

Bimanual Examination: Assess uterine size, mobility, and associated masses (e.g., fibroids).

POP-Q System: Measures specific points of vaginal and uterine descent for precise staging.

Neurological Assessment: Evaluate for pelvic floor muscle weakness or nerve damage (e.g., pudendal nerve).

3. Diagnostic Tests

Urinalysis/Culture: To rule out UTI in patients with urinary symptoms.

Urodynamic Testing: For complex urinary incontinence or voiding dysfunction.

Ultrasound: Transvaginal or transabdominal to assess uterine size, fibroids, or retained products.

MRI: For complex cases to evaluate pelvic floor anatomy or enterocele.

Cystoscopy/Colonoscopy: Rarely needed to assess bladder or bowel involvement.

Endometrial Biopsy: If abnormal uterine bleeding suggests malignancy.

4. Differential Diagnosis

Cystocele/Rectocele: Isolated prolapse of bladder or rectum.

Enterocele: Prolapse of small bowel into the vaginal vault.

Uterine Fibroids or Cervical Polyps: May mimic prolapse on examination.

Cervical/Endometrial Cancer: Must be ruled out in cases of bleeding or ulceration.

Vaginal Wall Cysts: Gartner's duct cysts or Bartholin gland cysts.

Management

Management depends on prolapse severity, symptoms, patient age, reproductive goals, and comorbidities.

1. Conservative Management (Preferred for mild cases or patients unfit for surgery)

Pelvic Floor Muscle Training (PFMT

Kegel exercises to strengthen levator ani muscles; effective for first-degree prolapse.

Supervised physiotherapy improves outcomes.

Pessary

Vaginal device (e.g., ring, Gellhorn, or donut pessary) to support the uterus.

Ideal for women desiring fertility preservation, elderly patients, or those unfit for surgery.

Requires regular cleaning and monitoring for vaginal erosion or infection.

Lifestyle Modifications

Weight loss to reduce intra-abdominal pressure.

Treatment of chronic cough or constipation.

Avoiding heavy lifting.

Hormonal Therapy

Topical oestrogen (e.g., vaginal oestrogen cream) in postmenopausal women to improve tissue strength and reduce irritation.

Contraindicated in patients with oestrogen-sensitive cancers

2. Surgical Management (For symptomatic second- or third-degree prolapse or procidentia):

a. Uterine-Preserving Procedures (For women desiring fertility or uterine preservation):

Sacrospinous Hysteropexy: Suspends the uterus to the sacrospinous ligament via vaginal approach.

Sacrocolpopexy: Uses mesh to attach the uterus or vaginal vault to the sacrum (abdominal or laparoscopic approach).

Manchester Procedure: Shortens cardinal ligaments and amputates part of the cervix (less common).

b. Hysterectomy

Vaginal Hysterectomy: Preferred for prolapse, often combined with vaginal wall repair (colporrhaphy).

Abdominal Hysterectomy: For large uteri or coexisting pathology (e.g., fibroids).

Post-hysterectomy, vaginal vault suspension (e.g., sacrocolpopexy) prevents vault prolapse.

c. Colporrhaphy

Anterior colporrhaphy for cystocele; posterior colporrhaphy for rectocele.

d. Obliterative Procedures

LeFort Colpocleisis: Closes the vaginal canal in elderly women unfit for major surgery who do not desire sexual activity.

Mesh Use: Controversial due to risks of erosion or chronic pain; used selectively in sacrocolpopexy.

3. Postoperative Care

Pelvic rest (avoid intercourse, tampons) for 6–8 weeks.

Monitor for complications (e.g., infection, mesh erosion, or recurrence).

Continue pelvic floor exercises to maintain support.

4. General Measures

Patient education on prolapse, treatment options, and recurrence prevention.

Regular follow-up to assess symptom resolution and pelvic floor integrity.

STI screening if infection is suspected as a contributing factor.

Complications

Urinary Dysfunction: Incontinence, retention, or recurrent UTIs.

Bowel Dysfunction: Constipation or faecal incontinence.

Sexual Dysfunction: Dyspareunia or reduced satisfaction.

Cervical Ulceration/Infection: In procidentia, due to exposure and irritation.

Recurrence: Common if risk factors (e.g., obesity, chronic straining) persist.

Surgical Complications: Bleeding, infection, mesh erosion, or vault prolapse post-hysterectomy.

Prevention

Pelvic Floor Exercises: Routine Kegels during and after pregnancy to strengthen pelvic muscles.

Obstetric Care: Minimize trauma during vaginal deliveries (e.g., avoid prolonged labor, optimize episiotomy use).

Lifestyle Modifications: Maintain healthy weight, treat chronic cough or constipation, and avoid heavy lifting.

Estrogen Therapy: Postmenopausal women may benefit from topical oestrogen to maintain tissue integrity.

Prophylactic Measures: Early intervention for mild prolapse to prevent progression.

Prognosis

Mild Prolapse: Excellent outcomes with conservative management (e.g., PFMT, pessary).

Severe Prolapse: Surgical correction has high success rates (80–90% symptom resolution), but recurrence is possible (10–20%) if risk factors persist.

Quality of Life: Significant improvement with appropriate treatment, though sexual or urinary symptoms may persist in some cases.

Regular follow-up is critical to monitor for recurrence or complications.

Special Considerations

1. Pregnancy

Prolapse often improves during pregnancy due to uterine enlargement but may worsen postpartum.

Pessaries are safe during pregnancy; surgery is deferred until after delivery.

2. Postmenopausal Women: Estrogen therapy and pessaries are first-line; surgery is considered for severe cases.

3. Young Women/Fertility Preservation: Uterine-sparing procedures (e.g., hysteropexy) are preferred.

4. Elderly/Frail Patients: Obliterative procedures or pessaries are suitable for those unfit for major surgery.

Common Uterine Pathologies

Mnemonic: “FAME CUP”

Letter	Condition	Description
F	Fibroid	Benign smooth muscle tumour
A	Adenomyosis	Endometrium in myometrium
M	Malignancy	Endometrial carcinoma, sarcoma
E	Endometritis	Infection/inflammation of endometrium
C	Congenital anomalies	Septate, bicornuate uterus
U	Uterine prolapse	Descent of uterus into vaginal canal
P	Polyps	Benign endometrial overgrowth

9.7 Inversion of Uterus

(Inqilab -i-Rahim)

Definition

Uterine inversion is a rare but potentially life-threatening obstetric and gynaecological condition in which the uterus turns inside out, partially or completely, with the uterine fundus collapsing into the endometrial cavity or protruding through the cervix into the vagina. It is classified as acute (occurring immediately postpartum) or chronic (developing gradually, often associated with tumours or other pathology). Prompt recognition and management are critical to prevent severe complications such as haemorrhage or shock.

Etiology

Uterine inversion is primarily associated with obstetric and gynaecological factors.

1. Obstetric Causes (Acute Inversion)

Mismanagement of the Third Stage of Labor

Excessive traction on the umbilical cord during placental delivery.

Inappropriate fundal pressure (Crede's manoeuvre) before placental separation.

Uterine Atony:Weak or poorly contracted myometrium fails to resist inversion.

Placenta Accreta or Abnormal Placental Implantation: Partial adherence of the placenta to the uterine wall increases risk during delivery.

Rapid Labor or Precipitous Delivery: Excessive intrauterine pressure may contribute.

Multiparity: Lax uterine ligaments and weakened myometrium increase susceptibility.

2. Non-Obstetric Causes (Chronic Inversion)

Uterine Tumours: Submucous fibroids or endometrial polyps pulling the fundus inward.

Endometrial Cancer or Sarcoma: Rarely, malignant tumours may initiate inversion.

Connective Tissue Weakness: Conditions like Ehlers-Danlos syndrome or congenital uterine anomalies.

3. Iatrogenic Causes

Aggressive manual removal of the placenta.

Improper use of uterotonic agents (e.g., oxytocin) before placental separation.

Epidemiology

Incidence

Acute postpartum uterine inversion occurs in approximately 1 in 2,000 to 1 in 20,000 deliveries, with higher rates in low-resource settings due to suboptimal obstetric care.

Chronic inversion is extremely rare, with incidence poorly documented.

Risk Factors

Multiparity.

Prolonged labor or rapid delivery.

Placenta accreta or abnormal placentation.

Previous uterine inversion.

Inexperienced birth attendants or mismanaged labor.

Pathophysiology

Uterine inversion occurs when the uterine fundus collapses inward, often due to a combination of mechanical forces and myometrial weakness.

Mechanism in Acute Inversion

During the third stage of labor, excessive traction on the umbilical cord or fundal pressure pulls the fundus through the cervix.

Uterine atony allows the fundus to invert, dragging the placenta (if still attached) and uterine walls into the endometrial cavity or vagina.

The inverted uterus may compress neurovascular structures, leading to severe pain, haemorrhage and neurogenic or hypovolemic shock.

Mechanism in Chronic Inversion

Gradual inversion is caused by intrauterine masses (e.g., fibroids) that exert traction on the fundus.

Chronic inflammation or tissue weakening may contribute.

Degrees of Inversion

First-degree (Incomplete): Fundus inverts into the endometrial cavity but does not reach the cervix.

Second-degree: Fundus reaches or protrudes through the cervical os into the vagina.

Third-degree: Fundus extends to or beyond the vaginal introitus.

Fourth-degree (Complete): Entire uterus and vagina are inverted, protruding externally (rare).

The inverted uterus disrupts normal blood flow, leading to ischemia, edema and potential necrosis if untreated. Vagal stimulation from cervical traction may cause bradycardia or shock.

Clinical Features

1. Acute Uterine Inversion

Symptoms

Severe pelvic or lower abdominal pain immediately postpartum.

Profuse vaginal bleeding (due to exposed endometrial surface or atony).

Symptoms of shock (hypotension, tachycardia, pallor or syncope).

Sensation of a mass in the vagina (if inversion extends beyond the cervix).

Signs

Absence of the uterine fundus on abdominal palpation (a hallmark sign).

Palpable or visible mass in the vagina or at the introitus (inverted uterus, often with attached placenta).

Signs of hypovolemic shock (tachycardia, hypotension) or neurogenic shock (bradycardia from vagal stimulation).

Cervical constriction or “dimple” felt abdominally in incomplete inversion.

2. Chronic Uterine Inversion

Symptoms

Chronic pelvic pain or discomfort.

Irregular or heavy vaginal bleeding.

Infertility or recurrent miscarriage (due to endometrial disruption).

Vaginal discharge (often foul-smelling if infection is present).

Signs

Palpable mass in the vagina on examination.

Uterine fundus not palpable abdominally.

Possible coexisting fibroid or polyp on imaging or hysteroscopy.

Diagnosis

Diagnosis is primarily clinical, with imaging to confirm or assess complications.

1. History and Physical Examination

History

Recent delivery with excessive cord traction or fundal pressure (acute).

Chronic symptoms (e.g., bleeding, infertility) in non-puerperal cases.

Examination

Abdominal: Absence of the uterine fundus or a “dimple” at the fundus site.

Vaginal/Speculum: Palpable or visible inverted uterus or mass in the vagina.

Bimanual: Confirms absence of normal uterine contour and presence of a mass.

2. Imaging

Ultrasound (Transvaginal or Transabdominal): Shows inverted uterine contour, with the fundus in the lower uterus or vagina. May identify associated masses (e.g., fibroids) or retained placenta.

MRI Provides detailed visualization of inversion, especially in chronic cases or when ultrasound is inconclusive.

CTS: Rarely used, but may detect inversion or complications in emergency settings.

3. Additional Tests

Hysteroscopy: Confirms chronic inversion or evaluates endometrial pathology.

Complete Blood Count (CBC): Assesses for anemia or infection (elevated white cell count).

Coagulation Studies: To evaluate for disseminated intravascular coagulation (DIC) in severe hemorrhagic cases.

4. Differential Diagnosis

Submucous Fibroid or Polyp: May protrude into the vagina, mimicking inversion.

Uterine Prolapse: Descent of the uterus without inversion.

Cervical or Endometrial Cancer: May cause vaginal bleeding or a mass.

Retained Products of Conception: Postpartum bleeding without inversion.

Vaginal Wall Mass: Gartner’s duct cyst or other vaginal pathology.

Management

Uterine inversion is a medical emergency in acute cases, requiring immediate intervention to prevent life-threatening complications. Management depends on the acuity and underlying cause.

1. Acute Uterine Inversion (Obstetric Emergency)

Initial Management

Call for Help: Involve obstetric, anaesthesia and surgical teams

Stabilize the Patient

Administer IV fluids and blood transfusion for hypovolemic shock.

Oxygen supplementation if hypoxic.

Monitor vital signs and urine output (Foley catheter).

Discontinue Uterotonics: Stop oxytocin or prostaglandins, as they may worsen cervical constriction.

Manual Repositioning (First-Line)

Attempt immediate manual reduction under adequate analgesia or anaesthesia (general or regional).

Johnson's Maneuver: Apply steady pressure to the inverted fundus through the vagina to push it back through the cervix. Avoid excessive force to prevent uterine rupture.

Administer tocolytics (e.g., terbutaline 0.25 mg IV or nitroglycerin 50–100 mcg IV) to relax the uterus and cervix.

If the placenta is still attached, do not remove it until after repositioning to avoid massive haemorrhage.

Post-Repositioning

Administer uterotonics (e.g., oxytocin 20–40 IU IV infusion) to promote uterine contraction and prevent re-inversion.

Antibiotics (e.g., ampicillin or clindamycin + gentamicin) to prevent infection, especially if prolonged manipulation occurred.

Monitor for haemorrhage, infection or re-inversion.

Surgical Intervention (If Manual Repositioning Fails):

Huntington Procedure: Abdominal approach; traction on round ligaments to pull the uterus back into position.

Haultain Procedure: Incision of the posterior cervical ring to facilitate repositioning.

Laparotomy: For complex cases or if ischemia/necrosis is suspected.

Hysterectomy: Last resort, if the uterus is non-viable or repositioning fails repeatedly.

2. Chronic Uterine Inversion

Evaluation: Identify underlying causes (e.g., fibroids, malignancy) via imaging or hysteroscopy.

Surgical Correction

Vaginal Approach: Spinelli or Kustner procedure to incise the cervical ring and reposition the uterus.

Abdominal Approach: Laparoscopic or open surgery to correct inversion and address underlying pathology (e.g., myomectomy for fibroids).

Hysterectomy: Considered if fertility is not desired or if malignancy is present.

Preoperative Preparation: Antibiotics to prevent infection; possible endometrial biopsy to rule out malignancy.

3. General Measures

Patient Counseling: Explain the condition, treatment options and recurrence risks.

Partner Notification: If infection (e.g., STI-related) contributed to chronic inversion.

Follow-Up: Regular gynaecological exams to monitor uterine position and fertility outcomes.

Fertility Preservation: Uterine-sparing procedures are prioritized in women desiring future pregnancies.

Complications

Acute Inversion

Severe postpartum haemorrhage (up to 90% of cases).

Hypovolemic or neurogenic shock.

Infection or sepsis (due to prolonged exposure or manipulation).

Uterine rupture or necrosis (rare, if untreated).

Chronic Inversion

Infertility or recurrent miscarriage due to endometrial scarring.

Asherman's syndrome (intrauterine adhesions).

Chronic pelvic pain or abnormal uterine bleeding.

Surgical Complications

Bleeding, infection or injury to adjacent organs (bladder, bowel).

Recurrence of inversion (rare with proper management).

Prevention

Proper Obstetric Management:

Avoid excessive traction on the umbilical cord during the third stage of labor.

Use controlled cord traction only after signs of placental separation.

Avoid fundal pressure before placental delivery.

Uterotonic Use: Administer oxytocin only after confirming placental separation.

Risk Assessment: Identify high-risk patients (e.g., placenta accreta, multiparity) and ensure experienced birth attendants.

Postpartum Monitoring: Prompt recognition of atony or abnormal bleeding to prevent inversion.

Gynecological Care: Early detection and removal of intrauterine masses (e.g., fibroids) to prevent chronic inversion.

Prognosis

Acute Inversion

With prompt recognition and manual repositioning, outcomes are excellent (>90% success rate).

Delayed treatment increases risks of haemorrhage, shock or hysterectomy.

Fertility is usually preserved if the uterus is repositioned without complications.

Chronic Inversion

Prognosis depends on the underlying cause and extent of endometrial damage.

Fertility may be compromised due to scarring or adhesions.

Surgical correction is effective, but hysterectomy may be required in severe cases.

Recurrence: Rare in subsequent pregnancies with proper obstetric management.

Special Cases

Postpartum Setting: Acute inversion is a medical emergency requiring immediate intervention in a controlled setting (e.g., operating room).

Pregnancy Planning: Women with a history of inversion should be monitored closely in future pregnancies; cesarean delivery may be considered if risk factors (e.g., placenta accreta) persist.

Chronic Cases: Rule out malignancy in non-puerperal inversion, especially in older women.

Low-Resource Settings: Higher incidence due to limited access to skilled obstetric care; training birth attendants is critical.

9.8 Adenomyosis

(*Rahmi daroon-i-rahmiyat / Uzal-i-Guddi*)

Definition

Adenomyosis is a benign gynaecological condition characterized by the presence of ectopic endometrial glands and stroma within the myometrium, the muscular layer of the uterus. This leads to uterine enlargement, pain and abnormal uterine bleeding. Adenomyosis is often associated with other gynaecological conditions, such as endometriosis and uterine fibroids, and can significantly impact quality of life and fertility.

Etiology

The exact cause of adenomyosis is not fully understood, but several factors are implicated.

1. Invasive Growth of Endometrium

Endometrial tissue invades the myometrium, possibly due to disruption of the endometrial-myometrial interface during menstruation, childbirth or uterine procedures.

Theories include invagination of the basal endometrium or migration along myometrial lymphatics.

2. Hormonal Influence

Estrogen-dependent condition; symptoms often worsen with high oestrogen states (e.g., reproductive years) and regress after menopause.

Dysregulation of oestrogen, progesterone, or prolactin signaling may promote ectopic endometrial growth.

3. Uterine Trauma or Procedures

Childbirth, cesarean section, dilation and curettage (D&C), or other uterine surgeries may disrupt the endometrial-myometrial barrier, facilitating invasion.

Multiparity is a significant risk factor.

4. Inflammation and Immune Dysregulation

Chronic endometrial inflammation or altered immune responses may contribute to ectopic tissue growth.

Increased expression of inflammatory cytokines (e.g., IL-6, IL-8) is observed.

5. Genetic and Environmental Factors

Family history of adenomyosis or endometriosis suggests a genetic predisposition.

Environmental exposures (e.g., endocrine disruptors) may play a role.

6. Associated Conditions

Endometriosis (30–50% of adenomyosis cases).

Uterine fibroids (common comorbidity).

History of infertility or miscarriage.

Epidemiology

Prevalence: Varies widely (10–60% in hysterectomy specimens), as diagnosis is often confirmed histologically. Incidence is likely underreported due to asymptomatic cases or diagnostic challenges.

Age: Most common in women aged 35–50 years, particularly multiparous women in their late reproductive years.

Risk Factors

Multiparity.

Previous uterine surgery (e.g., cesarean section, myomectomy).

Endometriosis or fibroids.

Obesity (due to increased oestrogen from adipose tissue).

Late menarche or short menstrual cycles (increased oestrogen exposure).

Geographic Variation: Higher prevalence in populations with access to advanced imaging or surgical diagnostics; underdiagnosed in low-resource settings.

Pathophysiology

Adenomyosis results from the infiltration of endometrial glands and stroma into the myometrium, leading to;

1. Myometrial Hypertrophy and Hyperplasia Reactive changes in surrounding muscle cause diffuse or focal uterine enlargement.

2. Ectopic Endometrial Activity: Ectopic tissue responds to hormonal cycles, causing localized bleeding, inflammation, and pain during menstruation.
3. Disrupted Uterine Contractility: Altered myometrial function impairs uterine peristalsis, contributing to dysmenorrhea and infertility.
4. Vascular Changes: Increased vascularity and microbleeding within the myometrium exacerbate heavy menstrual bleeding.

Types

1. Diffuse Adenomyosis Ectopic tissue is spread throughout the myometrium, causing uniform uterine enlargement.
2. Focal Adenomyosis (Adenomyoma): Localized nodules of adenomyotic tissue, resembling fibroids but histologically distinct.

Molecular Mechanisms

Overexpression of oestrogen receptors and aromatase increases local oestrogen production.

Dysregulation of apoptosis and proliferation pathways promotes ectopic tissue survival.

Inflammatory mediators (e.g., prostaglandins) contribute to pain and bleeding.

Clinical Features

1. Symptoms

Dysmenorrhea Severe, progressive menstrual pain, often described as deep pelvic or lower abdominal cramping.

Menorrhagia Heavy menstrual bleeding, leading to anemia in severe cases.

Metrorrhagia: Irregular or intermenstrual bleeding.

Chronic Pelvic Pain: Persistent, non-cyclic pain in some cases.

Dyspareunia: Painful intercourse, particularly deep dyspareunia.

Infertility or Subfertility: Due to impaired endometrial receptivity or uterine contractility.

Pressure Symptoms: In severe cases, uterine enlargement may cause bladder or bowel symptoms (e.g., urgency, constipation).

Asymptomatic: Up to 20–30% of cases, often discovered incidentally during imaging or surgery.

2. Signs

Uterine Enlargement: Palpable, soft, and tender uterus on bimanual examination, often described as “boggy.”

Uterine Tenderness: Especially during menstruation.

Associated Findings: Signs of endometriosis or fibroids (e.g., adnexal tenderness, nodules).

Diagnosis

Diagnosis is based on clinical suspicion, imaging, and, in some cases, histological confirmation.

1. History

Detailed menstrual history (onset, duration, and severity of bleeding or pain).

Obstetric history (parity, prior uterine procedures).

Assess for infertility, endometriosis, or fibroid symptoms.

2. Physical Examination

Bimanual Examination: Enlarged, tender, or boggy uterus; may mimic fibroids.

Speculum Examination: Normal cervix unless coexisting pathology (e.g., cervical erosion).

3. Imaging

Transvaginal Ultrasound (TVUS)

First-line imaging; sensitivity 70–85%.

Findings: Asymmetric myometrial thickening, heterogeneous echotexture, myometrial cysts, poorly defined endometrial-myometrial junction, or focal adenomyomas.

Magnetic Resonance Imaging (MRI)

Gold standard for non-invasive diagnosis; sensitivity >90%.

Findings: Thickened junctional zone (>12 mm), myometrial cysts, or high-signal foci on T2-weighted images.

Hysterosalpingography (HSG): May show diverticula or irregular endometrial contours but is not specific.

4. Histological Diagnosis

Definitive diagnosis requires hysterectomy with histopathological examination (endometrial glands/stroma within myometrium, >2.5 mm below the endometrial-myometrial junction).

Endometrial biopsy or D&C is not diagnostic due to superficial sampling.

Differential Diagnosis

1. Uterine Fibroids: Focal masses with distinct borders, unlike diffuse adenomyosis.
2. Endometriosis: Pelvic implants but may coexist with adenomyosis.
3. Endometrial Cancer: Irregular bleeding, especially in postmenopausal women; requires biopsy.
4. Chronic Endometritis: Inflammatory changes without myometrial invasion.
5. Uterine Sarcoma: Rare, but rapid uterine enlargement requires urgent evaluation.

Management

Management is tailored to symptoms, severity, reproductive goals, and patient age. Options include medical, surgical, and conservative approaches.

1. Medical Management (First-Line for Symptom Control).

Nonsteroidal Anti-Inflammatory Drugs (NSAIDs): Ibuprofen or naproxen for dysmenorrhea and pelvic pain.

Hormonal Therapies:

1. Combined Oral Contraceptives (COCs): Reduce menstrual flow and pain by suppressing ovulation.

2. Progestins - Levonorgestrel-releasing intrauterine system (LNG-IUS, e.g., Mirena): Highly effective for menorrhagia and pain; reduces uterine size. Oral progestins (e.g., norethindrone, medroxyprogesterone) for cycle regulation.

3. Gonadotropin-Releasing Hormone (GnRH) Agonists (e.g., leuprolide): Induce a hypoestrogenic state, reducing adenomyotic activity. Used short-term due to side effects (e.g., bone loss, menopausal symptoms).

4. GnRH Antagonists (e.g., elagolix): Emerging option for pain relief with fewer side effects.

5. Aromatase Inhibitors (e.g., letrozole): Use to suppress local oestrogen production.

Tranexamic Acid: Reduces heavy menstrual bleeding in non-hormonal candidates.

Danazol: Less commonly used due to androgenic side effects but effective for pain and bleeding.

2. Surgical Management

Hysterectomy

Definitive treatment for severe, refractory adenomyosis in women who have completed childbearing.

Vaginal, laparoscopic or abdominal approach depending on uterine size and comorbidities.

Total hysterectomy (removal of uterus and cervix) is preferred; subtotal hysterectomy may leave residual adenomyotic tissue.

Uterine-Sparing Procedures (For women desiring fertility):

Adenomyomectomy: Excision of focal adenomyomas; technically challenging and less effective for diffuse disease.

Uterine Artery Embolization (UAE): Reduces blood flow to adenomyotic tissue, alleviating symptoms (less effective than for fibroids).

High-Intensity Focused Ultrasound (HIFU): Non-invasive ablation of adenomyotic tissue; limited availability and long-term data.

Endometrial Ablation: May reduce bleeding but less effective for deep adenomyosis.

3. Conservative Management

Observation for asymptomatic or mild cases, especially in perimenopausal women, as symptoms often regress post-menopause.

Lifestyle modifications (e.g., weight management, stress reduction) to support overall health.

4. Fertility Management

Adenomyosis is associated with reduced implantation rates and increased miscarriage risk.

LNG-IUS or GnRH agonists may improve endometrial receptivity before assisted reproductive techniques (e.g., IVF).

Surgical excision (adenomyomectomy) may be considered in focal cases but carries risks of uterine rupture in pregnancy.

5. General Measures

Patient education on the condition, treatment options and impact on fertility.

Regular follow-up to monitor symptoms, response to therapy and complications (e.g., anemia).

Screen for coexisting conditions (e.g., endometriosis, fibroids)

Complications

Anemia: Due to chronic heavy menstrual bleeding.

Chronic Pelvic Pain Persistent pain impacting quality of life.

Infertility/Subfertility: Impaired endometrial receptivity or uterine contractility.

Pregnancy Complications Increased risk of miscarriage, preterm labor or abnormal placentation (e.g., placenta previa).

Psychosocial Impact Pain, bleeding, and infertility may lead to anxiety or depression.

Surgical Risks Hysterectomy or adenomyomectomy may cause bleeding, infection or adhesion formation.

Prevention

No specific preventive measures exist due to the unclear etiology.

Risk Reduction Strategies

Minimize unnecessary uterine procedures (e.g., excessive D&C).

Manage obesity and oestrogen-related conditions (e.g., polycystic ovary syndrome).

Early treatment of endometriosis or pelvic infections to reduce inflammation.

Screening: Routine gynaecological examinations and imaging in women with risk factors (e.g., multiparity, prior uterine surgery).

Prognosis

Symptom Control: Medical therapies (e.g., LNG-IUS, hormonal treatments) are effective in 60–80% of patients for pain and bleeding.

Fertility: Variable outcomes; adenomyosis may reduce IVF success rates, but targeted treatments can improve outcomes.

Post-Menopause: Symptoms typically resolve due to oestrogen decline, unless hormone replacement therapy is used.

Hysterectomy: Curative for women not desiring fertility, with excellent resolution of symptoms.

Recurrence Rare after hysterectomy; possible with uterine-sparing procedures if adenomyotic tissue remains.

Special Cases

Pregnancy

Adenomyosis may increase risks of preterm labor, placental abnormalities or cesarean delivery.

Hormonal treatments are contraindicated; NSAIDs or conservative measures are used for pain.

Infertility Patients

Adenomyosis is increasingly recognized as a cause of recurrent implantation failure.

Pretreatment with GnRH agonists or LNG-IUS may improve IVF outcome

Postmenopausal Women

Symptoms are rare unless on hormone replacement therapy; persistent bleeding warrants evaluation for malignancy.

Adolescents/Young Women

Rare but possible in those with early menarche or endometriosis; conservative management is preferred.

9.9 Polyps of Uterus

(*Bawasir-al-Rahim)*

Definition

Uterine polyps, also known as endometrial polyps, are benign growths that arise from the endometrium, the inner lining of the uterus. They are typically pedunculated or sessile masses attached to the endometrial surface, projecting into the uterine cavity. Uterine polyps are composed of endometrial glands, stroma and blood vessels, and may vary in size from a few millimetres to several centimetres.

Epidemiology

Prevalence: Uterine polyps are common, with a prevalence of 10–40% in women undergoing diagnostic evaluation for abnormal uterine bleeding. They are more frequent in perimenopausal and postmenopausal women but can occur at any age.

Age: Peak incidence occurs between 40 and 50 years, though they may be found in premenopausal and postmenopausal women.

Risk Factors

Increased oestrogen exposure (unopposed oestrogen, obesity, polycystic ovary syndrome [PCOS])

Hormone replacement therapy (HRT), particularly oestrogen-only regimens

Tamoxifen use (selective oestrogen receptor modulator with estrogenic effects on the endometrium)

Hypertension and diabetes mellitus

Nulliparity or low parity

Genetic predisposition (e.g., Lynch syndrome increases risk of malignant transformation)

Pathophysiology

Uterine polyps result from focal hyperplasia of the endometrium due to excessive or unopposed oestrogen stimulation. Key mechanisms include:

Hormonal Influence: Estrogen promotes endometrial proliferation, while progesterone counteracts this effect. An imbalance favouring oestrogen leads to localized overgrowth of endometrial tissue.

Molecular Factors: Overexpression of oestrogen and progesterone receptors, growth factors (e.g., vascular endothelial growth factor [VEGF]) and genetic alterations (e.g., in PTEN or KRAS genes) may contribute to polyp formation.

Structural Features:

Polyps may be single or multiple, pedunculated (attached by a stalk) or sessile (broad-based). Histologically, they consist of endometrial glands, fibrous or collagenous stroma, and thick-walled blood vessels. Some polyps may undergo cystic, hyperplastic or atrophic changes depending on hormonal status.

Malignant Potential: Although most uterine polyps are benign, approximately 0.5–1% may become malignant, such as endometrial adenocarcinoma, particularly in postmenopausal women or those with risk factors like Lynch syndrome.

Classification

Uterine polyps can be classified based on:

1. Location:

Endometrial polyps (arising from the endometrium, most common)

Cervical polyps (arising from the endocervical mucosa)

2. Histology:

Functional polyps: Respond to hormonal cycles, resembling normal endometrium.

Atrophic polyps: Seen in postmenopausal women, with inactive glands.

Hyperplastic polyps: Associated with endometrial hyperplasia, indicating excessive oestrogen exposure.

Adenomyomatous polyps: Contain smooth muscle fibers in addition to endometrial tissue.

Malignant polyps: Contain foci of endometrial carcinoma or sarcoma (rare).

3. Number: Single or multiple.

Clinical Features

Uterine polyps may be asymptomatic or symptomatic, depending on size, location and hormonal status. Common clinical presentations include:

a. Abnormal Uterine Bleeding (AUB):

Intermenstrual bleeding

Heavy menstrual bleeding (menorrhagia)

Postmenopausal bleeding

Irregular bleeding patterns

b. Infertility: Polyps may interfere with embryo implantation or sperm transport, contributing to subfertility.

c. Pelvic Pain or Discomfort: Rare, usually associated with large polyps or pedunculated polyps undergoing torsion or necrosis.

d. Asymptomatic: Many polyps are discovered incidentally during imaging or hysteroscopy for other indications.

Diagnosis

Accurate diagnosis of uterine polyps involves a combination of clinical evaluation, imaging and histopathological confirmation.

1. History and Physical Examination:

Detailed menstrual history, including bleeding patterns and associated symptoms.

Risk factor assessment (e.g., obesity, tamoxifen use, HRT).

Pelvic examination may reveal a polyp protruding through the cervix (more common with cervical polyps).

2. Imaging Modalities:

Transvaginal Ultrasound (TVUS)

First-line imaging modality.

Polyps appear as hyperechoic masses within the endometrial cavity, often with a feeding vessel visible on Doppler ultrasound.

Saline infusion sonohysterography (SIS) enhances visualization by distending the uterine cavity, improving sensitivity for detecting polyps (90–95%).

Hysteroscopy

Gold standard for diagnosis.

Allows direct visualization of the uterine cavity and polypectomy under vision.

Sensitivity and specificity approach 95–100%.

Magnetic Resonance Imaging (MRI)

Rarely used, reserved for complex cases or when malignancy is suspected.

Polyps appear as T2-hyperintense masses with enhancement on contrast.

3. Endometrial Sampling:

Endometrial biopsy or dilatation and curettage (D&C) may be performed to sample the endometrium, particularly in postmenopausal women with bleeding.

Limited sensitivity for detecting polyps (may miss focal lesions).

4. Histopathology:

Definitive diagnosis requires histological examination of resected polyp tissue.

Features include endometrial glands, stroma and blood vessels, with or without hyperplastic or malignant changes.

Differential Diagnosis

Submucosal leiomyomas (fibroids)

Endometrial hyperplasia

Endometrial carcinoma

Adenomyosis

Retained products of conception

Blood clots or debris in the uterine cavity

Management

Management of uterine polyps depends on symptoms, patient age, reproductive goals and risk of malignancy.

1. Conservative Management:

Asymptomatic polyps in premenopausal women with low malignancy risk may be monitored with periodic ultrasound.

Small polyps (<1 cm) may regress spontaneously, particularly after menopause or cessation of hormonal therapy.

2. Medical Management:

Limited role for medical therapy, as polyps are unlikely to resolve with hormonal treatment.

Progestins or gonadotropin-releasing hormone (GnRH) agonists may be considered in some cases to manage bleeding but are not curative.

Levonorgestrel-releasing intrauterine system (LNG-IUS) may reduce polyp recurrence in some patients.

3. Surgical Management:

Hysteroscopic Polypectomy: Preferred method for symptomatic polyps or those with high-risk features (e.g., postmenopausal bleeding). Performed under direct visualization using a hysteroscope, with resection via wire loop, scissors or morcellation.

Advantages: Minimally invasive, preserves fertility, allows histological evaluation.

Dilatation and Curettage (D&C): Less preferred due to lower diagnostic and therapeutic accuracy (blind procedure). May be combined with hysteroscopy in resource-limited settings.

Hysterectomy: Reserved for cases with confirmed malignancy, multiple recurrent polyps, or when fertility is not a concern. Considered in postmenopausal women with atypical hyperplasia or carcinoma.

4. Follow-Up:

Postmenopausal women or those with risk factors for malignancy require close monitoring after polypectomy. Recurrence rates are low (2–15%) but higher in women with ongoing oestrogen exposure or tamoxifen use.

Complications

Malignant Transformation: Rare (0.5–1%) but more common in postmenopausal women, those with Lynch syndrome, or polyps >1.5 cm.

Infertility: Polyps may obstruct the endometrial cavity or interfere with implantation, contributing to subfertility.

Recurrence: May occur, particularly in women with persistent risk factors (e.g., obesity, tamoxifen use).

Surgical Complications: Rare, including uterine perforation, infection or adhesion formation (Asherman syndrome) post-hysteroscopy.

Prognosis

Most uterine polyps are benign and resolve with surgical removal or, in some cases, spontaneously.

Symptomatic relief is achieved in 75–100% of patients after polypectomy.

Fertility outcomes improve in women with polyps causing infertility, with pregnancy rates increasing post-resection.

Malignant transformation, though rare, warrants careful evaluation, particularly in high-risk groups.

Prevention

Management of risk factors, such as obesity and unopposed oestrogen exposure, may reduce polyp formation. Routine screening for polyps is not recommended in asymptomatic women due to low malignancy risk. In high-risk groups (e.g., tamoxifen users, Lynch syndrome), periodic endometrial evaluation with ultrasound or hysteroscopy may be considered.

Key Points

Uterine polyps are common benign endometrial growths, often linked to oestrogen excess.

Abnormal uterine bleeding is the hallmark symptom, but many polyps are asymptomatic.

Transvaginal ultrasound with saline infusion sonohysterography and hysteroscopy are key diagnostic tools.

Hysteroscopic polypectomy is the treatment of choice for symptomatic or high-risk polyps.

Malignant transformation is rare but must be ruled out, especially in postmenopausal women or those with risk factors.

9.10 Cysts and Neoplasms of the Uterus

(*Akyas wa sal'a)*

Introduction

Cysts and neoplasms of the uterus encompass a range of benign and malignant conditions originating from the uterine tissues, including the endometrium, myometrium, and cervix. Cysts are fluid-filled sacs, while neoplasms include benign tumours (e.g., leiomyomas) and malignant tumours (e.g., endometrial carcinoma, uterine sarcomas). These conditions vary in prevalence, clinical presentation and management, with significant implications for reproductive health, fertility, and overall morbidity.

Uterine Cysts

Uterine cysts are rare, fluid-filled lesions within or associated with the uterine wall or cavity. Unlike ovarian cysts, true uterine cysts are uncommon and often misdiagnosed or confused with other uterine pathologies (e.g., Nabothian cysts of the cervix, cystic degeneration of leiomyomas, or endometrial cysts related to adenomyosis).

Types of Uterine Cysts

1. Nabothian Cysts:

Found in Cervix (endocervical glands).

Benign, mucus-filled cysts resulting from obstruction of endocervical glands, often due to chronic cervicitis or healing after cervical trauma.

Prevalence: Common, especially in reproductive-age women.

2. Cystic Degeneration of Uterine Leiomyomas:

Areas of cystic change within benign uterine fibroids due to hyaline degeneration or necrosis.

Prevalence: Occurs in 4–10% of leiomyomas, more common in larger tumours.

3. Endometrial Cysts (Adenomyosis-Related):

Cystic spaces within the myometrium caused by ectopic endometrial tissue in adenomyosis.

Prevalence: Rare, seen in severe adenomyosis cases.

4. Congenital Uterine Cysts:

Rare anomalies, such as Mullerian duct cysts, resulting from embryologic maldevelopment.

Prevalence: Extremely rare, often associated with uterine malformations.

Epidemiology

Nabothian Cysts: Common in women of reproductive age, particularly multiparous women or those with a history of cervical inflammation.

Cystic Leiomyomas: More frequent in women aged 30–50 years, aligning with the peak incidence of leiomyomas.

Endometrial Cysts: Seen in women with adenomyosis, typically aged 40–50 years.

Risk Factors

Chronic cervicitis (for Nabothian cysts).

Estrogen exposure, obesity and nulliparity (for leiomyomas and adenomyosis-related cysts).

Congenital anomalies (for Mullerian cysts).

Pathophysiology

Nabothian Cysts: Result from blockage of endocervical gland openings, leading to mucus accumulation. Chronic inflammation or squamous metaplasia contributes.

Cystic Degeneration of Leiomyomas: Occurs due to inadequate blood supply in large fibroids, leading to hyaline or cystic degeneration. The cystic areas contain gelatinous or fluid-filled spaces.

Endometrial Cysts: Form when ectopic endometrial tissue within the myometrium (adenomyosis) undergoes cyclic bleeding, creating small cystic cavities.

Congenital Cysts: Arise from incomplete fusion or resorption of Mullerian ducts during embryogenesis.

Clinical Features

Nabothian Cysts: Usually asymptomatic, discovered incidentally during pelvic examination or imaging. Rarely cause cervical enlargement or discomfort if large.

Cystic Leiomyomas: Heavy menstrual bleeding (menorrhagia). Pelvic pain or pressure, especially with large cysts. Infertility or pregnancy complications (e.g., miscarriage, preterm labor).

Endometrial Cysts (Adenomyosis): Dysmenorrhea (painful periods). Menorrhagia or irregular bleeding. Uterine enlargement or tenderness.

Congenital Cysts: May present with infertility, recurrent miscarriage, or symptoms related to associated uterine anomalies (e.g., dyspareunia, amenorrhea).

Diagnosis

1. History and Physical Examination:

Assess menstrual history, pain and fertility issues.

Pelvic examination may reveal a palpable mass (leiomyomas), uterine tenderness (adenomyosis), or visible cervical cysts (Nabothian).

2. Imaging:

Transvaginal Ultrasound (TVUS): First-line modality.

Nabothian cysts: Hypoechoic, well-defined cervical lesions.

Cystic leiomyomas: Heterogeneous masses with cystic areas within the myometrium.

Endometrial cysts: Small, hypoechoic areas within a diffusely enlarged myometrium (adenomyosis).

Saline Infusion Sonohysterography (SIS): Enhances visualization of intrauterine cysts.

Magnetic Resonance Imaging (MRI):

Gold standard for characterizing adenomyosis-related cysts and cystic leiomyomas. Shows T2-hyperintense cystic areas and distinguishes benign from malignant lesions.

Hysteroscopy: Useful for evaluating intrauterine cysts or associated endometrial pathology.

3. Histopathology:

Rarely required for Nabothian cysts (diagnosed clinically or via imaging).

Biopsy or surgical resection (e.g., myomectomy) confirms cystic degeneration in leiomyomas or adenomyosis.

Differential Diagnosis

Endometrial polyps

Submucosal leiomyomas

Endometrial hyperplasia or carcinoma

Ovarian cysts (misdiagnosed as uterine in imaging)

Uterine sarcomas (rare, but cystic degeneration can mimic benign cysts)

Management

1. Conservative Management:

Asymptomatic Nabothian cysts require no treatment.

Small, asymptomatic cystic leiomyomas or endometrial cysts may be monitored with serial imaging.

2. Medical Management:

Symptomatic relief for adenomyosis-related cysts: Nonsteroidal anti-inflammatory drugs (NSAIDs) for pain, hormonal therapy (e.g., oral contraceptives, progestins, or levonorgestrel-releasing intrauterine system [LNG-IUS]) to reduce bleeding.

GnRH agonists may shrink cystic leiomyomas temporarily but are not curative.

3. Surgical Management:

Nabothian Cysts: Rarely require intervention; large symptomatic cysts may be excised or drained via electrocautery or cryotherapy.

Cystic Leiomyomas:

Myomectomy (open, laparoscopic or hysteroscopic) for fertility preservation or symptomatic relief.

Uterine artery embolization (UAE) to reduce blood supply and shrink fibroids.

Hysterectomy for severe symptoms or when fertility is not a concern.

Endometrial Cysts (Adenomyosis):

Hysterectomy is definitive for severe cases.

Endometrial ablation or excision for focal adenomyosis (rarely performed).

Congenital Cysts: Surgical resection or correction of associated anomalies, depending on symptoms and reproductive goals.

4. Follow-Up:

Regular ultrasound monitoring for asymptomatic cysts.

Post-treatment follow-up for recurrence or complications.

Complications

Nabothian Cysts: Rare, but large cysts may cause cervical obstruction or infection.

Cystic Leiomyomas: Pain, infertility, pregnancy complications (e.g., preterm labor, malpresentation), or degeneration leading to acute abdomen.

Endometrial Cysts: Chronic pain, infertility or progression of adenomyosis.

Congenital Cysts: Associated with congenital anomalies, leading to infertility or obstetric complications.

Uterine Neoplasms

Definition

Uterine neoplasms are abnormal growths of uterine tissue, classified as benign (e.g., leiomyomas) or malignant (e.g., endometrial carcinoma, uterine sarcomas). They arise from the endometrium, myometrium or cervix and vary in clinical presentation, prognosis and management.

Types of Uterine Neoplasms

1. Benign Neoplasms

Leiomyomas (Uterine Fibroids):Most common benign uterine tumour, composed of smooth muscle and fibrous tissue.

Subtypes: Submucosal, intramural, subserosal or pedunculated.

Adenomyomas: Rare, benign tumours with endometrial glands and stroma within the myometrium, distinct from adenomyosis.

2. Malignant Neoplasms

Endometrial Carcinoma: Most common uterine malignancy, arising from the endometrium.

Subtypes: Type I (endometrioid, oestrogen-dependent, better prognosis) and Type II (non-endometrioid, e.g., serous, clear cell, poorer prognosis).

Uterine Sarcomas: Rare, aggressive tumours arising from the myometrium or endometrial stroma.

Subtypes: Leiomyosarcoma, endometrial stromal sarcoma, adenosarcoma.

Carcinosarcoma (Malignant Mixed Mullerian Tumour): Mixed epithelial and mesenchymal malignancy, often aggressive.

Epidemiology

Leiomyomas

Prevalence: 20–80% of women by age 50, highest in reproductive-age women (30–50 years).

Risk Factors: Africans, obesity, nulliparity, early menarche, late menopause, hypertension.

Endometrial Carcinoma

Prevalence: Most common gynaecological malignancy in developed countries, with a lifetime risk of ~3%.

Age: Peak incidence at 60–70 years (postmenopausal).

Risk Factors: Unopposed oestrogen exposure, obesity, diabetes, PCOS, Lynch syndrome, tamoxifen use, nulliparity.

Uterine Sarcomas

Prevalence: Rare, accounting for 3–7% of uterine malignancies.

Age: Typically postmenopausal, but leiomyosarcoma may occur in younger women.

Risk Factors: Prior pelvic radiation, tamoxifen use, Africans (for leiomyosarcoma).

Carcinosarcoma

Prevalence: <2% of uterine malignancies, typically in postmenopausal women.

Risk Factors: Similar to endometrial carcinoma, plus prior radiation exposure.

Pathophysiology

Leiomyomas

Arise from monoclonal proliferation of myometrial smooth muscle cells.

Estrogen and progesterone promote growth via upregulation of growth factors (e.g., TGF-β, VEGF).

Genetic alterations: MED12 mutations, HMGA2 rearrangements.

Endometrial Carcinoma

Type I: Driven by unopposed oestrogen, leading to endometrial hyperplasia and progression to endometrioid carcinoma. PTEN, KRAS and PIK3CA mutations are common.

Type II: Estrogen-independent, associated with p53 mutations, HER2 amplification and aggressive behavior (serous, clear cell subtypes).

Uterine Sarcomas

Leiomyosarcoma: Arises from myometrial smooth muscle, with complex karyotypes and TP53 mutations.

Endometrial stromal sarcoma: Characterized by JAZF1-SUZ12 gene fusions in low-grade tumours; high-grade tumours show YWHAE-NUTM2 fusions.

Adenosarcoma: Mixed tumour with benign glands and low-grade sarcomatous stroma.

Carcinosarcoma

Biphasic tumour with epithelial (carcinoma) and mesenchymal (sarcoma) components, often driven by epithelial-mesenchymal transition (EMT) and TP53 mutations.

Clinical Features

Leiomyomas

Heavy menstrual bleeding (menorrhagia), especially with submucosal fibroids.

Pelvic pain or pressure, urinary frequency, constipation (large fibroids).

Infertility or recurrent miscarriage.

Asymptomatic in up to 50% of cases.

Endometrial Carcinoma

Postmenopausal bleeding (hallmark symptom, present in 90% of cases).

Abnormal uterine bleeding in premenopausal women.

Pelvic pain, weight loss or systemic symptoms in advanced stages.

Uterine Sarcomas

Abnormal uterine bleeding (postmenopausal or irregular).

Rapidly enlarging pelvic mass.

Pain, weight loss or systemic symptoms in advanced disease.

Carcinosarcoma

Postmenopausal bleeding, pelvic mass or pain.

Systemic symptoms (e.g., weight loss, fatigue) in metastatic disease.

Diagnosis

1. History and Physical Examination

Detailed menstrual history, bleeding patterns and systemic symptoms.

Pelvic examination may reveal an enlarged uterus, palpable mass or cervical abnormalities.

2. Imaging:

Transvaginal Ultrasound (TVUS)

Leiomyomas: Well-defined, hypoechoic myometrial masses; cystic degeneration may be seen.

Endometrial carcinoma: Thickened endometrium (>4 mm in postmenopausal women), irregular masses.

Sarcomas: Heterogeneous, rapidly growing masses with necrosis or haemorrhage.

Saline Infusion Sonohysterography (SIS)

Enhances visualization of endometrial lesions (e.g., submucosal fibroids, endometrial carcinoma).

MRI

Gold standard for characterizing leiomyomas, sarcomas and adenomyosis.

Endometrial carcinoma: T2-hyperintense endometrial mass with myometrial invasion.

Sarcomas: Heterogeneous masses with necrosis, haemorrhage, or irregular borders.

CT/PET Scan

Used for staging malignant neoplasms (endometrial carcinoma, sarcomas, carcinosarcoma).

3. Endometrial Sampling

Endometrial biopsy or dilatation and curettage (D&C) for suspected endometrial carcinoma or sarcoma. Sensitivity: 90–95% for detecting endometrial carcinoma; lower for sarcomas (focal lesions).

4. Hysteroscopy

Direct visualization of endometrial cavity for polyps, submucosal fibroids or carcinoma. Allows targeted biopsy or resection.

5. Histopathology

Leiomyomas: Whorled bundles of smooth muscle cells with minimal atypia.

Endometrial carcinoma: Endometrioid (glandular) or non-endometrioid (serous, clear cell) patterns.

Sarcomas: High-grade spindle cells (leiomyosarcoma), stromal atypia (endometrial stromal sarcoma), or mixed features (adenosarcoma, carcinosarcoma).

6. Molecular Testing

Lynch syndrome testing (e.g., MMR immunohistochemistry) in endometrial carcinoma.

Genetic profiling (e.g., TP53, PTEN) for prognostic assessment in sarcomas or advanced carcinoma.

Differential Diagnosis

Uterine polyps

Endometrial hyperplasia

Adenomyosis

Cervical carcinoma

Metastatic tumours to the uterus (rare)

Ovarian tumours (may mimic uterine masses on imaging)

Management

1. Benign Neoplasms (Leiomyomas)

Conservative Management: Asymptomatic fibroids: Monitor with serial ultrasound.

Medical Management: NSAIDs for pain relief.

Hormonal therapy (e.g., oral contraceptives, progestins, LNG-IUS) to control bleeding.

GnRH agonists/antagonists or selective progesterone receptor modulators (e.g., ulipristal acetate) to shrink fibroids.

Surgical Management

Myomectomy (open, laparoscopic, or hysteroscopic) for fertility preservation or symptomatic relief.

Uterine artery embolization (UAE) or focused ultrasound surgery (FUS) for non-surgical candidates.

Hysterectomy for definitive treatment in non-fertility-preserving cases.

2. Malignant Neoplasms

Endometrial Carcinoma

Surgery: Total hysterectomy with bilateral salpingo-oophorectomy (TH/BSO) ± lymph node assessment (sentinel lymph node biopsy or lymphadenectomy).

Adjuvant Therapy

Radiation (vaginal brachytherapy or external beam) for intermediate/high-risk disease.

Chemotherapy (carboplatin/paclitaxel) for advanced or high-grade tumours.

Hormonal therapy (progestins) for fertility preservation in select early-stage cases (e.g., grade 1 endometrioid).

Targeted Therapy: Immunotherapy (e.g., pembrolizumab for MMR-deficient tumours) or PARP inhibitors in advanced cases.

Uterine Sarcoma

Surgery: TH/BSO, often without lymphadenectomy (sarcomas rarely metastasize to lymph nodes).

Adjuvant Therapy: Chemotherapy (e.g., doxorubicin, ifosfamide) or radiation for high-risk or metastatic disease.

Palliative Care: For advanced, unresectable tumours.

Carcinosarcoma

Surgery: TH/BSO with staging (peritoneal washings, omentectomy).

Adjuvant Therapy: Chemotherapy (carboplatin/paclitaxel) ± radiation for local control.

Prognosis: Poor due to aggressive behavior and high recurrence rates.

3. Follow-Up

Benign neoplasms: Monitor for recurrence or symptom progression.

Malignant neoplasms: Regular surveillance with imaging, tumour markers (e.g., CA-125 in sarcomas) and clinical evaluation for recurrence.

Complications

Leiomyomas

Infertility, miscarriage or obstetric complications (e.g., preterm labor, malpresentation).

Degeneration (hyaline, cystic, or red degeneration), causing acute pain.

Rarely, sarcomatous transformation (<0.5%, leiomyosarcoma).

Endometrial Carcinoma

Local invasion (myometrium, cervix) or distant metastasis (lungs, liver).

Recurrence, particularly in high-grade or Type II tumours.

Uterine Sarcomas/Carcinosarcoma:

Rapid metastasis (hematogenous spread to lungs, liver).

High mortality rates due to aggressive biology.

Prognosis

Leiomyomas: Excellent prognosis; symptoms resolve with treatment or menopause.

Endometrial Carcinoma:

Type I: 5-year survival >80% for early-stage disease (stage I/II).

Type II: Poorer prognosis, with 5-year survival ~30–60% for advanced stages.

Uterine Sarcomas: Poor prognosis; 5-year survival 20–50% depending on subtype and stage.

Carcinosarcoma: 5-year survival <30%, with high recurrence rates.

Prevention

Leiomyomas: Weight management, hormonal balance (e.g., oral contraceptives to reduce oestrogen excess).

Endometrial Carcinoma: Manage risk factors: Obesity, diabetes, unopposed oestrogen. Screening in high-risk groups (e.g., Lynch syndrome) with annual endometrial biopsy or TVUS starting at age 30–35.

Sarcomas/Carcinosarcoma: No specific preventive measures; avoid unnecessary pelvic radiation or tamoxifen in high-risk patients.

Key Points

Cysts

Uterine cysts are rare; Nabothian cysts (cervical) and cystic degeneration of leiomyomas are most common. Most are benign and asymptomatic, requiring no treatment unless symptomatic. Diagnosis relies on TVUS, MRI or hysteroscopy; histopathology confirms complex cases.

Neoplasms

Leiomyomas are the most common benign uterine tumours, managed conservatively or surgically based on symptoms. Endometrial carcinoma is the most common uterine malignancy, with postmenopausal bleeding as the hallmark symptom. Uterine sarcomas and carcinosarcomas are rare, aggressive and require prompt surgical intervention.

Diagnosis: TVUS, MRI, hysteroscopy and endometrial biopsy are done for evaluation.

Management: Plan according to fertility goals, symptom severity and malignancy risk, ranging from conservative monitoring to hysterectomy and adjuvant therapy.

Prognosis: Benign lesions have excellent outcomes; malignant neoplasms require early detection for optimal survival.

Endometrial Cancer

Definition

Endometrial cancer is a malignant neoplasm originating from the endometrium of the uterus. It is the most common gynaecological malignancy in developed countries and primarily affects postmenopausal women. Endometrial cancer is broadly classified into two types based on etiology, histopathology and prognosis: Type I (endometrioid, oestrogen-dependent) and Type II (non-endometrioid, oestrogen-independent).

Epidemiology

Prevalence: Endometrial cancer accounts for approximately 7% of all cancers in women and is the most common gynecologic cancer in developed countries, with a lifetime risk of ~3%.

Incidence: Approximately 66,000 new cases annually in the United States (2023 data), with rising incidence due to increasing obesity rates.

Age: Peak incidence occurs between 60 and 70 years, with >90% of cases in postmenopausal women. Rare in women under 40 years (<5%).

Geographic Variation: Higher incidence in developed countries (e.g., North America, Europe) due to obesity, low parity and longer life expectancy.

Risk Factors

Estrogen-Related: Unopposed oestrogen exposure (e.g., oestrogen-only hormone replacement therapy [HRT], obesity, polycystic ovary syndrome [PCOS], early menarche, late menopause, nulliparity).

Medical: Tamoxifen use (selective oestrogen receptor modulator with endometrial stimulation), diabetes mellitus, hypertension.

Genetic: Lynch syndrome (hereditary nonpolyposis colorectal cancer, HNPCC) increases risk by 40–60% (MLH1, MSH2, MSH6, PMS2 mutations).

Other: Family history of endometrial or colorectal cancer, previous breast or ovarian cancer.

Protective Factors

Combined oral contraceptives (reduce risk by 50% with >5 years of use).

Pregnancy and higher parity.

Progesterone therapy (e.g., levonorgestrel-releasing intrauterine system [LNG-IUS]).

Smoking (reduces oestrogen levels, though not recommended due to other risks).

Pathophysiology

Endometrial cancer arises from malignant transformation of endometrial cells, driven by hormonal, genetic and molecular alterations. The two main types differ in their pathogenesis:

1. Type I Endometrial Cancer (Endometrioid)

Etiology: Estrogen-driven, associated with unopposed oestrogen exposure leading to endometrial hyperplasia (simple, complex or atypical).

Histopathology: Endometrioid adenocarcinoma (grades 1–3 based on differentiation). Well-differentiated tumours (grade 1) resemble normal endometrium.

Precursor Lesion: Atypical endometrial hyperplasia, with 20–50% progression to carcinoma if untreated.

Prognosis: Favorable, with 5-year survival rates of 80–90% for early-stage disease.

2. Type II Endometrial Cancer (Non-Endometrioid)

Etiology: Estrogen-independent, often arising in atrophic endometrium.

Histopathology: Includes serous, clear cell, mucinous or undifferentiated carcinomas. Serous carcinoma is the most common subtype.

Precursor Lesion: Endometrial intraepithelial carcinoma (EIC) for serous subtype.

Prognosis: Poor, with aggressive behavior and 5-year survival rates of 30–60%.

3. Staging (FIGO 2023 Classification)

Stage I: Confined to the uterus (IA: <50% myometrial invasion; IB: ≥50% invasion).

Stage 2: Cervical stromal invasion.

Stage III: Local/regional spread (e.g., adnexa, lymph nodes, vagina).

Stage IV: Distant metastasis (e.g., lungs, liver, bones) or bladder/rectal invasion.

Clinical Features

Postmenopausal Bleeding (PMB)

Hallmark symptom, present in 90% of cases.

Any PMB warrants evaluation, as 10–15% of cases are due to endometrial cancer.

Abnormal Uterine Bleeding (AUB)

In premenopausal women: Irregular, heavy or intermenstrual bleeding.

Advanced Disease

Pelvic pain or pressure (due to myometrial invasion or extrauterine spread).

Weight loss, fatigue or anorexia.

Symptoms of metastasis (e.g., cough, dyspnea for lung metastases; abdominal distension for peritoneal spread).

Asymptomatic: Rare, detected incidentally during imaging or hysterectomy for other indications.

Diagnosis

Accurate diagnosis involves a combination of clinical evaluation, imaging and histopathological confirmation.

1. History and Physical Examination

Detailed menstrual history, risk factors (e.g., obesity, tamoxifen use, family history).

Pelvic examination: May reveal uterine enlargement, cervical abnormalities, or palpable masses in advanced disease.

General examination: Assess for signs of metastasis (e.g., lymphadenopathy, hepatomegaly).

2. Imaging

a. Transvaginal Ultrasound (TVUS)

First-line modality for evaluating PMB. Endometrial thickness >4 mm in postmenopausal women or >10–15 mm in premenopausal women prompts further evaluation.

Findings: Thickened, heterogeneous endometrium; irregular masses; myometrial invasion.

Sensitivity: 90–95% for detecting endometrial abnormalities.

b. Saline Infusion Sonohysterography (SIS)

Enhances visualization of focal endometrial lesions (e.g., polyps vs. carcinoma).

c. Magnetic Resonance Imaging (MRI)

Gold standard for assessing myometrial invasion and staging.

Findings: T2-hyperintense endometrial mass, disruption of junctional zone, lymph node involvement.

d. Computed Tomography (CT) or Positron Emission Tomography (PET)

Used for staging in advanced disease or suspected metastasis. Detects lymph node, peritoneal, or distant spread.

3. Endometrial Sampling

a. Endometrial Biopsy

OPD procedure using a Pipelle .

Sensitivity: 90–95% for detecting endometrial carcinoma.

Preferred for initial evaluation of AUB or PMB.

b. Dilatation and Curettage (D&C):

Performed under anaesthesia, if biopsy is inconclusive or insufficient tissue is obtained.

Often combined with hysteroscopy for direct visualization.

c. Hysteroscopy

Allows visualization of the endometrial cavity and targeted biopsy of suspicious lesions.

Sensitivity and specificity: 95–100%.

4. Histopathology

Confirms diagnosis and determines tumour type (endometrioid vs. non-endometrioid) and grade.

Endometrioid: Glandular structures resembling normal endometrium (grades 1–3).

Non-endometrioid: Papillary (serous), clear cell or undifferentiated patterns.

Immunohistochemistry: Assess for mismatch repair (MMR) proteins (Lynch syndrome), p53 or oestrogen/progesterone receptor status.

5. Molecular Testing

MSI testing or MMR immunohistochemistry for Lynch syndrome screening.

Next-generation sequencing (e.g., PTEN, TP53, POLE mutations) for prognostic and therapeutic guidance.

POLE-mutated tumours (5–10%) have an excellent prognosis; MMR-deficient tumours may respond to immunotherapy.

6. Staging

Surgical staging (FIGO system) involves total hysterectomy, bilateral salpingo-oophorectomy (TH/BSO), peritoneal washings, and lymph node assessment (sentinel lymph node biopsy or lymphadenectomy).

Differential Diagnosis

Endometrial hyperplasia (simple, complex, atypical)

Uterine polyps

Submucosal leiomyomas

Adenomyosis

Uterine sarcomas or carcinosarcoma

Cervical cancer

Metastatic tumours to the endometrium (e.g., breast, colon)

Management

Management of endometrial cancer is tailored to tumour type, stage, grade, patient age, comorbidities and fertility desires.

1. Surgical Management

a. Standard Treatment

Total hysterectomy with bilateral salpingo-oophorectomy (TH/BSO).

Sentinel lymph node biopsy (preferred) or pelvic/para-aortic lymphadenectomy for staging.

Peritoneal washings and omentectomy in high-risk or non-endometrioid tumours.

b. Minimally Invasive Surgery

Laparoscopic or robotic-assisted TH/BSO preferred for early-stage disease (stages I–II).

Reduces morbidity compared to open surgery.

c. Fertility-Sparing Treatment

Considered in young women with grade 1 endometrioid carcinoma confined to the endometrium (stage IA).

High-dose progestin therapy (e.g., megestrol acetate, LNG-IUS) with regular endometrial sampling every 3–6 months.

Requires complete response (no residual tumour) before attempting pregnancy; hysterectomy recommended post-childbearing.

2. Adjuvant Therapy

a. Radiation Therapy

Vaginal brachytherapy for stage I, intermediate-risk disease (e.g., grade 2–3, minimal myometrial invasion).

External beam radiation therapy (EBRT) for stage II or high-risk stage I (e.g., deep myometrial invasion, lymphovascular space invasion).

b. Chemotherapy

Indicated for stage III–IV or high-risk disease (e.g., serous, clear cell carcinomas).

Regimen: Carboplatin and paclitaxel (standard).

c. Hormonal Therapy

Progestins (e.g., megestrol acetate) for recurrent or metastatic endometrioid carcinoma with positive oestrogen/progesterone receptors.

d. Targeted Therapy

Immunotherapy (e.g., pembrolizumab, dostarlimab) for MMR-deficient or MSI-high tumours.

Lenvatinib (VEGF inhibitor) with pembrolizumab for advanced, non-MSI-high tumours.

PARP inhibitors (e.g., olaparib) under investigation for specific molecular subtypes.

3. Palliative Care

For advanced, unresectable or metastatic disease.

Focuses on symptom control (e.g., pain, bleeding) and quality of life.

4. Follow-Up

Surveillance every 3–6 months for 2–3 years, then annually.

Includes physical examination, symptom review and imaging (CT/MRI) if high-risk.

CA-125 levels may be monitored in advanced or serous carcinomas.

Complications

Local Invasion: Myometrium, cervix or adjacent structures (bladder, rectum).

Metastasis: Common sites include lymph nodes, lungs, liver and peritoneum.

Recurrence: 10–15% in early-stage disease; higher in advanced or Type II tumours (30–50%).

Vaginal cuff recurrence (common in stage I–II).

Distant recurrence (lungs, liver in stage III–IV).

Treatment-Related

Surgical: Lymphedema, infection or bowel/bladder injury.

Radiation: Vaginal stenosis, bowel toxicity or secondary malignancies.

Chemotherapy: Neutropenia, neuropathy or renal toxicity.

Prognosis

Stage I: 5-year survival 80–90% (Type I, endometrioid).

Stage II: 5-year survival 70–80%.

Stage III: 5-year survival 50–60%. Stage IV: 5-year survival 15–30%.

Type I vs. Type II:

Type I (endometrioid): Better prognosis due to early detection and lower grade.

Type II (non-endometrioid): Poor prognosis due to aggressive biology and late presentation.

Molecular Subtypes:

POLE-mutated: Excellent prognosis (5-year survival >90%).

MMR deficient: Intermediate prognosis, responsive to immunotherapy.

TP53 mutated: Poor prognosis, aggressive disease.

Copy number low: Favorable prognosis, typical of low-grade endometrioid tumours.

Prevention

Lifestyle Modifications

Weight management to reduce obesity-related oestrogen excess.

Control of diabetes and hypertension.

Hormonal Interventions

Combined oral contraceptives or LNG-IUS to reduce endometrial proliferation.

Avoid unopposed oestrogen HRT in women with an intact uterus.

Screening

No routine screening in the general population due to low prevalence and effective early detection via PMB evaluation.

High-risk groups (e.g., Lynch syndrome)

Annual endometrial biopsy or TVUS starting at age 30–35.

Advise prophylactic hysterectomy after childbearing.

Genetic Counseling

Recommended for patients with a family history of endometrial, colorectal or ovarian cancer to assess for Lynch syndrome.

Key Points

Endometrial cancer is the most common gynecologic malignancy, with postmenopausal bleeding as the hallmark symptom.

Type I (endometrioid, oestrogen-driven) accounts for 80–90% of cases and has a better prognosis than Type II (non-endometrioid, aggressive).

Risk factors include unopposed oestrogen, obesity, diabetes and Lynch syndrome.

Diagnosis involves TVUS, endometrial biopsy and hysteroscopy; MRI/CT for staging.

Surgical management (TH/BSO) is the cornerstone, with adjuvant radiation, chemotherapy or immunotherapy based on stage and molecular profile.

Fertility-sparing options are possible for select early-stage cases but require close monitoring.

Prognosis is excellent for early-stage Type I cancers but poor for advanced or Type II tumours.

Prevention focuses on managing risk factors and screening high-risk groups (e.g., Lynch syndrome).

Long Answer Questions

1. Classify uterine diseases, describe the clinical features and management of uterine fibroids.
2. Discuss the etiology, diagnosis and treatment of endometriosis and adenomyosis.
3. Explain abnormal uterine bleeding (AUB)—types, causes and therapeutic approach.
4. Describe chronic endometritis—pathophysiology, symptoms and treatment.
5. Elaborate on uterine prolapse—grades, causes and surgical management.

Short Answer Questions (2 Marks Each)

1. What is adenomyosis?
2. Name two causes of abnormal uterine bleeding.
3. Define endometritis.
4. Mention one complication of untreated fibroid.
5. What is the role of oestrogen in uterine pathology?

Multiple Choice Questions (1 Mark Each)

1. Most common benign tumour of the uterus:

a) Polyp b) Fibroid c) Adenoma d) Cyst

Ans: b) Fibroid

2. Endometriosis involves:

a) Cervix b) Endometrium c) Extrauterine endometrial tissue d) Myometrium

Ans: c) Extrauterine endometrial tissue

3. Adenomyosis is characterized by:

a) Endometrial tissue in myometrium b) Fibroid degeneration c) Cervical erosion d) Uterine atrophy

Ans: a) Endometrial tissue in myometrium

4. Common symptom of uterine fibroid:

a) Amenorrhea b) Menorrhagia c) Dyspareunia d) Vaginal dryness

Ans: b) Menorrhagia

5. Endometritis is commonly caused by:

a) Viral infection b) Bacterial infection c) Hormonal imbalance d) Trauma

Ans: b) Bacterial infection

6. Which condition may present with dysmenorrhea and infertility?

a) Fibroid b) Endometriosis c) Cervical polyp d) Vaginitis

Ans: b) Endometriosis

7. Uterine prolapse is graded based on:

a) Cervical length b) Vaginal depth c) Descent of uterus d) Menstrual history

Ans: c) Descent of uterus

8. Which hormone promotes endometrial proliferation?

a) Progesterone b) Estrogen c) FSH d) LH

Ans: b) Estrogen

9. Pyometra refers to:

a) Blood in uterus b) Pus in uterus c) Fluid in uterus d) Air in uterus

Ans: b) Pus in uterus

10. Which imaging modality is preferred for fibroid diagnosis?

a) X-ray b) CT scan c) Ultrasound d) MRI brain

Ans: c) Ultrasound

10

Diseases of the Fallopian Tubes & Ovaries

(Amrad-I Qadhifen wa Khusya al-Rahim)

10.1 *Iltihab-i-Qadhifain* (Salpingitis)
10.2 *Iltihab-i-Khusya-i-Rahim* (Oophritis)
10.3 *Batana-i-Rahmiyat/Darun-i-Rahmiyat* (Endometriois)
10.4 *Mutalazema takai-yasul-mabayez* (polycystic ovarian syndrome)
10.5 *Akyas wa Sal'a* (Cysts & Neopalsm)

Learning Objective (At the end of the session, the students should be able to):

Discuss the causes, types, diagnosis, management and complications of *Iltihab-e-Qazafain* (Salpingitis).
Describe briefly *Iltihab-e-Khusyatur-Rahim* (Oophoritis)
Discuss the causes, classify to sites, diagnosis, management and complications of *Batan-e-Rehmiyat* (Endometriosis)
Elaborate the etiopathogenesis, diagnosis, management and complications of PCOD
Explain the causes, stages, diagnosis and complications of *Daweera-wa-Sulaat* (Cysts & Neoplasm)

10.1 Salpingitis

(*Iltihab-i-Qadhifain*)

Definition

Salpingitis is the inflammation of the fallopian tubes, often resulting from an infectious process. It is a key component of pelvic inflammatory disease (PID), which involves inflammation of the upper female reproductive tract, including the uterus, fallopian tubes and ovaries. Salpingitis can be acute, subacute or chronic, and it is primarily caused by bacterial infections, with significant implications for reproductive health, including infertility and ectopic pregnancy.

Epidemiology

Prevalence: Salpingitis is a common manifestation of PID, affecting approximately 4–5% of reproductive-age women. Global prevalence varies, with higher rates in regions with limited access to healthcare.

Age: Most common in sexually active women aged 15–35 years, with peak incidence in the 20–24 age group.

Risk Factors

1. Sexual Behavior: Multiple sexual partners, new partners, or unprotected intercourse.
2. Infections: History of sexually transmitted infections (STIs), particularly Chlamydia trachomatis and Neisseria gonorrhoeae .
3. Obstetric/Gynecological History: Recent intrauterine procedures (e.g., insertion of intrauterine devices [IUDs], abortion, or endometrial biopsy).
4. Other: Poor genital hygiene, douching, smoking and low socioeconomic status.
5. Geographic Variation: Higher incidence in developing countries due to limited STI screening and treatment.

Etiology

Salpingitis is primarily infectious, with bacteria ascending from the lower genital tract (vagina and cervix) to the fallopian tubes. Common causative organisms include:

Sexually Transmitted Pathogens

Chlamydia trachomatis (most common, 50–60% of cases, often asymptomatic initially).

Neisseria gonorrhoeae (20–30% of cases, associated with acute, severe symptoms).

Polymicrobial Infections

Anaerobes (e.g., Bacteroides spp., Peptostreptococcus spp.).

Aerobic bacteria (e.g., Escherichia coli, Streptococcus spp.).

Mycoplasma genitalium (emerging cause).

Rare Causes

Mycobacterium tuberculosis (tuberculous salpingitis, common in endemic areas, often chronic).

Actinomyces spp. (associated with long-term IUD use).

Non-infectious causes (rare): Autoimmune disorders, chemical irritation (e.g., post-surgical).

Pathophysiology

Salpingitis results from the ascent of pathogens from the lower genital tract to the fallopian tubes, leading to inflammation and tissue damage. The process involves:

1. Infection and Inflammation

Pathogens breach the cervical mucus barrier, often facilitated by menstruation, sexual intercourse or intrauterine procedures.

Bacteria invade the fallopian tube mucosa, triggering an inflammatory response with neutrophil infiltration, edema and exudate formation.

Purulent exudate (pus) may accumulate in the tubal lumen, leading to pyosalpinx (pus-filled tube).

2. Tissue Damage

Acute inflammation causes ciliary dysfunction, mucosal ulceration and adhesions.

Chronic inflammation leads to fibrosis, tubal scarring, and occlusion, impairing ovum transport and increasing ectopic pregnancy risk.

3. Spread

Infection may spread to adjacent structures (e.g., ovaries, peritoneum), causing tubo-ovarian abscess (TOA) or peritonitis.

Hematogenous spread (e.g., in tuberculous salpingitis) is rare but possible.

4. Types

Acute Salpingitis: Characterized by intense inflammation, purulent discharge and systemic symptoms.

Chronic Salpingitis: Results from untreated or recurrent acute episodes, leading to adhesions, tubal occlusion or hydrosalpinx (fluid-filled tube).

Clinical Features

The presentation of salpingitis varies depending on its acuity and severity. Many cases, particularly those caused by Chlamydia, may be asymptomatic or subclinical, contributing to delayed diagnosis and complications.

1. Acute Salpingitis

Pelvic Pain: Bilateral lower abdominal or pelvic pain, often constant and worsening with movement or intercourse (dyspareunia).

Fever: Present in 30–50% of cases, often low-grade (38–39°C).

Vaginal Discharge: Purulent or mucopurulent cervical discharge, sometimes malodorous.

Abnormal Uterine Bleeding: Intermenstrual bleeding or postcoital bleeding.

Symptoms: Malaise, nausea or vomiting in severe cases.

Physical Examination

Cervical motion tenderness (chandelier sign).

Adnexal tenderness or mass (e.g., pyosalpinx, TOA).

Uterine tenderness on bimanual examination.

2. Chronic Salpingitis

Chronic Pelvic Pain: Dull, persistent pain, often unilateral.

Infertility: Due to tubal occlusion or adhesions.

Menstrual Irregularities: Dysmenorrhea or menorrhagia.

Asymptomatic: Common in chlamydial infections, detected during infertility evaluation.

Physical Examination: Adnexal thickening or masses (e.g., hydrosalpinx).

3. Tuberculous Salpingitis

Insidious onset with weight loss, night sweats and low-grade fever.

Infertility or amenorrhea as presenting complaints.

Often associated with pulmonary or extrapulmonary tuberculosis.

Diagnosis

Diagnosis of salpingitis is based on clinical criteria, laboratory tests, imaging and in some cases, invasive procedures. The goal is to confirm inflammation, identify the causative organism and assess complications.

1. Clinical Criteria (CDC Guidelines for PID):

Minimum criteria (presumptive diagnosis):

Lower abdominal or pelvic pain.

Cervical motion tenderness, uterine tenderness or adnexal tenderness.

Additional criteria (increase specificity):

Fever (>38°C).

Abnormal cervical or vaginal discharge.

Elevated inflammatory markers (e.g., C-reactive protein [CRP], erythrocyte sedimentation rate [ESR]).

Laboratory evidence of Chlamydia or Gonococcus infection.

Definitive criteria:

Endometrial biopsy showing endometritis.

Imaging or laparoscopy confirming salpingitis.

2. Laboratory Tests

Cervical/Vaginal Swabs: Nucleic acid amplification tests (NAATs) for Chlamydia trachomatis and Neisseria gonorrhoeae (gold standard).

Culture for gonorrhoea or other bacteria (less sensitive but useful for antibiotic sensitivity).

Blood Tests

Complete blood count (CBC): Leukocytosis in acute cases.

CRP/ESR: Elevated in acute inflammation.

HIV and syphilis testing (due to shared risk factors).

Urine Testing

Pregnancy test to rule out ectopic pregnancy.

Urinalysis to exclude urinary tract infection.

3. Imaging

Transvaginal Ultrasound (TVUS): First-line imaging modality.

Findings: Thickened, fluid-filled fallopian tubes (hydrosalpinx or pyosalpinx), tubo-ovarian abscess or free pelvic fluid.

Sensitivity: 80–90% for detecting tubal abnormalities.

Magnetic Resonance Imaging (MRI):

Used for complex cases or suspected TOA.

Shows tubal wall thickening, enhancement or abscess formation.

Computed Tomography (CT): Less specific but useful for detecting complications (e.g., abscess, peritonitis).

Hysterosalpingography (HSG):

Used in chronic cases to assess tubal patency during infertility evaluation.

Shows tubal occlusion or dilatation.

4. Laparoscopy

Gold standard for definitive diagnosis but rarely used due to invasiveness.

Findings: Tubal erythema, edema, purulent exudate or adhesions.

Reserved for atypical presentations, treatment failure or suspected complications.

5. Endometrial Biopsy

Confirms endometritis (often coexists with salpingitis).

Useful in chronic or subclinical cases.

6. Tuberculous Salpingitis

Tuberculin skin test or interferon-gamma release assays (e.g., QuantiFERON-TB).

Biopsy or culture of tubal tissue for Mycobacterium tuberculosis .

Chest X-ray or CT to evaluate pulmonary involvement.

Differential Diagnosis

1. Ectopic Pregnancy: Presents with unilateral pelvic pain and positive pregnancy test.
2. Ovarian Cyst/Torsion: Unilateral pain, adnexal mass on imaging.
3. Appendicitis: Right-sided pain, nausea and fever; diagnosed via CT or ultrasound.
4. Endometriosis: Chronic pelvic pain, dysmenorrhea and infertility; diagnosed via laparoscopy.

5. Uterine Pathology: Leiomyomas, adenomyosis or endometrial cancer (postmenopausal bleeding).
6. Urinary Tract Infection/Pyelonephritis: Dysuria, flank pain and positive urinalysis.
7. Bowel Disorders: Irritable bowel syndrome, inflammatory bowel disease or diverticulitis.

Management

Management of salpingitis focuses on eradicating infection, relieving symptoms and preventing complications. Treatment follows CDC or WHO guidelines for PID, with adjustments for severity and etiology.

1. Antibiotic Therapy

Empirical Treatment: Broad-spectrum antibiotics to cover Chlamydia, Gonococcus and polymicrobial infections.

Outpatient Regimen (mild to moderate cases):

Ceftriaxone: 500 mg intramuscularly (single dose) for gonorrhoea.

Doxycycline: 100 mg orally twice daily for 14 days for chlamydia.

Metronidazole: 500 mg orally twice daily for 14 days for anaerobes (optional).

Inpatient Regimen (severe cases, pregnancy, or complications):

Cefotetan: 2 g IV every 12 hours or cefoxitin 2 g IV every 6 hours.

Doxycycline: 100 mg IV or orally every 12 hours for 14 days.

Metronidazole: 500 mg IV every 8 hours for anaerobes.

Alternative Regimens: Azithromycin (for Mycoplasma or chlamydia) or levofloxacin (for resistant organisms). Adjust based on culture and sensitivity results.

Tuberculous Salpingitis:

Standard anti-tuberculous therapy: Isoniazid, rifampin, ethambutol and pyrazinamide for 6–9 months.

Duration: Continue antibiotics for at least 48 hours after clinical improvement in hospitalized patients; complete 14 days for outpatient treatment.

Partner Treatment: Treat sexual partners for STIs (e.g., ceftriaxone and azithromycin for gonorrhoea/chlamydia) to prevent reinfection.

2. Supportive Care

Analgesics (e.g., ibuprofen, acetaminophen) for pain relief.

Hydration and rest for systemic symptoms.

Avoid sexual intercourse until treatment completion and partner treatment.

3. Surgical Management

Indications

Tubo-ovarian abscess unresponsive to antibiotics.

Ruptured abscess or peritonitis.

Chronic salpingitis with persistent pain or infertility (e.g., tubal occlusion).

Procedures

Laparoscopy or laparotomy for abscess drainage or adhesiolysis.

Salpingectomy (removal of one or both fallopian tubes) for severe, unilateral disease.

Hysterectomy with bilateral salpingo-oophorectomy for refractory cases (rare, reserved for non-fertility-preserving scenarios).

Tuberculous Salpingitis: Surgical exploration may be needed for diagnosis or management of complications (e.g., adhesions, infertility).

4. Follow-Up

Reassess within 48–72 hours of starting antibiotics to confirm clinical improvement.

Repeat STI testing 3–6 months post-treatment to detect reinfection.

Evaluate tubal patency (e.g., HSG) in patients with infertility concerns.

Complications

1. Infertility: Occurs in 10–20% of women with PID due to tubal scarring or occlusion, more common with Chlamydia or recurrent episodes.
2. Ectopic Pregnancy: Risk increased 7–10 fold due to impaired tubal motility and adhesions.
3. Tubo-Ovarian Abscess (TOA): Occurs in 10–15% of acute PID cases; may rupture, causing peritonitis or sepsis.
4. Chronic Pelvic Pain: Seen in 20–30% of women post-salpingitis due to adhesions or fibrosis.
5. Hydrosalpinx: Fluid-filled, occluded fallopian tube, often asymptomatic but associated with infertility.
6. Perihepatitis (Fitz-Hugh-Curtis Syndrome): Liver capsule inflammation due to peritoneal spread, causing right upper quadrant pain.
7. Sepsis: Rare but life-threatening in untreated or severe cases.

Prognosis

1. Acute Salpingitis: With prompt antibiotic treatment, most patients recover fully within 2–3 weeks, with minimal long-term sequelae if treated early.
2. Chronic Salpingitis: Poorer prognosis for fertility, with 15–20% risk of infertility and 5–10% risk of ectopic pregnancy per episode.
3. Tuberculous Salpingitis: Good prognosis with anti-tuberculous therapy, but fertility outcomes are poor due to extensive tubal damage.

Prevention

STI Prevention

Promote safe sexual practices (e.g., condom use, monogamy).

Routine STI screening in sexually active women, especially those <25 years or with multiple partners.

Partner notification and treatment for confirmed STIs.

Gynecological Procedures

Use aseptic techniques during IUD insertion, endometrial biopsy or abortion.

Administer prophylactic antibiotics for high-risk procedures.

Education

Educate women on symptoms of PID and the importance of early medical attention.

Discourage douching, which disrupts vaginal flora and increases infection risk.

Tuberculosis Control

Screen and treat latent TB in endemic areas to prevent tuberculous salpingitis.

Vaccination

No specific vaccines for salpingitis, but HPV vaccination reduces risk of cervical infections that may predispose to PID.

Key Points

Salpingitis is inflammation of the fallopian tubes, often part of PID, primarily caused by Chlamydia trachomatis and Neisseria gonorrhoeae .

Risk factors include STIs, multiple sexual partners and intrauterine procedures; it is most common in young, sexually active women.

Clinical features include pelvic pain, cervical motion tenderness and discharge; many cases are asymptomatic, especially with chlamydia.

Diagnosis relies on clinical criteria, NAATs for STIs and imaging (TVUS, MRI); laparoscopy is definitive but rarely needed.

Treatment involves broad-spectrum antibiotics (e.g., ceftriaxone, doxycycline) for 14 days; severe cases require hospitalization.

Complications include infertility, ectopic pregnancy, tubo-ovarian abscess and chronic pelvic pain.

Prevention focuses on STI screening, safe sex practices and aseptic gynaecological procedures.

Early diagnosis and treatment are critical to preserve fertility and prevent long-term sequelae.

10.2 Oophritis

(*Iltihab-i-Khuṣya*-i-*Rahim*)

Definition

Oophritis is the inflammation of one or both ovaries, often occurring as part of pelvic inflammatory disease (PID), which also involves the fallopian tubes (salpingitis), uterus and other pelvic structures. Oophoritis can be acute, subacute or chronic and is typically caused by bacterial infections, though non-infectious causes are possible. It is a significant gynaecological condition due to its potential to cause pelvic pain, infertility and other reproductive complications.

Epidemiology

Prevalence: Oophoritis is less common as an isolated condition but frequently occurs in conjunction with salpingitis in PID. The true prevalence of isolated oophoritis is difficult to estimate due to underdiagnosis.

Age: Predominantly affects sexually active women aged 15–35 years, with peak incidence in the 20–24 age group.

Risk Factors

1. Sexual Behavior: Multiple sexual partners, new partners or unprotected intercourse.
2. Infections: History of sexually transmitted infections (STIs), particularly Chlamydia trachomatis and Neisseria gonorrhoeae .
3. Gynecological procedures: Recent intrauterine procedures (e.g., intrauterine device [IUD] insertion, abortion, endometrial biopsy).
4. Other: Poor genital hygiene, douching, smoking, low socioeconomic status and history of PID.
5. Geographic Variation: Higher incidence in developing countries due to limited access to STI screening and treatment.

Etiology

Oophoritis is primarily infectious, with bacteria ascending from the lower genital tract to the ovaries via the fallopian tubes or direct spread. Common causative organisms include:

1. Sexually Transmitted Pathogens

Chlamydia trachomatis (most common, 50–60% of PID cases, often subclinical).

Neisseria gonorrhoeae (20–30% of cases, associated with acute, severe symptoms).

2. Polymicrobial Infections

Anaerobes (e.g., Bacteroides spp., Peptostreptococcus spp.).

Aerobic bacteria (e.g., Escherichia coli, Streptococcus spp.).

Mycoplasma genitalium (emerging cause).

3. Rare Causes

Mycobacterium tuberculosis (tuberculous oophoritis, common in endemic areas, often chronic).

Actinomyces spp. (associated with long-term IUD use).

Non-infectious causes (rare): Autoimmune oophoritis (e.g., autoimmune oophoritis in premature ovarian failure), chemical irritation or post-surgical inflammation.

Pathophysiology

Oophoritis results from the spread of infection from the lower genital tract to the ovaries, typically via the fallopian tubes in the context of PID. The process involves:

1. Infection and Inflammation

Pathogens ascend from the vagina and cervix, often facilitated by menstruation, sexual intercourse or intrauterine procedures.

Bacteria invade the ovarian stroma or follicles, triggering an inflammatory response with neutrophil infiltration, edema and cytokine release.

Purulent exudate may form, leading to abscess formation (tubo-ovarian abscess, TOA).

2. Tissue Damage

Acute inflammation causes ovarian edema, follicular damage and cortical scarring.

Chronic inflammation leads to fibrosis, adhesions and potential ovarian dysfunction, impairing ovulation and hormone production.

3. Spread

Infection may involve adjacent structures (e.g., fallopian tubes, peritoneum), forming a tubo-ovarian complex or abscess.

Hematogenous spread (e.g., in tuberculous oophoritis) is rare but can occur, particularly in endemic areas.

4. Types

Acute Oophoritis: Intense inflammation with systemic symptoms, often associated with PID.

Chronic Oophoritis: Results from recurrent or untreated acute episodes, leading to adhesions, ovarian cysts or premature ovarian insufficiency.

Autoimmune Oophoritis: Lymphocytic infiltration of the ovaries, leading to follicular destruction and premature ovarian failure.

Clinical Features

The presentation of oophoritis varies depending on its acuity, severity and etiology. Many cases, particularly those caused by Chlamydia, may be asymptomatic or subclinical, contributing to delayed diagnosis and complications.

1. Acute Oophoritis

Pelvic Pain: Unilateral or bilateral lower abdominal or pelvic pain, often sharp or constant, exacerbated by movement or intercourse (dyspareunia).

Fever: Present in 30–50% of cases, typically low-grade (38–39°C).

Vaginal Discharge: Purulent or mucopurulent cervical discharge, often malodorous, due to concurrent cervicitis or endometritis.

Abnormal Uterine Bleeding: Intermenstrual or postcoital bleeding.

Systemic Symptoms: Malaise, nausea, vomiting or anorexia in severe cases.

Physical Examination

Adnexal tenderness or mass (e.g., swollen ovary or TOA).

Cervical motion tenderness (chandelier sign) in PID.

Uterine tenderness on bimanual examination.

2. Chronic Oophritis

Chronic Pelvic Pain: Dull, persistent pain, often unilateral, due to adhesions or scarring.

Infertility: Secondary to ovarian dysfunction or tubo-ovarian adhesions.

Menstrual Irregularities: Oligomenorrhea, amenorrhea or dysmenorrhea.

Asymptomatic: Common in chlamydial infections, detected during infertility evaluation.

Physical Examination: Adnexal thickening or palpable mass (e.g., ovarian cyst, TOA).

3. Tuberculous Oophritis

Insidious onset with weight loss, night sweats, low-grade fever and fatigue.

Infertility or amenorrhea as primary complaints.

Often associated with pulmonary or extrapulmonary tuberculosis.

Adnexal masses or ascites on examination.

4. Autoimmune Oophritis

Symptoms of premature ovarian insufficiency: Amenorrhea, hot flashes or infertility in women <40 years. Associated with autoimmune disorders (e.g., Addison's disease, thyroiditis).

Diagnosis

Diagnosis of oophoritis is challenging due to its overlap with other PID components and requires a combination of clinical evaluation, laboratory tests, imaging and in some cases, invasive procedures. The Centers for Disease Control and Prevention (CDC) criteria for PID are often used to guide diagnosis.

1. Clinical Criteria (CDC Guidelines for PID)

Minimum Criteria (presumptive diagnosis)

Lower abdominal or pelvic pain.

Adnexal tenderness, cervical motion tenderness or uterine tenderness.

Additional Criteria (increase specificity)

Fever (>38°C).

Abnormal cervical or vaginal discharge.

Elevated inflammatory markers (e.g., C-reactive protein [CRP], erythrocyte sedimentation rate [ESR]).

Laboratory evidence of Chlamydia or Gonococcus infection.

Definitive Criteria

Laparoscopic evidence of ovarian inflammation or tubo-ovarian abscess.

Endometrial biopsy showing endometritis (coexists in PID).

2. Laboratory Tests

1. Cervical/Vaginal Swabs: Nucleic acid amplification tests (NAATs) for Chlamydia trachomatis and Neisseria gonorrhoeae (gold standard, sensitivity >95%).

Culture for gonorrhoea or other bacteria (for antibiotic sensitivity).

2. Blood Tests: Complete blood count (CBC): Leukocytosis in acute cases.

CRP/ESR: Elevated in acute inflammation.

HIV and syphilis testing (due to shared risk factors).

Anti-Mullerian hormone (AMH) or follicle-stimulating hormone (FSH) in suspected autoimmune oophoritis to assess ovarian reserve.

3. Urine Testing: Pregnancy test to rule out ectopic pregnancy.

Urinalysis to exclude urinary tract infection.

3. Imaging

Transvaginal Ultrasound (TVUS)

First-line imaging modality.

Findings: Enlarged, edematous ovaries, tubo-ovarian abscess (complex, thick-walled mass), or free pelvic fluid.

Sensitivity: 85–90% for detecting ovarian abnormalities in PID.

Magnetic Resonance Imaging (MRI)

Used for complex cases or suspected TOA.

Shows ovarian enlargement, enhancement, or abscess formation.

Computed Tomography (CT)

Less specific but useful for detecting complications (e.g., abscess, peritonitis).

Hysterosalpingography (HSG)

Used in chronic cases to assess tubal patency during infertility evaluation, though not specific for oophoritis.

4. Laparoscopy

Gold standard for definitive diagnosis but rarely used due to invasiveness.

Findings: Ovarian erythema, edema, purulent exudate or adhesions; tubo-ovarian complex or abscess. Reserved for atypical presentations, treatment failure, or suspected complications.

5. Endometrial Biopsy

Confirms endometritis (often coexists with oophoritis in PID).

Useful in chronic or subclinical cases.

6. Tuberculous Oophoritis

Tuberculin skin test or interferon-gamma release assays (e.g., QuantiFERON-TB).

Biopsy or culture of ovarian/tubal tissue for Mycobacterium tuberculosis.

Chest X-ray or CT to evaluate pulmonary involvement.

7. Autoimmune Oophoritis

Autoantibody testing: Anti-ovarian antibodies, anti-adrenal antibodies (e.g., 21-hydroxylase), or anti-thyroid antibodies.

Hormonal profile: Elevated FSH, low AMH or low estradiol indicating ovarian failure.

Differential Diagnosis

1. Ectopic Pregnancy: Unilateral pelvic pain, positive pregnancy test and adnexal mass.
2. Ovarian Cyst/Torsion: Acute unilateral pain, cystic mass on imaging.

Often coexists but primarily affects fallopian tubes; distinguished by tubal findings on imaging.

3. Endometriosis: Chronic pelvic pain, dysmenorrhea and infertility; diagnosed via laparoscopy.
4. Appendicitis: Right-sided pain, nausea and fever; diagnosed via CT or ultrasound.
5. Uterine Pathology: Leiomyomas, adenomyosis or endometrial cancer (postmenopausal bleeding).
6. Urinary Tract Infection/Pyelonephritis: Dysuria, flank pain and positive urinalysis.
7. Autoimmune Disorders: Addison's disease or thyroiditis in autoimmune oophoritis.

Management

Management of oophoritis focuses on treating infection, relieving symptoms and preventing complications. Treatment aligns with CDC or WHO guidelines for PID, with adjustments for severity and etiology.

1. Antibiotic Therapy

Empirical Treatment: Broad-spectrum antibiotics for Chlamydia, Gonococcus and polymicrobial infections.

Outpatient Regimen (mild to moderate cases)

Ceftriaxone: 500 mg intramuscularly (single dose) for gonorrhoea.

Doxycycline: 100 mg orally twice daily for 14 days for chlamydia.

Metronidazole: 500 mg orally twice daily for 14 days for anaerobes (optional).

Inpatient Regimen (severe cases, pregnancy or complications)

Cefotetan: 2 g IV every 12 hours or cefoxitin 2 g IV every 6 hours.

Doxycycline: 100 mg IV or orally every 12 hours for 14 days.

Metronidazole: 500 mg IV every 8 hours for anaerobes.

Alternative Regimens

Azithromycin (for Mycoplasma or chlamydia) or levofloxacin (for resistant organisms).

Adjust antibiotics based on culture and sensitivity results.

Tuberculous Oophoritis

Standard anti-tuberculous therapy: Isoniazid, rifampicin, ethambutol and pyrazinamide for 6–9 months.

Autoimmune Oophoritis

No specific antimicrobial therapy; immunosuppressive therapy (e.g., corticosteroids) may be considered in confirmed autoimmune cases, though evidence is limited.

Duration: Continue antibiotics for at least 48 hours after clinical improvement in hospitalized patients; complete 14 days for outpatient treatment.

Partner Treatment: Treat sexual partners for STIs (e.g., ceftriaxone and azithromycin for gonorrhoea/chlamydia) to prevent reinfection.

2. Supportive Care

Analgesics (e.g., ibuprofen, acetaminophen) for pain relief.

Hydration and rest for systemic symptoms.

Avoid sexual intercourse until treatment completion and partner treatment.

3. Surgical Management

Indications

Tubo-ovarian abscess unresponsive to antibiotics.

Ruptured abscess or peritonitis.

Chronic oophoritis with persistent pain or infertility (e.g., adhesions, ovarian cysts).

Procedures

Laparoscopy or laparotomy for abscess drainage, adhesiolysis or oophorectomy.

Salpingo-oophorectomy (removal of ovary and fallopian tube) for unilateral, severe disease.

Hysterectomy with bilateral salpingo-oophorectomy for refractory cases (rare, reserved for non-fertility-preserving scenarios).

Tuberculous Oophritis: Surgical exploration may be needed for diagnosis or management of complications (e.g., adhesions, infertility).

Autoimmune Oophritis: Surgery rarely indicated; oophorectomy considered only in severe, refractory cases.

4. Management of Autoimmune Oophritis

Hormone replacement therapy (HRT) for premature ovarian insufficiency (oestrogen and progesterone).

Fertility preservation (e.g., oocyte cryopreservation) in early-stage disease.

Treat underlying autoimmune conditions (e.g., Addison's disease).

5. Follow-Up

Reassess within 48–72 hours of starting antibiotics to confirm clinical improvement.

Repeat STI testing 3–6 months post-treatment to detect reinfection.

Evaluate ovarian function (e.g., AMH, FSH) and tubal patency (e.g., HSG) in patients with infertility concerns.

Complications

1. Infertility: Occurs in 10–20% of women with PID due to ovarian scarring, adhesions or follicular damage; more common with recurrent episodes.
2. Tubo-Ovarian Abscess (TOA): Occurs in 10–15% of acute PID cases; may rupture, causing peritonitis or sepsis.

3. Chronic Pelvic Pain: Seen in 20–30% of women post-oophoritis due to adhesions or fibrosis.
4. Ectopic Pregnancy: Increased risk (7–10-fold) due to tubal damage from coexisting salpingitis.
5. Premature Ovarian Insufficiency: In autoimmune oophoritis or severe chronic cases, leading to amenorrhea and infertility.
6. Perihepatitis (Fitz-Hugh-Curtis Syndrome): Liver capsule inflammation due to peritoneal spread, causing right upper quadrant pain.
7. Sepsis: Rare but life-threatening in untreated or severe cases.

Prognosis

Acute Oophoritis: With prompt antibiotic treatment, most patients recover fully within 2–3 weeks, with minimal long-term sequelae if treated early.

Chronic Oophoritis: Poorer prognosis for fertility, with 15–20% risk of infertility and increased risk of ectopic pregnancy.

Tuberculous Oophoritis: Good prognosis with anti-tuberculous therapy, but fertility outcomes are poor due to extensive ovarian and tubal damage.

Autoimmune Oophoritis: Poor prognosis for ovarian function, with high risk of premature ovarian insufficiency; fertility preservation is challenging.

Recurrent Episodes: Increase risk of complications exponentially; each episode doubles infertility risk.

Prevention

STI Prevention:

Promote safe sexual practices (e.g., condom use, monogamy).

Routine STI screening in sexually active women, especially those <25 years or with multiple partners.

Partner notification and treatment for confirmed STIs.

Gynecological Procedures:

Use aseptic techniques during IUD insertion, endometrial biopsy or abortion.

Administer prophylactic antibiotics for high-risk procedures.

Education:

Educate women on symptoms of PID and the importance of early medical attention.

Discourage douching, which disrupts vaginal flora and increases infection risk.

Tuberculosis Control: Screen and treat latent TB in endemic areas to prevent tuberculous oophoritis.

Autoimmune Oophoritis: Early detection of autoimmune disorders through screening (e.g., anti-ovarian antibodies) in women with premature ovarian insufficiency or related conditions.

Vaccination: No specific vaccines for oophoritis, but HPV vaccination reduces risk of cervical infections that may predispose to PID.

Key Points

Oophoritis is inflammation of the ovaries, often part of PID, primarily caused by *Chlamydia trachomatis* and *Neisseria gonorrhoeae.*

Risk factors include STIs, multiple sexual partners and intrauterine procedures; it is most common in young, sexually active women.

Clinical features include pelvic pain, adnexal tenderness and discharge; many cases are asymptomatic, especially with chlamydia.

Diagnosis relies on clinical criteria, NAATs for STIs and imaging (TVUS, MRI); laparoscopy is definitive but rarely needed.

Treatment involves broad-spectrum antibiotics (e.g., ceftriaxone, doxycycline) for 14 days; severe cases require hospitalization.

Complications include infertility, tubo-ovarian abscess, chronic pelvic pain and ectopic pregnancy.

Autoimmune oophoritis is rare and associated with premature ovarian insufficiency, requiring hormonal and immunosuppressive therapy.

Prevention focuses on STI screening, safe sex practices and aseptic gynecologic procedures.

Early diagnosis and treatment are critical to preserve fertility and prevent long-term sequelae.

10.3 Endometriosis

(Batana-*i- Rahimiyat / Darun- i- Rahimiyat*)

Definition

Endometriosis is a chronic, oestrogen-dependent gynaecological condition characterized by the presence of endometrial-like tissue (glands and stroma) outside the uterine cavity. These ectopic implants are commonly found in the pelvic cavity but can occur in distant sites, leading to inflammation, scarring and symptoms such as pelvic pain, dysmenorrhea and infertility. Endometriosis significantly impacts quality of life and is a leading cause of gynaecological morbidity.

Etiology

The exact cause of endometriosis remains unclear, but several theories and contributing factors are proposed:

1. Retrograde Menstruation (Sampson's Theory)

Menstrual blood containing endometrial cells flows backward through the fallopian tubes into the pelvic cavity, where these cells implant and grow.

Most widely accepted theory, supported by the high prevalence in women with heavy menstrual flow or anatomical obstructions.

2. Coelomic Metaplasia

Peritoneal mesothelium transforms into endometrial-like tissue under hormonal or inflammatory stimuli, particularly in the pelvis.

3. Embryonic Rest Theory

Mullerian duct remnants differentiate into endometrial tissue outside the uterus during embryonic development.

4. Lymphatic/Vascular Spread

Endometrial cells disseminate via lymphatic or blood vessels, explaining rare extrapelvic sites (e.g., lungs, brain).

5. Immune Dysregulation

Impaired immune clearance of ectopic endometrial cells allows implantation and proliferation.

Increased inflammatory cytokines (e.g., IL-6, IL-8, TNF-α) and altered natural killer cell function are implicated.

6. Hormonal Influence

Estrogen promotes growth of ectopic endometrial tissue.

Progesterone resistance in endometriotic lesions contributes to persistence.

7. Genetic and Epigenetic Factors

Family history (first-degree relatives have a 7–10-fold increased risk).

Genetic polymorphisms (e.g., in oestrogen receptor genes) and epigenetic changes (e.g., DNA methylation) may predispose.

8. Environmental Factors

Exposure to endocrine-disrupting chemicals (e.g., dioxins, bisphenol A) may increase risk.

9. Risk Factors

Early menarche, short menstrual cycles or prolonged menstruation.

Nulliparity or low parity.

Obstructive uterine anomalies (e.g., cervical stenosis).

Obesity (increased oestrogen production).

Family history of endometriosis.

Epidemiology

Prevalence: Affects approximately 6–10% of reproductive-age women (176 million women worldwide). Higher prevalence (20–50%) in women with infertility or chronic pelvic pain.

Age: Most common in women aged 25–35 years, though it can occur in adolescents and rarely, postmenopausal women (with hormone therapy).

Geographic Variation: Higher detection in developed countries due to better diagnostic access; likely underdiagnosed in low-resource settings.

Associated Conditions: Adenomyosis, uterine fibroids, irritable bowel syndrome and autoimmune disorders.

Pathophysiology

Ectopic Implants: Endometrial-like tissue implants on pelvic structures (e.g., ovaries, peritoneum, uteroacral ligaments) or rarely, extrapelvic sites (e.g., diaphragm, lungs).

Hormonal Response: Implants are oestrogen-responsive, undergoing cyclic proliferation, bleeding and inflammation, mimicking the endometrium.

Inflammatory Cascade: Ectopic tissue produces prostaglandins, cytokines and chemokines, leading to chronic inflammation. Fibrosis, adhesions and scarring distort pelvic anatomy, causing pain and organ dysfunction.

Types of Endometriosis

1. Superficial Peritoneal Endometriosis: Small implants on the peritoneal surface.

2. Ovarian Endometriomas: Cystic lesions ("chocolate cysts") filled with blood.

3. Deep Infiltrating Endometriosis (DIE): Nodules infiltrating >5 mm into pelvic structures (e.g., rectovaginal septum, bladder).

Infertility Mechanisms

Adhesions distort tubal anatomy, impairing oocyte transport.

Inflammatory environment disrupts ovulation, fertilization and implantation.

Altered endometrial receptivity and progesterone resistance.

Extrapelvic Endometriosis: Rare, involving sites like the lungs (catamenial pneumothorax), diaphragm, or abdominal wall (e.g., cesarean scar endometriosis).

Clinical Features

1. Symptoms

Dysmenorrhea: Severe, progressive menstrual pain, often radiating to the lower back or thighs.

Chronic Pelvic Pain: Non-cyclic pain, worsen during menstruation or ovulation.

Dyspareunia: Deep pelvic pain during intercourse, particularly with deep infiltrating endometriosis.

Menorrhagia or Menometrorrhagia: Heavy or irregular menstrual bleeding.

Infertility: Seen in 30–50% of women with endometriosis; often the presenting complaint.

Bowel/Bladder Symptoms (with DIE)

Dyschezia (painful defecation), diarrhea or constipation during menses.

Dysuria, hematuria or urgency if bladder is involved.

Extrapelvic Symptoms:

Catamenial pneumothorax or hemoptysis (lung involvement).

Cyclic pain or swelling in scar tissue (abdominal wall endometriosis).

Asymptomatic: Up to 20–25% of cases, diagnosed incidentally during infertility evaluation or surgery.

2. Signs

Pelvic Examination

Tenderness in the posterior fornix or uterosacral ligaments.

Fixed retroverted uterus (due to adhesions).

Palpable nodules in the rectovaginal septum (DIE).

Adnexal mass (endometrioma).

Speculum Examination: Usually normal unless cervical or vaginal endometriosis is present.

Systemic Signs: Rare, but fatigue or weight loss may occur in chronic cases.

Diagnosis

Diagnosis combines clinical evaluation, imaging and in some cases, surgical confirmation. Definitive diagnosis requires laparoscopy with biopsy.

1. History

Detailed menstrual history, pain and obstetric history.

Family history of endometriosis or related conditions.

Assess for cyclic symptoms or extrapelvic manifestations.

2. Physical Examination

Bimanual Examination: Detects tenderness, nodules or adnexal masses.

Rectovaginal Examination: Identifies deep nodules in the rectovaginal septum.

Speculum Examination: Rules out cervical or vaginal pathology.

3. Imaging

Transvaginal Ultrasound (TVUS)

First-line for ovarian endometriomas; sensitivity 80–90%.

Findings: Homogeneous, hypoechoic ovarian cysts ("chocolate cysts") with ground-glass appearance.

Limited for superficial or deep infiltrating endometriosis.

Magnetic Resonance Imaging (MRI)

Preferred for deep infiltrating endometriosis; sensitivity >90%.

Findings: High-signal foci (hemorrhagic cysts) on T1-weighted images, adhesions or rectovaginal nodules.

CT Scan: Rarely used; may detect extrapelvic disease or complications (e.g., bowel obstruction).

Hysterosalpingography (HSG): May show tubal occlusion in infertility cases but is not specific.

4. Laparoscopy

Gold standard for definitive diagnosis.

Visualizes peritoneal implants (red, blue-black, or white lesions), endometriomas or adhesions.

Biopsy confirms endometrial glands/stroma; negative biopsy does not rule out endometriosis.

Staging (American Society for Reproductive Medicine [ASRM]):

Stage I (Minimal): Superficial implants, few adhesions.

Stage II (Mild): More implants, minimal adhesions.

Stage III (Moderate): Endometriomas, moderate adhesions.

Stage IV (Severe): Extensive implants, dense adhesions, large endometriomas.

5. Biomarkers

CA-125: Elevated in some cases but non-specific; not routinely used.

Emerging biomarkers (e.g., microRNAs) are under investigation but not yet validated.

6. Differential Diagnosis

Pelvic Inflammatory Disease (PID): Acute onset, fever and cervical motion tenderness.

Uterine Fibroids: Focal masses, less cyclic pain.

Adenomyosis: Diffuse uterine enlargement, often coexists.

Ovarian Cysts or Tumours: Non-cyclic pain, different imaging characteristics.

Irritable Bowel Syndrome (IBS): Bowel symptoms without cyclic pattern.

Endometrial/Cervical Cancer: Postmenopausal bleeding or abnormal discharge.

Management

Management is individualized based on symptoms, fertility goals, disease severity and patient age. Goals are symptom relief, fertility preservation and prevention of progression.

1. **Medical Management** (First-Line for Pain and Symptom Control):

a. Nonsteroidal Anti-Inflammatory Drugs (NSAIDs).

Ibuprofen or naproxen for dysmenorrhea and pelvic pain.

b. Hormonal Therapies

Combined Oral Contraceptives (COCs)

Continuous or cyclic use reduces menstrual flow and pain by suppressing ovulation. First-line for adolescents and women not desiring pregnancy.

Progestins

Levonorgestrel-releasing intrauterine system (LNG-IUS, e.g., Mirena): Reduces pain and bleeding; effective for 3–5 years.

Oral progestins (e.g., dienogest, norethindrone): Suppress endometrial growth.

Gonadotropin-Releasing Hormone (GnRH) Agonists (e.g., leuprolide, goserelin)

Induce hypoestrogenic state, reducing implant activity.

Used for 3–6 months due to side effects (hot flashes, bone loss); add-back therapy (low-dose oestrogen/progestin) minimizes risks.

GnRH Antagonists (e.g., elagolix, relugolix)

Oral agents for pain relief with fewer side effects than agonists.

Aromatase Inhibitors (e.g., letrozole)

Off-label use for refractory cases; suppress local oestrogen production.

Danazol: Rarely used due to androgenic side effects but effective for pain.

Analgesics

Adjunct for refractory pain; rarely, opioids for severe cases under specialist care.

2. **Surgical Management**

Indications: Refractory pain, large endometriomas (>4 cm), infertility or suspected malignancy.

a. Laparoscopy

Excision or ablation of implants and adhesiolysis improves pain and fertility.

Cystectomy for endometriomas preserves ovarian function better than drainage.

Preferred over laparotomy for minimal invasiveness.

b. Hysterectomy with or without Oophorectomy

Definitive treatment for severe, refractory cases in women who have completed childbearing.

Bilateral salpingo-oophorectomy (BSO) induces menopause, reducing recurrence but requiring hormone replacement therapy (HRT) in premenopausal women.

Hysterectomy alone may not eliminate symptoms if extrauterine implants remain.

c. Presacral Neurectomy or Uterosacral Nerve Ablation: For severe dysmenorrhea, though less commonly performed.

d. Extrapelvic Endometriosis: Specialized surgery (e.g., thoracic or colorectal) for rare sites.

3. Fertility Management

a. Laparoscopic Surgery: Improves spontaneous pregnancy rates in mild-to-moderate endometriosis (ASRM Stages I–II).

b. Assisted Reproductive Technologies (ART)

In vitro fertilization (IVF) is first-line for infertility in moderate-to-severe cases.

Pretreatment with GnRH agonists or LNG-IUS may improve IVF outcomes.

c. Ovulation Induction: Clomiphene or gonadotropins for mild cases, though less effective in advanced disease.

4. Conservative Management

Observation for asymptomatic or minimal disease, particularly in perimenopausal women.

Lifestyle modifications: Weight management, anti-inflammatory diet and stress reduction may alleviate symptoms.

5. General Measures

Patient Education: Discuss chronic nature of disease, treatment options and fertility implications.

Multidisciplinary Care: Involve gynaecologists, obstetricians and psychologists for comprehensive management.

Follow-Up: Regular monitoring for symptom recurrence, complications or fertility outcomes.

Complications

1. Infertility: 30–50% of women with endometriosis; due to adhesions, ovarian damage or endometrial dysfunction.

2. Chronic Pelvic Pain: Persistent pain impacts quality of life and mental health.
3. Adhesions and Organ Dysfunction: Bowel obstruction, hydronephrosis or bladder dysfunction in deep infiltrating endometriosis.
4. Ovarian Reserve Reduction: Endometriomas or repeated ovarian surgeries may impair ovarian function.
5. Malignancy Risk: Rare (1–2%) association with endometrioid or clear cell ovarian carcinoma, particularly with endometriomas.
6. Psychosocial Impact: Anxiety, depression or relationship strain due to chronic pain and infertility.

Prevention

No definitive preventive measures due to unclear etiology.

Risk Reduction

Early treatment of heavy menstrual flow or uterine anomalies.

Use of COCs or progestins to reduce retrograde menstruation.

Regular gynaecological screening in high-risk women (e.g., family history).

Minimize exposure to other hormonal drugs.

Prognosis

1. Symptom Control: Medical and surgical treatments relieve pain in 70–90% of patients, though recurrence is common (20–50% within 5 years).
2. Fertility: Spontaneous pregnancy rates improve with surgery in mild cases; IVF is effective for advanced disease.
3. Post-Menopause Symptoms typically regress due to oestrogen decline, unless HRT is used.
4. Chronic Nature: Endometriosis is a lifelong condition requiring long-term management, especially in severe cases.

Special Considerations

Adolescents

Early-onset endometriosis may present with acyclic pain; early diagnosis prevents progression.

COCs or LNG-IUS are first-line; surgery is reserved for refractory cases.

Pregnancy

Symptoms may improve due to progesterone dominance, but complications (e.g., miscarriage, preterm labor) are increased.

Hormonal treatments are contraindicated; NSAIDs should be used cautiously.

Postmenopausal Women

Rare unless on HRT; persistent symptoms need evaluation for malignancy.

Infertility Patients

Early laparoscopy or ART is recommended to optimize fertility outcomes.

Extrapelvic Endometriosis

Requires multidisciplinary care (e.g., thoracic surgeons for lung involvement).

Definitions

Hydrosalpinx ➤ Serous fluid accumulation in blocked fallopian tube; often post-PID.

Pyosalpinx ➤ Pus-filled fallopian tube due to severe infection.

Tubo-Ovarian Abscess ➤ Encapsulated infectious mass involving tube and ovary; complication of PID.

Follicular Cyst ➤ Functional ovarian cyst from unruptured follicle; usually self-resolving.

Dermoid Cyst (Teratoma) ➤ Germ cell tumour containing hair, teeth, fat; often benign.

PCOS ➤ Endocrine disorder with anovulation, hyperandrogenism, polycystic ovaries.

10.4 Polycystic Ovarian Syndrome (PCOS)

(*Mutalazema takai-yasul- mabayez*)

Definition

Polycystic Ovarian Syndrome (PCOS) is a common endocrine and metabolic disorder characterized by a combination of hyperandrogenism, ovulatory dysfunction and polycystic ovarian morphology. It affects women of reproductive age and is associated with reproductive, metabolic and psychological complications, including infertility, insulin resistance and increased cardiovascular risk. PCOS is a heterogeneous condition, with variable clinical presentations and no single diagnostic criterion.

Epidemiology

Prevalence: PCOS affects 6–20% of women of reproductive age worldwide, depending on diagnostic criteria (e.g., Rotterdam, NIH). Prevalence is higher in certain populations, such as South Asian and Indigenous women (up to 25%).

Age: Typically diagnosed in adolescence or early adulthood (15–35 years), though symptoms may persist into perimenopause.

Geographic Variation: Higher prevalence in regions with high rates of obesity and insulin resistance (e.g., South Asia, Middle East).

Risk Factors

Genetic: Family history of PCOS (50–70% heritability); associated with gene variants (e.g., FTO, DENND1A).

Environmental: Obesity, sedentary lifestyle, high-calorie diets and stress.

Endocrine: Insulin resistance, hyperinsulinemia and prenatal androgen exposure.

Etiology

The exact cause of PCOS is multifactorial, involving genetic, environmental and hormonal factors.

Genetic Factors

Polygenic inheritance with variants in genes regulating androgen biosynthesis (e.g., CYP17, CYP11A1), insulin signaling and ovarian function.

Familial clustering: First-degree relatives of women with PCOS have a higher risk of hyperandrogenism or metabolic dysfunction.

Hormonal Imbalance

Hyperandrogenism: Increased ovarian and adrenal androgen production (e.g., testosterone, androstenedione) due to dysregulation of steroidogenesis.

Insulin Resistance: Present in 50–70% of women with PCOS, leading to compensatory hyperinsulinemia, which stimulates ovarian theca cells to produce androgens.

Gonadotropin Dysregulation: Elevated luteinizing hormone (LH) to follicle-stimulating hormone (FSH) ratio, promoting androgen production and impairing ovulation.

Environmental Factors

Obesity exacerbates insulin resistance and hyperandrogenism.

Poor diet (high glycemic index foods) and lack of physical activity worsen metabolic features.

Prenatal exposure to androgens or endocrine disruptors may predispose to PCOS-like phenotypes.

Other Factors

Chronic low-grade inflammation linked to obesity and insulin resistance.

Dysbiosis of gut microbiota (emerging research).

Pathophysiology

PCOS is characterized by a complex interplay of hormonal, metabolic and ovarian abnormalities:

1. Hyperandrogenism

Increased androgen production by ovarian theca cells, driven by hyperinsulinemia and elevated LH.

Inhibits follicular maturation, leading to anovulation and accumulation of small antral follicles (polycystic morphology).

Manifests as hirsutism, acne and androgenic alopecia.

2. Ovulatory Dysfunction

Disrupted hypothalamic-pituitary-ovarian axis with elevated LH:FSH ratio.

Arrest of follicular development at the antral stage, preventing dominant follicle selection and ovulation.

Results in oligomenorrhea or amenorrhea.

3. Polycystic Ovarian Morphology

Multiple small cysts (2–9 mm) in the ovaries due to arrested folliculogenesis.

Increased ovarian stroma and volume, visible on ultrasound.

4. Insulin Resistance

Impairs glucose uptake in peripheral tissues, leading to hyperinsulinemia.

Hyperinsulinemia enhances ovarian androgen production and reduces sex hormone-binding globulin (SHBG), increasing free androgen levels.

5. Inflammation

Chronic low-grade inflammation (elevated C-reactive protein, cytokines) contributes to insulin resistance and cardiovascular risk.

6. Neuroendocrine Dysregulation

Increased gonadotropin-releasing hormone (GnRH) pulse frequency stimulates LH secretion, exacerbating hyperandrogenism.

7. Metabolic Dysfunction

Dyslipidaemia (elevated triglycerides, low HDL).

Increased risk of type 2 diabetes and cardiovascular disease.

Clinical Features

PCOS presents with a spectrum of symptoms, reflecting its heterogeneous nature. The Rotterdam criteria categorize features into three domains: hyperandrogenism, ovulatory dysfunction and polycystic ovarian morphology.

1. Hyperandrogenism

Hirsutism: Excessive hair growth in androgen-dependent areas (e.g., face, chest, back), affecting 60–80% of women.

Acne: Common in adolescence and adulthood, often resistant to standard treatments.

Androgenic Alopecia: Male-pattern hair loss or thinning.

Virilization (rare): Clitoromegaly, deepening of voice or increased muscle mass (suggests severe hyperandrogenism or other conditions, e.g., adrenal tumours).

2. Ovulatory Dysfunction

Oligomenorrhea: Menstrual cycles >35 days or <8 cycles per year (70–80% of cases).

Amenorrhea: Absence of menstruation for ≥3 months.

Infertility: Due to anovulation, a leading cause of female infertility.

Dysfunctional Uterine Bleeding: Irregular or heavy menstrual bleeding.

3. Metabolic Features

Obesity: Present in 40–80% of women, often central (visceral) obesity.

Acanthosis Nigricans: Dark, velvety skin patches (neck, axillae), a marker of insulin resistance.

Metabolic Syndrome: Hypertension, dyslipidaemia and impaired glucose tolerance in 30–40% of women.

4. Psychological Features

Anxiety and depression (30–50% prevalence, higher than the general population).

Body image concerns due to hirsutism, acne or obesity.

Reduced quality of life.

5. Other

Sleep apnea: More common in obese women with PCOS.

Fatigue: Linked to insulin resistance or sleep disturbances.

Diagnosis

Diagnosis of PCOS is based on the Rotterdam Criteria (2003), requiring at least two of the following three features after excluding other causes:

1. Oligo- or Anovulation: Irregular or absent menstrual cycles.

2. Clinical or Biochemical Hyperandrogenism

Clinical: Hirsutism (Ferriman-Gallwey score ≥8), acne or androgenic alopecia.

Biochemical: Elevated total testosterone, free testosterone or androstenedione.

3. Polycystic Ovarian Morphology

≥12 follicles (2–9 mm) in one or both ovaries or ovarian volume >10 cm^3 on ultrasound.

Exclusion of Other Conditions:

Thyroid disorders (TSH, free T4).

Hyperprolactinemia (prolactin levels).

Congenital adrenal hyperplasia (17-hydroxyprogesterone).

Cushing's syndrome (cortisol levels, dexamethasone suppression test).

Androgen-secreting tumours (rapid-onset virilization, markedly elevated testosterone).

Premature ovarian insufficiency (elevated FSH, low estradiol).

Diagnostic Tools

1. History and Physical Examination

Menstrual history, symptoms of hyperandrogenism and metabolic risk factors.

Assess for hirsutism (Ferriman-Gallwey score), acanthosis nigricans and obesity (BMI, waist circumference).

2. Laboratory Tests

Hormonal Profile

Total and free testosterone, SHBG, androstenedione.

LH:FSH ratio (often >2 in PCOS).

AMH (elevated in PCOS due to increased follicular count).

Metabolic Profile

Fasting glucose, HbA1c or oral glucose tolerance test (OGTT) for diabetes risk.

Lipid profile (triglycerides, HDL, LDL).

Exclusion Tests

TSH, prolactin, 17-hydroxyprogesterone, cortisol.

3. Imaging

Transvaginal Ultrasound (TVUS): Preferred for assessing ovarian morphology. Findings: ≥12 follicles per ovary (2–9 mm), increased ovarian volume (>10 cm^3), or stromal prominence. Transabdominal ultrasound in adolescents or virgins.

MRI/CT: Rarely used, reserved for suspected ovarian/adrenal tumours.

4. Other

Endometrial biopsy in women with prolonged amenorrhea to rule out endometrial hyperplasia.

Screening for depression/anxiety using validated tools (e.g., PHQ-9).

Differential Diagnosis

Thyroid Dysfunction: Hypothyroidism or hyperthyroidism (menstrual irregularities).

Hyperprolactinemia: Amenorrhea and galactorrhea.

Congenital Adrenal Hyperplasia: 21-hydroxylase deficiency (elevated 17-hydroxyprogesterone).

Cushing's Syndrome: Central obesity, moon face and striae.

Androgen-Secreting Tumours: Rapid-onset virilization, markedly elevated androgens.

Premature Ovarian Insufficiency: Elevated FSH, low estradiol, amenorrhea.

Hypothalamic Amenorrhea: Low BMI, stress or excessive exercise.

Management

Management of PCOS is individualized, focusing on symptom control, fertility restoration and prevention of long-term complications. A multidisciplinary approach involving gynaecologists, endocrinologists, dietitians and psychologists is ideal.

1. **Lifestyle Modifications**

Weight Loss: 5–10% weight reduction improves insulin sensitivity, ovulation and hirsutism.

Diet: Low glycemic index, high-fiber diet; calorie restriction in obese patients.

Exercise: 150 minutes/week of moderate aerobic activity (e.g., brisk walking, cycling).

Behavioral Interventions: Stress management, smoking cessation and sleep hygiene.

2. **Medical Management**

Menstrual Regulation

Combined oral contraceptives (COCs): First-line for oligomenorrhea and hyperandrogenism.

Reduces androgen levels, increases SHBG and regulates cycles.

Preferred: Low-dose ethinyl estradiol with non-androgenic progestins (e.g., drospirenone).

Progestin therapy (e.g., medroxyprogesterone acetate 10 mg for 10–14 days every 1–2 months) for women unable to take COCs.

Levonorgestrel-releasing intrauterine system (LNG-IUS) for endometrial protection.

Hyperandrogenism

COCs: Reduce hirsutism and acne (6–12 months for noticeable improvement).

Anti-androgens

Spironolactone (50–100 mg daily): Reduces hirsutism; monitor for hyperkalaemia.

Finasteride or flutamide (less commonly used due to side effects).

Topical treatments: Eflornithine cream for facial hirsutism.

Infertility

Ovulation Induction

Clomiphene citrate (50–150 mg daily for 5 days): First-line, induces ovulation in 70–80% of women.

Letrozole (2.5–7.5 mg daily for 5 days): Aromatase inhibitor, superior to clomiphene in some studies.

Metformin (1500–2000 mg daily): Improves ovulation in insulin-resistant women, often combined with clomiphene.

Gonadotropins (FSH injections): For clomiphene-resistant cases, under supervision.

Assisted Reproductive Technology (ART)

In vitro fertilization (IVF) for persistent anovulation or tubal factors.

Risk of ovarian hyperstimulation syndrome (OHSS) in PCOS patients.

Metabolic Management

Metformin: Improves insulin sensitivity, reduces androgen levels and lowers diabetes risk.

Statins or fibrates for dyslipidaemia (rarely needed in reproductive age).

Screening and management of hypertension and glucose intolerance.

3. **Surgical Management**

Laparoscopic Ovarian Drilling (LOD): Indicated for clomiphene-resistant anovulation.

Uses laser or diathermy to puncture ovarian stroma, reducing androgen production and restoring ovulation.

Risks: Adhesions, premature ovarian insufficiency (rare).

Bariatric Surgery: Considered in morbidly obese women (BMI >40) to improve metabolic and reproductive outcomes.

4. **Psychological Support**

Counseling or cognitive-behavioral therapy (CBT) for anxiety, depression or body image issues.

Counsel to improve quality of life.

5. **Follow-Up**

Regular monitoring (every 3–6 months) for menstrual regularity, metabolic parameters (glucose, lipids) and psychological health.

Endometrial ultrasound or biopsy in women with prolonged amenorrhea to assess for hyperplasia.

Complications

Reproductive

Infertility: Due to anovulation (leading cause of female infertility).

Increased risk of miscarriage (30–50% in first trimester).

Metabolic syndrome

30–40% prevalence in PCOS.

Type 2 diabetes: 5–10-fold increased risk.

Cardiovascular disease: Increased risk due to dyslipidaemia, hypertension and insulin resistance.

Endometrial: Endometrial hyperplasia and carcinoma: 2–3-fold increased risk due to unopposed oestrogen from anovulation.

Psychological: Depression, anxiety and eating disorders (e.g., binge eating due to body image concerns).

Obstetric: Gestational diabetes, preeclampsia and preterm birth in pregnant women with PCOS.

Other: Obstructive sleep apnea (5–10-fold increased risk in obese women).

Non-alcoholic fatty liver disease (NAFLD) due to insulin resistance.

Prognosis

With treatment (e.g., ovulation induction, lifestyle changes), 70–80% of women achieve ovulation; pregnancy rates vary (50–70% with ART).

Lifelong risk of diabetes and cardiovascular disease requires ongoing monitoring and lifestyle management.

Regular menstrual cycles or progestin therapy reduces hyperplasia/carcinoma risk.

Psychological and cosmetic symptoms (e.g., hirsutism) may persist, impacting well-being.

Prevention

Lifestyle

Maintain healthy weight to reduce insulin resistance and hyperandrogenism.

Regular physical activity and balanced diet (low glycemic index) to prevent obesity.

Screening

Early screening for PCOS in adolescents with irregular menses or hirsutism.

Regular metabolic screening (glucose, lipids) in women with PCOS to detect diabetes or dyslipidaemia.

Endometrial Protection

Use COCs or progestins to induce regular withdrawal bleeds and prevent hyperplasia.

Education

Counsel women on long-term risks (diabetes, endometrial cancer) and the importance of lifestyle modification.

Genetic Counseling

Consider in women with strong family history of PCOS or related conditions (e.g., diabetes).

Key Points

PCOS is a common endocrine disorder characterized by hyperandrogenism, ovulatory dysfunction and polycystic ovarian morphology, diagnosed using Rotterdam criteria (2 of 3 features).

It affects 6–20% of reproductive-age women, with genetic, hormonal and environmental contributors.

Clinical features include hirsutism, irregular menses, infertility, obesity and acanthosis nigricans; psychological comorbidities are common.

Diagnosis involves clinical assessment, hormonal testing (testosterone, LH:FSH) and transvaginal ultrasound; rule out other causes (e.g., thyroid dysfunction, adrenal hyperplasia).

Management includes lifestyle changes, COCs for menstrual regulation, anti-androgens for hirsutism and ovulation induction for infertility.

Complications include infertility, endometrial hyperplasia/carcinoma, type 2 diabetes and cardiovascular disease.

Prevention focuses on weight management, regular screening and endometrial protection.

A multidisciplinary approach is essential for addressing reproductive, metabolic and psychological aspects.

Diagnostic Clues

Symptom	Likely Diagnosis
Fever + pelvic tenderness	PID / TOA
Irregular cycles + acne	PCOS
Sudden pain + mass	Ovarian torsion / cyst
Infertility + tubal dilation	Hydrosalpinx
Curdy discharge + itching	Candidiasis (ovarian/vaginal)

Common Tubo-Ovarian Pathologies

Mnemonic: “HOT COPS”

Letter ----Condition --------------Description

H --------Hydrosalpinx ------------Fluid-filled fallopian tube

O -------- Ovarian Cyst -------------Functional or neoplastic

T ----Tubo-Ovarian Abscess ----- Pus-filled mass, PID complication

C ------ Chlamydia Infection ------STI causing tubal damage

O ------- Oophoritis ---------------- Ovarian inflammation

P --------- PCOS ---------------------Hormonal disorder, infertility

S ------- Salpingitis ------------------Tubal inflammation, PID component

10.5 Cysts & Neoplasm

(*Akyas wa sal'a*)

Introduction

Cysts and neoplasms of the fallopian tubes and ovaries encompass a wide spectrum of benign, borderline and malignant conditions. These structures are integral to female reproductive function, and their pathologies can significantly impact fertility, hormonal balance and overall health. Cysts are typically fluid-filled sacs, often benign, while neoplasms range from benign tumours to aggressive malignancies. Accurate diagnosis and management are essential due to the potential for malignancy and complications such as torsion, rupture or infertility.

Fallopian Tube Cysts and Neoplasms

Cysts of the Fallopian Tubes

Definition

Fallopian tube cysts are fluid-filled lesions associated with the fallopian tubes, often resulting from inflammatory or congenital processes. Common types include hydrosalpinx, paratubal cysts, and tubo-ovarian cysts, which are frequently linked to pelvic inflammatory disease (PID) or developmental anomalies.

Types

1. Hydrosalpinx:

Fluid-filled, dilated fallopian tube due to distal obstruction, often secondary to PID or endometriosis.

2. Paratubal Cysts (Paraovarian Cysts):

Benign cysts arising from mesonephric (Wolffian) or paramesonephric (Mullerian) duct remnants, located adjacent to the fallopian tube or ovary.

3. Tubo-Ovarian Cysts:

Cystic masses involving both the fallopian tube and ovary, typically associated with PID or tubo-ovarian abscess (TOA).

4. Congenital Cysts:

Rare, resulting from Mullerian duct anomalies.

Epidemiology

Prevalence: Hydrosalpinx is common in women with a history of PID (10–20% of PID cases). Paratubal cysts occur in 5–10% of women undergoing pelvic imaging. Tubo-ovarian cysts are less frequent, linked to severe PID.

Age: Reproductive-age women (20–40 years) are most affected, though paratubal cysts may be found in adolescents.

Risk Factors:

PID, STIs (Chlamydia trachomatis, Neisseria gonorrhoeae).

Endometriosis, prior pelvic surgery or adhesions.

Infertility or history of tubal ligation.

Pathophysiology

1. Hydrosalpinx: Distal tubal obstruction (e.g., from PID or adhesions) leads to accumulation of serous fluid, dilating the tube. Chronic inflammation causes ciliary damage and mucosal scarring.
2. Paratubal Cysts: Arise from embryonic remnants; typically thin-walled and filled with clear fluid.
3. Tubo-Ovarian Cysts: Result from inflammatory fusion of the tube and ovary, often with purulent or serous fluid due to infection or abscess resolution.
4. Congenital Cysts: Form from incomplete regression of Mullerian or Wolffian ducts during embryogenesis.

Clinical Features

Asymptomatic: Many cysts are incidental findings on imaging.

Pelvic Pain: Dull or acute pain, especially if complicated by torsion or rupture.

Infertility: Hydrosalpinx or tubo-ovarian cysts may impair tubal function.

Menstrual Irregularities: Associated with coexisting PID or endometriosis.

Palpable Mass: Large cysts may be detected on pelvic examination.

Systemic Symptoms: Fever or malaise in tubo-ovarian cysts linked to infection.

Diagnosis

Imaging

Transvaginal Ultrasound (TVUS): First-line; shows dilated, fluid-filled tubes (hydrosalpinx), thin-walled paratubal cysts or complex tubo-ovarian masses.

MRI: Differentiates cystic from solid masses; useful for complex cases.

Hysterosalpingography (HSG): Detects hydrosalpinx or tubal occlusion in infertility evaluation.

Laboratory Tests

Inflammatory markers (CRP, ESR) if infection suspected.

CA-125: Mildly elevated in inflammatory cysts but non-specific.

Laparoscopy: Confirms diagnosis and assesses tubal patency or adhesions.

Differential Diagnosis

Ovarian cysts or neoplasms.

Ectopic pregnancy.

Endometrioma.

Appendiceal abscess or diverticulitis.

Neoplasms of the Fallopian Tubes

Definition

Fallopian tube neoplasms are rare, with primary malignancies accounting for <1% of gynecologic cancers. Benign tumours and secondary metastases (e.g., from ovarian or endometrial cancer) are more common.

Types

1. Benign Neoplasms

Adenomatoid Tumours: Most common benign tumour, arising from mesothelial cells.

Leiomyomas: Rare, similar to uterine fibroids.

Teratomas: Extremely rare, containing multiple tissue types.

2. Malignant Neoplasms

Primary Fallopian Tube Carcinoma (PFTC): Rare adenocarcinoma, often serous subtype.

Borderline Tumours: Low malignant potential, rare.

Metastatic Tumours: From ovary, endometrium or gastrointestinal tract.

Epidemiology

Prevalence: PFTC accounts for 0.3–1% of gynecologic malignancies, with 1,500–2,000 cases annually worldwide.

Age: Peak incidence at 50–60 years (postmenopausal).

Risk Factors

BRCA1/BRCA2 mutations (10–15% of PFTC cases).

Chronic salpingitis or tubal tuberculosis.

Nulliparity, infertility or history of PID.

Protective: Oral contraceptive use, pregnancy, salpingectomy.

Pathophysiology

Benign Neoplasms: Adenomatoid tumours arise from mesothelial proliferation; leiomyomas from smooth muscle cells.

PFTC: High-grade serous carcinoma often originates from the fimbrial end, linked to TP53 mutations and serous tubal intraepithelial carcinoma (STIC). Recent evidence suggests many ovarian serous carcinomas originate in the fallopian tube.

Metastatic Tumours: Spread via direct extension, peritoneal spread or lymphatics.

Clinical Features

PFTC:

Latzko's Triad: Pelvic pain, vaginal discharge (serosanguinous) and a pelvic mass (present in <15% of cases).

Hydrops Tubae Profluens: Intermittent discharge relieved by a gush of fluid (pathognomonic but rare).

Postmenopausal bleeding or abnormal uterine bleeding.

Often asymptomatic until advanced stages.

Benign Tumours: Usually asymptomatic; incidental findings during surgery or imaging.

Metastatic Tumours: Symptoms of primary cancer (e.g., abdominal distension, weight loss).

Diagnosis

Imaging

TVUS: Detects tubal masses or fluid; PFTC appears as a solid or cystic mass with vascularity.

MRI/CT: Assesses mass characteristics and staging (lymph nodes, peritoneal spread).

HSG: May show tubal filling defects but is non-specific.

Laboratory Tests

CA-125: Elevated in 80–90% of PFTC cases, useful for monitoring.

HE4 (Human Epididymis Protein 4): Emerging biomarker for malignancy.

Laparoscopy/Surgery: Biopsy or salpingectomy for histological confirmation.

Histopathology

PFTC: Serous adenocarcinoma with papillary or glandular patterns.

Metastatic tumours: Mesothelial-lined tubules.

Differential Diagnosis

Ovarian carcinoma (often indistinguishable from PFTC).

Hydrosalpinx or pyosalpinx.

Endometrial cancer with tubal metastasis.

Tubo-ovarian abscess.

Ovarian Cysts and Neoplasms

Ovarian Cysts

Definition

Ovarian cysts are fluid-filled sacs within or on the surface of the ovary, often benign and functional (related to ovulation). Non-functional cysts include benign neoplasms or pathological conditions.

Types

1. Functional Cysts

Follicular Cysts: Result from failure of follicle rupture during ovulation.

Corpus Luteum Cysts: Form from persistent corpus luteum, sometimes hemorrhagic.

2. Non-Functional Cysts:

Endometriomas: Cysts filled with old blood (“chocolate cysts”) due to endometriosis.

Dermoid Cysts (Mature Cystic Teratomas): Benign tumours containing multiple tissue types (e.g., hair, fat, teeth).

Cystadenomas: Benign epithelial tumours (serous or mucinous).

Polycystic Ovaries: Multiple small follicles in PCOS, not true cysts.

3. Pathological Cysts

Tubo-Ovarian cysts/abscesses (PID-related).

Hemorrhagic cysts.

Epidemiology

Prevalence: Functional cysts are common, affecting 10–20% of reproductive-age women. Dermoid cysts occur in 10–15% of ovarian masses; endometriomas in 5–10% of women with endometriosis.

Age: Functional cysts and PCOS in reproductive age; dermoid cysts in adolescents and young adults; cystadenomas and endometriomas in older women (30–50 years).

Risk Factors

Ovulation (functional cysts).

Endometriosis (endometriomas).

PCOS (polycystic morphology).

Family history of ovarian cysts or cancer.

Pathophysiology

Functional Cysts: Follicular cysts arise from unruptured follicles; corpus luteum cysts from persistent luteal tissue, often with haemorrhage.

Endometriomas: Ectopic endometrial tissue bleeds cyclically, forming hemorrhagic cysts.

Dermoid Cysts: Arise from pluripotent germ cells, forming heterogeneous tissues.

Cystadenomas: Epithelial proliferation (serous or mucinous), often with clear or viscous fluid.

Tubo-Ovarian Cysts: Inflammatory fusion of ovary and tube, often post-PID.

Clinical Features

Asymptomatic: Many cysts are incidental findings.

Pelvic Pain: Dull or acute, especially with torsion, rupture or haemorrhage.

Menstrual Irregularities: Common with endometriomas or PCOS.

Abdominal Distension: Large cysts (>5 cm) may cause bloating.

Infertility: Associated with endometriomas or PCOS.

Acute Symptoms: Severe pain, nausea or fever with torsion or rupture.

Diagnosis

Imaging

TVUS: First-line; distinguishes simple (functional) from complex (neoplastic) cysts.

Simple cysts: Thin-walled, anechoic.

Complex cysts: Septations, solid components or irregular walls (e.g., dermoid, endometrioma).

MRI: Characterizes complex cysts; fat or blood components in dermoids/endometriomas.

CT: Used for staging or suspected malignancy.

Laboratory Tests

CA-125: Mildly elevated in endometriomas or inflammation; significantly elevated in malignancy.

Beta-hCG: Rule out ectopic pregnancy.

AMH: Elevated in PCOS.

Laparoscopy: Diagnostic and therapeutic for complex or symptomatic cysts.

Differential Diagnosis

Fallopian tube cysts or neoplasms.

Ectopic pregnancy.

Appendiceal abscess.

Gastrointestinal cysts (e.g., mesenteric cysts).

Ovarian Neoplasms

Definition

Ovarian neoplasms are tumours arising from ovarian tissue, classified as benign, borderline or malignant. They originate from epithelial, germ cell or sex cord-stromal cells.

Types

1. Benign Neoplasms

Serous/Mucinous Cystadenomas: Epithelial tumours, often cystic.

Mature Cystic Teratomas (Dermoids): Germ cell tumours, benign.

Fibromas/Thecomas: Sex cord-stromal tumours, solid.

2. Borderline Tumours

Low malignant potential, epithelial (serous or mucinous), with atypical cells but no stromal invasion.

3. Malignant Neoplasms

Epithelial Ovarian Cancer (EOC): Most common (90%), includes high-grade serous (70%), endometrioid, clear cell and mucinous carcinomas.

Germ Cell Tumours: Dysgerminoma, yolk sac tumour, immature teratoma (young women).

Sex Cord-Stromal Tumours: Granulosa cell tumours, Sertoli-Leydig cell tumours.

Metastatic Tumours: From breast, colon or stomach (Krukenberg tumors).

Epidemiology

Prevalence: Ovarian cancer is the 5th leading cause of cancer death in women. Benign tumors are more common, especially cystadenomas and dermoids.

Age

Benign: Reproductive age (dermoids, cystadenomas).

Malignant: Postmenopausal (50–70 years for EOC); germ cell tumors in adolescents/young adults.

Risk Factors

BRCA1/BRCA2 mutations (15–40% lifetime risk of ovarian cancer).

Family history of ovarian, breast or endometrial cancer.

Nulliparity, late menopause or infertility.

Endometriosis (increases risk of endometrioid/clear cell carcinoma).

Protective Factors: Oral contraceptives, pregnancy, breastfeeding, tubal ligation, salpingectomy.

Pathophysiology

Benign Neoplasms

Cystadenomas: Epithelial proliferation with cystic fluid accumulation.

Dermoids: Germ cell differentiation into ectodermal, mesodermal and endodermal tissues.

Fibromas: Stromal cell proliferation, often hormonally inactive.

Malignant Neoplasms

EOC: High-grade serous carcinoma often arises from fallopian tube fimbriae (STIC) or

ovarian surface epithelium; TP53 mutations common.

Germ Cell Tumors: Arise from primordial germ cells; dysgerminomas are highly radiosensitive.

Sex Cord-Stromal Tumors: Granulosa cell tumors produce estrogen, leading to endometrial hyperplasia.

Metastatic Tumors: Hematogenous or peritoneal spread to ovaries.

Clinical Features

Benign Neoplasms

Asymptomatic or mild pelvic pain.

Palpable mass or bloating with large tumors.

Hormonal effects (e.g., estrogen production in thecomas).

Malignant Neoplasms

Vague symptoms: Abdominal bloating, early satiety, pelvic pain.

Ascites, weight loss or bowel obstruction in advanced stages.

Paraneoplastic syndromes (e.g., hypercalcemia in dysgerminoma).

Hormonal effects (e.g., precocious puberty in granulosa cell tumors).

Diagnosis

Imaging

TVUS: Differentiates benign (simple cysts) from malignant (solid components, septations, ascites).

MRI/CT: Staging and characterization of complex masses.

PET-CT: Detects metastasis in malignant cases.

Laboratory Tests

Tumor Markers

CA-125: Elevated in Epithelial ovarian cancer (80–90% of advanced cases).

AFP, hCG, LDH: For germ cell tumors.

Inhibin, estradiol: For granulosa cell tumors.

Genetic Testing: BRCA1/2 mutations in suspected hereditary cases.

Histopathology

Surgical biopsy or resection confirms tumor type and grade.

Frozen section intraoperatively guides surgical extent.

Laparoscopy/Laparotomy: Diagnostic and therapeutic for staging or resection.

Differential Diagnosis

Functional ovarian cysts.

Fallopian tube pathology (hydrosalpinx, PFTC).

Endometriomas.

Metastatic cancer (e.g., Krukenberg tumors).

Non-gynecologic masses (e.g., appendiceal, mesenteric).

Management

Fallopian Tube Cysts

1. Conservative Management

Asymptomatic small cysts (e.g., paratubal): Monitor with serial ultrasound.

Hydrosalpinx in infertility: May resolve with antibiotic treatment, if PID-related.

2. Medical Management

Antibiotics for tubo-ovarian cysts with infection (e.g., ceftriaxone, doxycycline, metronidazole).

Analgesics for pain.

3. Surgical Management

Laparoscopy: Cystectomy for paratubal cysts or salpingostomy for hydrosalpinx.

Salpingectomy: For persistent hydrosalpinx or infertility (improves IVF outcomes).

Drainage: For tubo-ovarian cysts/abscesses unresponsive to antibiotics.

Fallopian Tube Neoplasms

1. Benign Neoplasms

Surgical excision (e.g., salpingectomy) for symptomatic or large tumors.

Observation for small, asymptomatic adenomatoid tumors.

2. Malignant Neoplasms (PFTC)

Surgery: Total hysterectomy, bilateral salpingo-oophorectomy (TH/BSO), omentectomy, lymph node dissection and peritoneal washings (FIGO staging).

Chemotherapy: Platinum-based (carboplatin/paclitaxel) for stage I–IV disease.

Targeted Therapy: PARP inhibitors (e.g., olaparib) for BRCA-mutated cases.

Radiation: Rarely used, reserved for palliation.

Ovarian Cysts

1. Conservative Management

Functional cysts (<5 cm): Monitor with ultrasound; most resolve within 1–3 cycles.

Asymptomatic simple cysts: Observation in premenopausal women.

2. Medical Management

Oral contraceptives to prevent new functional cysts (no effect on existing cysts).

Analgesics for pain.

Antibiotics for infected tubo-ovarian cysts.

3. Surgical Management

Laparoscopy: Cystectomy for benign cysts (e.g., dermoids, endometriomas) to preserve ovarian tissue.

Oophorectomy: For large, complex or recurrent cysts in postmenopausal women.

Drainage: For tubo-ovarian abscesses, often image-guided.

Ovarian Neoplasms

1. Benign Neoplasms

Laparoscopic cystectomy or oophorectomy for symptomatic or large tumors.

Observation for small, asymptomatic tumors in premenopausal women.

2. Borderline Tumors

Fertility-sparing surgery (unilateral salpingo-oophorectomy) in young women.

TH/BSO for postmenopausal women or advanced disease.

Adjuvant chemotherapy rarely needed.

3. Malignant Neoplasms

Surgery

Early-Stage (I–II): TH/BSO, omentectomy, lymph node sampling; fertility-sparing surgery in select cases (e.g., germ cell tumors).

Advanced-Stage (III–IV): Cytoreductive surgery to achieve minimal residual disease, followed by chemotherapy.

Chemotherapy

Platinum-based (carboplatin/paclitaxel) for EOC.

BEP (bleomycin, etoposide, cisplatin) for germ cell tumors.

Targeted Therapy

PARP inhibitors (e.g., olaparib, niraparib) for BRCA-mutated or HRD-positive EOC.

Bevacizumab (anti-VEGF) for advanced EOC.

Hormonal Therapy: For low-grade serous or granulosa cell tumors.

Radiation: Rarely used, except in dysgerminomas or palliation.

Complications

Fallopian Tube Cysts

Infertility (hydrosalpinx impairs tubal function).

Torsion or rupture (rare, causes acute pain).

Chronic pelvic pain due to adhesions.

Fallopian Tube Neoplasms

Metastasis (PFTC spreads to peritoneum, lymph nodes).

Recurrence (20–30% in early-stage PFTC).

Bowel obstruction or ascites in advanced disease.

Ovarian Cysts

Torsion (5–10% of dermoids or large cysts).

Rupture (hemorrhage, peritonitis).

Infertility (endometriomas, PCOS).

Ovarian Neoplasms

Metastasis (EOC spreads to peritoneum, liver, lungs).

Ascites, pleural effusion, or bowel obstruction.

Infertility or premature ovarian insufficiency post-treatment.

Prognosis

Fallopian Tube Cysts: Excellent with appropriate management; hydrosalpinx may impair fertility unless treated.

Fallopian Tube Neoplasms

Benign: Excellent prognosis post-resection.

PFTC: Poor prognosis; 5-year survival 50–60% for stage I–II, 10–20% for stage III–IV.

Ovarian Cysts: Functional cysts resolve spontaneously; benign cysts (e.g., dermoids) have excellent outcomes post-surgery.

Ovarian Neoplasms

Benign/Borderline: Near 100% 5-year survival.

EOC: 5-year survival 90% for stage I, 30–40% for stage III, <20% for stage IV.

Germ Cell Tumors: >90% 5-year survival with chemotherapy.

Sex Cord-Stromal Tumors: Variable; granulosa cell tumors have 80–90% survival for early stages.

Prevention

Fallopian Tube Cysts

STI prevention (condoms, screening) to reduce PID risk.

Early treatment of PID with antibiotics.

Manage endometriosis to prevent adhesions.

Fallopian Tube Neoplasms

Opportunistic salpingectomy during hysterectomy or sterilization to reduce PFTC risk.

Genetic counselling and prophylactic salpingo-oophorectomy for BRCA1/2 carriers.

Ovarian Cysts

Oral contraceptives to suppress ovulation and prevent functional cysts.

Manage endometriosis and PCOS to reduce endometrioma risk.

Ovarian Neoplasms

Oral contraceptives (reduce EOC risk by 50% with 5+ years of use).

Prophylactic salpingo-oophorectomy for BRCA1/2 mutations after childbearing.

Regular screening in high-risk women (TVUS, CA-125, though limited efficacy).

Key Points

1. Fallopian Tube Cysts: Include hydrosalpinx, paratubal cysts, and tubo-ovarian cysts, often linked to PID or congenital anomalies; managed conservatively or surgically.
2. Fallopian Tube Neoplasms: Rare; PFTC is a high-grade serous carcinoma with poor prognosis, treated with surgery and chemotherapy.
3. Ovarian Cysts: Functional (follicular, corpus luteum) or non-functional (endometriomas, dermoids, cystadenomas); most are benign and resolve spontaneously or with surgery.
4. Ovarian Neoplasms: Epithelial (EOC, most common), germ cell, or sex cord-stromal; EOC has poor prognosis unless detected early.
5. Diagnosis: Relies on TVUS, MRI/CT, tumor markers (CA-125, AFP, inhibin), and histopathology; laparoscopy is definitive.
6. Management: Ranges from observation for benign cysts to surgery and chemotherapy for malignancies; fertility-sparing options for young women.
7. Complications: Include infertility, torsion, rupture, metastasis, and chronic pain.
8. Prevention: Focuses on STI control, oral contraceptives, and prophylactic surgery in high-risk groups.

Diagnostic Approach to Tubo-Ovarian Disorders

Patient Presents with Pelvic Pain / Infertility / Mass

↓

History Taking
(Menstrual irregularity, discharge, fever, infertility)

↓

Physical Examination
(Bimanual palpation, speculum exam)

↓

Initial Investigations:

↓ ↓ ↓

USG Pelvis   CBC & Hormones   Vaginal Swabs / Cultures

↓

Identify Likely Condition:

↓

PID → Fever, tenderness, discharge

PCOS → Irregular cycles, hirsutism, ↑ LH

Ovarian Cyst → Mass on USG, pain

Hydrosalpinx → Tubal dilation, infertility

↓

Confirm Diagnosis → Begin Targeted Treatment

Ovarian Cancer

Definition

Ovarian cancer is a malignant neoplasm originating from the ovaries or related structures, such as the fallopian tubes or peritoneum. It is the most lethal gynaecological cancer due to its late presentation and aggressive nature. The most common type is epithelial ovarian cancer, but germ cell and sex cord-stromal tumors also occur.

Epidemiology

Prevalence: Ovarian cancer is the 5th leading cause of cancer death in women, with ~20,000 new cases annually in the U.S. (2023 data).

Age: Primarily affects postmenopausal women (peak incidence: 50–70 years); germ cell tumors occur in younger women (15–30 years).

Geographic Variation: Higher incidence in developed countries (e.g., North America, Europe) due to longer life expectancy and lower parity.

Risk Factors

Family history of ovarian, breast, or endometrial cancer.

BRCA1/BRCA2 mutations (15–40% lifetime risk).

Nulliparity, late menopause, or infertility.

Endometriosis (increases risk of endometrioid/clear cell types).

Obesity and hormone replacement therapy (HRT).

Protective Factors

Oral contraceptives (reduce risk by 50% with 5+ years of use).

Pregnancy, breastfeeding, tubal ligation or salpingectomy.

Etiology

Genetic: BRCA1/BRCA2 mutations and Lynch syndrome (HNPCC) increase risk. TP53 mutations are common in high-grade serous carcinoma.

Hormonal: Prolonged estrogen exposure (e.g., nulliparity, late menopause) promotes epithelial proliferation.

Environmental: Obesity, smoking and talc exposure (controversial) may contribute.

Inflammatory: Chronic inflammation (e.g., from endometriosis or PID) may trigger malignant transformation.

Pathophysiology

Ovarian cancer arises from different ovarian cell types:

1. Epithelial Ovarian Cancer (EOC (90%):

Subtypes: High-grade serous (70%), endometrioid, clear cell, mucinous, low-grade serous.

Often originates from fallopian tube fimbriae (serous tubal intraepithelial carcinoma, STIC) or ovarian surface epithelium.

Spreads early to peritoneum, omentum or lymph nodes.

2. Germ Cell Tumors (5%)

Arise from primordial germ cells (e.g., dysgerminoma, yolk sac tumor, teratoma).

Common in young women; highly treatable.

3. Sex Cord-Stromal Tumors (2–5%)

Arise from ovarian stroma or granulosa cells (e.g., granulosa cell tumors, Sertoli-Leydig tumors).

May produce hormones (estrogen or androgens).

4. Metastatic Tumors (5%)

Spread from breast, colon, or stomach (Krukenberg tumors).

Staging (FIGO 2023)

Stage I: Confined to ovaries/ fallopian tubes.

Stage II: Spread to pelvic structures (e.g., uterus, bladder).

Stage III: Spread to peritoneum, omentum or lymph nodes.

Stage IV: Distant metastases (e.g., liver, lungs).

Clinical Features

Ovarian cancer is often called a “silent killer” due to vague symptoms and late presentation:

Early-Stage (I–II)

Often asymptomatic, found incidentally on imaging or surgery.

Mild pelvic pain, bloating or urinary frequency.

Advanced Stage (III–IV)

Abdominal bloating or distension (due to ascites).

Early satiety, nausea or weight loss.

Pelvic or abdominal pain.

Bowel changes (e.g., constipation, obstruction).

Shortness of breath (pleural effusion).

Other

Abnormal uterine bleeding (hormone-producing tumors).

Paraneoplastic syndromes (e.g., hypercalcemia in dysgerminoma).

Physical exam: Palpable pelvic mass, ascites or omental caking.

Diagnosis

Ovarian cancer diagnosis involves clinical evaluation, imaging, tumor markers and histopathology.

1. History and Physical Examination

Assess symptoms, family history and risk factors.

Pelvic exam: Palpable adnexal mass or ascites.

2. Imaging

Transvaginal Ultrasound (TVUS):

First-line; shows complex ovarian masses (solid areas, septations, irregular walls).

Sensitivity: 85–90% for detecting malignancy.

CT/MRI: For staging, detects peritoneal implants, lymph nodes or metastases.

PET-CT: Identifies distant metastases in advanced cases.

3. Tumor Markers

CA-125: Elevated in 80–90% of advanced EOC; less specific in early stages or non-epithelial tumors.

HE4: More specific for EOC, used with CA-125.

AFP, hCG, LDH: For germ cell tumors.

Inhibin, Estradiol: For granulosa cell tumors.

4. Histopathology

Surgical biopsy or resection confirms tumor type and grade.

Frozen section intraoperatively guides surgical extent.

5. Genetic Testing

BRCA1/BRCA2 testing for hereditary risk (10–15% of cases).

Tumor profiling for homologous recombination deficiency (HRD) to guide therapy.

6. Laparoscopy/Laparotomy

Confirms diagnosis, stages disease and guides surgical resection.

Risk of Malignancy Index (RMI)

Combines CA-125, ultrasound findings and menopausal status to predict malignancy risk.

RMI >200 suggests high risk, prompting surgical referral.

Differential Diagnosis

Benign ovarian cysts (functional, dermoid, endometrioma).

Fallopian tube carcinoma or hydrosalpinx.

Endometrial cancer with ovarian metastasis.

Non-gynaecological masses (e.g., appendiceal abscess, mesenteric cysts).

Metastatic cancer (e.g., Krukenberg tumors).

Management

Management depends on tumor type, stage, patient age and fertility desires. A multidisciplinary approach (gynecologic oncologist, medical oncologist, pathologist) is essential.

1. Surgical Management

Early-Stage (I–II)

Total hysterectomy, bilateral salpingo-oophorectomy (TH/BSO), omentectomy, lymph node sampling and peritoneal washings.

Fertility-sparing surgery (unilateral salpingo-oophorectomy) for young women with stage I germ cell tumors or low-grade EOC.

Advanced-Stage (III–IV)

Cytoreductive (debulking) surgery to remove all visible tumor (optimal if <1 cm residual disease).

Includes TH/BSO, omentectomy, peritonectomy and bowel resection if needed.

Neoadjuvant chemotherapy (before surgery) for unresectable disease.

Germ Cell/Sex Cord-Stromal Tumors

Fertility-sparing surgery often possible due to younger age and chemosensitivity.

2. Chemotherapy

Epithelial Ovarian Cancer

Platinum-based regimen: Carboplatin + paclitaxel (6 cycles, every 3 weeks).

Intraperitoneal chemotherapy for stage III with optimal debulking.

Germ Cell Tumors

BEP (bleomycin, etoposide, cisplatin) for 3–4 cycles; highly effective.

Sex Cord-Stromal Tumors

Chemotherapy (BEP or paclitaxel/carboplatin) for advanced or recurrent cases.

Metastatic Tumors: Treat primary cancer (e.g., colon, breast).

3. Targeted Therapy

PARP Inhibitors: Olaparib, niraparib for BRCA-mutated or HRD-positive EOC, used as maintenance therapy.

Anti-Angiogenic Agents: Bevacizumab for advanced EOC to reduce ascites and delay progression.

Immunotherapy: Under investigation (e.g., checkpoint inhibitors).

4. Hormonal Therapy

Tamoxifen or aromatase inhibitors for low-grade serous or granulosa cell tumors.

5. Palliative Care

For advanced, unresectable or recurrent disease.

Manages symptoms (e.g., ascites, bowel obstruction) and improves quality of life.

6. Follow-Up

Monitor every 3–6 months with CA-125, physical examination and imaging (CT/MRI).

Recurrence detected by rising CA-125 or new symptoms.

Complications

Metastasis: Spread to peritoneum, liver, lungs or lymph nodes.

Ascites: Common in advanced stages, causes abdominal distension.

Bowel Obstruction: Due to peritoneal carcinomatosis.

Pleural Effusion: Leads to shortness of breath.

Treatment-Related Chemotherapy: Neutropenia, neuropathy, renal toxicity. Infection, adhesions or infertility.

Prognosis

Early-Stage (I–II): 5-year survival >90% for stage I, 70–80% for stage II.

Advanced-Stage (III–IV): 5-year survival 30–40% for stage III, <20% for stage IV.

Germ Cell Tumors: >90% 5-year survival, even in advanced stages.

Sex Cord-Stromal Tumors: 80–90% for early stages; worse for advanced disease.

Factors

Stage at diagnosis.

Tumor type (serous worse than mucinous).

Optimal debulking and response to chemotherapy improve outcomes.

BRCA mutations: Better response to PARP inhibitors but higher recurrence risk.

Prevention

Maintain healthy weight to reduce risk.

Avoid prolonged HRT in postmenopausal women.

Pharmacological

Oral contraceptives (5+ years reduce risk by 50%).

Surgical

Opportunistic salpingectomy during hysterectomy or sterilization.

Prophylactic bilateral salpingo-oophorectomy for BRCA1/BRCA2 carriers after childbirth. (reduces risk by 80–90%).

Screening

No effective population-based screening (TVUS, CA-125 lack specificity).

High-risk women (BRCA mutations, family history):Annual TVUS and CA-125 starting at age 30-35.

Genetic Counseling

Recommended for women with family history of ovarian or breast cancer.

Key Points

Ovarian cancer is the worst gynecologic malignancy, primarily epithelial (high-grade serous), with germ cell and sex cord-stromal types less common.

Risk factors include BRCA mutations, nulliparity and endometriosis; oral contraceptives are protective.

Symptoms are vague (bloating, pelvic pain, ascites), leading to late diagnosis (70% stage III–IV).

Diagnosis uses TVUS, CA-125, and surgical biopsy; staging is surgical (FIGO).

Treatment involves cytoreductive surgery and platinum-based chemotherapy; PARP inhibitors for BRCA-mutated cases.

Complications include metastasis, ascites and bowel obstruction.

Prognosis is poor for advanced stages (5-year survival <40%) but excellent for early stages and germ cell tumors.

Prevention includes oral contraceptives, salpingectomy and prophylactic surgery for high-risk women.

Early detection is challenging; high-risk screening is critical for BRCA carriers.

Long Answer Questions

1. Classify diseases of the fallopian tubes and describe the clinical features and management of pelvic inflammatory disease (PID).
2. Discuss the etiology, diagnosis and treatment of hydrosalpinx and pyosalpinx.
3. Explain the types, symptoms and management of ovarian cysts.
4. Describe the pathophysiology and treatment of polycystic ovarian syndrome (PCOS).
5. Elaborate on tubo-ovarian abscess—causes, complications and surgical approach.

Short Answer Questions

1. What is salpingitis?
2. Name two complications of PID.
3. Define hydrosalpinx.
4. Mention one hormonal feature of PCOS.
5. What is the function of the fallopian tube?

Multiple Choice Questions (1 Mark Each)

1. Hydrosalpinx refers to:

a) Blood in tube b) Pus in tube c) Fluid in tube d) Air in tube

Ans: c) Fluid in tube

2. Most common cause of tubal infertility:

a) Fibroid b) PID c) PCOS d) Endometriosis

Ans: b) PID

3. Which hormone is elevated in PCOS?

a) FSH b) LH c) Estrogen d) Progesterone

Ans: b) LH

4. Ovarian cysts are commonly diagnosed by:

a) X-ray b) CT scan c) Ultrasound d) MRI brain

Ans: c) Ultrasound

5. Tubo-ovarian abscess is a complication of:

a) Fibroid b) PID c) PCOS d) Menopause

Ans: b) PID

6. Which ovarian disorder presents with multiple small follicles on USG?

a) Endometrioma b) PCOS c) Dermoid cyst d) Corpus luteum cyst

Ans: b) PCOS

7. Pyosalpinx contains:

a) Blood b) Pus c) Serous fluid d) Air

Ans: b) Pus

8. Which of the following is a functional ovarian cyst?

a) Dermoid b) Follicular c) Endometrioma d) Serous cystadenoma

Ans: b) Follicular

9. Most common benign ovarian tumor in reproductive age:

a) Serous cystadenoma b) Dermoid cyst c) Mucinous cystadenoma d) Endometrioma

Ans: b) Dermoid cyst

10. Which test is used to assess tubal patency?

a) Pap smear b) Hysterosalpingography c) USG abdomen d) CT pelvis

Ans: b) Hysterosalpingography

11

Pelvic Infections

(Ta'diya-e-aana)

11.1 *Zanana A'da Tanasuliyya ka Tbi i Dafi- Nizam* (Defence of genital tract)

11.2 Zanana A'da Tanasuliyya se mutalliq Asbab sitta Daruriyya wa Ghayr Daruriyya ka kirdar (Role of Six Essential & Non Essential Factors in maintaining genital health)

11.3 *Marad-I Iltihab-i-hauz e-aana* (Pelvic inflammatory Diseases)

11.4 *Amrad-i-manqoola Jinsiyya* (Sexually transmitted Diseases)

11.5 *Tadrriun A'da' Tanasuliyya zanana* (Genital Tuberculosis)

11.6 Waja'hauz-e-aana aur Waja'al Khasira (Pelvic Pain & Low Backache)

Learning Objective (At the end of the session, the students should be able to)-

Explain the defence mechanism of the genital tract & Role of *Asbab sitta zarooria & ghair zarooriya* in maintaining genital health.

Describe & discuss the etiopathogenesis, diagnosis, management and complications of Pelvic Inflammatory Disease.

Discuss the causes, diagnosis, management and complications of Sexually Transmitted Diseases.

Describe the etiopathogenesis, diagnosis, management and complications of Genital Tuberculosis.

Enumerate the causes of Pelvic Pain & Low Backache and describe its management.

11.1 Defence of genital tract

(Zanana A'da Tanasuliyya ka Tbi i Dafi- Nizam)

The defence mechanisms of the female genital tract are an essential component of reproductive health, protecting against infections and maintaining a balanced microbial environment. These mechanisms are multifaceted, involving anatomical, physiological, immunological and microbiological factors that work together to protect the genital tract from pathogens during reproductive life.

Defence/ Mechanisms of the Female Genital Tract

The female genital tract, comprising the vulva, vagina, cervix, uterus, fallopian tubes and ovaries, is equipped with a dynamic and integrated defence system to protect against infections, maintain homeostasis and ensure reproductive health. These defences can be categorized into anatomical and physical barriers, physiological and chemical defences, microbial defences, immunological defences and hormonal influences. Each component plays a distinct yet complementary role.

1. Anatomical and Physical Barriers

The anatomical structure of the female genital tract provides the first line of defence against pathogens.

Vulva and Perineum: The external genitalia, including the labia majora and minora, act as a physical barrier, protecting the vaginal introitus from external contaminants. The skin of the vulva contains sebaceous and sweat glands that secrete antimicrobial substances, such as sebum and lysozyme, which inhibit microbial growth.

Vaginal Structure: The vagina is a muscular, collapsible tube lined with stratified squamous epithelium, which is thick and resistant to microbial invasion. The vaginal walls are closely apposed, limiting the entry of pathogens and reducing exposure to external irritants.

Cervical Mucus Plug: The cervix produces a mucus plug that acts as a physical barrier, particularly during pregnancy. This plug is viscous and rich in antimicrobial peptides, preventing the ascent of pathogens from the vagina into the upper genital tract (uterus and fallopian tubes).

Uterine and Tubal Anatomy: The narrow cervical canal and the tortuous fallopian tubes create anatomical barrier that limit pathogen migration. The ciliated epithelium of the fallopian tubes facilitates the clearance of debris and pathogens toward the peritoneal cavity or back to the uterus.

2. Physiological and Chemical Defences

The female genital tract maintains a chemical environment that inhibits pathogen growth and supports a healthy microbiome.

Acidic Vaginal pH: The vaginal environment is maintained at an acidic pH (3.5–4.5) primarily due to the production of lactic acid by Lactobacillus species. This acidic environment inhibits the growth of many pathogenic bacteria and fungi, such as Escherichia coli, Staphylococcus aureus and Candida albicans. The low pH is a critical defence mechanism, disrupted in conditions like bacterial vaginosis, where pH rises, allowing opportunistic pathogens to proliferate.

Cervical Mucus: Cervical mucus, produced by endocervical glands, contains antimicrobial agents such as lysozyme, lactoferrin and defensins. These substances neutralize or kill pathogens. The mucus also traps microorganisms, preventing their ascent into the upper genital tract. The consistency of cervical mucus varies with the menstrual cycle, becoming thinner during ovulation to facilitate sperm passage but remaining thick and viscous at other times to act as a barrier.

Vaginal Secretions: Vaginal transudate and secretions contain enzymes (e.g., lysozyme, proteases) and antimicrobial peptides (e.g., defensins, cathelicidins) that target bacterial cell walls and membranes, enhancing pathogen clearance.

Shedding of Epithelium: The vaginal epithelium undergoes cyclical turnover, particularly under hormonal influence. Desquamation of superficial epithelial cells removes adherent pathogens, preventing colonization.

3. Microbial Defences: The Vaginal Microbiome

The vaginal microbiome, dominated by Lactobacillus species (e.g., Lactobacillus crispatus, L. jensenii, L. gasseri, L. iners), is a cornerstone of genital tract defence.

Lactobacillus Dominance: Lactobacilli ferment glycogen (produced by vaginal epithelial cells under estrogen influence) into lactic acid, maintaining the acidic vaginal pH. They also produce hydrogen peroxide (H_2O_2) and bacteriocins, which are antimicrobial peptides that inhibit the growth of pathogenic bacteria and fungi.

Competitive Exclusion: Lactobacilli compete with pathogens for nutrients and adhesion sites on the vaginal epithelium, preventing colonization by harmful microbes. A healthy Lactobacillus-dominated microbiome is associated with a reduced risk of infections such as bacterial vaginosis, yeast infections and sexually transmitted infections (STIs).

Microbiome Dysbiosis: Disruption of the vaginal microbiome (e.g., due to antibiotics, douching, or hormonal changes) can lead to dysbiosis, characterized by overgrowth of anaerobic bacteria (e.g., Gardnerella vaginalis, Prevotella spp.). This increases susceptibility to infections and complications like pelvic inflammatory disease (PID) and preterm birth.

4. Immunological Defences

The female genital tract has a strong immune system that balances pathogen defence with immune tolerance to support reproduction (e.g., preventing rejection of sperm or the fetus).

Innate Immunity

Antimicrobial Peptides: The vaginal and cervical epithelia produce defensins (e.g., human β-defensin-1, -2), cathelicidins and secretory leukocyte protease inhibitor (SLPI), which directly kill or inhibit pathogens.

Toll-Like Receptors (TLRs): TLRs on epithelial and immune cells recognize pathogen-associated molecular patterns (PAMPs) and trigger inflammatory responses, recruiting immune cells to sites of infection.

Phagocytic Cells: Neutrophils, macrophages, and dendritic cells in the vaginal and cervical mucosa phagocytose pathogens and present antigens to initiate adaptive immune responses.

Natural Killer (NK) Cells: NK cells in the endometrium and decidua (during pregnancy) provide surveillance against viral infections and abnormal cells while maintaining immune tolerance to the fetus.

Adaptive Immunity

Mucosal Immunity: The genital tract is part of the mucosal immune system, producing immunoglobulin A (IgA) and immunoglobulin G (IgG). Secretory IgA in cervical mucus neutralizes pathogens and prevents their adhesion to mucosal surfaces.

Lymphocytes: T and B lymphocytes in the genital tract mount specific immune responses against recurrent or persistent infections. However, the adaptive immune response is tightly regulated to avoid excessive inflammation, which could impair fertility or pregnancy.

Immune Tolerance: During pregnancy, the genital tract and decidua suppress excessive immune responses to prevent rejection of the semi-allogeneic fetus, mediated by regulatory T cells (Tregs) and anti-inflammatory cytokines (e.g., IL-10, TGF-β).

Endometrial Immune Dynamics: The endometrium undergoes cyclical immune changes under hormonal control. During the secretory phase, immune cell populations (e.g., uterine NK cells, macrophages) increase to prepare for potential pregnancy while maintaining defence against pathogens.

5. Hormonal Influences

Hormonal fluctuations, particularly estrogen and progesterone, profoundly influence the genital tract's defense mechanisms.

Estrogen: High estrogen levels (e.g., during the follicular phase or pregnancy) promote:

Thickening of the vaginal epithelium, enhancing its barrier function.

Increased glycogen production, supporting Lactobacillus growth and maintaining acidic pH.

Enhanced cervical mucus production, which supports the mucus plug's protective role.

Upregulation of antimicrobial peptide production.

Progesterone: High progesterone levels (e.g., during the luteal phase or pregnancy) modulate immune responses to favor tolerance, reducing inflammation to support implantation and pregnancy. However, this can temporarily increase susceptibility to certain infections, such as Candida albicans.

Menstrual Cycle Variations: The cyclical changes in hormone levels lead to variations in immune activity, mucus viscosity and microbiome composition, influencing susceptibility to infections at different cycle phases.

6. Clinical Implications and Pathology

Disruptions to the genital tract's defence mechanisms can lead to infections and reproductive complications. Key conditions include:

1. Bacterial Vaginosis (BV): Characterized by a shift from Lactobacillus dominance to anaerobic bacteria, leading to elevated vaginal pH and increased risk of STIs, PID and preterm birth.

2. Vulvovaginal Candidiasis: Overgrowth of Candida albicans, often triggered by hormonal changes, antibiotics or immunosuppression, disrupting the vaginal microbiome.

3. Sexually Transmitted Infections (STIs): Pathogens like Chlamydia trachomatis, Neisseria gonorrhoeae and human papillomavirus (HPV) can destroy the genital tract defences, leading to complications like PID, infertility or cervical cancer.

4. Pelvic Inflammatory Disease (PID): Ascending infections from the lower genital tract to the uterus and fallopian tubes can cause chronic inflammation, scarring and infertility.

Pregnancy-Related Infections: The immune suppression required for fetal tolerance increases susceptibility to infections, necessitating healthy lower genital tract defences.

7. Therapeutic and Preventive Strategies

Understanding the defence mechanisms informs clinical management and prevention of genital tract infections:

Probiotics: Oral or vaginal probiotics containing Lactobacillus species can restore a healthy microbiome and prevent BV or candidiasis.

Hormonal Therapy: Estrogen therapy (e.g., in postmenopausal women) can restore vaginal epithelial thickness and acidity, reducing infection risk.

Antimicrobial Agents: Targeted antibiotics or antifungals treat infections while minimizing microbiome disruption.

Vaccinations: Vaccines against HPV and hepatitis B reduce the burden of STIs and associated complications.

Hygiene Practices: Avoiding douching and using pH-balanced products preserve the vaginal microbiome and pH.

Barrier Methods: Condoms and diaphragms reduce STI transmission, supporting anatomical defences.

Conclusion

The defence of the female genital tract is a complex interplay of anatomical, physiological, microbial, immunological and hormonal mechanisms. These systems work synergistically to protect against pathogens while maintaining an environment favourable to reproduction.

Definitions

Pelvic Inflammatory Disease (PID) ➤ Infection of upper genital tract—endometrium, tubes, ovaries—often due to STIs.

Genital Tuberculosis ➤ Secondary TB spread to reproductive organs via blood or lymphatics; causes infertility.

Tubo-Ovarian Abscess ➤ Encapsulated pus-filled mass involving tube and ovary; complication of PID.

Actinomyces Infection ➤ Chronic PID associated with IUCD use; diagnosed via Pap smear or biopsy.

11.2 Role of Six Essential & Non Essential Factors in maintaining genital health

(*Zanana A'da Tanasuliyya se mutalliq Asbab sitta Daruriyya wa Ghayr Daruriyya ka kirdar*)

The concept of *Asbaabe Sitta Zarooriya wa Ghayr Zarooriya* (the six essential and non-essential causes) originates from Unani medicine, a traditional system rooted in Greco-Arabic principles, which emphasizes holistic health maintenance and disease prevention. In the context of female genital health, these six factors—comprising essential (*Zarooriya)* and non-essential (*Ghayr Zarooriya*) components—play a pivotal role in maintaining the physiological balance, immune defences and overall well-being of the female genital tract.

Overview of *Asbaabe Sitta Zarooriya wa Ghayr Zarooriya*

The *Asbaabe Sitta Zarooriya* (six essential causes) are fundamental to life and health, and their balance is critical for maintaining the homeostasis of the female genital tract. These include:

1. *Hawa-e-Muheet* (Atmospheric Air): The quality of the surrounding air and environment.

2. *Makool wa Mashroob* (Food and Drink): Dietary intake and hydration.

3. *Harkat wa Sukoon-e-Badani* (Physical Activity and Rest): Balance of exercise and rest.

4. *Harkat wa Sukoon-e-Nafsani* (Mental Activity and Repose): Emotional and psychological balance.

5. *Naum wa Yaqza* (Sleep and Wakefulness): Adequate sleep and wakeful periods.

6. *Ihtibaas wa Istifraagh* (Retention and Evacuation): Proper retention and elimination of bodily wastes.

The *Ghayr Zarooriya* (non-essential causes) include factors like personal hygiene, lifestyle habits and environmental influences that, though not vital for survival, significantly impact health when optimized or neglected.

Each of these factors contributes to maintain the female genital tract's defences, including its anatomical barriers, vaginal microbiome, immune responses and hormonal balance.

Role of *Asbaabe Sitta Zarooriya wa Ghayr Zarooriya* in Female Genital Health

1. *Hawa-e-Muheet* (Atmospheric Air)

The quality of the surrounding environment directly affects the female genital tract's health by influencing microbial exposure and mucosal integrity.

Role in Genital Health

Clean, well-ventilated air reduces exposure to pollutants, allergens and airborne pathogens that could irritate the vulvar or vaginal mucosa, potentially leading to infections like vulvovaginal candidiasis or bacterial vaginosis.

Poor air quality, high humidity or exposure to damp environments can promote fungal growth (e.g., Candida albicans) or disrupt the vaginal microbiome by altering pH and epithelial health.

In Unani medicine, the concept of Hawa-e-Muheet emphasizes maintaining a temperate environment to support the body's Mizaj (temperament), which, for the female genital tract, explains preserving the warm and moist atmosphere making to a healthy vaginal ecosystem.

Clinical Implications

Women living in polluted or humid environments are at higher risk of genital infections due to microbial proliferation. Advising patients to maintain dry, clean genital areas and avoid synthetic clothing aligns with Unani principles of optimizing environmental air.

Avoiding chemical irritants (e.g., scented hygiene products) supports mucosal health, preventing disruption of the vaginal epithelium's barrier function.

2. *Makool wa Mashroob* (Food and Drink)

Diet and hydration are essential for maintaining the female genital tract's physiological and immunological defences.

Role in Genital Health

A balanced diet rich in vitamins (e.g., A, C, E), zinc and probiotics supports the vaginal epithelium's integrity and immune function. For instance, vitamin A promotes epithelial cell turnover, while vitamin C enhances immune responses against pathogens.

Adequate hydration ensures proper cervical mucus production, which contains antimicrobial peptides (e.g., defensins, lactoferrin) that protect against ascending infections.

In Unani medicine, foods are classified based on their *Mizaj* (hot, cold, wet, dry), and a diet planned according to an individual's temperament could supports genital health. For example, cold foods (e.g., yogurt, cucumber) may be recommended to balance excessive heat (*Hararat*), which could manifest as inflammation or infections in the genital tract.

Probiotic-rich foods (e.g., yogurt, fermented foods) promote a Lactobacillus dominated vaginal microbiome, maintaining an acidic pH (3.5–4.5) that inhibits pathogens like Gardnerella vaginalis or Escherichia coli.

Clinical Implications

Diets high in sugars or refined carbohydrates can predispose to candidiasis by providing substrates for Candida albicans growth. Unani dietary advice emphasizes moderation and natural foods to prevent such imbalances.

Dehydration or poor nutrition can reduce cervical mucus production, weakening the mucus plug's barrier function and increasing susceptibility to infections like pelvic inflammatory disease (PID).

Nutritional deficiencies (e.g., zinc or vitamin D) may impair immune responses, increasing STI risk. Unani physicians may recommend specific foods (e.g., nuts, seeds) to correct these deficiencies.

3. *Harkat wa Sukoon-e-Badani* (Physical Activity and Rest)

Physical activity and rest influence blood circulation, hormonal balance and immune function, all of which are vital for genital health.

Role in Genital Health

Moderate physical activity improves pelvic blood flow, enhancing nutrient transport to the vaginal and cervical tissues, which supports epithelial health and antimicrobial peptide production.

Exercise strengthens systemic immunity, reducing susceptibility to infections like bacterial vaginosis or STIs by enhancing neutrophil and macrophage activity.

Adequate rest prevents stress-induced cortisol elevations, which can suppress immune responses and disrupt hormonal balance, potentially leading to vaginal dysbiosis or increased infection risk.

In Unani medicine, excessive physical exertion (*Harkat-e-Zayeda*) or inadequate rest (*Sukoon-e-Naqis*) disrupts the body's *Quwa* (vital faculties), weakening the genital tract's defenses. Balanced activity is recommended to maintain *Tabiyat* (the body's self-healing capacity).

Clinical Implications

Sedentary lifestyles may impair pelvic circulation, increasing the risk of vaginal atrophy or infections, particularly in postmenopausal women with low estrogen levels.

Overexertion can exacerbate conditions like endometriosis or chronic pelvic pain, which compromise genital health. Unani principles advocate for moderate exercise (e.g., walking, other exercises) according to the patient's Mizaj.

4. *Harkat wa Sukoon-e-Nafsani* (Mental Activity and Repose)

Emotional and psychological balance significantly impacts female genital health through neuroendocrine pathways.

Role in Genital Health

Chronic stress or emotional distress elevates cortisol and catecholamines, which suppress immune function and disrupt the hypothalamic-pituitary-ovarian axis. This can lead to hormonal imbalances, altering vaginal pH and microbiome composition, thus increasing infection susceptibility. Psychological stress may exacerbate conditions like recurrent vulvovaginal candidiasis or vaginismus, as it affects immune regulation and pelvic muscle tone.

In Unani medicine, mental repose (*Sukoon-e-Nafsani*) is essential to maintain *Ruh* (vital spirit) and prevent *Amraz-e-Nafsani* (psychosomatic disorders). Positive emotions and stress management are believed to support the genital tract's *Mizaj* and immune defenses.

Clinical Implications

Stress management techniques (e.g., counselling) can reduce cortisol levels, supporting immune function and hormonal balance, thus preventing infections or exacerbations of chronic conditions.

Unani practitioners may recommend calming therapies (e.g., aromatherapy, nutool therapy) to restore mental repose, aligning with modern psychoneuroimmunology principles that link emotional health to mucosal immunity.

5. *Naum wa Yaqza* (Sleep and Wakefulness)

Adequate sleep is essential for hormonal regulation, immune function and tissue repair, all of which influence genital health.

Role in Genital Health

Sleep supports the production of melatonin, which has antioxidant and immunomodulatory effects, enhancing the genital tract's ability to combat oxidative stress and infections.

Adequate sleep regulates estrogen and progesterone levels, which are needed for vaginal epithelial thickness, glycogen production (for Lactobacillus growth) and cervical mucus function.

In Unani medicine, sleep (*Naum*) is considered a restorative process that strengthens *Tabiyat* and supports the body's *Hararat-e-Ghariziya* (innate heat), essential for maintaining the genital tract's warm and moist environment.

Sleep deprivation disrupts immune responses, increasing susceptibility to infections like Chlamydia trachomatis or Candida albicans by reducing NK cell activity and antimicrobial peptide production.

Clinical Implications

Chronic sleep disturbances (e.g., in shift workers) may increase the risk of genital infections or exacerbate conditions like polycystic ovary syndrome (PCOS), which affects hormonal balance.

Unani recommendations for regular sleep schedules and a peaceful sleep environment (e.g., dark, quiet rooms) align with modern advice to optimize circadian rhythms for reproductive health.

6. *Ihtibaas wa Istifraagh* (Retention and Evacuation)

Proper retention and elimination of bodily wastes are essential for preventing infections and maintaining genital health.

Role in Genital Health

Urinary and Bowel Elimination: Regular urination and bowel movements prevent the accumulation of pathogens in the perineal area, reducing the risk of ascending infections (e.g., urinary tract infections progressing to PID).

Menstrual Flow: Normal menstruation serves as a natural cleansing mechanism, expelling endometrial debris and potential pathogens from the uterus. In Unani terms, menstruation is a form of *Istifraagh* that removes excess *Akhlat* (humors), maintaining uterine health.

Hygiene Practices: Proper genital hygiene (e.g., cleaning from front to back) prevents fecal contamination of the vaginal introitus, reducing the risk of infections like bacterial vaginosis or E. coli-related vaginitis.

In Unani medicine, imbalances in *Ihtibaas* (retention) or *Istifraagh* (evacuation) can lead to *Sudda* (obstruction) or accumulation of harmful *Madda* (matter), predisposing to infections or inflammatory conditions in the genital tract.

Clinical Implications

Constipation or urinary retention can increase perineal microbial load, promoting infections. Unani therapies like dietary fiber or laxatives drugs may be used to restore regular evacuation.

Menstrual irregularities (e.g., amenorrhea or menorrhagia) may indicate humoral imbalances, requiring dietary or drug interventions to restore normal *Istifraagh*. Overuse of douching or harsh soaps disrupts the vaginal microbiome, impairing *Ihtibaas* of beneficial Lactobacillus species. Thus Unani emphasizes gentle, natural hygiene practices to maintain genital health.

Non-Essential Causes (*Ghayr Zarooriya*)

While not vital for survival, *Ghayr Zarooriya* factors like personal hygiene, clothing and lifestyle habits significantly influence female genital health.

Personal Hygiene: In Unani medicine, cleanliness (*Tanqiya*) is essential to prevent the accumulation of *Madda-e-Fasida* (morbid matter) in the genital area. Modern gynaecology supports this by recommending pH-balanced, fragrance-free products to avoid disrupting the vaginal microbiome.

Clothing and Lifestyle: Tight, non-breathable clothing can create a moist environment, promoting fungal or bacterial growth. Unani medicine advises loose, natural fabrics to maintain a temperate *Mizaj* in the genital region, aligning with modern advice to wear cotton undergarments.

Sexual Practices: Safe sexual practices (e.g., condom use) reduce STI transmission, supporting the genital tract's defences. Unani emphasizes moderation in sexual activity to avoid weakening the body's *Quwa* or disrupting humoral balance.

Environmental and Occupational Factors: Exposure to occupational hazards (e.g., chemicals) or prolonged sitting can affect genital health. Unani recommends lifestyle adjustments to minimize such risks, complementing modern preventive strategies.

Integration with Modern Gynecology

The *Asbaabe Sitta Zarooriya wa Ghayr Zarooriya* align closely with modern gynaecological principles for maintaining female genital health.

Microbiome Health: The emphasis on diet, hygiene, and evacuation supports a Lactobacillus-dominated vaginal microbiome, critical for maintaining acidic pH and preventing infections.

Hormonal Balance: Sleep, stress management, and physical activity regulate estrogen and progesterone, which influence vaginal epithelial health and cervical mucus production.

Immune Function: A balanced lifestyle (diet, exercise, sleep, mental health) enhances innate and adaptive immunity, protecting against pathogens like Chlamydia, HPV, or Candida.

Preventive Care: Unani's focus on hygiene and environmental factors complements modern recommendations for STI prevention, regular screenings, and lifestyle modifications.

Clinical Applications

Preventive Strategies: Educate patients on balanced diets, stress management, adequate sleep and proper hygiene to support genital health, drawing from both Unani and modern principles.

Management of Infections: Combine Unani dietary and lifestyle interventions (e.g., probiotic-rich foods, stress reduction) with modern treatments (e.g., antibiotics, antifungals) to restore vaginal health.

Chronic Conditions: For conditions like recurrent vaginitis or PCOS, integrate Unani principles (e.g., correcting humoral imbalances through diet and rest) with hormonal therapies or probiotics.

Patient Counseling: Use the holistic framework of *Asbaabe Sitta* to provide comprehensive lifestyle advice, addressing environmental, dietary and psychological factors that impact genital health.

Conclusion

The *Asbaabe Sitta Zarooriya wa Ghayr Zarooriya* provide a holistic framework for understanding and maintaining female genital health, emphasizing the interplay of environmental, dietary, physical, psychological and hygienic factors. By supporting the vaginal microbiome, hormonal balance and immune defences, these principles align with modern gynaecological approaches to prevent infections, promote reproductive health and can manage gynaecological disorders.

11.3 Pelvic inflammatory Diseases

(*Marad-I Iltihab-i-hauz e-aana)*

Definition

Pelvic inflammatory disease refers to a spectrum of inflammatory disorders of the upper female genital tract, including endometritis, salpingitis, tubo-ovarian abscess and pelvic peritonitis, usually caused by ascending infections from the vagina or cervix. PID can be acute, subacute or chronic, with varying degrees of severity and clinical presentation.

Epidemiology

Prevalence: PID is a common gynaecological condition, particularly among sexually active women of reproductive age (15–44 years). The exact prevalence is difficult to determine due to underdiagnosis and varying diagnostic criteria, but it is estimated to affect 4–12% of women in developed countries and has a higher incidence in developing regions.

Risk Factors

Sexual Behavior: Multiple sexual partners, unprotected intercourse and history of sexually transmitted infections (STIs) increase risk.

Age: Most common in women under 25 years due to higher rates of STIs and a less developed cervical mucus barrier.

Contraceptive Use: Intrauterine device (IUD) insertion, particularly within the first 3–6 weeks, carries a small risk of PID due to introduction of bacteria.

Other Factors: Douching, recent pelvic procedures (e.g., endometrial biopsy, abortion), smoking and low socioeconomic status are associated with increased risk.

Global Burden: PID is a leading cause of infertility and ectopic pregnancy worldwide, with significant healthcare costs and long-term sequelae.

Etiology

PID is typically a polymicrobial infection caused by the ascent of pathogens from the lower genital tract. The primary causative organisms include:

1. Sexually Transmitted Pathogens

Chlamydia trachomatis: The most common cause, responsible for 30–50% of PID cases, often leading to subclinical or “silent” PID.

Neisseria gonorrhoeae: Causes 20–40% of cases, often associated with acute, symptomatic PID.

2. Polymicrobial Flora

Anaerobic bacteria (e.g., Bacteroides fragilis, Prevotella spp.).

Aerobic gram-negative bacilli (e.g., Escherichia coli).

Facultative anaerobes (e.g., Gardnerella vaginalis, Streptococcus spp.).

Mycoplasma and Ureaplasma species (e.g., Mycoplasma genitalium).

3. Less Common Pathogens: Tuberculosis (Mycobacterium tuberculosis) in endemic areas, and rarely, actinomycosis associated with long-term IUD use.

Pathogenesis of Ascent: Pathogens ascend from the vagina or cervix to the upper genital tract, facilitated by:

Disruption of cervical mucus barrier (e.g., during menstruation or post-procedure).

Sexual intercourse, which may introduce or propel pathogens.

Douching, which disrupts the vaginal microbiome and facilitates bacterial ascent.

Pathophysiology

The pathogenesis of PID involves a complex interplay of microbial invasion, inflammation and tissue damage:

1. Initiation of Infection: Pathogens colonize the vaginal or cervical mucosa, often following disruption of the vaginal microbiome (e.g., in bacterial vaginosis) or cervical mucus barrier. Chlamydia trachomatis and Neisseria gonorrhoeae adhere to and invade endocervical epithelial cells, triggering an inflammatory response.
2. Ascending Spread: Bacteria ascend through the cervical canal to the endometrium, fallopian tubes and peritoneal cavity, causing endometritis, salpingitis and peritonitis. The fallopian tubes are particularly vulnerable due to their delicate mucosal lining and ciliated epithelium, which can be damaged by inflammation.
3. Inflammatory Response: Infection triggers an innate immune response, with recruitment of neutrophils, macrophages and release of pro-inflammatory cytokines (e.g., IL-1, IL-6, TNF-α). This leads to tissue edema, pus formation and potential abscesses (e.g., tubo-ovarian abscess).
4. Tissue Damage and Scarring: Chronic or recurrent inflammation causes fibrosis and scarring of the fallopian tubes, leading to tubal occlusion, hydrosalpinx or adhesions. Damage to ciliated epithelium impairs ovum transport, increasing the risk of infertility and ectopic pregnancy.
5. Polymicrobial Involvement: Initial STI pathogens may facilitate secondary infections by vaginal flora, leading to polymicrobial PID, which exacerbates tissue damage and complications.

Clinical Features

PID presents with a wide spectrum of symptoms, ranging from mild to severe, and may be asymptomatic in up to 60% of cases (especially with Chlamydia).

Symptoms

Lower Abdominal Pain: Bilateral, dull or cramping pain is the hallmark symptom, often worsening during menstruation or intercourse.

Abnormal Vaginal Discharge: Purulent or mucopurulent discharge due to cervicitis or endometritis.

Dysmenorrhea: Painful menstruation.

Dyspareunia: Painful intercourse, particularly deep dyspareunia.

Fever: Present in severe cases (e.g., with tubo-ovarian abscess).

Menstrual Irregularities: Intermenstrual bleeding or postcoital bleeding due to endometritis or cervicitis.

Systemic Symptoms: Malaise, nausea or vomiting in severe cases.

Asymptomatic PID: Common in chlamydial infections, leading to delayed diagnosis and increased risk of complications.

Physical Examination

Cervical Motion Tenderness: Pain on moving the cervix during bimanual examination (classic sign).

Adnexal Tenderness: Unilateral or bilateral tenderness on palpation of the fallopian tubes or ovaries.

Uterine Tenderness: Pain on uterine palpation.

Fever: Temperature >38°C in acute cases.

Pelvic Mass: May indicate tubo-ovarian abscess or hydrosalpinx.

Associated Findings

Mucopurulent cervical discharge or friable cervix on speculum examination.

Right upper quadrant pain (Fitz-Hugh-Curtis syndrome) due to perihepatitis from peritoneal spread of infection.

Diagnosis

PID diagnosis is primarily clinical due to the lack of a single definitive test and the need for prompt treatment to prevent complications. The Centres for Disease Control and Prevention (CDC) provides diagnostic criteria.

CDC Diagnostic Criteria (2021)

Minimum Criteria (presumptive diagnosis, initiate treatment):

Lower abdominal or pelvic pain AND

Cervical motion tenderness OR uterine tenderness OR adnexal tenderness.

Additional Criteria (increase specificity): Fever (>38°C).

Abnormal cervical or vaginal discharge (mucopurulent).

Elevated white blood cell count (leukocytosis).

Elevated erythrocyte sedimentation rate (ESR) or C-reactive protein (CRP).

Laboratory evidence of Chlamydia trachomatis or Neisseria gonorrhoeae (e.g., nucleic acid amplification tests [NAAT]).

Definitive Criteria (rarely required): Endometrial biopsy showing endometritis.

Imaging (e.g., transvaginal ultrasound, MRI or CT) showing thickened, fluid-filled fallopian tubes, tubo-ovarian abscess or free pelvic fluid. Laparoscopy confirming salpingitis or tubo-ovarian abscess.

Diagnostic Tests

Microbiological Testing: NAAT for Chlamydia trachomatis and Neisseria gonorrhoeae (cervical or vaginal swab).Vaginal wet mount or Gram stain to assess for bacterial vaginosis or other pathogens. Culture or NAAT for Mycoplasma genitalium if available.

Complete blood count (CBC) for leukocytosis.

ESR or CRP for inflammation.

Transvaginal ultrasound to detect tubo-ovarian abscess, hydrosalpinx or pelvic free fluid.

CT/MRI for complex cases or suspected abscess.

Laparoscopy: Gold standard for definitive diagnosis but rarely used due to invasiveness.

Endometrial Biopsy: Histological evidence of endometritis (plasma cell infiltration).

Differential Diagnosis

Appendicitis, ectopic pregnancy, ovarian cyst rupture, endometriosis, urinary tract infection, inflammatory bowel disease or gastroenteritis.

Careful history and examination are crucial to rule out these conditions.

Management

Prompt treatment of PID is essential to prevent complications. Management includes antimicrobial therapy, supportive care and, in severe cases, surgical intervention.

Antimicrobial Therapy (CDC 2021 Guidelines)

Outpatient Treatment (for mild to moderate PID)

Regimen A: Ceftriaxone 500 mg IM single dose + Doxycycline 100 mg orally twice daily for 14 days ± Metronidazole 500 mg orally twice daily for 14 days.

Regimen B: Cefoxitin 2 g IM single dose + Probenecid 1 g orally + Doxycycline 100 mg orally twice daily for 14 days ± Metronidazole 500 mg orally twice daily for 14 days.

Metronidazole is added to cover anaerobic bacteria, especially in cases with bacterial vaginosis or recent pelvic procedures.

Inpatient Treatment (for severe PID, pregnancy, tubo-ovarian abscess, or intolerance to oral therapy)

Regimen A: Cefotetan 2 g IV every 12 hours OR Cefoxitin 2 g IV every 6 hours + Doxycycline 100 mg IV/orally every 12 hours.

Regimen B: Clindamycin 900 mg IV every 8 hours + Gentamicin 2 mg/kg IV loading dose followed by 1.5 mg/kg every 8 hours.

Transition to oral doxycycline (100 mg twice daily) ± metronidazole for a total of 14 days after clinical improvement (usually within 48–72 hours).

Alternative Conditions

Azithromycin may be used for Mycoplasma genitalium or in doxycycline intolerance.

Fluoroquinolones are avoided due to resistance in Neisseria gonorrhoeae.

Supportive Care

Analgesics (e.g., ibuprofen) for pain relief.

Hydration and rest for systemic symptoms.

Removal of IUD, if PID develops within 3–6 weeks of insertion, after initiating antibiotics.

Surgical Management

Indicated for tubo-ovarian abscess: Unresponsive to antibiotics, ruptured abscess or severe peritonitis.

Procedures include ultrasound-guided abscess drainage, laparoscopy or laparotomy for abscess resection or salpingectomy/oophorectomy in severe cases.

Partner Treatment

Sexual partners from the past two months should be evaluated and treated for Chlamydia and Gonorrhea to prevent reinfection.

Abstinence from sexual intercourse until treatment completion and symptom resolution.

Follow-Up: Reassess within 48–72 hours to ensure clinical improvement (resolution of fever, pain and tenderness). Repeat STI testing after 3–6 months to rule out reinfection.

Complications

PID can lead to significant long-term sequelae, particularly if untreated or inadequately treated:

1. Infertility: Occurs in 10–20% of women with PID due to tubal scarring and occlusion. Risk increases with recurrent episodes (up to 40% after three episodes).
2. Ectopic Pregnancy: Tubal damage increases the risk by 7–10-fold, due to impaired ovum transport.
3. Chronic Pelvic Pain: Seen in 15–30% of cases, due to adhesions, fibrosis or recurrent infections.
4. Tubo-Ovarian Abscess: Occurs in 10–15% of severe cases, potentially leading to sepsis or rupture.
5. Fitz-Hugh-Curtis Syndrome: Perihepatitis causing right upper quadrant pain and liver capsule adhesions.

Psychosocial Impact: Chronic pain and infertility can lead to psychological distress and reduced quality of life.

Prevention: Preventing PID involves addressing risk factors and promoting early intervention.

STI Prevention: Promote consistent condom use to reduce Chlamydia and Gonorrhea transmission. Routine STI screening in sexually active women under 25 years or with risk factors. Vaccination against human papillomavirus (HPV) and hepatitis B to reduce STI-related complications.

Education: Counsel patients on safe sexual practices and the risks of douching, which disrupts the mucosal integrity. Educate about symptoms of PID to encourage early presentation.

Special Populations

Pregnancy: PID is rare in pregnancy due to the cervical mucus plug but requires aggressive inpatient treatment to prevent maternal and fetal complications (e.g., preterm labor, chorioamnionitis).

Postmenopausal Women: PID is uncommon but may occur with tubo-ovarian abscess or non-STI pathogens (e.g., E. coli). Consider alternative diagnoses like malignancy.

Conclusion

Pelvic inflammatory disease is a common gynaecological condition with significant implications for reproductive health. Its polymicrobial etiology, often driven by Chlamydia trachomatis and Neisseria gonorrhoeae, underscores the importance of early diagnosis and treatment to prevent complications like infertility, ectopic pregnancy and chronic pelvic pain. A strong clinical suspicion, combined with clinical and laboratory evaluation, is essential for accurate diagnosis. Comprehensive management, including broad-spectrum antibiotics, supportive care and partner treatment is necessary to stop acute symptoms and long-term sequelae. Preventive strategies, including STI screening, safe sexual practices and public health interventions, are all needed to minimize the burden of PID.

Common Pelvic Pathogens

Letter	Pathogen	Associated Infection
C	Chlamydia trachomatis	PID, tubal damage
G	Gonorrhea	Cervicitis, PID
O	Other anaerobes	Polymicrobial PID
T	Trichomonas vaginalis	Vaginitis, strawberry cervix
M	Mycoplasma genitalium	PID, endometritis
A	Actinomyces israelii	IUCD-related PID
P	Prevotella species	Bacterial vaginosis, PID
S	Streptococcus species	Postpartum pelvic infections

Pathogenesis of Pelvic Inflammatory Disease (PID)

Initial Infection (Vagina/Cervix)

↓

Disruption of Endocervical Barrier

↓

Ascends of Pathogens
(Chlamydia, Gonorrhea, Anaerobes)

↓

Infection of Upper Genital Tract:

↓

Endometrium → Endometritis
Fallopian Tubes → Salpingitis
Ovaries → Oophoritis
Pelvic Peritoneum → Peritonitis

↓

Inflammation, Adhesions, Scarring

↓

Complications:
Infertility, Ectopic Pregnancy, Chronic Pelvic Pain

Spread of Genital Tuberculosis

Primary TB Infection (Lungs or GI Tract)

↓

Hematogenous or Lymphatic Spread

↓

Genital Organs Involved:

↓

Fallopian Tubes → Salpingitis

Endometrium → Endometritis

Ovaries → Oophoritis

Peritoneum → Peritonitis

↓

Granuloma Formation, Caseation, Fibrosis

↓

Clinical Manifestations:

Infertility, Amenorrhea, Pelvic Mass, Pain

11.4 Sexually Transmitted Diseases

(*Amrad-i-manqoola Jinsiyya*)

Sexually transmitted diseases (STDs), also known as sexually transmitted infections (STIs), are infections primarily transmitted through sexual contact, including vaginal, anal or oral intercourse. They represent a significant public health concern due to their prevalence, potential for serious complications and impact on reproductive health. In the context of gynaecology, STDs are important because they can affect the female genital tract, leading to conditions such as pelvic inflammatory disease (PID), infertility, ectopic pregnancy and increased risk of HIV transmission.

Definition

STDs are infections caused by bacteria, viruses, parasites or fungi transmitted through sexual activity, including vaginal, anal or oral sex, and occasionally through non-sexual routes (e.g., vertical transmission, bloodborne spread). They primarily affect the genital tract but can involve systemic manifestations and long-term sequelae.

Epidemiology

Global Burden: The World Health Organization (WHO) estimates over 1 million new STI cases daily worldwide, with more than 374 million new cases annually of curable STIs (Chlamydia, Gonorrhea, Syphilis and Trichomoniasis). Viral STIs, such as human papillomavirus (HPV) and herpes simplex virus (HSV), affect millions more.

Prevalence in Women: Women are disproportionately affected due to anatomical factors (e.g., larger mucosal surface area, cervical ectopy in adolescents), hormonal influences and socioeconomic barriers to healthcare. Approximately 50% of new STI cases occur in women aged 15–24 years.

Risk Factors: Unprotected sexual intercourse.

Multiple sexual partners or high-risk partners (e.g., commercial sex workers, individuals with STIs).

Young age (<25 years), due to biological (immature cervical barrier) and behavioral factors.

History of STIs, substance abuse.

Socioeconomic factors, including limited access to healthcare, poverty and lack of health education.

Regional Variations: Higher incidence in low- and middle-income countries due to limited screening, treatment and prevention programs. In developed countries, rising STI rates are noted due to changes in sexual behavior and reduced barrier usage.

Etiology

STDs are caused by a diverse group of pathogens, each with distinct characteristics and clinical implications. The major STDs affecting the female genital tract include:

1. Bacterial STIs

Chlamydia trachomatis: A common cause of cervicitis and PID; often asymptomatic ("silent" infection).

Neisseria gonorrhoeae: Causes gonorrhea, leading to cervicitis, urethritis and PID.

Treponema pallidum: Causes syphilis, with genital and systemic manifestations.

Mycoplasma genitalium: An emerging cause of cervicitis and PID.

2. Viral STIs

Human Papillomavirus (HPV): Associated with genital warts, cervical dysplasia and cervical cancer.

Herpes Simplex Virus (HSV): Causes genital herpes, with recurrent painful lesions.

Human Immunodeficiency Virus (HIV): Affects immune function, increasing susceptibility to other STIs.

Hepatitis B Virus (HBV): Transmitted sexually and perinatally, causing liver disease.

3. Parasitic STIs

Trichomonas vaginalis: Causes trichomoniasis, a common cause of vaginitis.

4. Fungal STIs

Candida albicans: While not always sexually transmitted, recurrent candidiasis may be linked to sexual activity.

Pathophysiology

The pathophysiology of STDs involves microbial invasion, host immune response and tissue damage, with specific mechanisms caused by pathogens:

Bacterial STIs

1. Chlamydia trachomatis: Obligate intracellular bacterium that infects columnar epithelial cells of the cervix, causing inflammation (cervicitis). Ascending infection leads to endometritis, salpingitis or PID, with scarring and fibrosis causing infertility or ectopic pregnancy.
2. Neisseria gonorrhoeae: Attaches to cervical mucosa via pili, triggering acute inflammation and purulent discharge. Ascending infection causes PID or disseminated gonococcal infection (DGI).

3. Treponema pallidum: Invades mucosal surfaces, leading to localized chancre (primary syphilis), followed by systemic dissemination via hematogenous spread, causing secondary and tertiary syphilis.
4. Mycoplasma genitalium: Adheres to epithelial cells, causing chronic inflammation and contributing to cervicitis or PID.

Viral STIs

1. HPV: Infects basal epithelial cells, leading to cellular proliferation (warts) or dysplasia (high-risk HPV types, e.g., 16, 18). Persistent infection is a major risk factor for cervical cancer.
2. HSV: Infects epithelial cells, causing vesicular lesions and establishes latency in sensory ganglia, leading to recurrent outbreaks triggered by stress or immunosuppression.
3. HIV: Targets CD4+ T-cells, impairing immune function and increasing susceptibility to opportunistic infections and other STIs.
4. HBV: Infects hepatocytes, causing acute or chronic hepatitis, with sexual transmission facilitated by mucosal contact with infected fluids.

Parasitic STIs

Trichomonas vaginalis: Adheres to vaginal epithelium, causing inflammation and frothy discharge. It disrupts the vaginal microbiome, increasing susceptibility to bacterial STIs and HIV.

General Mechanisms

Ascending Infection: Pathogens breach the cervical mucus barrier, facilitated by menstruation, douching or sexual activity, leading to upper genital tract involvement.

Immune Evasion: Pathogens like Chlamydia and HSV evade host immunity through intracellular survival or latency, respectively.

Microbiome Disruption: STIs often alter the vaginal microbiome, reducing Lactobacillus dominance and increasing pH, which promotes secondary infections.

Clinical features

STDs present with a spectrum of symptoms, from asymptomatic to severe, depending on the pathogen and host factors. Women may be asymptomatic in up to 50–70% of cases, particularly with Chlamydia and HPV.

1. Chlamydia (Chlamydia trachomatis)

Symptoms: Asymptomatic in 70–80% of women; when present, mucopurulent cervical discharge, postcoital bleeding, dysuria or lower abdominal pain (if PID develops).

Signs: Cervicitis with mucopurulent discharge, cervical friability, or cervical motion tenderness in PID.

2. Gonorrhea (Neisseria gonorrhoeae)

Symptoms: Asymptomatic in 50% of women; purulent vaginal discharge, dysuria, intermenstrual bleeding or pelvic pain.

Signs: Purulent cervical discharge, cervicitis or signs of PID (e.g., adnexal tenderness).

3. Syphilis (Treponema pallidum)

Primary: Painless genital chancre (ulcer) at the site of inoculation (vulva, vagina, cervix).

Secondary: Systemic symptoms (rash, lymphadenopathy, fever, mucosal lesions) 4–8 weeks after chancre.

Latent: Asymptomatic phase, detectable only by serology.

Tertiary: Rare, with gummatous lesions, neurosyphilis or cardiovascular involvement.

Signs: Chancre, condyloma lata (secondary syphilis), or systemic findings.

4. Genital Herpes (HSV-1 or HSV-2)

Symptoms: Painful genital vesicles or ulcers, dysuria, inguinal lymphadenopathy or flu-like symptoms (primary infection). Recurrent episodes are milder.

Signs: Vesicular or ulcerative lesions on vulva, vagina or cervix; tender lymphadenopathy.

5. Human Papillomavirus (HPV)

Symptoms: Often asymptomatic; genital warts (condyloma acuminata) with low-risk types (e.g., HPV 6, 11). High-risk types (e.g., HPV 16, 18) may cause abnormal cervical cytology.

Signs: Warty growths on vulva, vagina or cervix; abnormal Pap smear findings.

6. HIV

Symptoms: Acute retroviral syndrome (fever, rash, lymphadenopathy) 2–4 weeks post-exposure; asymptomatic chronic phase until AIDS develops.

Signs: Opportunistic infections, cervical dysplasia (due to HPV co-infection) or lymphadenopathy.

7. Trichomoniasis (Trichomonas vaginalis)

Symptoms: Frothy, yellow-green vaginal discharge, vaginal irritation, dysuria or dyspareunia; asymptomatic in 50% of cases.

Signs: “Strawberry cervix” (punctate hemorrhages), vaginal erythema.

8. Hepatitis B

Symptoms: Often asymptomatic; acute hepatitis with jaundice, fatigue or abdominal pain.

Signs: Hepatomegaly, jaundice or abnormal liver function tests.

Diagnosis

Accurate diagnosis of STDs requires a combination of clinical evaluation, laboratory testing and imaging when indicated. Asymptomatic infections necessitate routine screening in high-risk populations.

General Diagnostic Approach

History: Sexual history (partners, condom use, prior STIs), symptoms and risk factors.

Physical Examination: Speculum and bimanual examination to assess for discharge, lesions or tenderness.

Laboratory Tests

Nucleic Acid Amplification Tests (NAAT): Gold standard for Chlamydia, Gonorrhea and Mycoplasma genitalium (cervical/vaginal swab, urine).

Serology: Syphilis (RPR, VDRL, or treponemal-specific tests like FTA-ABS); HIV (ELISA, Western blot, or rapid tests); HBV (HBsAg, anti-HBc).

Viral Culture or PCR: HSV diagnosis from lesion swabs.

Wet Mount: Trichomonas vaginalis (motile trichomonads) or clue cells (bacterial vaginosis).

Pap Smear/HPV Testing: Detects HPV-related cervical dysplasia; co-testing for high-risk HPV types.

Imaging: Ultrasound or CT for complications (e.g., PID, tubo-ovarian abscess).

Specific Diagnostic Criteria

Chlamydia/Gonorrhea: NAAT positive from cervical/vaginal swab or urine.

Syphilis: Positive non-treponemal (RPR/VDRL) and treponemal tests; dark-field microscopy for primary chancre.

HSV: PCR or culture from lesions; serology for past exposure (IgG).

HPV: Visual inspection for warts; Pap smear or HPV DNA testing for cervical abnormalities.

HIV: Positive ELISA confirmed by Western blot or PCR; CD4 count and viral load for staging.

Trichomoniasis: Wet mount, NAAT or culture from vaginal discharge.

HBV: HBsAg positive; HBV DNA for active infection.

Screening Recommendations (CDC, 2021)

Annual Chlamydia and Gonorrhea screening for sexually active women <25 years or with risk factors.

HPV screening (co-testing with Pap smear) every 3–5 years for women aged 21–65 years.

HIV screening at least once for all adults; annually for high-risk groups.

Syphilis and HBV screening in high-risk populations or during pregnancy.

Management

Treatment of STDs aims to eradicate the infection, alleviate symptoms, prevent complications and reduce transmission. Management follows CDC or WHO guidelines.

1. Chlamydia

Treatment: Azithromycin 1 g orally single dose OR Doxycycline 100 mg orally twice daily for 7 days. Partner Treatment: Treat all sexual partners from the past two months; abstain from sex for 7 days post-treatment.

2. Gonorrhea

Treatment: Ceftriaxone 500 mg IM single dose (or 1 g for weight >150 kg) ± Doxycycline 100 mg twice daily for 7 days (if co-infection with Chlamydia suspected). Partner Treatment: As above; address rising antibiotic resistance (e.g., cephalosporin-resistant strains).

3. Syphilis

Primary/Secondary/Early Latent: Benzathine penicillin G 2.4 million units IM single dose.

Late Latent/Tertiary: Benzathine penicillin G 2.4 million units IM weekly for 3 weeks.

Neurosyphilis: Aqueous penicillin G 18–24 million units IV daily for 10–14 days.

Partner Treatment: Evaluate and treat partners based on stage and exposure history.

4. Genital Herpes

Primary Infection: Acyclovir 400 mg orally three times daily for 7–10 days OR Valacyclovir 1 g orally twice daily for 7–10 days.

Recurrent Episodes: Acyclovir 800 mg orally three times daily for 2 days OR Valacyclovir 500 mg twice daily for 3 days.

Suppressive Therapy: Valacyclovir 500–1000 mg daily for high-risk patients (e.g., frequent recurrences, HIV-positive).

Counseling: Educate on transmission risk during asymptomatic shedding.

5. HPV

Genital Warts: Topical therapies (imiquimod, podophyllotoxin) or surgical removal (cryotherapy, excision).

Cervical Dysplasia: Colposcopy, biopsy and treatment (e.g., loop electrosurgical excision procedure [LEEP]) for high-grade lesions.

Vaccination: HPV vaccine (9-valent) for prevention.

6. HIV

Treatment: Antiretroviral therapy (ART) initiated immediately, according to viral load and CD4 count.

Prevention: Pre-exposure prophylaxis (PrEP) for high-risk individuals; post-exposure prophylaxis (PEP) within 72 hours of exposure.

7. Trichomoniasis

Treatment: Metronidazole 2 g orally single dose OR Tinidazole 2 g orally single dose.

Partner Treatment: Treat all partners; abstain from sex until therapy.

8. Hepatitis B

Treatment: Antiviral therapy (e.g., tenofovir, entecavir) for chronic HBV; supportive care for acute infection.

Vaccination: HBV vaccine for prevention.

General Principles

Treat empirically for co-infections (e.g., Chlamydia with Gonorrhea).

Follow up to confirm cure (test of cure for Gonorrhea, Trichomoniasis or persistent symptoms).

Counsel on abstinence or condom use during treatment to prevent reinfection.

Address complications (e.g., PID, infertility) with appropriate referral.

Complications

STDs can lead to significant gynaecological and systemic complications, particularly in women.

Pelvic Inflammatory Disease (PID): Caused by Chlamydia, Gonorrhea or Mycoplasma, leading to endometritis, salpingitis or tubo-ovarian abscess.

Infertility: Tubal scarring from PID (Chlamydia, Gonorrhea) affects 10–20% of untreated cases.

Ectopic Pregnancy: Increased risk (7–10-fold) due to tubal damage.

Chronic Pelvic Pain: Resulting from adhesions or recurrent infections.

Cervical Cancer: High-risk HPV types (16, 18) cause 99% of cervical cancers.

HIV Transmission: Genital ulcers (HSV, syphilis) and inflammation increase HIV acquisition risk.

Pregnancy Complications: Vertical transmission (Syphilis, HIV, HBV), preterm birth or low birth weight.

Disseminated Infections: Gonorrhea, neurosyphilis or chronic HBV.

Prevention

Preventing STDs is essential to reduce their burden on female genital health:

Behavioral Interventions

Promote consistent condom use (male or female condoms).

Encourage monogamy or reduced number of sexual partners.

Educate on avoiding douching, which disrupts vaginal defence.

Vaccinations

HPV vaccine (9-valent) for ages 9–45 years to prevent HPV-related warts and cancers.

HBV vaccine for all infants and high-risk adults.

Screening and Early Treatment

Routine STI screening for sexually active women <25 years or with risk factors.

Partner notification and treatment to prevent reinfection.

Prophylaxis

PrEP for HIV prevention in high-risk women.

PEP for HIV exposure (within 72 hours).

Public Health Measures

Community-based education and STI clinics.

Access to affordable condoms and healthcare services.

Special Populations

Pregnant Women: Screen for Chlamydia, Gonorrhea, Syphilis, HIV and HBV to prevent vertical transmission and adverse outcomes (e.g., congenital syphilis, neonatal HIV).

Adolescents: Higher biological susceptibility (cervical ectopy) and behavioural risks; emphasize education and vaccination.

Menopausal Women: Increased risk of vaginal atrophy and STI transmission due to thinning of mucosa; screen for HPV and HIV.

HIV-Positive Women: Higher risk of HPV-related cervical dysplasia and recurrent HSV; regular monitoring and ART adherence are needed.

Conclusion

Sexually transmitted diseases are a major cause of morbidity in women, with significant implications for gynecological and reproductive health. Their diverse etiologies—bacterial, viral and parasitic—require a planned approach to diagnosis, treatment and prevention. Asymptomatic infections, particularly Chlamydia and HPV, underscore the importance of routine screening in high-risk populations. Prompt treatment with appropriate antimicrobial or antiviral therapies, combined with partner management and patient education, is essential to prevent complications such as PID, infertility and cervical cancer. Preventive strategies, including vaccinations, use of barrier contraceptives and public health interventions, are necessary to reduce the global burden of STD.

11.5 Genital Tuberculosis

(*Tadrriun A'da' Tanasuliyya zanana*)

Genital tuberculosis (TB) is a form of extrapulmonary tuberculosis that affects the female genital tract, often as a result of hematogenous or lymphatic spread from a primary focus, typically pulmonary TB. It is a significant cause of infertility and chronic pelvic pain in endemic areas and is frequently underdiagnosed due to its insidious presentation and diagnostic challenges.

Definition

Genital tuberculosis is an infection of the female genital tract caused by Mycobacterium tuberculosis or rarely, *Mycobacterium bovis*. It primarily affects the fallopian tubes, endometrium and ovaries, but can involve the cervix, vagina or vulva. It is a form of extrapulmonary TB and is often associated with infertility, menstrual irregularities and chronic pelvic pain.

Epidemiology

Global Burden: Genital TB accounts for 5–10% of extrapulmonary TB cases and is more prevalent in TB-endemic regions, such as South Asia, Sub-Saharan Africa and parts of Eastern Europe. In high-burden countries like India, it is estimated to cause 10–20% of infertility cases in women.

Prevalence: Exact prevalence is unknown due to underdiagnosis, but studies suggest it affects 1–2% of women undergoing infertility evaluation in endemic areas. It is less common in low-TB-incidence countries but can occur in immigrant populations or immunocompromised individuals.

Risk Factors

Residence in or travel to TB-endemic areas.

History of pulmonary or extrapulmonary TB.

Immunosuppression (e.g., HIV, diabetes, malnutrition, or immunosuppressive therapy).

Socioeconomic factors (poverty, overcrowding, poor healthcare access).

Close contact with active TB cases.

Age: Most common in women of reproductive age (20–40 years), reflecting the peak incidence of TB and its impact on fertility.

Etiology

Causative Organism: Mycobacterium tuberculosis is the primary pathogen. Mycobacterium bovis is rare and typically associated with unpasteurized dairy consumption.

Mode of Spread

Hematogenous Spread: The most common route, where TB bacilli disseminate from a primary focus (usually pulmonary TB) to the genital tract during the initial bacteremia.

Lymphatic Spread: Less common, from regional lymph nodes (e.g., abdominal or pelvic nodes).

Direct Spread: Rare, from adjacent organs (e.g., peritoneal TB or intestinal TB).

Sexual Transmission: Extremely rare but reported in cases of male partner with genitourinary TB.

Site of Involvement

Fallopian Tubes: Affected in 90–100% of cases, often bilaterally, leading to tubal scarring and infertility.

Endometrium: Involved in 50–60% of cases, causing endometrial adhesions or menstrual irregularities.

Ovaries: Affected in 20–30% of cases, often as tubo-ovarian masses or abscesses.

Cervix, Vagina, Vulva: Rare (<5%), presenting as ulcers or hypertrophic lesions.

Associated Conditions: Genital TB is often associated with pulmonary TB (active or latent) or other extrapulmonary sites (e.g., peritoneal TB, lymph node TB). Co-infection with HIV increases the risk and severity.

Pathophysiology

The pathogenesis of genital TB involves the following stages.

1. Primary Infection

Mycobacterium tuberculosis typically enters the body via inhalation, establishing a primary focus in the lungs. In 5–15% of cases, bacilli spread hematogenously during primary or reactivation phases to the genital tract.

The fallopian tubes are the primary site due to their rich vascular supply, with bacilli lodging in the submucosa or muscularis layers.

2. Inflammatory Response

The bacilli trigger a granulomatous inflammatory response, characterized by caseating granulomas with epithelioid cells, Langhans giant cells and lymphocytes.

Chronic inflammation leads to tissue destruction, fibrosis and adhesions, particularly in the fallopian tubes and endometrium.

3. Tubal Involvement

Tubal infection causes salpingitis, with mucosal edema, ulceration and caseation. Fibrosis leads to tubal occlusion, hydrosalpinx or pyosalpinx, impairing ovum transport and causing infertility.

Adhesions may form between the tubes, ovaries and adjacent structures, leading to tubo-ovarian masses.

4. Endometrial Involvement

Endometrial TB causes granulomatous endometritis, with caseation and synechiae (intrauterine adhesions) leading to Asherman's syndrome.

Disruption of endometrial vasculature and hormonal responsiveness results in menstrual irregularities or amenorrhea.

5. Ovarian and Peritoneal Involvement

Ovaries may develop granulomas or abscesses, often as part of tubo-ovarian complexes.

Peritoneal TB (pelvic peritonitis) causes ascites, adhesions, or "frozen pelvis," mimicking malignancy.

6. Immune Response

The host immune response, mediated by T-helper cells and cytokines (e.g., IFN-γ, TNF-α), controls infection but also contributes to tissue damage.

Immunosuppression (e.g., HIV) leads to atypical, disseminated disease with less granuloma formation.

Clinical Features

Genital TB is often insidious, with 20–30% of cases asymptomatic, detected during infertility evaluations. Symptoms vary depending on the site and severity of involvement.

Symptoms

Infertility: The most common presentation (70–80% of cases), due to tubal occlusion, endometrial adhesions or ovulatory dysfunction.

Menstrual Irregularities: Oligomenorrhea, hypomenorrhea or amenorrhea (due to endometrial destruction or Asherman's syndrome); menorrhagia in early stages.

Chronic Pelvic Pain: Dull, persistent pain due to adhesions, tubo-ovarian masses or pelvic peritonitis.

Abnormal Vaginal Discharge: Serosanguinous or purulent discharge in cervical or vaginal TB.

Systemic Symptoms: Low-grade fever, night sweats, weight loss or fatigue in active TB.

Postcoital Bleeding: Rare, associated with cervical TB.

Mass Effect: Palpable pelvic mass (tubo-ovarian abscess) or ascites in peritoneal TB.

Signs

Pelvic Examination: Adnexal tenderness, fixed or enlarged uterus or palpable tubo-ovarian masses.

Cervical Lesions: Ulcers or hypertrophic growths (rare).

General Examination: Signs of pulmonary TB (e.g., cough, hemoptysis) or lymphadenopathy in disseminated disease.

Peritoneal TB: Ascites, abdominal distension or "doughy abdomen" due to adhesions.

Special Conditions

Asymptomatic cases are common, especially in early stages, leading to delayed diagnosis.

HIV co-infection may present with atypical or severe manifestations, such as disseminated TB or tubo-ovarian abscess.

Diagnosis

Diagnosing genital TB is challenging due to its nonspecific symptoms, low bacterial load and need for invasive testing. A high index of suspicion is required, especially in endemic areas or infertility cases.

Diagnostic Approach

History: Infertility, menstrual irregularities, history of TB exposure or residence in endemic areas.

Physical Examination: Pelvic and systemic examination for signs of TB or complications.

Laboratory Tests

Microbiological Tests

Acid-fast bacilli (AFB) staining of endometrial biopsy, menstrual blood or cervical discharge (low sensitivity due to paucibacillary disease).

Culture for Mycobacterium tuberculosis (gold standard but slow; 4–6 weeks).

Nucleic acid amplification tests (NAAT), for rapid detection and rifampicin resistance.

Tuberculin Skin Test (TST) or Interferon-Gamma Release Assays (IGRA): Indicate TB exposure but not active disease; less specific in endemic areas or BCG-vaccinated individuals.

Complete Blood Count (CBC): Anemia, leukocytosis or elevated erythrocyte sedimentation rate (ESR).

HIV Testing: Recommended due to high co-infection rates.

Histopathology

Endometrial biopsy or curettage showing caseating granulomas with epithelioid cells and Langhans giant cells.

Sensitivity is low (10–40%) due to cyclical endometrial shedding.

Imaging

Ultrasound: Transvaginal ultrasound may show tubal thickening, hydrosalpinx, tubo-ovarian masses, or endometrial synechiae.

Hysterosalpingography (HSG): Beaded or rigid tubes, tubal occlusion or intrauterine adhesions (Asherman's syndrome).

CT/MRI: Detects pelvic masses, ascites or peritoneal thickening; useful for peritoneal TB.

Chest X-ray: Screens for pulmonary TB (active or healed lesions in 50% of cases).

Laparoscopy/Hysteroscopy

Gold standard for visualization; findings include tubal granulomas, adhesions, caseous nodules, or "frozen pelvis."

Hysteroscopy may reveal endometrial adhesions or caseation.

Biopsies can be taken for histopathology and culture.

Other Tests

Ascitic fluid analysis (in peritoneal TB): High protein, low glucose and AFB staining or culture.

CA-125: Elevated in peritoneal TB, mimicking ovarian malignancy.

Diagnostic Criteria

Definitive: Positive AFB culture, NAAT or histopathologic evidence of granulomas from genital tract tissue.

Presumptive: Clinical features (infertility, pelvic pain), imaging findings and positive TST/IGRA in endemic areas or high-risk patients.

Differential Diagnosis

Pelvic inflammatory disease (PID) due to other pathogens (Chlamydia, Gonorrhea).

Endometriosis, ovarian malignancy or ectopic pregnancy.

Chronic appendicitis or inflammatory bowel disease.

Sarcoidosis or other granulomatous diseases.

Management

The management of genital TB focuses on eradicating the infection, preventing complications and addressing infertility or other sequelae. Treatment follows WHO or National TB guidelines.

Antitubercular Therapy (ATT): Standard Regimen (WHO, 2023)

Intensive Phase (2 months): Isoniazid (H), Rifampicin (R), Pyrazinamide (Z), and Ethambutol (E) daily.

Continuation Phase (4 months): Isoniazid and Rifampicin daily.

Total duration: 6 months for drug-sensitive TB.

Dosing

Isoniazid: 5 mg/kg (max 300 mg/day).

Rifampicin: 10 mg/kg (max 600 mg/day).

Pyrazinamide: 25 mg/kg (max 2 g/day).

Ethambutol: 15 mg/kg (max 1.6 g/day).

Modifications

Multidrug-resistant TB (MDR-TB): Requires second-line drugs (e.g., fluoroquinolones, bedaquiline) for 9–18 months, guided by drug susceptibility testing.

HIV co-infection: Coordinate ATT with antiretroviral therapy (ART), adjusting for drug interactions (e.g., rifampicin reduces ART efficacy).

Monitoring

Monthly follow-up for clinical response (resolution of symptoms, weight gain).

Liver function tests (LFTs) due to hepatotoxicity risk.

Repeat endometrial biopsy or imaging to assess treatment response in complex cases.

Supportive Care

Nutritional support to address malnutrition, a common comorbidity.

Analgesics (e.g., NSAIDs) for pelvic pain.

Psychological counseling for infertility-related distress.

Surgical Management

Indications

Persistent tubo-ovarian abscess or pyosalpinx unresponsive to ATT.

Severe adhesions causing chronic pain or infertility.

Suspected malignancy requiring diagnostic surgery

Procedures

Laparoscopic adhesiolysis or drainage of abscesses.

Salpingectomy or hysterectomy in severe cases (e.g., destroyed tubes, endometrial scarring).

Hysteroscopic adhesiolysis for Asherman's syndrome.

Surgery is avoided during active infection due to risk of dissemination; ATT should be initiated first.

Infertility Management

ATT may restore fertility in early cases, but tubal or endometrial damage is often irreversible.

Assisted reproductive technologies (ART), such as in vitro fertilization (IVF), may be considered after ATT completion, but success rates are lower due to tubal and endometrial pathology.

Hysteroscopic adhesiolysis may improve endometrial receptivity in Asherman's syndrome.

Partner and Contact Tracing

Screen sexual partners and household contacts for TB (pulmonary or genitourinary).

Treat latent TB infection with isoniazid prophylaxis (6–9 months) in high-risk contacts.

Follow-Up

Monitor for clinical improvement (e.g., resolution of pain, menstrual regularity) and complications.

Repeat imaging or hysteroscopy to assess structural damage post-treatment.

Long-term follow-up for infertility or recurrence in endemic areas.

Complications

Genital TB can lead to significant gynecological and systemic complications:

Infertility: The most common complication, affecting 70–80% of cases due to tubal occlusion, endometrial adhesions (Asherman's syndrome) or ovulatory dysfunction.

Chronic Pelvic Pain: Caused by adhesions, tubo-ovarian masses or pelvic peritonitis.

Ectopic Pregnancy: Increased risk due to tubal scarring and impaired ciliary function.

Tubo-Ovarian Abscess: Occurs in advanced cases, potentially leading to sepsis or rupture if untreated.

Asherman's Syndrome: Intrauterine adhesions causing amenorrhea or infertility due to endometrial destruction.

Ectopic Pregnancy: Increased risk due to tubal scarring and impaired ciliary function.

Chronic Pelvic Pain: Persistent pain from adhesions, tubo-ovarian masses or pelvic peritonitis.

Disseminated TB: Rare but serious, with spread to other organs (e.g., peritoneum, lymph nodes) in immunocompromised patients.

Malignancy Mimicry: Tubo-ovarian masses or peritoneal TB may mimic ovarian or endometrial cancer, leading to diagnostic challenges.

Psychosocial Impact: Infertility and chronic pain can cause significant emotional distress and reduced quality of life.

Prevention

Preventing genital TB involves addressing the broader epidemiology of tuberculosis and reducing risk factors for genital tract involvement.

TB Control Programs

Early diagnosis and treatment of pulmonary TB to prevent hematogenous spread.

BCG vaccination in endemic areas to reduce primary TB infection, though its efficacy against extrapulmonary TB is limited.

Screening and Contact Tracing

Screen high-risk populations (e.g., HIV-positive individuals, those in TB-endemic areas) for latent or active TB using TST, IGRA, or chest X-ray.

Prophylactic treatment (e.g., isoniazid for 6–9 months) for latent TB infection in contacts of active TB cases.

Infertility Evaluation

Routine screening for TB in women presenting with infertility in endemic areas, using endometrial biopsy, NAAT or laparoscopy.

Public Health Measures

Improve access to healthcare and TB diagnostics .

Address socioeconomic factors (e.g., malnutrition, overcrowding) that increase TB risk.

HIV Management

Early initiation of ART in HIV-positive women to reduce susceptibility to TB.

Regular TB screening in HIV-positive populations.

Education

Raise awareness among healthcare providers about genital TB as a cause of infertility and pelvic pain in endemic areas.

Educate patients on TB symptoms and the importance of early treatment.

Special Populations

HIV-Positive Women

Higher risk of genital TB due to immunosuppression, with atypical presentations (e.g., disseminated disease, non-caseating granulomas).

Requires coordinated ATT and ART, with careful monitoring for drug interactions (e.g., rifampicin reduces efficacy of certain antiretrovirals).

Pregnant Women

Genital TB is rare in pregnancy but can cause congenital TB or adverse outcomes (e.g., preterm birth, low birth weight).

ATT is safe in pregnancy (avoid streptomycin due to ototoxicity); rifampicin, isoniazidn and ethambutol are preferred.

Infertile Women

Genital TB is a leading cause of infertility in endemic areas; routine screening (endometrial biopsy, HSG or laparoscopy) is recommended for unexplained infertility.

ART (e.g., IVF) may be considered post-treatment, but its success is limited by tubal and endometrial damage.

Postmenopausal Women

Rare presentation, often as tubo-ovarian masses or endometrial abnormalities mimicking malignancy.

Requires careful diagnostic workup to differentiate from ovarian or endometrial cancer.

Conclusion

Genital tuberculosis is an important yet underdiagnosed cause of infertility and chronic pelvic pain, particularly in TB-endemic regions. Its insidious presentation, often asymptomatic or mimicking other gynecological conditions, necessitates a high clinical suspicion and a comprehensive diagnostic approach, including microbiological, histopathological and imaging modalities. Antitubercular therapy is highly effective, but irreversible tubal and endometrial damage often limits fertility. Complications such as infertility, ectopic pregnancy and chronic pelvic pain highlight the importance of early diagnosis and treatment. Preventive strategies, including TB control programs, screening in high-risk populations, and addressing socioeconomic factors, are essential to reduce the burden of genital TB.

Complications

PID → Infertility, ectopic pregnancy, chronic pain, Fitz-Hugh-Curtis syndrome

Genital TB → Asherman's syndrome, tubal block, amenorrhea

TOA (Tubo-Ovarian Abscess) → Rupture, sepsis

STDs → Cervical cancer (HPV), pelvic adhesions

11.6 Pelvic Pain & Low Backache

(*Waja 'hauz-e-aana aur Waja'al Khasira*)

Definition

Pelvic Pain: Pain perceived in the lower abdomen or pelvis, below the umbilicus and above the inguinal ligaments, encompassing the reproductive organs (uterus, fallopian tubes, ovaries), bladder, distal ureters, rectum and pelvic peritoneum. It may be acute (sudden onset, <6 months) or chronic (persistent or recurrent for ≥6 months).

Low Backache: Pain localized to the lumbar or sacral region, often radiating to the pelvis or lower extremities. In women, it may be referred from pelvic pathology or arise from musculoskeletal or neurological causes.

Classification

Acute Pelvic Pain: Sudden onset, often indicating emergency conditions (e.g., ectopic pregnancy, ovarian torsion).

Chronic Pelvic Pain (CPP): Persistent or recurrent pain for ≥6 months, often multifactorial, affecting 15–20% of women.

Cyclical Pain: Related to the menstrual cycle (e.g., dysmenorrhea, endometriosis).

Non-Cyclical Pain: Unrelated to menstruation, often due to non-gynecological causes.

Epidemiology

Prevalence

Pelvic pain affects 15–25% of women of reproductive age, with chronic pelvic pain (CPP) reported in 10–20% of women globally. Low backache is reported in 50–80% of women at some point, with 20–30% experiencing chronic low back pain.

In gynecological OPDs, 30–50% of women presenting with pelvic pain have a gynecological etiology, while the others have urological, gastrointestinal or musculoskeletal causes.

Age Distribution

Reproductive age (15–45 years): Common causes include endometriosis, PID and dysmenorrhea.

Postmenopausal women: Malignancies, pelvic organ prolapse or musculoskeletal issues predominate.

Risk Factors

Gynecological: History of sexually transmitted infections (STIs), endometriosis, pelvic surgery or infertility.

Lifestyle: Sedentary behavior, obesity, smoking or poor posture.

Psychosocial: Stress, depression or history of sexual abuse (common in CPP).

Socioeconomic: Limited healthcare access increases risk of untreated conditions (e.g., PID, genital TB).

Etiology

Pelvic pain and low backache in women can arise from gynecological, non-gynecological or mixed causes.

1. Gynecological Causes

Menstrual-Related

Primary Dysmenorrhea: Painful menstruation due to prostaglandin-mediated uterine contractions.

Secondary Dysmenorrhea: Pain due to underlying pathology (e.g., endometriosis, adenomyosis).

Endometriosis: Ectopic endometrial tissue causing cyclical pelvic pain, dyspareunia and infertility.

Adenomyosis: Endometrial tissue within the myometrium, leading to heavy, painful menses and chronic pelvic pain.

Pelvic Inflammatory Disease (PID): Ascending infection (Chlamydia, Gonorrhea) causing endometritis, salpingitis or tubo-ovarian abscess.

Genital Tuberculosis: Chronic granulomatous infection of the fallopian tubes or endometrium, leading to infertility and chronic pelvic pain.

Ovarian Pathology

Ovarian cysts (functional or neoplastic): Pain from rupture, torsion or mass effect.

Ovarian torsion: Acute pain due to twisting of the ovary, often with an adnexal mass.

Uterine Pathology

Uterine fibroids (leiomyomas): Pain from degeneration, torsion or pressure on adjacent structures.

Asherman's syndrome: Intrauterine adhesions causing pelvic pain and amenorrhea (e.g., post-TB).

Pelvic Congestion Syndrome: Dilated pelvic veins causing chronic, dull pelvic pain, often post-coital.

Pelvic Organ Prolapse: Descent of uterus, bladder or rectum, causing pelvic heaviness or low backache.

Ectopic Pregnancy: Acute pelvic pain with risk of rupture, often unilateral.

Endometrial or Cervical Cancer: Postmenopausal pain or bleeding, rare in younger women.

2. Non-Gynecological Causes

Urological

Urinary tract infections (UTIs): Cystitis or pyelonephritis causing suprapubic or flank pain.

Urolithiasis: Renal or ureteral stones causing referred pelvic or back pain.

Interstitial cystitis: Chronic bladder pain with urinary frequency.

Gastrointestinal

Irritable bowel syndrome (IBS): Cramping, bloating and pelvic pain.

Appendicitis: Acute right lower quadrant pain, mimicking gynecological conditions.

Inflammatory bowel disease (IBD): Crohn's disease or ulcerative colitis causing pelvic or referred pain.

Diverticulitis: Left-sided pelvic pain in older women.

Musculoskeletal

Lumbar disc disease: Herniation or degeneration causing low backache radiating to the pelvis.

Sacroiliac joint dysfunction: Pain in the lower back or pelvis, exacerbated by movement.

Myofascial pain syndrome: Trigger points in pelvic or lumbar muscles.

Neurological

Pudendal nerve irritation: Chronic pelvic pain with burning or neuropathic features.

Referred pain from spinal pathology (e.g., radiculopathy).

Psychosomatic: Chronic pelvic pain associated with psychological stress, depression or history of trauma.

3. Mixed or Multifactorial Causes

Chronic pelvic pain often involves overlapping gynecological (e.g., endometriosis) and non-gynecological (e.g., IBS, musculoskeletal) factors, with psychosocial factors.

Pathophysiology

The pathophysiology of pelvic pain and low backache depends on the underlying etiology, but involves common mechanisms:

1. Inflammation: Conditions like PID, endometriosis or genital TB trigger inflammatory mediators (e.g., prostaglandins, cytokines), causing pain and tissue damage. Endometriotic implants release inflammatory cytokines (e.g., IL-1, TNF-α), leading to adhesions and fibrosis.

2. Visceral Pain: Uterine or ovarian pathology (e.g., dysmenorrhea, ovarian cysts) causes visceral pain via stimulation of nociceptors in pelvic organs, often poorly localized.

3. Referred Pain: Pelvic pathology (e.g., endometriosis, PID) can refer pain to the lower back due to shared innervation (e.g., T10–L1 spinal segments).

4. Adhesions and Fibrosis: Chronic inflammation (e.g., PID, genital TB) leads to adhesions, causing mechanical pain and restricted organ mobility.

5. Vascular Congestion: Pelvic congestion syndrome results from dilated pelvic veins, causing dull, aching pain exacerbated by standing or coitus.

6. Urological: Bladder inflammation (e.g., interstitial cystitis) or ureteral obstruction (e.g., stones) stimulates visceral nociceptors, causing suprapubic or referred back pain.

7. Gastrointestinal: Bowel inflammation or distension (e.g., IBS, diverticulitis) activates visceral pain pathways, referring to the pelvis or back.

8. Musculoskeletal: Mechanical stress (e.g., disc herniation, sacroiliac dysfunction) or muscle spasms cause somatic pain, often radiating to the pelvis.

9. Neuropathic: Nerve compression or irritation (e.g., pudendal nerve) causes burning or shooting pain in the pelvic or sacral region.

10. Chronic pain increases central sensitization, lowering pain thresholds and perpetuating pain perception.

11. Stress or trauma activates the hypothalamic-pituitary-adrenal axis, increasing cortisol and exacerbating pain perception.

Unani Perspective (*Asbaabe Sitta Zarooriya*)

Hawa-e-Muheet: Poor environmental conditions (e.g., dampness) may exacerbate infections like PID or TB, contributing to pain.

Makool wa Mashroob: Malnutrition weakens Tabiyat (self-healing capacity), increasing susceptibility to chronic conditions like genital TB or PID.

Harkat wa Sukoon-e-Badani: Sedentary lifestyle or overexertion can cause musculoskeletal pain or impair pelvic circulation, worsening conditions like pelvic congestion syndrome.

Harkat wa Sukoon-e-Nafsani: Stress or emotional distress (Amraz-e-Nafsani) amplifies pain perception in CPP, disrupting Ruh (vital spirit).

Naum wa Yaqza: Poor sleep impairs Hararat-e-Ghariziya (innate heat), reducing immune response and exacerbating chronic pain.

Ihtibaas wa Istifraagh: Retention of Akhlat (humors) or improper elimination (e.g., constipation) may contribute to pelvic inflammation or pain.

Clinical Evaluation

A systematic approach is essential to identify the cause of pelvic pain and low backache.

History

Pain Characteristics: Onset (acute vs. chronic), location (unilateral, bilateral, suprapubic, sacral), duration, quality (dull, sharp, burning) and aggravating/relieving factors (e.g., menstruation, posture).

Associated Symptoms: Menstrual irregularities, abnormal vaginal discharge, dyspareunia, infertility, urinary symptoms (dysuria, frequency), gastrointestinal symptoms (bloating, diarrhea) or systemic symptoms (fever, weight loss).

Gynecological History: Menstrual cycle patterns, obstetric history, STI history, pelvic surgeries or IUD use.

Risk Factors: Sexual history, TB exposure, smoking, obesity or psychosocial stressors.

Unani Perspective: Assess lifestyle factors (diet, sleep, stress, hygiene) to identify imbalances in *Asbaabe Sitta Zarooriya* .

Physical Examination

General Examination: Assess for systemic signs (e.g., fever, lymphadenopathy, weight loss) suggestive of TB or malignancy.

Abdominal Examination: Palpate for masses, tenderness or distension (e.g., ascites in peritoneal TB).

Pelvic Examination: Per speculum: Assess for discharge (PID, trichomoniasis), cervical lesions (TB, cancer), or “strawberry cervix” (trichomoniasis).

Bimanual: Check for uterine/adnexal tenderness, masses (fibroids, ovarian cysts) or cervical motion tenderness (PID).

Musculoskeletal Examination: Evaluate posture, lumbar spine, sacroiliac joints or trigger points for musculoskeletal causes.

Neurological Examination: Assess for sensory changes or radiculopathy in neuropathic pain.

Diagnosis

Diagnosis requires a combination of clinical evaluation, laboratory tests, imaging and invasive procedures when indicated.

Laboratory Tests

Complete Blood Count (CBC): Leukocytosis in PID or appendicitis; anemia in malignancy or TB.

Erythrocyte Sedimentation Rate (ESR)/C-Reactive Protein (CRP): Elevated in inflammatory conditions (PID, TB, endometriosis).

STI Testing: Nucleic acid amplification tests (NAAT) for Chlamydia, Gonorrhea or

Mycoplasma genitalium; wet mount for Trichomonas vaginalis.

TB Testing: Endometrial biopsy for AFB staining, culture or NAAT (e.g., GeneXpert); TST/IGRA for exposure.

Tumor Markers: CA-125 elevated in ovarian malignancy or peritoneal TB; not specific for diagnosis.

Urinalysis/Culture: Rule out UTI or pyelonephritis.

Pregnancy Test: Mandatory in reproductive-age women to exclude ectopic pregnancy.

Imaging

Transvaginal Ultrasound: Detects ovarian cysts, fibroids, tubo-ovarian abscess, hydrosalpinx or endometrial abnormalities.

Hysterosalpingography (HSG): Identifies tubal occlusion or adhesions in TB or PID-related infertility.

CT/MRI: Evaluates complex masses, peritoneal TB or musculoskeletal pathology.

X-ray: Lumbar spine X-ray for disc disease; chest X-ray for TB screening.

Invasive Procedures

Endometrial Biopsy: Diagnoses endometrial TB or malignancy.

Laparoscopy: Gold standard for endometriosis, PID, TB or adhesions; allows biopsy and adhesiolysis.

Hysteroscopy: Assesses intrauterine adhesions (Asherman's syndrome) or endometrial pathology.

Cystoscopy/Colonoscopy: For urological or gastrointestinal causes (e.g., interstitial cystitis, IBD).

Differential Diagnosis

Gynecological: Endometriosis, PID, genital TB, ovarian torsion, ectopic pregnancy, fibroids.

Urological: UTI, urolithiasis, interstitial cystitis.

Gastrointestinal: IBS, appendicitis, IBD, diverticulitis.

Musculoskeletal: Lumbar disc disease, sacroiliac dysfunction.

Neurological: Pudendal nerve irritation, radiculopathy.

Psychosomatic: Chronic pain aggravated by stress or trauma.

Management

Management of pelvic pain and low backache depends on the underlying cause, with a multidisciplinary approach often required.

1. Gynecological Causes

a. Primary Dysmenorrhea

NSAIDs (e.g., ibuprofen 400–800 mg every 6–8 hours) for prostaglandin inhibition.

Combined oral contraceptives (COCs) to suppress ovulation and reduce menstrual pain.

b. Endometriosis

Medical: NSAIDs, COCs, progestins (e.g., levonorgestrel IUD), or GnRH agonists (e.g., leuprolide).

Surgical: Laparoscopic excision or ablation of endometriotic implants; adhesiolysis.

c. PID

Antibiotics: Ceftriaxone 500 mg IM single dose + Doxycycline 100 mg twice daily for 14 days ± Metronidazole 500 mg twice daily (CDC, 2021).

Inpatient therapy for severe cases or tubo-ovarian abscess.

d. Genital TB

Antitubercular therapy (ATT): Isoniazid, Rifampicin, Pyrazinamide, Ethambutol for 2 months, followed by Isoniazid and Rifampicin for 4 months.

Surgical intervention for abscesses or severe adhesions.

e. Ovarian Cysts

Functional cysts: Observation or COCs to prevent recurrence.

Torsion or rupture: Surgical intervention (laparoscopy/laparotomy).

f. Fibroids

Medical: NSAIDs, tranexamic acid for menorrhagia, or GnRH agonists.

Surgical: Myomectomy or hysterectomy for severe cases.

g. Pelvic Congestion Syndrome

Medical: Medroxyprogesterone.

Interventional: Embolization of pelvic veins.

h. Ectopic Pregnancy

Medical: Methotrexate for stable, unruptured cases.

Surgical: Salpingectomy or salpingostomy for rupture or large ectopic.

2. Non-Gynecological Causes

Urological

UTI: Antibiotics (e.g., nitrofurantoin, fosfomycin).

Urolithiasis: Analgesics, hydration or urological intervention (e.g., lithotripsy).

Interstitial cystitis: Dietary modification, pentosan polysulfate, or bladder instillations.

Gastrointestinal

IBS: Dietary changes, antispasmodics (e.g., hyoscyamine).

IBD: Anti-inflammatory drugs.

Musculoskeletal

Physical therapy, NSAIDs or muscle relaxants for lumbar disc disease or sacroiliac dysfunction.

Trigger point injections for myofascial pain.

Neurological

Gabapentin or amitriptyline for neuropathic pain.

Pudendal nerve blocks for pudendal nerve irritation.

3. Chronic Pelvic Pain (CPP)

Pain management: NSAIDs, acetaminophen, or low-dose tricyclic antidepressants (e.g., amitriptyline 10–25 mg nightly).

Psychological therapy: Cognitive-behavioral therapy (CBT) for psychosomatic components.

Physical therapy: Pelvic floor exercises for myofascial pain or pelvic floor dysfunction.

Laparoscopy: Diagnostic and therapeutic for endometriosis or adhesions.

Hormonal Therapy: Combined oral contraceptives or progestins for cyclical pain.

4. Unani Medicine Approach

Hawa-e-Muheet: Ensure clean, ventilated environments to reduce infection risk (e.g., PID, TB).

Makool wa Mashroob: Balanced diet (e.g., anti-inflammatory foods, probiotics) to support Tabiyat and reduce inflammation.

Harkat wa Sukoon-e-Badani: Moderate exercise (e.g., yoga) to improve pelvic circulation; avoid overexertion.

Harkat wa Sukoon-e-Nafsani: Stress reduction (e.g., Unani aromatherapy, counseling) to mitigate CPP.

Naum wa Yaqza: Adequate sleep to restore Hararat-e-Ghariziya and support pain management.

Ihtibaas wa Istifraagh: Promote regular elimination (e.g., fiber-rich diet) and hygiene to prevent infections or Sudd (obstruction).

Complications

Infertility (endometriosis, PID, genital TB).

Ectopic pregnancy (PID, TB).

Chronic pelvic pain syndrome due to adhesions or central sensitization.

Malignancy progression if untreated (e.g., cervical/endometrial cancer).

Chronic kidney disease (recurrent urolithiasis).

Bowel obstruction or fistulae (IBD, diverticulitis).

Permanent disability from untreated musculoskeletal or neurological conditions.

Psychosocial: Depression, anxiety or reduced quality of life from chronic pain.

Prevention

STI prevention: Condom use, routine screening for Chlamydia and Gonorrhea .

Early treatment of infections (e.g., PID, TB) to prevent adhesions or infertility.

HPV vaccination to reduce cervical cancer risk.

Urological: Adequate hydration, prompt UTI treatment.

Gastrointestinal: Dietary modification for IBS, regular screening for IBD.

Musculoskeletal: Maintain healthy posture, regular exercise and weight management.

Special Populations

1. Adolescents: Higher risk of PID and primary dysmenorrhea; emphasize education and STI screening.
2. Pregnant Women: Ectopic pregnancy and appendicitis are emergencies; avoid teratogenic drugs (e.g., methotrexate).
3. Postmenopausal Women: Malignancy and pelvic organ prolapse are more common; consider musculoskeletal causes for low backache.
4. HIV-Positive Women: Increased risk of PID, TB and HPV-related dysplasia; regular screening and ART adherence are necessary.

Conclusion

Pelvic pain and low backache in women are complex symptoms with diverse gynecological and non-gynecological etiologies, requiring a systematic, multidisciplinary approach to diagnosis and management. Gynecological causes, such as endometriosis, PID and genital TB, are common, but urological, gastrointestinal, musculoskeletal and psychosomatic factors must also be noted. A thorough history, physical examination and targeted investigations (e.g., ultrasound, laparoscopy) are essential for accurate diagnosis. Management involves addressing the underlying cause, relieving pain and preventing complications through medical, surgical and lifestyle interventions.

Long Answer Questions

1. Define pelvic inflammatory disease (PID) and describe its etiology, clinical features and management.
2. Discuss sexually transmitted infections (STIs) causing pelvic infections with examples and treatment.
3. Explain genital tuberculosis—pathogenesis, symptoms, diagnosis and treatment.
4. Describe the differential diagnosis of chronic pelvic pain and low backache in gynecological infections.
5. Elaborate on complications of untreated pelvic infections including infertility and ectopic pregnancy.

Short Answer Questions

1. What is the most common cause of PID?
2. Name two STDs that can lead to pelvic infections.
3. Define genital tuberculosis.

4. Mention one complication of PID.
5. What is the role of laparoscopy in diagnosing pelvic infections?

Multiple Choice Questions (1 Mark Each)

1. Most common pathogen in PID:

a) Candida b) Chlamydia trachomatis c) HPV d) Trichomonas

Ans: b) Chlamydia trachomatis

2. Genital TB most commonly affects:

a) Vulva b) Cervix c) Fallopian tubes d) Vagina

Ans: c) Fallopian tubes

3. Pelvic pain + low backache + fever may suggest:

a) Fibroid b) PID c) PCOS d) Menopause

Ans: b) PID

4. Gold standard for diagnosing genital TB:

a) Pap smear b) Endometrial biopsy c) USG pelvis d) Wet mount

Ans: b) Endometrial biopsy

5. Which STD may present with strawberry cervix?

a) Gonorrhea b) Trichomoniasis c) Syphilis d) HPV

Ans: b) Trichomoniasis

6. Pelvic infection after IUCD insertion is commonly due to:

a) Candida b) Gonorrhea c) Actinomyces d) HPV

Ans: c) Actinomyces

7. Which of the following is NOT a symptom of PID?

a) Fever b) Vaginal dryness c) Purulent discharge d) Pelvic tenderness

Ans: b) Vaginal dryness

8. Tuberculosis of endometrium may lead to:

a) Menorrhagia b) Asherman's syndrome c) Dysmenorrhea d) Fibroid

Ans: b) Asherman's syndrome

9. Which test detects clue cells in vaginal discharge?

a) Gram stain b) Wet mount c) KOH prep d) Pap smear

Ans: b) Wet mount

10. Chronic pelvic pain with infertility may suggest:

a) Endometriosis b) PID c) PCOS d) Fibroid

Ans: b) PID

12

Infertility

(Uqr)

12.1 Zanan 'Uqr (Female infertility)
12.2 Mardana 'Uqr (Male infertility)
12.3 Tawlid ke imdadi Ta'riqe (Assisted Reproductive Techniques)

Learning Objective (At the end of the session, the students should be able to)-

Define female infertility, classify the causes and describe briefly its diagnosis, management and complications.
Explain the causes of male infertility.
Describe in brief various types of Assisted Reproductive Techniques.

12.1 Female infertility

(*Zanan 'Uqr*)

Introduction

Female infertility is defined as the inability to conceive after 12 months of regular, unprotected sexual intercourse in women under 35 years, or 6 months in women over 35, or the inability to carry a pregnancy to term (primary or secondary infertility). It affects approximately 10–15% of couples worldwide, with female factors contributing to 35–40% of cases, either alone or in combination with male factors. Infertility is a significant public health issue, with social, psychological and economic implications.

Epidemiology

Global Prevalence: Infertility affects 1 in 6 couples of reproductive age globally, with female infertility contributing to 37% of cases in developed nations and up to 67% in resource-limited settings, according to the World Health Organization (WHO, 2024).

Regional Variations: Higher prevalence in areas with high rates of untreated sexually transmitted infections (STIs) or delayed childbearing .

Demographic Trends: Increasing infertility rates due to delayed motherhood (fertility declines significantly after age 35), obesity (BMI >30 increases risk), and environmental exposures.

Cause	Percentage of Cases
Ovulatory Disorders	25–30%
Tubal/Pelvic Factors	11–67%
Uterine Factors	10–15%
Endometriosis	25–40%
Unexplained Infertility	10–15%

Prevalence of Female Infertility by Cause (Estimated Global Distribution)

Pathophysiology

Female fertility requires coordinated function of the hypothalamic-pituitary-ovarian (HPO) axis, healthy reproductive organs and optimal systemic health. Key processes include:

Ovulation: Regulated by gonadotropin-releasing hormone (GnRH) stimulating follicle-stimulating hormone (FSH) and luteinizing hormone (LH), leading to follicular development and ovulation.

Tubal Function: Patent fallopian tubes for gamete transport and fertilization.

Uterine Environment: Normal endometrial receptivity for implantation.

Cervical Factors: Adequate cervical mucus for sperm transport.

Disruptions at any level result in infertility

Ovulatory Dysfunction: Anovulation or oligo-ovulation due to HPO axis dysregulation (e.g., PCOS, hypothalamic amenorrhea).

Tubal Damage: Scarring or obstruction from PID or endometriosis impairs gamete transport.

Uterine Abnormalities: Fibroids, polyps or adhesions disrupt implantation.

Systemic Factors: Endocrine disorders (e.g., thyroid dysfunction, hyperprolactinemia) or metabolic syndromes alter reproductive function.

Pathophysiological Mechanisms

Oxidative Stress: Increased reactive oxygen species in endometriosis or obesity damage oocytes and embryos.

Inflammation: Chronic pelvic inflammation (e.g., PID, endometriosis) alters the peritoneal environment, affecting fertilization.

Hormonal Imbalance: Elevated androgens in PCOS or low AMH in POI reduce oocyte quality and quantity.

Causes of Female Infertility

Female infertility arises from multiple etiologies, categorized by anatomical or functional components:

Ovulatory Disorders (25–30% of cases)

Polycystic Ovary Syndrome (PCOS): Most common cause (70% of anovulatory infertility). Characterized by oligo-ovulation, hyperandrogenism and polycystic ovaries on ultrasound. Associated with insulin resistance.

Hypothalamic Dysfunction: Functional hypothalamic amenorrhea due to stress, excessive exercise or low body weight.

Premature Ovarian Insufficiency (POI): Loss of ovarian function before age 40 (1% of women), often idiopathic or genetic (e.g., FMR1 premutation).

Endocrine Disorders: Hypothyroidism (2–3%), hyperprolactinemia (13%), or Cushing's syndrome disrupt ovulation.

Luteal Phase Defect: Inadequate progesterone production, though controversial as alone cause.

Tubal and Pelvic Factors (11–67%)

Pelvic Inflammatory Disease (PID): Chlamydia or gonorrhea infections cause tubal scarring or hydrosalpinges.

Endometriosis: Affects 25–40% of infertile women, causing pelvic adhesions, inflammation and altered oocyte quality.

Previous Pelvic Surgery: Adhesions from appendicectomy or cesarean section.

Uterine Factors (10–15%)

Fibroids: Submucosal or intramural fibroids distort the uterine cavity, reducing implantation rates .

Endometrial Polyps: Interfere with implantation.

Congenital Anomalies: Septate uterus (most common, 35% of anomalies) increases miscarriage risk.

Asherman's Syndrome: Intrauterine adhesions from curettage or infection.

Cervical Factors

Cervical stenosis or hostile mucus (e.g., antisperm antibodies) impedes sperm transport.

Unexplained Infertility (10–15%)

No identifiable cause after standard evaluation, possibly due to subtle endometrial or immunological defects.

Lifestyle and Environmental Factors

Obesity: BMI >27 increases infertility risk via hormonal imbalances.

Smoking: Reduces ovarian reserve and implantation rates

Environmental Toxins: Endocrine disruptors (e.g., BPA, pesticides) impair oocyte quality.

Age: Fertility declines after age 35 due to reduced oocyte quantity and quality (live birth rate per cycle: 40% at age 30 vs. 15% at age 40).

Cause	**Mechanism**	**Prevalence**
PCOS	Anovulation, hyperandrogenism	70% of ovulatory disorders
Endometriosis	Inflammation, adhesions	25–40% of infertile women
Tubal Blockage	Scarring from PID	11–67%
Uterine Fibroids	Distorted cavity, impaired implantation	10–15%

Common Causes of Female Infertility and Their Mechanisms

Diagnostic Evaluation

Diagnosis requires a systematic approach, initiated after 12 months of infertility (6 months for women >35 or with risk factors). The goal is to identify the cause while minimizing invasive testing.

History

Menstrual History: Irregular cycles (<21 or >35 days) suggest anovulation.

Reproductive History: Prior pregnancies, miscarriages or abortions.

Medical/Surgical History: PID, endometriosis, diabetes, thyroid disease or pelvic surgery.

Lifestyle: Smoking, alcohol, BMI, exercise and occupational exposures.

Sexual History: Frequency, timing and sexual dysfunction.

Physical Examination

General: BMI, hirsutism (PCOS), galactorrhea (hyperprolactinemia) or thyroid enlargement.

Pelvic: Assess for uterine/cervical abnormalities, ovarian masses or tenderness (endometriosis).

Laboratory Tests

Ovarian Reserve

Day 3 FSH (>10–15 mIU/mL indicates poor reserve).

Anti-Mullerian Hormone (AMH, <1.66 ng/mL predicts low response).

Antral follicle count (AFC) via ultrasound (<5–7 follicles suggests diminished reserve).

Ovulation

Mid-luteal progesterone (>3 ng/mL confirms ovulation).

Basal body temperature charting (less common due to variability).

Endocrine

TSH, free T4 for thyroid function.

Prolactin for hyperprolactinemia.

Androgens (e.g., testosterone, DHEAS) for PCOS.

Imaging

Transvaginal Ultrasound: Assesses ovarian morphology, AFC and uterine abnormalities

Hysterosalpingography (HSG): Evaluates tubal patency and uterine cavity .

Saline Infusion Sonography (SIS): Detects intrauterine lesions .

Specialized Tests

Laparoscopy: Gold standard for endometriosis or pelvic adhesions (diagnostic yield 40–60% in unexplained infertility).

Hysteroscope: Confirms intrauterine pathology (e.g., polyps, septum).

Genetic Testing: Karyotyping or FMR1 testing for POI or recurrent miscarriage.

Test	Indication	Sensitivity/Specificity
HSG	Tubal patency, uterine cavity	65%/83%
Transvaginal Ultrasound	Ovarian reserve, uterine anomalies	80–90%/90%
Laparoscopy	Endometriosis, adhesions	90%/95%

Diagnostic Tests and Their Indications

Management

Management is done according to the cause, patient age and preferences, ranging from lifestyle changes to ART.

Lifestyle Modifications

Weight Management: 10–15% weight loss in obese women with PCOS restores ovulation in 50–70% of cases.

Smoking Cessation: Improves live birth rates .

Stress Reduction: Counseling improve outcomes.

Medical Management

Ovulation Induction

Clomiphene Citrate: 50–150 mg/day for 5 days; live birth rate 24–31% over 3 cycles with IUI, multiple pregnancy risk 7–12.5% .

Letrozole: 2.5–7.5 mg/day for 5 days; preferred for PCOS

Gonadotropins: FSH or HMG (37.5–200 IU/day); live birth rate 32–33% with IUI, >65% with IVF, multiple pregnancy risk up to 36%.

Pulsatile GnRH: For hypothalamic amenorrhea; pregnancy rate 70–100% over 6 months.

Adjunctive Therapies

Metformin for PCOS with insulin resistance .

Dopamine agonists (e.g., cabergoline) for hyperprolactinemia.

Surgical Management

Laparoscopy: Excision of endometriosis improves spontaneous pregnancy rates.

Hysteroscopy: Polypectomy increases IUI pregnancy rates .

Tubal Surgery: Salpingectomy for hydrosalpinges before IVF .

Assisted Reproductive Technologies (ART)

Intrauterine Insemination (IUI): For unexplained infertility or mild male factor; live birth rate 19.1% over 5 cycles with ovulation induction.

In Vitro Fertilization (IVF): For tubal factor, severe male factor or failed treatments; live birth rate 30–40% per cycle (age <35).

Intracytoplasmic Sperm Injection (ICSI): For severe male factor or fertilization failure.

Oocyte Donation: For POI or poor ovarian response.

Treatment Options and Outcomes

Treatment	**Indication**	**Success Rate**
Clomiphene + IUI	Anovulation, unexplained infertility	24–31% over 3 cycles
IVF	Tubal factor, severe male factor	30–40% per cycle
Laparoscopy	Endometriosis	50–60% spontaneous pregnancy

Complications

Infertility and its treatments causes physical, psychological and long-term risks:

Psychological Impact: Anxiety, depression and social stigma (reported in 50–60% of infertile women, WHO 2024). Counseling reduces stress .

Ovarian Hyperstimulation Syndrome (OHSS): Occurs in 1–5% of ART cycles; severe cases (0.1–0.2%) involve ascites, thromboembolism.

Multiple Pregnancies: Risk 7–12.5% with clomiphene/letrozole, 13–36% with gonadotropins, 32% with ART. Increases preterm birth.

Ectopic Pregnancy: 1.3% after IVF, up to 30% post-tubal surgery.

Long-term Health Risks

PCOS: Increased risk of diabetes, metabolic syndrome and endometrial cancer.

POI: Osteoporosis, cardiovascular disease .

Birth Defects: Slightly increased with IVF/ICSI .

Complication	Risk Estimate	Notes
OHSS	1–5% of ART cycles	Severe cases rare
Multiple Pregnancy	7–36% depending on treatment	Higher with ART
Ectopic Pregnancy	1.3–30%	Tubal factor increases risk

Complications and Risk Estimates

Prevention and Counseling

Preventive Measures

Early treatment of STIs to prevent PID and tubal damage.

Weight management and smoking cessation to optimize fertility.

Fertility preservation (e.g., oocyte cryopreservation) for women delaying childbearing or undergoing gonadotoxic treatments.

Counseling

Psychological support to address emotional distress.

Genetic Couinseling for couples with recurrent miscarriage or genetic disorders.

Education on age-related fertility decline and treatment options.

Conclusion

Female infertility is a multifactorial condition requiring a multidisciplinary approach involving gynecologists, reproductive endocrinologists and mental health professionals. Advances in ART, such as improved embryo selection and personalized protocols, have enhanced success rates, but challenges remain in addressing unexplained infertility and ensuring access to care in low-resource settings.

References

World Health Organization. (2024). Infertility Prevalence Estimates, 1990–2021.

StatPearls. (2020). Female Infertility. NCBI Bookshelf.

ASRM Practice Committee. (2021). Guidelines on Infertility Evaluation and Treatment.

Recent RCTs and meta-analyses (e.g., NEJM, Lancet, Fertility and Sterility).

Definitions

Primary Infertility ➤ Inability to conceive despite regular intercourse for one year without prior pregnancies.

Secondary Infertility ➤ Failure to conceive after previous live birth or pregnancy.

Oligospermia ➤ Low sperm count in semen analysis.

Anovulation ➤ Failure of ovulation due to hormonal or systemic causes.

ART (Assisted Reproductive Technology) ➤ Techniques like IUI, IVF, ICSI to help achieve pregnancy.

Causes of Infertility		
Mnemonic: "HORMONES CUP"		
Letter	**Female Factor**	**Male Factor**
H	Hormonal imbalance (PCOS)	Hypogonadism
O	Ovulatory disorders	Obstructive azoospermia
R	Reproductive tract anomaly	Retrograde ejaculation
M	Menstrual irregularity	Motility defects
O	Ovarian failure	Oligospermia
N	No fertilization (tubal)	Necrozoospermia
E	Endometriosis	Erectile dysfunction
S	Structural defects (septate uterus)	Sperm morphology issues

12.2 Male infertility

(*Mardana 'Uqr*)

Definition

Male infertility is defined as the inability of a male partner to contribute to conception after one year of regular, unprotected sexual intercourse with a fertile female partner. It accounts for approximately 40–50% of infertility cases in couples, either as a sole factor or in combination with female factors.

Epidemiology

Infertility affects 10–15% of couples globally, with male factors contributing to 40–50% of cases.

Prevalence varies by region, with higher rates in areas with environmental exposures, lifestyle factors or limited access to healthcare.

Approximately 7% of men worldwide experience fertility issues, with azoospermia affecting 1% of the male population and 10–15% of infertile men.

Etiology

Male infertility results from abnormalities in sperm production, function or transport or from systemic factors affecting reproductive health. Causes can be broadly classified as follows.

1. Pre-testicular Causes (Hypothalamic-Pituitary Axis Dysfunction)

Hypogonadotropic hypogonadism: Congenital (e.g., Kallmann syndrome) or acquired (e.g., pituitary tumors, trauma or radiation).

Hyperprolactinemia: Prolactin-secreting pituitary adenomas suppress gonadotropin-releasing hormone (GnRH) and luteinizing hormone (LH).

Endocrine disorders: Hypothyroidism, hyperthyroidism or adrenal disorders (e.g., congenital adrenal hyperplasia).

Exogenous factors: Anabolic steroids, testosterone replacement therapy or medications (e.g., chemotherapy, opiates) suppressing gonadotropin secretion.

2. Testicular Causes (Primary Testicular Failure)

Genetic disorders

Klinefelter syndrome (47,XXY): Small testes, azoospermia and elevated follicle-stimulating hormone (FSH).

Y-chromosome microdeletions (e.g., AZF regions): Impaired spermatogenesis.

Cryptorchidism: Undescended testes leading to impaired spermatogenesis.

Varicocele: Dilated veins in the scrotum causing elevated testicular temperature and oxidative stress; the most common treatable cause of male infertility (present in ~40% of infertile men).

Testicular trauma or torsion: Physical damage impairing spermatogenesis.

Infections: Orchitis (e.g., mumps, epididymitis) causing testicular atrophy or obstruction.

Toxins and environmental factors: Radiation, chemotherapy, pesticides, heavy metals or heat exposure impairing spermatogenesis.

Idiopathic: Up to 30–40% of cases have no identifiable cause.

3. Post-testicular Causes (Obstructive or Ejaculatory Dysfunction)

Obstructive azoospermia

Congenital bilateral absence of the vas deferens (CBAVD): Often associated with cystic fibrosis gene mutations.

Epididymal or vasal obstruction: Due to infections, surgery (e.g., vasectomy) or trauma.

Ejaculatory dysfunction

Retrograde ejaculation: Semen enters the bladder due to bladder neck dysfunction (e.g., diabetes, spinal cord injury or alpha-blockers).

Premature ejaculation or anejaculation: Neurological or psychological causes.

Sexual dysfunction: Erectile dysfunction or low libido due to psychological, vascular or neurological factors.

4. Systemic and Lifestyle Factors

Chronic illnesses: Diabetes, renal failure, liver disease or cancer.

Obesity: Associated with hypogonadism and reduced sperm quality due to aromatization of testosterone to estrogen.

Lifestyle factors: Smoking, excessive alcohol, recreational drugs (e.g., marijuana, cocaine) and anabolic steroids.

Environmental exposures: Heat (e.g., saunas, tight clothing), pollutants or endocrine affectors.

Pathophysiology

Sperm production (spermatogenesis) occurs in the seminiferous tubules of the testes, regulated by the hypothalamic-pituitary-gonadal (HPG) axis:

GnRH from the hypothalamus stimulates LH and FSH secretion from the pituitary.

LH stimulates Leydig cells to produce testosterone, essential for spermatogenesis.

FSH supports Sertoli cells, which support developing sperm.

Obstructions at any level (pre-testicular, testicular or post-testicular) impair sperm count, motility, morphology or transport, leading to infertility.

Clinical Evaluation

A thorough evaluation is indicated to identify the cause of male infertility. The approach includes:

1. History

Reproductive history: Duration of infertility, previous pregnancies or miscarriages.

Medical history: Chronic illnesses, infections (e.g., mumps, STIs), surgeries (e.g., vasectomy, hernia repair) or medications.

Lifestyle: Smoking, alcohol, drug use, occupational exposures or heat exposure.

Sexual history: Libido, erectile function, ejaculation issues or frequency of intercourse.

Family history: Genetic disorders, infertility or congenital anomalies.

2. Physical Examination

General examination: Assess for obesity, secondary sexual characteristics or signs of systemic disease.

Genital examination

Testicular size and consistency (normal testicular volume: ~15–25 mL).

Presence of varicocele (palpable "bag of worms" in scrotum).

Epididymal or vas deferens abnormalities.

Signs of infection or masses.

3. Semen Analysis

The mainstay of male infertility evaluation, performed after 2–5 days of abstinence.

World Health Organization (WHO) 2021 reference values

```
Volume: ≥1.4 mL
Sperm concentration: ≥16 million/mL
Total sperm count: ≥39 million per ejaculate
Motility: ≥42% total motility, ≥30% progressive motility
Morphology: ≥4% normal forms
Vitality: ≥54% live sperm
```

Abnormalities:

Azoospermia: No sperm in ejaculate (obstructive or non-obstructive).

Oligospermia: Low sperm concentration (<16 million/mL).

Asthenospermia: Reduced motility.

Teratospermia: Abnormal morphology.

Oligoasthenoteratospermia: Combined defects in count, motility and morphology.

4. Laboratory and Hormonal Testing

Hormonal profile

FSH: Elevated in testicular failure; low in hypogonadotropic hypogonadism.

LH: Elevated in primary hypogonadism; low in secondary hypogonadism.

Testosterone: Low levels indicate hypogonadism.

Prolactin: Elevated in pituitary dysfunction.

Estradiol: Elevated in obesity or testicular tumors.

Genetic testing

Karyotyping for Klinefelter syndrome or translocations.

Y-chromosome microdeletion analysis.

CFTR gene testing for CBAVD.

Other tests: Fructose in semen (absent in obstructive azoospermia), antisperm antibodies or infection screening.

5. Imaging

Scrotal ultrasound: To assess testicular size, varicocele or epididymal abnormalities.

Transrectal ultrasound (TRUS): To evaluate for ejaculatory duct obstruction or seminal vesicle abnormalities.

MRI/CT: For suspected pituitary or hypothalamic lesions.

6. Specialized Tests

Sperm function tests: DNA fragmentation, acrosome reaction or sperm penetration assays (rarely used). Testicular biopsy: Indicated in azoospermia to distinguish obstructive from non-obstructive causes.

Management

Management depends on the underlying cause, ranging from lifestyle modifications to surgical interventions or assisted reproductive technologies (ART).

1. Lifestyle Modifications

Smoking cessation, reduced alcohol intake and avoidance of illicit or off label drugs.

Weight loss in obese patients to improve testosterone levels and sperm quality.

Avoidance of heat exposure (e.g., tight clothing).

Antioxidant supplements (e.g., vitamin C, E or coenzyme Q10) may improve sperm parameters in select cases.

2. Medical Management

Hormonal therapy

Gonadotropin therapy (hCG, hMG) for hypogonadotropic hypogonadism.

Dopamine agonists (e.g., cabergoline) for hyperprolactinemia.

Clomiphene citrate or aromatase inhibitors (off-label) for low testosterone-to-estradiol ratio.

Infections: Antibiotics for epididymitis or prostatitis.

Ejaculatory dysfunction: Alpha-agonists (e.g., pseudoephedrine) for retrograde ejaculation or psychotherapy for psychogenic causes.

3. Surgical Management

Varicocelectomy: Microsurgical repair for clinically significant varicoceles; improves semen parameters in 60–70% of cases.

Vasectomy reversal: Microsurgical vasovasostomy or vasoepididymostomy for post-vasectomy infertility.

Transurethral resection of ejaculatory ducts (TURED): For ejaculatory duct obstruction.

Testicular sperm extraction (TESE) or aspiration (TESA): For obstructive or non-obstructive azoospermia, used in conjunction with ART.

4. Assisted Reproductive Technologies (ART)

Intrauterine insemination (IUI): For mild oligospermia or ejaculatory dysfunction.

In vitro fertilization (IVF): For moderate to severe male factor infertility.

Intracytoplasmic sperm injection (ICSI): Direct injection of a single sperm into an oocyte; highly effective for severe oligospermia or azoospermia (using retrieved sperm).

Donor sperm: Considered when no viable sperm is available or in cases of genetic disorders.

5. Counseling and Support

Psychological counseling for couples to address emotional stress and relationship strain.

Genetic counseling for couples with identified genetic abnormalities to discuss risks to offspring.

Prognosis

Prognosis depends on the cause and severity of infertility.

Correctable causes (e.g., varicocele, obstruction) have better outcomes with targeted interventions.

ART, particularly ICSI, has revolutionized outcomes for severe male infertility, with pregnancy rates of 30–50% per cycle.

Idiopathic infertility and non-obstructive azoospermia carry a poorer prognosis, with limited treatment options.

Prevention

Early treatment of infections (e.g., STIs, mumps).

Avoidance of environmental toxins and lifestyle risk factors.

Timely repair of cryptorchidism in childhood to preserve testicular function.

Education on reproductive health and fertility preservation (e.g., sperm banking before chemotherapy).

Evaluation of Infertility

Couple Presents with ≥1 Year of Infertility
↓
Step 1: History & Clinical Examination
(Menstrual, sexual, medical history)
↓
Step 2: Basic Investigations
↓ ↓
Female Workup   Male Workup
↓ ↓
- USG pelvis   - Semen analysis
- Hormone assays   - Hormone profile (FSH, LH, Testosterone)
- HSG for tubal patency
- Ovarian reserve tests
↓
Step 3: Identify Cause:
↓ ↓ ↓
Anovulation   Tubal Factor   Male Factor
↓ ↓ ↓
Start Targeted Therapy:
Ovulation Induction / Surgical / ART
`

Types of ART Techniques

Infertility Diagnosis
↓
Is Natural Conception Possible?
↓ ↓
Yes   No → ART Required
↓
Choose ART Technique Based on Etiology

IUI	IVF	ICSI	GIFT/ZIFT
↓	↓	↓	↓
Mild Male Factor	Tubal / Ovulatory Disorders	Severe Male Factor	Advanced Options (Transfer methods)

`

12.3 Assisted Reproductive Techniques

(*Tawlid ke imdadi Ta'riqe*)

Introduction

Assisted Reproductive Techniques (ART) refer to medical interventions that facilitate pregnancy by manipulating gametes (sperm or oocytes) or embryos, typically involving in vitro processes. As defined by the World Health Organization (WHO, 2024), ART includes all treatments handling human oocytes, sperm or embryos for reproduction. ART addresses infertility, which affects 10–15% of couples globally, with female factors contributing to 35–40% and male factors to 40–50% of cases. Since the birth of Louise Brown, the first in vitro fertilization (IVF) baby in 1978, ART has transformed reproductive medicine, with over 8 million ART-conceived children born by 2024. These techniques are critical for managing complex infertility cases, including tubal factor, severe male factor and unexplained infertility, offering hope to diverse populations, including same-sex couples and single individuals.

History and Evolution of ART

1978: First successful IVF by Robert Edwards and Patrick Steptoe, a landmark achievement.

1980s: Development of controlled ovarian stimulation (COS) with gonadotropins and embryo cryopreservation.

1992: Introduction of intracytoplasmic sperm injection (ICSI) for severe male infertility.

2000s: Preimplantation genetic testing (PGT) and vitrification improved embryo survival and selection.

2010s–2020s: Advances in time-lapse imaging, artificial intelligence (AI) for embryo selection, and non-invasive diagnostics enhanced outcomes.

Types of ART

ART encompasses a range of procedures, each tailored to specific infertility causes:

a. Intrauterine Insemination (IUI)

Involves injecting washed, concentrated sperm directly into the uterus during ovulation.

Often combined with ovulation induction (e.g., clomiphene citrate, letrozole).

b. In Vitro Fertilization (IVF)

Oocytes are retrieved, fertilized in vitro, and embryos transferred to the uterus.

Standard for complex infertility cases.

c. Intracytoplasmic Sperm Injection (ICSI)

A single sperm is injected into an oocyte, addressing severe male factor infertility.

d. Gamete Intrafallopian Transfer (GIFT) and Zygote Intrafallopian Transfer (ZIFT)

Rarely used; involve transferring gametes or zygotes into fallopian tubes.

e. Donor Gametes and Embryos

Use of donated oocytes, sperm, or embryos for ovarian failure, genetic disorders, or same-sex couples.

f. Surrogacy

Gestational surrogacy involves embryo transfer to a surrogate's uterus for uterine factor infertility or medical contraindications.

g. Fertility Preservation: Oocyte or embryo cryopreservation for women facing gonadotoxic treatments or social reasons.

Procedure	Description	Key Indications
IUI	Sperm insemination into uterus	Mild male factor, cervical factor, unexplained infertility
IVF	In vitro fertilization, embryo transfer	Tubal factor, severe male factor, endometriosis
ICSI	Single sperm injection into oocyte	Severe oligospermia, azoospermia
Donor Gametes	Use of donated oocytes/sperm	Premature ovarian insufficiency, genetic concerns
Surrogacy |	Embryo transfer to surrogate	Uterine factor, medical contraindications

Overview of ART Procedures

Indications for ART

ART is indicated for a variety of infertility causes, often after initial treatments fails:

Female Factors

Tubal Factor: Bilateral tubal occlusion or hydrosalpinges (IVF live birth rate 30–40% per cycle).

Ovulatory Dysfunction: Failed ovulation induction in PCOS or hypothalamic amenorrhea (live birth rate after clomiphene/IUI 24–31%).

Endometriosis: Moderate to severe cases or post-surgical failure (IVF success 25–35%).

Diminished Ovarian Reserve: Low AMH (<1.66 ng/mL) or age >38 (donor oocytes for POI).

Uterine Factors: Severe Asherman's syndrome or congenital anomalies (surrogacy).

Unexplained Infertility: After 3–6 failed IUI cycles (IVF live birth rate 30–35%).

Male Factors

Severe Oligospermia or Azoospermia: Sperm concentration <5 million/mL or obstructive/non-obstructive azoospermia (ICSI success 30–40%).

Ejaculatory Dysfunction: Retrograde ejaculation or anejaculation (ICSI with retrieved sperm).

Genetic Concerns: Y-chromosome microdeletions or Klinefelter syndrome (ICSI with PGT).

Other Indications

Recurrent Pregnancy Loss: With chromosomal abnormalities.

Same-Sex Couples/Single Women: Using donor gametes or surrogacy.

Fertility Preservation: Oocyte freezing before chemotherapy or for delayed childbearing.

Indication	Preferred ART	Live Birth Rate (Age <35)
Tubal Factor	IVF	30–40% per cycle
Severe Male Factor	ICSI	30–40% per cycle
Unexplained Infertility	IVF after failed IUI	30–35% per cycle
POI	Donor Oocytes	50–60% per cycle

Indications and Preferred ART

ART Procedures

1. Intrauterine Insemination (IUI)

Process

Ovulation induction (optional) with clomiphene (50–150 mg/day) or letrozole (2.5–7.5 mg/day).

Semen preparation to isolate motile sperm (WHO 2021: ≥16 million/mL optimal).

Catheter-based insemination timed with ovulation (monitored via ultrasound or LH surge).

Success Rate: 10–20% per cycle; cumulative live birth rate 19.1% over 5 cycles with stimulation.

Considerations: Low cost, minimally invasive, but less effective for severe infertility.

2. In Vitro Fertilization (IVF)

Ovarian Stimulation: Gonadotropins (FSH, hMG, 150–300 IU/day) for 8–12 days to achieve 7–15 follicles. GnRH agonists (e.g., leuprolide) or antagonists (e.g., cetrorelix) to prevent premature ovulation. Trigger with hCG (5,000–10,000 IU) or GnRH agonist for oocyte maturation.

Oocyte Retrieval: Transvaginal ultrasound-guided aspiration under sedation (34–36 hours post-trigger).

Fertilization: Conventional IVF (sperm-oocyte incubation) or ICSI (60–80% fertilization rate).

Embryo Culture: Day 3 (cleavage stage) or day 5 (blastocyst) culture; blastocyst transfer preferred.

Embryo Transfer: 1–2 embryos transferred via catheter under ultrasound guidance.

Single embryo transfer (SET): Reduces multiple pregnancies (ASRM guideline).

Luteal Phase Support: Progesterone (vaginal, intramuscular, 50–100 mg/day) or hCG to support implantation.

3. Intracytoplasmic Sperm Injection (ICSI)

Process: Microinjection of a single sperm into an oocyte using micromanipulation.

Indications: Sperm concentration <5 million/mL, poor motility/morphology (<4% normal forms), or prior IVF failure.

Sperm Retrieval: Testicular sperm extraction (TESE) or aspiration (TESA) for azoospermia.

Success Rate: Comparable to IVF (30–40% live birth per cycle).

4. Preimplantation Genetic Testing (PGT)

PGT-A: Screens for aneuploidy, improving implantation .

PGT-B: For monogenic disorders (e.g., cystic fibrosis, CFTR mutations).

PGT-SR: For chromosomal rearrangements.

Process: Biopsy of 5–10 trophectoderm cells on day 5/6, followed by next-generation sequencing.

5. Cryopreservation

Vitrification: Rapid freezing of oocytes or embryos; survival rate >90%.

Indications: Excess embryos, fertility preservation or delayed transfer (e.g., OHSS risk).

Outcomes: Frozen embryo transfer (FET) live birth rate 25–35%.

6. Donor Gametes and Surrogacy

Oocyte Donation: For POI or poor ovarian response; live birth rate 50–60%.

Sperm Donation: For azoospermia or genetic concerns.

Surrogacy: Embryo transfer to a gestational carrier; success depends on embryo quality.

Outcomes and Success Rates

ART success varies by age, cause of infertility and technique:

IUI: Live birth rate 10–20% per cycle; cumulative 19.1% over 5 cycles with clomiphene/letrozole .

IVF: Live birth rate 30–40% per cycle for women <35, 25–30% at 35–37, 15–20% at 38–40, <10% at >40 (CDC 2023 data).

ICSI: Similar to IVF (30–40% for severe male factor).

Donor Oocytes: 50–60% live birth rate, independent of recipient age.

FET: Comparable to fresh transfer (25–35% live birth rate).

PGT-A: Increases implantation rate.

Factors Influencing Success

Age: Oocyte quality declines after 35 (AMH <1.66 ng/mL predicts poor response).

Embryo Quality: Blastocyst-stage embryos improve outcomes.

Lifestyle: Obesity (BMI >30) reduces success .

Indication	ART Type	Live Birth Rate (Age <35)
Tubal Factor	IVF	30–40% per cycle
Male Factor	ICSI	30–40% per cycle
Endometriosis	IVF	25–35% per cycle
Unexplained	IVF/IUI	30–35%/10–20% per cycle

ART Success Rates by Indication

Complications

1. Ovarian Hyperstimulation Syndrome (OHSS)

Incidence: 1–5% of IVF cycles; severe in 0.1–0.2%.

Symptoms: Ovarian enlargement, ascites, thromboembolism.

Risk Factors: Young age, PCOS, high AMH, >15 follicles.

Management: Cabergoline, GnRH antagonist protocols or cycle cancellation .

2. Multiple Pregnancies

Incidence: 7–12.5% with clomiphene/letrozole, 13–36% with gonadotropins, 20–30% with multi-embryo IVF transfer.

Risks: Preterm birth, low birth weight, maternal hypertension.

Prevention: Single embryo transfer (SET) reduces risk to <5%.

3. Ectopic Pregnancy

Incidence: 1.3–2% in IVF, higher with tubal factor (up to 30% post-tubal surgery).

Management: Methotrexate or surgical intervention.

4. Birth Defects

Slightly increased with IVF/ICSI , primarily due to multiple births or underlying infertility.

5. Psychological Impact

Anxiety and depression in 50–60% of patients (WHO, 2024). Counseling reduces stress .

Long-term Risks

No definitive link between ART and ovarian/endometrial cancer, but PCOS patients have elevated endometrial cancer risk. Cardiovascular risks in women with infertility .

Complication	Incidence	Management
OHSS	1–5%	Cabergoline, cycle cancellation
Multiple Pregnancy |	7–36%	Single embryo transfer
Ectopic Pregnancy	1.3–2%	Methotrexate, surgery
Birth Defects	-	PGT, SET

ART Complications and Risk Estimates

Ethical and Legal Considerations

Access and Equity: High costs limit access in low-resource settings. WHO advocates for universal ART coverage.

Donor Gametes/Surrogacy: Issues of anonymity, informed consent and compensation.

Embryo Disposition: Ethical debates over unused embryos (donation, research, or destruction).

PGT: Concerns about “designer babies” or eugenics with non-medical trait selection.

Conclusion

ART has revolutionized infertility treatment, offering solutions for complex male and female factors, including tubal occlusion, severe oligospermia and genetic disorders. Success rates have improved with advances in ICSI, PGT and cryopreservation, but challenges remain in managing complications, ensuring equitable access and addressing ethical concerns.

References

World Health Organization. (2024). Infertility Prevalence Estimates.

CDC. (2023). ART Success Rates Report.

ASRM Practice Committee. (2021). Guidelines on ART.

Peer-reviewed studies (e.g., NEJM, Lancet, Fertility and Sterility).

Technique	Full Form	Indication
IUI	Intrauterine insemination	Mild male factor, unexplained infertility
IVF	In-vitro fertilization	Tubal blockage, failed ovulation
ICSI	Intracytoplasmic sperm injection	Severe male infertility, azoospermia
GIFT	Gamete intrafallopian transfer	Functional tubes, religious concerns
ZIFT	Zygote intrafallopian transfer	Failed IVF implantation

Long Answer Questions

1. Define infertility and classify its types. Discuss causes and management of male infertility.
2. Explain female infertility—etiology, diagnostic approach and treatment modalities.
3. Describe assisted reproductive technologies (ART) and their role in infertility management.
4. Discuss hormonal evaluation and imaging techniques used in infertility diagnosis.
5. Elaborate on psychosocial impact of infertility and the role of counseling.

Short Answer Questions

1. What is primary infertility?
2. Name two causes of male infertility.
3. Mention one ovulation-inducing drug.
4. Define ICSI.
5. What is the role of hysterosalpingography in infertility?

Multiple Choice Questions (1 Mark Each)

1. Infertility is defined as failure to conceive after:

a) 6 months b) 12 months c) 18 months d) 24 months

Ans: b) 12 months

2. Most common cause of male infertility:

a) Erectile dysfunction b) Varicocele c) Low sperm count d) Retrograde ejaculation

Ans: c) Low sperm count

3. Ovulation induction drug commonly used in PCOS:

a) Metformin b) Clomiphene citrate c) Progesterone d) Bromocriptine

Ans: b) Clomiphene citrate

4. Which test assesses tubal patency?

a) Pap smear b) HSG c) USG abdomen d) CT pelvis

Ans: b) HSG

5. ICSI stands for:

a) Intrauterine sperm injection b) Intracytoplasmic sperm injection c) Intra-cervical sperm insemination d) In-vitro sperm culture

Ans: b) Intracytoplasmic sperm injection

6. Which hormone is most useful to assess ovarian reserve?

a) LH b) FSH c) Estrogen d) Progesterone

Ans: b) FSH

7. Which ART technique involves fertilization outside the body?

a) IUI b) IVF c) GIFT d) ZIFT

Ans: b) IVF

8. Common cause of tubal infertility:

a) Fibroid b) PID c) PCOS d) Endometriosis

Ans: b) PID

9. Which ART method is preferred in severe male factor infertility?

a) IUI b) IVF c) ICSI d) GIFT

Ans: c) ICSI

10. Which condition may require donor sperm?

a) PCOS b) Azoospermia c) Endometriosis d) Fibroid

Ans: b) Azoospermia

13

Diseases of Breast

(Amrad-i-Thadyayn)

13.1 *Waja-i-Thadi* (Mastalgia)
13.2 Iltehab-i-thadyayn (Mastitis)
13.3 Khuraj-i-Thadi (Breast Abscess)
13.4 Kathra-i-Laban (Galactorrhoea)
13.5 Akyas aur Sal'at-i-Thadi (Cysts & tumours of Breast)

Learning Objective (At the end of the session, the students should be able to)-

Elaborate causes, diagnosis, treatment & complications of *waja e saddi* (Mastalgia)
Explain causes, diagnosis, treatment & complications of *Iltihab- e-Saddiyain* (Mastitis)
Describe the causes, diagnosis, management & complications of *Khuraj-Saddi* (Breast Abscess).
Enumerate the causes of Galactorrhoea & describe its management
Discuss in Brief *Daweera-wa-Sulaat-e-Saddi* (Cysts & Tumours of Breast)

13.1 Mastalgia

(Waja-i-Thadi)

Definition

Mastalgia, or breast pain, is discomfort or pain in one or both breasts, often associated with hormonal fluctuations, benign breast conditions or rarely, malignancy. It is classified as:

1. Cyclical Mastalgia: Pain related to the menstrual cycle, typically bilateral and diffuse.
2. Non-Cyclical Mastalgia: Pain unrelated to the menstrual cycle, often localized and associated with structural or inflammatory causes.
3. Extramammary Pain: Referred pain from non-breast sources (e.g., chest wall, musculoskeletal).

Epidemiology

Prevalence: Affects 50–70% of women at some age, with 10–30% experiencing moderate to severe pain affecting daily activities.

Age: Most common in women of reproductive age (20–40 years); cyclical mastalgia is more prevalent in premenopausal women, while non-cyclical mastalgia may occur at all ages.

Risk Factors: Hormonal imbalances, high caffeine intake, stress, obesity or history of benign breast disease.

Etiology

1. Cyclical Mastalgia

Hormonal fluctuations (estrogen and progesterone) during the menstrual cycle.

Fibrocystic breast changes (e.g., cysts, fibrosis, ductal hyperplasia).

2. Non-Cyclical Mastalgia

Benign conditions: Breast cysts, fibroadenomas, ductal ectasia or mastitis.

Trauma or surgery (e.g., post-biopsy pain).

Musculoskeletal: Costochondritis, pectoral muscle strain or cervical radiculopathy.

Rarely, breast cancer (1–5% of cases).

3. Extramammary Causes: Angina, gastroesophageal reflux disease (GERD) or pleuritis.

Unani Perspective: Imbalance in *Mizaj* (temperament), particularly excess *Hararat* (heat) or *Rutubaat* (moisture) or disruption in *Asbaabe Sitta Zarooriya* (e.g., poor diet, stress) may contribute to breast pain.

Pathophysiology

1. Cyclical Mastalgia

Estrogen excess or progesterone deficiency in the luteal phase increases breast tissue sensitivity, leading to ductal dilatation, stromal edema and inflammation.

Prolactin may enhance breast tissue sensitivity to hormonal changes.

Fibrocystic changes cause localized tenderness due to cyst formation or fibrosis.

2. Non-Cyclical Mastalgia

Localized inflammation or mechanical pressure (e.g., cysts, fibroadenomas) stimulates nociceptors.

Musculoskeletal causes involve nerve irritation or muscle strain, referring pain to the breast.

Central Sensitization: Chronic mastalgia may lead to heightened pain perception due to neuroplastic changes in the central nervous system.

Unani Perspective: Accumulation of *Akhlat-e-Fasida* (morbid humors) or impaired *Quwa* (vital faculties) disrupts breast tissue homeostasis, contributing to pain.

Clinical Features

1. Cyclical Mastalgia

Bilateral, diffuse breast pain or heaviness, peaking in the luteal phase (days before menstruation).

Associated with breast swelling, nodularity or tenderness.

Resolves post-menses.

2. Non-Cyclical Mastalgia

Unilateral, localized pain (e.g., burning, stabbing, or aching). May be constant or intermittent, unrelated to menstrual cycle. Associated with palpable masses, trauma or musculoskeletal symptoms.

Extramammary Pain: Pain radiating from chest wall, shoulder or abdomen; no breast tenderness on palpation.

Red Flags: Persistent unilateral pain, palpable mass, skin changes (e.g., dimpling, peau d'orange) or nipple discharge (rule out malignancy).

Diagnosis

History

Pain characteristics: Onset, duration, location, cyclical vs. non-cyclical and aggravating/relieving factors.

Menstrual history, hormonal therapy use, caffeine intake or trauma.

Psychosocial factors: Stress, anxiety or history of abuse (common in chronic pain).

Physical Examination

Breast: Inspect for asymmetry, skin changes or nipple abnormalities; palpate for masses, tenderness or nodularity.

Chest wall: Assess for costochondritis or musculoskeletal tenderness.

Lymph nodes: Check axillary and supraclavicular nodes for lymphadenopathy.

Investigations

Ultrasound: First-line imaging for women <40 years to evaluate cysts or masses.

Mammography: For women >40 years or with red flags (e.g., mass, skin changes).

MRI: For complex cases or suspected malignancy.

Biopsy: Fine-needle aspiration (FNA) or core biopsy for palpable masses or suspicious imaging findings.

Hormonal Profile: Rarely needed; prolactin or thyroid function tests if indicated.

Differential Diagnosis

Benign breast disease (fibrocystic changes, fibroadenoma).

Mastitis or breast abscess.

Musculoskeletal (costochondritis, pectoral strain).

Breast cancer (rare but need to be excluded).

Extramammary causes (angina, GERD).

Management

General Measures

Reassurance: Most of the time, mastalgia is benign and self-limiting.

Lifestyle: Reduce caffeine, wear supportive bras and maintain a healthy weight.

Pain relief: NSAIDs (e.g., ibuprofen 400–800 mg as needed) or acetaminophen.

Cyclical Mastalgia

First-Line: Evening primrose oil (1–3 g daily, containing gamma-linolenic acid) for 3–6 months (limited evidence).

Hormonal Therapy

Combined oral contraceptives (COCs) or progestins to stabilize hormonal fluctuations.

Danazol (100–200 mg daily): Effective but limited by side effects (e.g., weight gain, hirsutism).

Tamoxifen (10 mg daily): For severe cases, short-term use due to risks (e.g., endometrial hyperplasia).

Other: Low-dose diuretics (e.g., spironolactone) for premenstrual edema.

Non-Cyclical Mastalgia

Treat underlying cause (e.g., aspiration for cysts, antibiotics for infection).

Local measures: Warm/cold compresses or topical NSAIDs.

Musculoskeletal: Physical therapy or trigger point injections.

Chronic Mastalgia

Multidisciplinary: Pain management, psychological counseling or low-dose antidepressants (e.g., amitriptyline 10–25 mg nightly) for neuropathic pain.

Complications

Psychosocial: Anxiety, depression or reduced quality of life in chronic cases.

Failure to identify malignancy or serious pathology. (e.g., abscess).

Treatment Side Effects: Hormonal therapies may cause weight gain, mood changes or endometrial risks.

Prevention

Lifestyle modifications: Reduce caffeine, maintain healthy weight and manage stress.

Regular breast self-examinations and screening (mammography for age >40) to detect abnormalities early.

Optimize *Asbaabe Sitta Zarooriya*: Balanced diet, exercise, sleep and emotional well-being to prevent humoral imbalances.

13.2 Mastitis

(*Iltehab-i-thadyayn*)

Definition

Mastitis is inflammation of the breast tissue, typically infectious, most commonly occurring during lactation (lactational mastitis) but also in non-lactating women (non-puerperal mastitis). It is usually caused by bacterial infection but can be non-infectious (e.g., granulomatous mastitis).

Epidemiology

Prevalence: Affects 10–20% of breastfeeding women, typically within the first 6 weeks postpartum. Non-puerperal mastitis is less common, occurring in 1–5% of women.

Age: Lactational mastitis is common in women aged 20–35 years; non-puerperal mastitis may occur across all ages.

Risk Factors

Lactational: Poor breastfeeding technique, milk stasis, cracked nipples or maternal stress.

Non-puerperal: Smoking, diabetes, immunosuppression or breast trauma.

Etiology

Lactational Mastitis

Infectious: Staphylococcus aureus (most common, including MRSA), Streptococcus spp., or Escherichia coli entering through cracked nipples or milk ducts.

Non-Infectious: Milk stasis due to blocked ducts or inadequate milk removal.

Non-Puerperal Mastitis

Infectious: Polymicrobial (e.g., S. aureus, anaerobes, Corynebacterium spp.).

Non-Infectious: Idiopathic granulomatous mastitis (autoimmune/inflammatory), associated with smoking or hyperprolactinemia.

Rare Causes: Tuberculosis, fungal infections or actinomycosis.

Pathophysiology

Lactational Mastitis

Milk stasis creates a favorable environment for bacterial growth, leading to infection.

Bacteria enter via cracked nipples or ductal openings, causing localized inflammation, edema and pain. Inflammatory cytokines (e.g., IL-1, TNF-α) exacerbate tissue swelling and systemic symptoms (e.g., fever).

Non-Puerperal Mastitis

Subareolar infection or ductal obstruction leads to periductal inflammation.

Granulomatous mastitis involves autoimmune-mediated granuloma formation, mimicking malignancy.

Progression: Untreated mastitis may lead to abscess formation or chronic inflammation.

Clinical Features

Lactational Mastitis

Unilateral breast pain, tenderness or warmth.

Erythema, swelling or a firm, indurated area.

Systemic symptoms: Fever (>38°C), chills, malaise or myalgia.

Nipple discharge (purulent if infection progresses).

Non-Puerperal Mastitis

Localized pain, often subareolar, with erythema or swelling.

Recurrent abscesses or fistulae in chronic cases.

Granulomatous mastitis: Painful mass, skin changes or nipple retraction, mimicking cancer.

Red Flags: Persistent mass, skin ulceration or lymphadenopathy (rule out malignancy or TB).

Diagnosis

History

Breastfeeding status, nipple trauma or milk stasis (lactational).

Smoking, diabetes or prior breast surgery (non-puerperal).

Systemic symptoms or recurrence.

Physical Examination

Inspect for erythema, warmth or skin changes.

Palpate for tenderness, masses or fluctuance (abscess).

Check axillary lymph nodes.

Investigations

Ultrasound: To detect abscess or mass; differentiates inflammatory from neoplastic lesions.

Mammography: For women >40 years or suspected malignancy.

Culture: Milk, nipple discharge or abscess, aspirate to identify pathogens and guide antibiotics.

Biopsy: Core biopsy for granulomatous mastitis or suspected malignancy.

TB Testing: AFB staining, culture or NAAT for suspected tuberculous mastitis.

Differential Diagnosis

Breast abscess, inflammatory breast cancer, fibrocystic changes or granulomatous mastitis.

Extramammary causes (e.g., costochondritis).

Management

Lactational Mastitis

Supportive Care

Continue breastfeeding or pumping to relieve milk stasis.

Warm compresses and massage to promote milk flow.

NSAIDs (e.g., ibuprofen) for pain and inflammation.

Antibiotics (for infectious mastitis):

Dicloxacillin or flucloxacillin 500 mg orally four times daily for 10–14 days.

Cephalexin 500 mg four times daily for penicillin-allergic patients.

Clindamycin 300 mg three times daily for suspected MRSA or anaerobes.

Follow-Up: Reassess in 48–72 hours; persistent symptoms suggest abscess.

Non-Puerperal Mastitis

Antibiotics: Broad-spectrum (e.g., amoxicillin-clavulanate 875/125 mg twice daily) for 10–14 days.

Granulomatous Mastitis

Corticosteroids (e.g., prednisone 0.5–1 mg/kg daily) for 4–6 weeks.

Methotrexate or azathioprine for refractory cases.

Surgical excision for persistent masses.

Abscess: Drainage

Complications

Breast Abscess: Progression of untreated infection.

Chronic Mastitis: Recurrent infections or granulomatous changes.

Fistulae: In non-puerperal mastitis or granulomatous mastitis.

Sepsis: Rare but life-threatening in severe cases.

Psychosocial: Anxiety or avoidance of breastfeeding due to pain.

Prevention

Lactational Mastitis

Proper breastfeeding technique, frequent feeding or pumping to prevent milk stasis. Treat cracked nipples promptly with lanolin or barrier creams.

Non-Puerperal Mastitis

Smoking cessation and glycemic control in diabetes. Early treatment of subareolar infections.

13.3 Breast Abscess

(*Khuraj-i-Thadi*)

Definition

A breast abscess is a localized collection of pus in the breast tissue, typically resulting from untreated or severe mastitis. It can be lactational (postpartum) or non-lactational, often requiring drainage.

Epidemiology

Prevalence: Occurs in 3–11% of women with lactational mastitis; less common in non-lactating women (1–2% of breast infections).

Age: Lactational abscesses are common in women aged 20–35 years; non-lactational abscesses occur across all ages.

Risk Factors

Lactational: Untreated mastitis, milk stasis or cracked nipples.

Non-lactational: Smoking, diabetes, immunosuppression or prior breast surgery.

Etiology

Lactational Abscess

Staphylococcus aureus (most common, including MRSA).

Streptococcus spp. or Escherichia coli (less common).

Non-Lactational Abscess

Polymicrobial: S. aureus, anaerobes (Bacteroides, Peptostreptococcus), or Corynebacterium spp..

Rare: Tuberculous abscess (in endemic areas).

Pathophysiology

Bacterial invasion leads to tissue necrosis and pus formation, covered by a fibrous capsule.

In lactational abscesses, milk stasis provides a nutrient-rich medium for bacterial proliferation.

Non-lactational abscesses often arise from ductal obstruction or periductal mastitis, with secondary infection.

Inflammatory mediators cause localized edema, pain and systemic symptoms (e.g., fever).

Clinical Features

Symptoms

Localized, severe breast pain often throbbing.

Swelling, warmth or fluctuant mass.

Fever, chills or malaise.

Nipple discharge (purulent) or skin erythema.

Signs

Tender, fluctuant mass with overlying erythema or induration.

Axillary lymphadenopathy in severe cases.

Skin breakdown or fistulae in chronic abscesses.

Diagnosis

History: Recent mastitis, breastfeeding status or risk factors (e.g., smoking, diabetes).

Physical Examination: Palpate for fluctuance, erythema or warmth; assess lymph nodes.

Investigations

Ultrasound: Confirms abscess (hypoechoic collection with irregular margins); guides drainage.

Mammography: For women >40 years or suspected malignancy.

Culture: Aspirate or pus culture to identify pathogens and antibiotic sensitivity.

Biopsy: For recurrent or non-resolving abscesses to exclude malignancy or TB.

TB Testing: AFB staining, culture or NAAT for suspected tuberculous abscess.

Differential Diagnosis

Mastitis, granulomatous mastitis, inflammatory breast cancer or tuberculous mastitis.

Management

Antibiotics

Empirical: Flucloxacillin 500 mg four times daily or clindamycin 300 mg three times daily (for MRSA or penicillin allergy) for 10–14 days.

Adjust based on culture results.

Drainage

Ultrasound-Guided Aspiration: Preferred for small (<3 cm) or superficial abscesses; may require repeated aspirations.

Incision and Drainage: For large (>3 cm), multiloculated or recurrent abscesses.

Surgical Excision: Rarely needed for chronic or abscesses with fistula.

Supportive Care

Continue breastfeeding or pumping (lactational abscess) to prevent milk stasis.

NSAIDs for pain and inflammation.

Warm compresses to promote drainage.

Complications

Recurrence: Common in non-lactational abscesses or inadequate drainage.

Fistulae: Chronic abscesses may form mammary fistulae.

Sepsis: Rare but life-threatening if untreated.

Scarring: Cosmetic or functional impairment post-drainage.

Prevention

Early treatment of mastitis to prevent progression.

Proper breastfeeding technique and nipple care.

Smoking cessation and glycemic control in non-lactational cases.

13.4 Galactorrhoea

(*Kathra-i-Laban*)

Definition

Galactorrhea is the spontaneous or expressible discharge of milk or milky fluid from the breast, unrelated to pregnancy or breastfeeding, persisting for >6 months after cessation of lactation or in non-pregnant women.

Epidemiology

Prevalence: Affects 1–10% of women, depending on the population studied; more common in reproductive-age women (20–35 years).

Risk Factors

Hyperprolactinemia (e.g., prolactinoma, medications).

Hypothyroidism, chronic renal failure or stress.

Nipple stimulation or breast trauma.

Etiology

Physiological

Postpartum or post-lactation (up to 6 months).

Excessive nipple stimulation (e.g., sexual activity, clothing irritation).

Pathological

Hyperprolactinemia

Prolactinoma (pituitary adenoma).

Medications: Antipsychotics (e.g., risperidone), antidepressants (e.g., SSRIs), antihypertensives (e.g., methyldopa) or metoclopramide.

Hypothyroidism (elevated TRH stimulates prolactin).

Endocrine: Polycystic ovary syndrome (PCOS), adrenal tumors or chronic renal failure.

Breast-Related: Duct ectasia, intraductal papilloma or breast cancer (rare).

Neurological: Chest wall trauma, surgery or herpes zoster (stimulates prolactin release).

Idiopathic: Normal prolactin levels with no identifiable cause.

Pathophysiology

Hyperprolactinemia: Prolactin stimulates mammary gland lactogenesis, leading to milk production.

Causes include pituitary tumors (prolactinoma), dopamine inhibition (e.g., medications) or TRH stimulation (hypothyroidism).

Local Stimulation: Reflexive prolactin release due to nipple or chest wall irritation.

Pathological Discharge: Intraductal lesions (e.g., papilloma) or malignancy may cause serous or bloody discharge mimicking galactorrhea.

Clinical Features

Symptoms

Milky or serous nipple discharge (unilateral or bilateral), spontaneous or expressible.

Associated symptoms: Menstrual irregularities, infertility or hirsutism (hyperprolactinemia); headache or visual changes (prolactinoma).

Breast tenderness or nodularity (if associated with fibrocystic changes).

Signs

Milky discharge on nipple compression.

Palpable breast masses (if papilloma or malignancy).

Signs of hypothyroidism (e.g., goiter, lethargy) or pituitary tumor (e.g., bitemporal hemianopsia).

History

Duration, nature (milky vs. serous/bloody) of discharge.

Menstrual history, medications or recent breast trauma.

Symptoms of hyperprolactinemia (e.g., amenorrhea, infertility) or hypothyroidism.

Physical Examination

Breast: Inspect for discharge; palpate for masses or tenderness.

General: Assess for signs of hypothyroidism, pituitary dysfunction or systemic disease.

Investigations

Prolactin Levels: Elevated (>25 ng/mL) suggests hyperprolactinemia; repeat fasting levels to confirm.

Thyroid Function Tests: TSH and free T4 to rule out hypothyroidism.

Renal Function Tests: To exclude chronic renal failure.

Imaging

MRI brain: For suspected prolactinoma, if prolactin >100 ng/mL or neurological symptoms present.

Ultrasound/Mammography: For unilateral discharge, palpable mass or age >40 years.

Cytology/Biopsy: For bloody or suspicious discharge to rule out papilloma or malignancy.

Differential Diagnosis

Physiological galactorrhea (post-lactation, nipple stimulation).

Prolactinoma, hypothyroidism or medication-induced.

Intraductal papilloma, duct ectasia or breast cancer.

Management

Physiological Galactorrhea

Reassurance and observation, if mild and self-limiting.

Avoid excessive nipple stimulation or tight clothing.

Hyperprolactinemia

Prolactinoma

Dopamine agonists: Cabergoline (0.25–1 mg twice weekly) or bromocriptine (2.5–10 mg daily).

Surgery or radiation for macroadenomas unresponsive to medical therapy.

Medication-Induced: Discontinue drug if possible; switch to alternatives (e.g., aripiprazole for antipsychotics).

Hypothyroidism: Levothyroxine to normalize TSH and prolactin.

Pathological Discharge

Surgical excision for intraductal papilloma or malignancy.

Antibiotics for associated infections (e.g., duct ectasia with secondary infection).

Supportive Care

Treat underlying conditions (e.g., renal failure, PCOS).

Psychological support for infertility or chronic symptoms.

Complications

Infertility: Due to hyperprolactinemia-induced ovulatory dysfunction.

Osteoporosis: Chronic hyperprolactinemia reduces estrogen, increasing bone loss.

Malignancy: Missed diagnosis of breast cancer in cases of bloody discharge.

Psychosocial: Distress from cosmetic concerns or infertility.

Prevention

Regular breast screening to detect abnormalities early.

Avoid medications which cause hyperprolactinemia .

Manage underlying conditions (e.g., hypothyroidism, stress) promptly.

Conclusion

Mastalgia, mastitis, breast abscess and galactorrhea are distinct but overlapping breast disorders frequently encountered in gynecological practice. Mastalgia is often benign but requires evaluation to rule out malignancy. Mastitis and breast abscess, primarily infectious, demand prompt antibiotic therapy and, in the case of abscesses, drainage to prevent complications. Galactorrhea reflects underlying hormonal or structural issues, necessitating a thorough endocrine and breast evaluation.

13.5 Cysts & tumours of Breast

(*Akyas aur Sal'at-i-Thadi*)

Introduction

Breast cysts and tumors encompass a spectrum of lesions ranging from benign, non-neoplastic conditions to malignant neoplasms. These conditions are common in clinical practice and require accurate diagnosis to guide appropriate management. Breast cysts are fluid-filled sacs, typically benign, while tumors include benign and malignant growths.

Epidemiology

Breast Cysts

Predominantly affect premenopausal women aged 30–50 years.

Incidence peaks in perimenopause due to hormonal fluctuations.

Less common after menopause unless associated with hormone replacement therapy (HRT).

Estimated prevalence: 50–70% of women may develop cysts during their lifetime.

Benign Breast Tumors

Fibroadenomas are the most common benign tumors, typically occurring in women aged 15–35 years.

Phyllodes tumors are rare, with an incidence of 2–3 per 100,000 women, often in the 40–50 age group.

Intraductal papillomas and lipomas are less frequent.

Malignant Breast Tumors

Breast cancer is the most common malignancy in women globally, with an estimated 2.3 million new cases annually (WHO, 2020).

Incidence increases with age, peaking in women over 50, though younger women can be affected, especially with genetic predispositions (e.g., BRCA1/2 mutations).

Risk factors include family history, nulliparity, early menarche, late menopause, obesity and alcohol use.

Pathophysiology

Breast Cysts

Definition: Fluid-filled sacs within the breast, typically arising from terminal duct lobular units (TDLUs).

Etiology: Result from hormonal imbalances, particularly estrogen excess, leading to ductal dilatation and fluid accumulation.

Types

Simple cysts: Thin-walled, fluid-filled, no solid components.

Complicated cysts: Contain debris or thick walls but lack malignant features.

Complex cysts: Contain solid components, requiring further evaluation for malignancy.

Pathogenesis

Hormonal stimulation causes proliferation and dilatation of ductal epithelium.

Cyst formation may result from obstruction of ducts or excessive secretion by epithelial cells.

Benign Breast Tumors

Fibroadenoma

Arises from stromal and epithelial proliferation within the terminal duct lobular unit.

Hormone sensitive, often enlarging during pregnancy or menstrual cycles.

Histologically, composed of fibrous stroma and glandular elements.

Phyllodes Tumor

Biphasic tumor with stromal and epithelial components.

Subtypes: Benign (most common), borderline and malignant.

Malignant phyllodes tumors may metastasize, unlike fibroadenomas.

Intraductal Papilloma

Arises from epithelial proliferation within ducts.

May cause nipple discharge (bloody or serous).

Rarely associated with malignancy unless atypical features are present.

Lipoma: Benign tumor of adipose tissue, soft and mobile.

Malignant Breast Tumors

Invasive Ductal Carcinoma (IDC)

Accounts for 70–80% of breast cancers.

Originates from ductal epithelium, invades surrounding stroma.

Subtypes include tubular, mucinous, medullary and papillary carcinomas.

Invasive Lobular Carcinoma (ILC)

Accounts for 10–15% of breast cancers.

Characterized by single-file infiltration of tumor cells due to loss of E-cadherin.

Ductal Carcinoma In Situ (DCIS)

Non-invasive, confined to ducts.

High risk of progression to invasive carcinoma if untreated.

Pathogenesis

Driven by genetic mutations (e.g., BRCA1/2, TP53), hormonal stimulation (estrogen/progesterone), and environmental factors. Tumor microenvironment, angiogenesis and immune evasion play key roles.

Clinical Features

Breast Cysts

Symptoms

Palpable, smooth, mobile lump, often tender.

May fluctuate in size with menstrual cycle.

Usually unilateral but can be multiple or bilateral.

Asymptomatic: Often detected incidentally on imaging.

Benign Breast Tumors

Fibroadenoma: Painless, well-defined, rubbery, mobile mass ("breast mouse").Typically 1–5 cm in size. Rarely associated with nipple discharge or skin changes.

Phyllodes Tumor: Larger, rapidly growing mass, often >5 cm. May cause skin stretching or ulceration in advanced cases.

Intraductal Papilloma: Nipple discharge (bloody or serous). Small, subareolar mass in some cases.

Lipoma: Soft, non-tender, mobile mass.

Malignant Breast Tumors

Symptoms: Painless, hard, irregular, fixed mass.

Skin changes: Dimpling, peau d'orange or ulceration.

Nipple retraction, discharge (bloody) or Paget's disease of the nipple.

Axillary lymphadenopathy in advanced cases.

Systemic Features (metastatic disease)

Bone pain, weight loss, respiratory symptoms or jaundice.

Diagnostic Evaluation

Clinical Assessment

History: Age, menstrual history, family history of breast/ovarian cancer, HRT use and symptoms (pain, discharge, lump characteristics).

Physical Examination

Inspection: Skin changes, nipple abnormalities.

Palpation: Mass characteristics (size, mobility, consistency), axillary/supraclavicular lymph nodes.

Triple Assessment (for any breast lump)

1. Clinical examination.
2. Imaging (mammography, ultrasound or MRI).
3. Tissue sampling (Fine needle aspiration cytology [FNAC] or core biopsy).

Imaging

Ultrasound: Preferred in women <40 years or for evaluating palpable lumps.

Cysts: Anechoic, well-defined, posterior acoustic enhancement.

Fibroadenomas: Hypoechoic, well-circumscribed, homogenous.

Malignant tumors: Irregular margins, hypoechoic, microcalcifications.

Mammography: Standard for women >40 years or with suspicious findings.

Features of malignancy: Mass, microcalcifications, architectural distortion.

MRI: Used for high-risk patients, dense breasts or equivocal findings. Assesses tumor extent, multifocality and contralateral breast.

Other Modalities

Ductography for nipple discharge.

PET-CT for staging metastatic disease.

Tissue Diagnosis

Fine Needle Aspiration Cytology (FNAC)

Useful for cysts (fluid aspiration) and solid masses.

Limited by inability to assess tissue architecture.

Core Biopsy

Gold standard for histological diagnosis.

Provides information on tumor type, grade and receptor status (ER, PR, HER2).

Excisional Biopsy

For indeterminate lesions or when core biopsy is inconclusive.

Staging (Malignant Tumors)

TNM staging (AJCC 8th edition)

T: Tumor size and extent.

N: Lymph node involvement.

M: Metastasis.

Management

Breast Cysts

1. Simple Cysts

Asymptomatic: Observation, no intervention needed.

Symptomatic: Aspiration for relief (fluid typically clear or yellow).

Complicated/Complex Cysts

Further evaluation with biopsy or imaging to rule out malignancy.

2. Recurrent Cysts

Consider hormonal therapy (e.g., oral contraceptives) or surgical excision in rare cases.

Benign Breast Tumors

1. Fibroadenoma

Observation: if small, asymptomatic and confirmed benign.

Excision if large, symptomatic or patient preference.

2. Phyllodes Tumor

Wide local excision with 1 cm margins.

Malignant phyllodes may require mastectomy or adjuvant therapy.

3. Intraductal Papilloma

Excision if symptomatic, atypical or associated with nipple discharge.

4. Lipoma

Observation unless symptomatic or cosmetically concerning.

Malignant Breast Tumors

Surgery

Breast-Conserving Surgery (BCS): Lumpectomy with negative margins, followed by radiotherapy.

Mastectomy: For large tumors, multifocal disease or patient preference.

Sentinel lymph node biopsy or axillary lymph node dissection for nodal staging.

Adjuvant Therapy

Chemotherapy: Anthracyclines, taxanes, or platinum-based regimens for high-risk or node-positive disease.

Hormonal Therapy: Tamoxifen (premenopausal) or aromatase inhibitors (postmenopausal) for ER/PR-positive tumors.

Targeted Therapy: Trastuzumab for HER2-positive tumors.

Radiotherapy: Post-BCS or in node-positive cases to reduce local recurrence.

Neoadjuvant Therapy

Used to shrink large tumors before surgery, particularly in locally advanced or inflammatory breast cancer.

Metastatic Disease

Systemic therapy (chemotherapy, hormonal therapy, targeted agents).

Palliative care to manage symptoms and improve quality of life.

Prognosis

Breast Cysts

Excellent prognosis; no malignant potential for simple cysts.

Complex cysts require careful evaluation to rule out malignancy.

Benign Tumors

Fibroadenomas: No increased cancer risk unless atypical hyperplasia is present.

Phyllodes tumors: Benign subtype has excellent prognosis; malignant subtype has a risk of recurrence or metastasis.

Malignant Tumors

Prognosis depends on stage, grade, receptor status and patient factors.

Early-stage breast cancer (Stage I–II): 5-year survival >90%.

Metastatic breast cancer (Stage IV): Median survival 2–3 years, though targeted therapies improve outcomes.

Special Conditions

High-Risk Patients: Genetic mutations (BRCA1/2, PALB2) need more screening (annual MRI and mammography) and consideration of prophylactic mastectomy or oophorectomy.

Pregnancy-Associated Breast Cancer: Rare, diagnosed in 1–3 per 10,000 pregnancies.

Management depends on maternal and fetal conditions.

Screening Recommendations: Mammography every 1–2 years for women aged 40–74 (varies by guideline).

High-risk women: Start screening earlier (age 30) with MRI.

Differential Diagnosis

Benign Conditions: Mastitis, abscess, fat necrosis, fibrocystic changes.

Malignant conditions: Lymphoma, sarcoma, metastasis from other primaries (e.g., melanoma).

Prevention and Patient Education

Risk Reduction

Maintain healthy weight, limit alcohol, regular exercise and breastfeeding.

Chemoprevention (tamoxifen or raloxifene) for high-risk women.

Patient Counseling

Encourage breast self-examination and awareness of changes.

Discuss benefits and limitations of screening.

Address psychological impact of diagnosis, especially for malignant tumors.

Conclusion

Breast cysts and tumors represent a diverse group of conditions requiring a systematic approach to diagnosis and management. Gynecologists role lies in early detection, counseling and coordinating multidisciplinary care. Advances in imaging, molecular profiling and targeted therapies continue to improve outcomes, particularly for malignant tumors.

References

1. Fisher B, et al. (2005). Tamoxifen for prevention of breast cancer: Report of the NSABP P-1 Study. J Natl Cancer Inst.

2. WHO (2020). Global Cancer Observatory: Breast Cancer Statistics.
3. American Joint Committee on Cancer (AJCC) 8th Edition Staging Manual.
4. Rosen PP. (2014). Rosen's Breast Pathology 4th ed.

Breast Carcinoma

1. Introduction

Breast carcinoma is the most common malignancy in women worldwide and a leading cause of cancer-related mortality. It encompasses a heterogeneous group of tumors with varying histological, molecular and clinical characteristics.

2. Epidemiology

Approximately 2.3 million new cases annually (WHO, 2020). Accounts for 25% of all cancers in women. Leading cause of cancer death in women globally (627,000 deaths annually).

Incidence

Highest in developed countries (e.g., North America, Western Europe) due to screening and lifestyle factors. Increasing in low- and middle-income countries due to changing risk profiles.

Age

Incidence rises with age, peaking in women aged 50–70 years.

Younger women (<40 years) account for 5–10% of cases, often with aggressive tumors.

Risk Factors

Non-modifiable: Female sex, age, family history, genetic mutations (BRCA1/2, TP53, PALB2), personal history of breast cancer or atypical hyperplasia.

Modifiable: Obesity, alcohol consumption, nulliparity, early menarche, late menopause, hormone replacement therapy (HRT), lack of physical activity.

Other: Radiation exposure, high breast density.

Protective Factors: Breastfeeding, early parity, regular physical activity.

Pathophysiology

Histological Types

Invasive Ductal Carcinoma (IDC)

Most common (70–80% of cases).

Arises from ductal epithelium, invades stroma.

Subtypes: Tubular, mucinous, medullary, papillary, metaplastic.

Invasive Lobular Carcinoma (ILC)

10–15% of cases.

Characterized by single-file infiltration due to E-cadherin loss.

Often bilateral or multifocal.

Ductal Carcinoma In Situ (DCIS)

Non-invasive, confined to ducts.

Accounts for 15–20% of screen-detected cancers.

High risk of progression to invasive carcinoma if untreated.

Other Types

Inflammatory breast cancer (rare, aggressive, presents with skin changes).

Paget's disease of the nipple (1–3%, often associated with underlying DCIS or IDC).

Rare tumors: Angiosarcoma, lymphoma, phyllodes tumor (malignant subtype).

Staging

TNM System (AJCC 8th Edition)

T (Tumor): Size and extent (T1–T4).

N (Node): Regional lymph node involvement (N0–N3).

M (Metastasis): Distant spread (M0–M1).

Incorporates biomarker status (ER, PR, HER2, grade) for prognostic staging.

Stages

Stage 0: DCIS.

Stage I–II: Early-stage, localized.

Stage III: Locally advanced.

Stage IV: Metastatic.

Clinical Features

Symptoms

Early-Stage

Painless, hard, irregular, fixed mass.

Often asymptomatic, detected via screening.

Locally Advanced

Skin changes: Dimpling, peau d'orange, ulceration.

Nipple retraction, bloody discharge, or Paget's disease.

Axillary lymphadenopathy.

Metastasis

Bone pain (bone metastases), dyspnea (lung metastases), jaundice (liver metastases), neurological symptoms (brain metastases).

Inflammatory Breast Cancer

Rapid onset of breast swelling, erythema, warmth and peau d'orange without a distinct mass.

Special Populations

Pregnancy-Associated Breast Cancer: Diagnosed during pregnancy or within 1 year postpartum. Often presents at a later stage due to delayed diagnosis.

Male Breast Cancer

<1% of cases, typically IDC.

Presents as a subareolar mass, often with nipple involvement.

Diagnostic Evaluation

Clinical Assessment

History: Age, family history, reproductive history (menarche, menopause, parity), HRT use, symptoms (lump, pain, discharge).

Physical Examination

Inspection: Skin changes, nipple abnormalities, asymmetry.

Palpation: Mass characteristics (size, mobility, consistency), axillary/supraclavicular lymph nodes.

Triple Assessment (gold standard for any breast lump):

1. Clinical examination.
2. Imaging (mammography, ultrasound, or MRI).
3. Tissue sampling (FNAC or core biopsy).

Imaging

Mammography

Standard for women >40 years or with suspicious findings.

Features of malignancy: Spiculated mass, microcalcifications, architectural distortion.

Sensitivity lower in dense breasts.

Ultrasound

Preferred in women <40 years or for palpable lumps.

Features of malignancy: Irregular margins, hypoechoic, increased vascularity.

Useful for guiding biopsies.

MRI

Indicated for high-risk patients, dense breasts or to assess tumor extent/multifocality.

High sensitivity for detecting contralateral disease.

Other Modalities

PET-CT for staging metastatic disease.

Ductography for nipple discharge (rarely used).

Tissue Diagnosis: Fine Needle Aspiration Cytology (FNAC)- Quick, less invasive, but limited by inability to assess tissue architecture.

Core Biopsy: Gold standard for histological diagnosis. Provides tumor type, grade and receptor status (ER, PR, HER2, Ki-67).

Excisional Biopsy: Rarely needed, used for indeterminate lesions.

Sentinel Lymph Node Biopsy (SLNB): Assesses axillary node status in clinically node-negative patients. Avoids morbidity of full axillary dissection.

Staging Workup

For locally advanced or metastatic disease:

CT chest/abdomen/pelvis, bone scan or PET-CT.

Liver function tests, tumor markers (CA 15-3, CEA; limited specificity).

Management

Management is multidisciplinary, involving surgeons, medical oncologists, radiation oncologists and gynecologists. Management is done according to tumor stage, subtype and patient factors.

Surgery

Breast-Conserving Surgery (BCS)

Lumpectomy with negative margins.

Indicated for early-stage disease (Stage I–II).

Followed by radiotherapy to reduce local recurrence.

Mastectomy

Indicated for large tumors, multifocal disease, patient preference or contraindications to radiotherapy.

Options: Simple, modified radical, or skin/nipple-sparing mastectomy.

Axillary Management

SLNB for clinically node-negative disease.

Axillary lymph node dissection (ALND) for node-positive disease or failed SLNB.

Surgery

Offered post-mastectomy (implants or autologous tissue flaps).

Adjuvant Therapy

Chemotherapy

Indicated for node-positive, high-risk or triple-negative/HER2+ tumors.

Regimens: Anthracyclines (doxorubicin), taxanes (paclitaxel), cyclophosphamide.

Neoadjuvant chemotherapy for locally advanced disease to downstage tumors.

Hormonal Therapy

For ER/PR-positive tumors.

Premenopausal: Tamoxifen (5–10 years) ± ovarian suppression (goserelin).

Postmenopausal: Aromatase inhibitors (anastrozole, letrozole) or tamoxifen.

Radiotherapy

Post-BCS to reduce local recurrence.

Post-mastectomy in node-positive or high-risk cases.

Palliative for symptomatic metastases (e.g., bone).

Neoadjuvant Therapy

Used to shrink tumors before surgery in locally advanced or inoperable cases.

Includes chemotherapy, hormonal therapy or HER2-targeted agents.

Allows assessment of tumor response and facilitates BCS.

Metastatic Disease (Stage IV)

Goal: Palliation, prolong survival, improve quality of life.

Systemic Therapy

Hormonal therapy for ER+ disease.

Chemotherapy or targeted therapy for TNBC or HER2+ disease.

Supportive Care

Bisphosphonates or denosumab for bone metastases.

Pain management, psychological support.

Prognosis

Early-Stage (Stage I–II): 5-year survival >90% with modern therapy. Luminal A tumors have the best prognosis.

Locally Advanced (Stage III): 5-year survival 50–70%, depending on response to therapy.

Metastatic (Stage IV): Median survival 2–3 years, improved with targeted therapies. TNBC and HER2+ tumors historically worse, but outcomes improving.

Special Conditions

High-Risk Patients

Genetic Predisposition

BRCA1/2 mutations: 50–80% lifetime risk of breast cancer.

Other mutations: TP53 (Li-Fraumeni syndrome), PTEN (Cowden syndrome).

Management: Enhanced screening (MRI + mammography from age 30), chemoprevention (tamoxifen), or prophylactic mastectomy/oophorectomy.

Screening Recommendations

General population: Mammography every 1–2 years for women aged 40–74 (varies by guideline).

High-risk: Annual MRI + mammography starting at age 30.

Pregnancy-Associated Breast Cancer

Incidence: 1–3 per 10,000 pregnancies.

Challenges: Delayed diagnosis due to breast changes in pregnancy.

Management

Surgery safe in all trimesters.

Chemotherapy safe after first trimester.

Radiotherapy and hormonal therapy deferred until postpartum.

Male Breast Cancer

Risk factors: BRCA2 mutations, Klinefelter syndrome, radiation exposure.

Management mirrors as per guidelines of female breast cancer but often diagnosed at a later stage.

Gynecological Implications

Fertility Preservation: Discuss egg/embryo cryopreservation before chemotherapy in young women.

Menopausal Symptoms: Hormonal therapy may induce menopausal symptoms; manage with non-hormonal options (e.g., SSRIs).

Ovarian Suppression: Used in premenopausal ER+ breast cancer to reduce recurrence risk.

Differential Diagnosis

Benign Conditions: Fibroadenoma, cysts, mastitis, fat necrosis, intraductal papilloma.

Other Malignancies: Lymphoma, sarcoma, metastasis (e.g., melanoma, lung cancer).

Prevention and Patient Education

Primary Prevention

Lifestyle: Maintain healthy weight, limit alcohol, regular exercise.

Chemoprevention: Tamoxifen or raloxifene for high-risk women.

Prophylactic surgery for BRCA carriers.

Secondary Prevention

Screening mammography reduces mortality by 20–30%.

Breast self-examination promotes awareness but not a substitute for screening.

Patient Counseling

Educate on risk factors, screening benefits and early detection.

Address psychological impact (anxiety, body image concerns).

Support and care (monitoring for recurrence, managing long-term side effects).

Conclusion

Breast carcinoma is a complex disease requiring a multidisciplinary approach. Gynecologists are integral to early detection, counselling and managing reproductive health implications. Advances in molecular subtyping, targeted therapies and immunotherapy have transformed outcomes, particularly for early-stage and HER2+ or ER+ tumors.

References

1. Bray F, et al. (2020). Global cancer statistics 2020: GLOBOCAN estimates. CA Cancer J Clin.
2. American Joint Committee on Cancer (AJCC) 8th Edition Staging Manual.
3. Harbeck N, et al. (2019). Breast cancer. Nat Rev Dis Primers.
4. NCCN Guidelines: Breast Cancer (Version 2025).

Long Answer Questions

1. Define mastitis and describe its types, clinical features and management.
2. Discuss mastalgia—classification, causes and therapeutic approach.
3. Explain breast abscess—etiology, diagnosis and treatment.
4. Describe benign breast cysts and neoplasms with differential diagnosis.
5. Elaborate on galactorrhea—causes, hormonal profile and management.

Short Answer Questions

1. What is cyclical mastalgia?
2. Name two causes of galactorrhea.
3. Define fibroadenoma.
4. Mention one complication of untreated breast abscess.
5. What is the role of prolactin in breast physiology?

Multiple Choice Questions (1 Mark Each)

1. Most common cause of mastitis in lactating women:

a) Candida b) Staphylococcus aureus c) E. coli d) HPV

Ans: b) Staphylococcus aureus

2. Cyclical mastalgia is associated with:

a) Menopause b) Ovulation c) Luteal phase d) Pregnancy

Ans: c) Luteal phase

3. Galactorrhea is caused by elevated levels of:

a) Estrogen b) Progesterone c) Prolactin d) LH

Ans: c) Prolactin

4. Most common benign breast tumor in young women:

a) Fibroadenoma b) Lipoma c) Papilloma d) Cystadenoma

Ans: a) Fibroadenoma

5. Breast abscess is a complication of:

a) Mastalgia b) Mastitis c) Galactorrhea d) Fibroadenoma

Ans: b) Mastitis

6. Which of the following is NOT a feature of fibrocystic breast disease?

a) Nodularity b) Cyclical pain c) Bloody discharge d) Premenstrual swelling

Ans: c) Bloody discharge

7. Galactorrhea may be associated with:

a) Hypothyroidism b) Hyperthyroidism c) Diabetes d) PCOS

Ans: a) Hypothyroidism

8. Which imaging modality is preferred for breast cyst evaluation in women <30 years?

a) CT scan b) Mammogram c) Ultrasound d) MRI

Ans: c) Ultrasound

9. Which drug is used to treat hyperprolactinemia-induced galactorrhea?

a) Danazol b) Bromocriptine c) Tamoxifen d) GnRH agonist

Ans: b) Bromocriptine

10. Which breast condition may mimic carcinoma on mammography due to calcifications?

a) Mastalgia b) Fat necrosis c) Galactorrhea d) Mastitis

Ans: b) Fat necrosis

14

Family Planning & Contraceptive Measures

(Khandani Mansuba Bandi aur Mani-aat-i-Haml Tadabir wa Adwiya)

14.1 *Mani-i-Haml Adwiya* (Contraceptives Medicines)
14.2 *Mani'-i-Haml Tadabir* (Contraceptives Measures)

Learning Objective (At the end of the session, the students should be able to)-

Describe the small family norms & their importance & Discuss the criteria for ideal contraceptives
Describe Contraceptive measures & its mechanism of action, types, doses, side effects of *Mana'e Hamal Advia* (contraceptive measures)
Demonstrate the correct technique to insert & remove IUCDs, use of cervical cap and diaphragm.

Family Planning & Contraceptive Measures

(*Khandani Mansuba Bandi aur Mani-aat-i-Haml Tadabir wa Adwiya*)

Family Planning and Contraceptive Measures

Family planning is an important component of reproductive health, empowering individuals and couples to make decisions about the number, timing and spacing of their children. It encompasses a range of strategies and interventions aimed at promoting reproductive health, reducing unintended pregnancies and improving maternal and child health outcomes. Family planning encompasses a broad spectrum of strategies, including the use of contraceptive methods, fertility awareness and counselling.

Contraceptive measures, the practical tool of family planning, include range of methods designed to prevent pregnancy by interfering with the reproductive process. These methods-hormonal, barrier, intrauterine, surgical and natural-offer options according to individual needs, preferences and medical conditions. Advances in medical technology and research have expanded the availability, safety and efficacy of contraceptives, making them integral to modern healthcare.

Selection of Contraceptive Method Based on Patient Profile

Patient Evaluation (Age, Marital Status, Parity, Medical History)

↓

Assess Needs:

↓ ↓ ↓

Spacing Limiting Emergency

↓ ↓ ↓

Barrier Sterilization ECP / Copper-T

Hormonal Vasectomy LNG Pills

IUCD Tubectomy

Natural

↓

Consider Contraindications

(Hypertension, Diabetes, Smoking, Breast Cancer)

↓

Counseling + Informed Consent

↓

Initiate Method + Follow-up

14.1 Contraceptives Medicines

(*Mani -i-Haml Adwiya*)

Contraceptive medicines represent a critical component of family planning and reproductive health, offering safe, effective and reversible options to prevent unintended pregnancies. These pharmacological interventions, primarily hormonal in nature, are designed to interfere with the reproductive process by altering ovulation, fertilization or implantation.

Overview of Contraceptive Medicines

Contraceptive medicines primarily consist of hormonal methods that utilize synthetic estrogens, progestins or a combination of both to regulate reproductive physiology. These medications are available in various forms, including oral pills, injectables, implants, transdermal patches, vaginal rings and emergency contraception. Non-hormonal pharmacological options, such as ulipristal acetate for emergency contraception, also play a role. The choice of method depends on patient preferences, medical history, lifestyle and reproductive goals.

Types of Contraceptive Medicines

Combined Hormonal Contraceptives (CHCs)

CHCs contain synthetic estrogen (e.g., ethinyl estradiol) and progestin (e.g., levonorgestrel, norethindrone or drospirenone). They work by suppressing ovulation, thickening cervical mucus to impede sperm penetration and thinning the endometrial lining to prevent implantation.

Oral Contraceptive Pills (COCs)

Formulations: Monophasic (fixed hormone dose), multiphasic (variable doses), or extended-cycle regimens.

Efficacy: ~99% with perfect use; ~91% with typical use.

Administration: Daily pill, typically in 21/7 or 24/4 cycles (active pills/placebo).

Examples: Levonorgestrel-ethinyl estradiol, drospirenone-ethinyl estradiol.

Benefits: Regulates menstrual cycles, reduces dysmenorrhea and lowers risk of ovarian/endometrial cancers.

Side Effects: Nausea, breast tenderness, breakthrough bleeding and rare risks like venous thromboembolism (VTE).

Contraindications: History of VTE, stroke, myocardial infarction, uncontrolled hypertension, smoking (>35 years) or estrogen-sensitive cancers.

Transdermal Patch

Example: Ortho Evra (norelgestromin-ethinyl estradiol).

Administration: Weekly patch application for 3 weeks, followed by a patch-free week.

Efficacy: Similar to COCs.

Advantages: Reduced daily compliance; steady hormone delivery.

Risks: Slightly higher VTE risk compared to COCs due to higher estrogen exposure.

Vaginal Ring

Example: NuvaRing (etonogestrel-ethinyl estradiol).

Administration: Inserted vaginally for 3 weeks, removed for 1 week.

Efficacy: Comparable to COCs.

Advantages: User-controlled, localized hormone delivery.

Side Effects: Vaginal irritation, discharge or discomfort.

Progestin-Only Contraceptives (POCs)

POCs contain only progestin and are suitable for patients with contraindications to estrogen, such as breastfeeding mothers or those with cardiovascular risks.

Progestin-Only Pills (POPs, 'Mini-Pills')

Examples: Norethindrone, drospirenone.

Mechanism: Thickens cervical mucus, inhibits ovulation (in ~50% of cycles) and alters endometrium.

Efficacy: ~99% with perfect use; ~91% with typical use.

Administration: Daily, with strict timing (within 3-hour window).

Advantages: Safe for patients with estrogen contraindications.

Side Effects: Irregular bleeding, weight gain, mood changes.

Contraindications: Active liver disease, breast cancer, undiagnosed abnormal uterine bleeding.

Injectables

Example: Depot medroxyprogesterone acetate (DMPA, Depo-Provera).

Administration: Intramuscular or subcutaneous injection every 12–14 weeks.

Efficacy: >99% with perfect use; ~94% with typical use.

Advantages: Long-acting, no daily compliance.

Side Effects: Irregular bleeding, weight gain, delayed return to fertility (up to 18 months), and potential bone density loss with prolonged use.

Contraindications: Similar to POPs; caution in patients at risk for osteoporosis.

Implants

Example: Nexplanon (etonogestrel).

Administration: Subdermal rod inserted in the upper arm, effective for up to 3 years.

Efficacy: >99%, one of the most effective methods.

Advantages: Long-acting, reversible, minimal user compliance.

Side Effects: Irregular bleeding, insertion/removal complications.

Contraindications: Similar to other POCs.

Emergency Contraceptive Pills (ECPs)

ECPs are used post-coitally to prevent pregnancy after unprotected intercourse or contraceptive failure.

Levonorgestrel ECPs

Example: Plan B One-Step.

Mechanism: Delays ovulation; may alter endometrium.

Dose: 1.5 mg single dose within 72 hours of intercourse (efficacy decreases with time).

Efficacy: Reduces pregnancy risk by 75–89%.

Side Effects: Nausea, fatigue, irregular bleeding.

Ulipristal Acetate

Example: Ella.

Mechanism: Selective progesterone receptor modulator; delays ovulation more effectively than levonorgestrel.

Dose: 30 mg single dose within 120 hours.

Efficacy: More effective than levonorgestrel, especially in overweight/obese patients.

Contraindications: Known or suspected pregnancy, breastfeeding (avoid for 36 hours post-dose).

Mechanisms of Action

Contraceptive medicines act through one or more of the following mechanisms:

Suppression of Ovulation: Estrogen and progestin inhibit the hypothalamic-pituitary-ovarian axis, preventing follicle development and ovulation.

Cervical Mucus Thickening: Progestins increase mucus viscosity, impeding sperm penetration.

Endometrial Alteration: Hormonal changes create an unfavorable environment for implantation.

Tubal Motility Changes: Progestins may slow ovum transport, reducing chances of fertilization.

Clinical Conditions

Patient Selection and Counseling

Medical History: Assess for contraindications (e.g., cardiovascular disease, liver dysfunction, breast cancer).

Lifestyle Factors: Consider adherence, frequency of intercourse and reproductive goals.

Counseling: Educate on correct use, side effects and non-contraceptive benefits (e.g., acne reduction, menstrual regulation).

Discuss efficacy, reversibility and patient preferences to optimize adherence.

Efficacy and Failure Rates

Perfect Use: Assumes correct and consistent use (e.g., 0.3% failure rate for COCs).

Typical Use: Accounts for human error (e.g., 9% failure rate for COCs).

Counseling Tip: Emphasize adherence to improve efficacy, especially for POPs and COCs.

Side Effects and Risks

Common: Breakthrough bleeding, nausea, breast tenderness, mood changes.

Serious (Rare): VTE, stroke, myocardial infarction (CHCs); bone density loss (DMPA).

Monitoring: Regular follow-up to assess side effects, blood pressure and patient satisfaction.

Drug Interactions

Certain medications (e.g., anticonvulsants, rifampicin) induce cytochrome P450 enzymes, reducing hormonal contraceptive efficacy.

Counseling: Advise backup contraception (e.g., condoms) when initiating interacting drugs.

Special Populations

Adolescents: Require confidentiality and education on adherence.

Postpartum/Breastfeeding: POCs preferred; CHCs avoided until 6 weeks postpartum (non-breastfeeding) or 6 months (breastfeeding).

Perimenopause: Low-dose CHCs or POCs may be used if no contraindications.

Chronic Conditions: POCs for patients with cardiovascular or thrombotic risks; avoid CHCs in high-risk groups.

Non-Contraceptive Benefits

Menstrual Regulation: Reduced dysmenorrhea, menorrhagia and irregular cycles.

Gynecologic Conditions: Management of endometriosis, polycystic ovary syndrome (PCOS) and acne.

Cancer Risk Reduction: CHCs lower risks of ovarian, endometrial and colorectal cancers.

Bone Health: DMPA may protect against endometrial hyperplasia but requires monitoring for bone density.

Contraindications and Precautions

Absolute Contraindications (CHCs): VTE, stroke, ischemic heart disease, migraine with aura, breast cancer, severe liver disease.

Relative Contraindications: Smoking (>35 years), hypertension, diabetes with complications.

POCs: Fewer contraindications but avoid in active breast cancer or severe liver disease.

Emerging Trends and Innovations

New Formulations: Low-dose estrogen pills, novel progestins (e.g., drospirenone-only POPs).

New- Cycle Regimens: Continuous COC use to reduce menstrual frequency.

Non-Hormonal Advances: Research into non-hormonal oral contraceptives targeting sperm function or ovulation.

Digital Health: Apps for tracking cycles and adherence reminders.

Clinical Management and Follow-Up

Initiation: Screen for contraindications; provide starter packs and instructions.

Follow-Up: Monitor at 3–6 months initially, then annually; assess side effects and adherence.

Discontinuation: Counsel on return to fertility (immediate for most methods, delayed for DMPA).

Complications: Manage breakthrough bleeding with dose adjustments or reassurance; refer for serious adverse events.

Key References

World Health Organization. (2020). Medical Eligibility Criteria for Contraceptive Use.

American College of Obstetricians and Gynecologists. (2023). Contraception Guidelines.

14.2 Contraceptives Measures

(Mani'-i-Haml Tadabir)

Contraceptive measures are broadly categorized as reversible (temporary) or irreversible (permanent), with further subdivisions based on mechanism and delivery.

Government-Supported Contraceptives (India)

1. Chhaya - Non-hormonal pill -Free under RMNCH+A
2. Antara -Injectable DMPA -Govt FP Scheme
3. Copper-T -IUCD -Available via ASHA
4. Condoms - Barrier - Janani Shishu Suraksha
5. Tubectomy -Surgical -Incentivized at PHCs

Hormonal Contraceptives

Hormonal contraceptives use synthetic estrogens and/or progestins to alter reproductive physiology, primarily by suppressing ovulation, thickening cervical mucus and modifying the endometrial lining.

Combined Hormonal Contraceptives (CHCs): described in previous chapter.

Intrauterine Devices (IUDs)

IUDs are long-acting reversible contraceptives (LARCs) inserted into the uterus by trained clinicians.

1. Copper IUD (e.g., ParaGard):

Mechanism: Copper ions impair sperm motility and viability; induces sterile inflammatory response preventing fertilization.

Duration: 10–12 years.

Efficacy: >99%.

Advantages: Non-hormonal, immediate reversibility, emergency contraception (if inserted within 5 days of intercourse).

Side Effects: Heavy menstrual bleeding, dysmenorrhea (especially initially).

Contraindications: Wilson's disease, uterine anomalies, acute pelvic infection, unexplained uterine bleeding.

Insertion: Requires sterile technique; mild cramping common.

2. Hormonal IUD (e.g., Mirena, Kyleena):

Composition: Levonorgestrel-releasing devices (13.5–52 mg).

Mechanism: Thickens cervical mucus, thins endometrium, may suppress ovulation.

Duration: 3–8 years, depending on device (e.g., Mirena: 8 years)

Efficacy: >99%.

Advantages: Reduces menstrual bleeding (amenorrhea in ~20% of Mirena users), treats menorrhagia and endometriosis.

Side Effects: Irregular bleeding (initial 3–6 months), ovarian cysts (usually benign), rare expulsion/ perforation.

Contraindications: Breast cancer, active pelvic infection, uterine anomalies.

Barrier Methods

Barrier methods physically or chemically prevent sperm from reaching the ovum.

1. Male Condom

Materials: Latex, polyurethane, or nitrile.

Efficacy: 98% (perfect use); 82% (typical use due to incorrect use).

Advantages: Protects against sexually transmitted infections (STIs), widely accessible.

Disadvantages: User-dependent, may reduce sensation, risk of breakage/slippage.

Counseling: Teach correct use .

2. Female Condom

Material: Polyurethane or nitrile.

Efficacy: 95% (perfect use); 79% (typical use).

Advantages: Female-controlled, STI protection.

Disadvantages: Higher cost, less widely available, insertion challenges.

3. Diaphragm/Cervical Cap

Use: Silicone devices used with spermicide, inserted before intercourse.

Efficacy: 94% (perfect use); 88% (typical use).

Advantages: Reusable, female-controlled.

Disadvantages: Requires fitting by trained one, user-dependent, no STI protection.

Contraindications: Latex allergy (for some diaphragms), recurrent urinary tract infections.

4. Spermicide (e.g., Nonoxynol-9):

Mechanism: Immobilizes sperm.

Efficacy: 82% (perfect use); 72% (typical use).

Disadvantages: Low efficacy alone, may irritate mucosa, increasing HIV transmission risk.

Counseling: Recommend combination with barrier methods.

Surgical (Permanent) Methods

1.Tubal Ligation/Occlusion

Procedure: Cutting, sealing or blocking fallopian tubes (e.g., via laparoscopy, clips, or hysteroscopic occlusion).

Efficacy: >99% (failure rate ~0.5% due to recanalization).

Advantages: Permanent, no ongoing compliance.

Risks: Surgical complications (e.g., infection, bleeding), not suited for (young/nulliparous patients).

Counseling: Discuss irreversibility, alternatives like LARCs.

2. Vasectomy

Procedure: Cutting or sealing vas deferens, typically outpatient.

Efficacy: >99% (confirm azoospermia post-procedure).

Advantages: Simpler, lower risk than tubal ligation.

Risks: Rare hematoma, chronic scrotal pain.

Counseling: Emphasize need for backup contraception until sterility confirmed (8–12 weeks).

Natural and Behavioral Methods

1. Fertility Awareness-Based Methods (FABMs)

Techniques: Calendar method, basal body temperature (BBT), cervical mucus monitoring, symptothermal method.

Mechanism: Identify fertile window to abstain or use barriers.

Efficacy: 95–99% (perfect use); 76–88% (typical use).

Advantages: Non-invasive, no cost, aligns with cultural/religious preferences.

Disadvantages: Requires training, regular cycles, abstinence during fertile days.

Contraindications: Irregular cycles, perimenopause, postpartum.

2. Lactational Amenorrhea Method (LAM)

Criteria: Exclusive breastfeeding, amenorrhea, <6 months postpartum.

Efficacy: 98% (perfect use).

Advantages: Temporary, no cost.

Disadvantages: Strict criteria, short-term.

3. Withdrawal (Coitus Interruptus)

Mechanism: Male partner withdraws before ejaculation.

Efficacy: 96% (perfect use); 78% (typical use).

Disadvantages: High failure rate, no STI protection, relies on male control.

Mechanisms of Action

Hormonal Methods: Suppress gonadotropin release (FSH/LH), preventing ovulation; thicken cervical mucus; alter endometrium.

Copper IUD: Creates spermicidal environment via copper ion release; induces endometrial inflammation.

Hormonal IUD: Local progestin effects on cervical mucus and endometrium; occasional ovulation suppression.

Barrier Methods: Physically block sperm (condoms, diaphragms) or immobilize sperm (spermicides).

Surgical Methods: Prevent gamete transport by occluding fallopian tubes or vas deferens.

Natural Methods: Avoid intercourse during fertile periods or use physiological infertility (e.g., LAM).

Clinical Considerations

Patient Assessment

Medical History: Screen for contraindications (e.g., cardiovascular disease, cancer, liver dysfunction, bleeding disorders).

Reproductive Goals: Assess desire for temporary vs. permanent methods, future fertility plans.

Lifestyle Factors: Evaluate adherence ability, sexual frequency, STI risk and cultural/religious preferences.

Physical Examination: Check for uterine anomalies (IUDs), blood pressure (CHCs), or pelvic abnormalities.

Efficacy Comparison

Highly Effective (>99%): IUDs, implants, surgical methods.

Moderately Effective (91–99%): CHCs, POCs, ECPs.

Less Effective (76–88%): Barrier methods, FABMs, withdrawal.

Counseling: Emphasize LARCs for patients seeking high efficacy with low user effort.

Patient Counseling

Discuss efficacy, side effects, non-contraceptive benefits and reversibility.

Align method with patient preferences, medical needs and lifestyle.

Provide support tools (e.g., apps for pill reminders, calendars for FABMs).

STI Prevention: Recommend condoms alongside non-protective methods (e.g., IUDs, hormonal methods).

Side Effects and Complications

1. Hormonal Methods

Common: Breakthrough bleeding, nausea, mood changes, weight gain.

Serious: VTE , bone density loss (DMPA), liver adenoma (rare).

2. IUDs

Common: Cramping, irregular bleeding (hormonal IUD), heavy menses (copper IUD).

Serious: Expulsion (2–10%), perforation (<1/1,000), pelvic inflammatory disease (PID, <1% if screened).

3. Barrier Methods: Allergic reactions, urinary tract infections (diaphragms), mucosal irritation (spermicides).

4. Surgical Methods: Infection, bleeding.

Management: NSAIDs for IUD-related pain, hormonal adjustments for bleeding, referral for serious complications.

Drug Interactions

Hormonal Methods: Enzyme-inducing drugs (e.g., rifampin, carbamazepine) reduce efficacy via cytochrome P450 induction.

Management: Use backup contraception (e.g., condoms) or switch to non-hormonal methods (e.g., copper IUD).

Special Populations

Adolescents: Prioritize LARCs (IUDs, implants) for high efficacy; ensure confidentiality per local laws.

Postpartum/Breastfeeding: POCs, copper IUDs, or LAM recommended.

CHCs avoided until 6 weeks postpartum (non-breastfeeding) or 6 months (breastfeeding) due to VTE risk and milk supply concerns.

Perimenopause: Low-dose COCs or POCs for contraception and symptom management; avoid in high-risk patients.

Chronic Conditions

Cardiovascular Disease/Hypertension: Use POCs, copper IUDs; avoid COCs.

Diabetes: POCs or IUDs preferred if vascular complications present.

Obesity: Ulipristal acetate preferred for emergency contraception; implants/IUDs for long-term use.

Non-Contraceptive Benefits

Hormonal Methods: Menstrual regulation, reduced dysmenorrhea/menorrhagia, acne improvement.

Decreased risk of ovarian (50% reduction), endometrial (40% reduction) and colorectal cancers (COCs).Management of endometriosis, polycystic ovary syndrome (PCOS) and premenstrual syndrome.

Hormonal IUDs: Treatment for heavy menstrual bleeding, endometrial hyperplasia, adenomyosis.

Copper IUD: Non-hormonal option for patients with hormone-related contraindications.

Contraindications

CHCs: Absolute: VTE, stroke, ischemic heart disease, migraine with aura, breast cancer, smoking (>35 years), severe hypertension. Relative: Obesity, diabetes, smoking (<35 years).

POCs/Hormonal IUDs: Breast cancer, active liver disease, undiagnosed uterine bleeding.

Copper IUD: Wilson’s disease, active pelvic infection, uterine anomalies.

Surgical Methods: Patient uncertainty, coerced decision-making.

FABMs: Irregular cycles, inability to track fertility signs.

Clinical Management

Initiation

Screen for pregnancy (urine/serum hCG if indicated).

Perform baseline assessments (e.g., blood pressure for CHCs, pelvic exam for IUDs).

Provide method-specific instructions (e.g., timing for POPs, insertion for IUDs).

Follow-Up

CHCs/POCs: Check at 3–6 months, then annually; monitor side effects, adherence.

IUDs: Confirm placement (string check) 4–6 weeks post-insertion; annual exams.

Barrier/FABMs: Reinforce correct use, address challenges.

Discontinuation

Fertility Return: Immediate for most methods; delayed for DMPA (6–18 months).

Counseling: Discuss alternative methods, preconception care if pregnancy desired.

Complications

Bleeding: NSAIDs for copper IUD; short-term estrogen or NSAIDs for hormonal IUD/POC bleeding.

IUD Issues: Ultrasound for missing strings; removal for expulsion/perforation.

Serious Events: Refer for VTE, PID or surgical complications.

Emerging Trends and Innovations

Hormonal Advances: Ultra-low-dose COCs, drospirenone-only POPs, novel delivery systems (e.g., microneedle patches, biodegradable implants).

Non-Hormonal Research: Sperm function inhibitors, ovulation suppressants, reversible male contraceptives (e.g., hormonal gels).

Digital Health: Apps for FABM tracking, telehealth for counseling, adherence reminders.

Access Improvements: Over-the-counter COCs (approved in some regions), pharmacy-based ECP provision.

Conclusion

Contraception is a dynamic field in gynecology, offering a spectrum of methods to meet diverse patient needs. Gynecologists must integrate scientific knowledge, clinical skills and patient-centered counseling to optimize outcomes.

Key References

World Health Organization. (2020). Medical Eligibility Criteria for Contraceptive Use, 5th Edition.

American College of Obstetricians and Gynecologists. (2023). Practice Bulletin: Contraception.

Curtis, K. M., et al. (2016). U.S. Medical Eligibility Criteria for Contraceptive Use. MMWR Recommendations and Reports, 65(3), 1–103.

Trussell, J. (2011). Contraceptive efficacy. In Contraceptive Technology, 20th Edition.

Classification of Contraceptive Methods

Contraceptive Methods
↓
Classify by Duration & Reversibility
↓ ↓ ↓
Temporary Permanent Emergency
↓ ↓ ↓

Temporary	Permanent	Emergency
Barrier	Sterilization	IUCD (Copper T)
Hormonal	Vasectomy	ECP Pills
IUCD	Tubectomy	LNG Pills
Natural		

	Types of Contraception	
	Mnemonic: "FAMILY STOP"	
Letter	**Method Type**	**Example**
F	Fertility awareness	Rhythm method, basal temp chart
A	Abstinence	Natural spacing
M	Male condom	Barrier method
I	Injectable contraceptive	DMPA (Antara Program)
L	Long-acting reversible	Copper-T, Implants
Y	Young-age suitability	Centchroman, condoms
S	Surgical (Permanent)	Tubectomy, Vasectomy
T	Temporary hormonal	OCPs, POPs
O	Oral emergency pills	Levonorgestrel
P	Postcoital IUCD use	Copper-T within 120 hours

Common Side Effects

OCPs	Nausea, weight gain, mood swings
Injectable	Menstrual irregularity
IUCD	Bleeding, expulsion, PID risk
Barrier	Allergy, discomfort
Emergency Pill	Nausea, delayed menses

Emergency Contraception

Emergency contraception (EC) refers to methods used to prevent pregnancy after unprotected or inadequately protected sexual intercourse, contraceptive failure (e.g., condom breakage) or sexual assault. It is a critical component of reproductive health, offering a time-sensitive intervention to reduce the risk of unintended pregnancy.

Emergency contraception is designed for use within a specific timeframe after unprotected intercourse, typically 72–120 hours, depending on the method. It is not intended for routine contraception but serves as a backup option to prevent pregnancy when primary methods fail or are not used. EC methods include oral medications (hormonal and non-hormonal) and the copper intrauterine device (IUD).

Types of Emergency Contraception

1. Oral Emergency Contraceptive Pills (ECPs)

ECPs are the most commonly used form of emergency contraception, available as hormonal (levonorgestrel) or non-hormonal (ulipristal acetate) formulations.

a. Levonorgestrel (LNG) ECPs

Examples: Plan B One-Step, Next Choice, Levonelle.

Composition: 1.5 mg levonorgestrel (single dose) or 0.75 mg taken 12 hours apart (older regimens).

Mechanism of Action: Primarily delays or inhibits ovulation by suppressing luteinizing hormone (LH) surge. May alter cervical mucus to impede sperm penetration. Limited evidence suggests possible endometrial changes, but not abortifacient.

Timing: Most effective within 72 hours of unprotected intercourse; efficacy decreases over time.

Efficacy: Reduces pregnancy risk by 75–89% when taken within 72 hours. ~2% failure rate if taken within 24 hours; higher with delay. Less effective in women with higher body mass index (BMI >30 kg/m^2).

Administration: Single 1.5 mg oral dose; no need for split dosing in modern formulations.

Side Effects: Nausea (15–25%), vomiting (5%), fatigue, headache, irregular bleeding.

Contraindications: Known pregnancy (no harm to fetus, but ineffective); hypersensitivity to levonorgestrel.

Availability: Over-the-counter in many countries; no prescription required for adults in most settings.

b. Ulipristal Acetate (UPA)

Example: Ella, EllaOne.

Composition: 30 mg ulipristal acetate, a selective progesterone receptor modulator (SPRM).

Mechanism of Action: Delays ovulation by inhibiting or postponing LH surge, even after follicle development begins. More effective than levonorgestrel near ovulation. May alter endometrial receptivity, but not abortifacient.

Timing: Effective within 120 hours (5 days) of unprotected intercourse.

Efficacy: Reduces pregnancy risk by ~85–90%; more effective than levonorgestrel, especially at 72–120 hours or in women with BMI >30 kg/m^2. Failure rate ~1–2% within 120 hours.

Administration: Single 30 mg oral dose.

Side Effects: Nausea, headache, abdominal pain, delayed menses (due to ovulation delay).

Contraindications

Known pregnancy (ineffective, no teratogenic risk).

Breastfeeding (avoid breastfeeding for 36 hours post-dose due to milk excretion).

Severe liver disease or hypersensitivity.

Availability: Prescription required in some areas; over-the-counter in others.

c. Combined Oral Contraceptive Pills (Yuzpe Regimen)

Composition: High-dose ethinyl estradiol (100–120 mcg) and levonorgestrel (0.5–0.6 mg) per dose, repeated 12 hours apart.

Mechanism: Similar to levonorgestrel ECPs; delays ovulation, may alter cervical mucus/endometrium.

Efficacy: 56–75% reduction in pregnancy risk; less effective than LNG or UPA.

Use: Rarely used due to lower efficacy and higher side effects (nausea, vomiting).

Contraindications: Same as combined hormonal contraceptives (e.g., VTE, stroke, breast cancer).

Copper Intrauterine Device (IUD)

Example: ParaGard, other copper-bearing IUDs.

Mechanism of Action

Copper ions impair sperm motility and viability, preventing fertilization.

Induces sterile inflammatory response in endometrium, inhibiting implantation.

Most effective EC method; not abortifacient.

Timing: Inserted within 120 hours (5 days) of unprotected intercourse; may be effective up to 7 days in some cases.

Efficacy: >99% reduction in pregnancy risk; failure rate <0.1%.

Advantages

Most effective EC method, unaffected by BMI or timing within 120 hours.

Provides long-term contraception (up to 10–12 years).

Side Effects

Insertion-related cramping, bleeding.

Heavier menses and dysmenorrhea post-insertion.

Contraindications

Active pelvic infection, uterine anomalies, Wilson's disease, unexplained uterine bleeding.

Known pregnancy (though no harm if inadvertently inserted).

Procedure: Requires trained clinician; sterile technique; ultrasound if placement uncertain.

Availability: Limited by need for clinical insertion and access to trained providers.

Clinical Conditions

Indications

Unprotected intercourse or contraceptive failure (e.g., condom breakage, missed pills).

Sexual assault.

Incorrect or inconsistent use of regular contraception (e.g., late DMPA injection).

Efficacy Comparison

Copper IUD: Most effective (>99%), BMI-independent, long-term contraception option.

Ulipristal Acetate: More effective than levonorgestrel, especially at 72–120 hours or BMI >30 kg/m^2.

Levonorgestrel: Effective within 72 hours; less effective in obese patients or near ovulation.

Yuzpe Regimen: Least effective, rarely used.

Key Points

EC does not cause abortion or harm an existing pregnancy.

Does not protect against STIs; recommend testing/counseling if at risk.

Discuss resumption or initiation of regular contraception (e.g., start COCs/POPs immediately after ECPs).

Follow-Up

Advise pregnancy test if menses delayed >7 days post-EC.

Monitor for side effects (e.g., irregular bleeding).

Copper IUD: Check placement 4–6 weeks post-insertion.

Side Effects and Management

ECPs

Nausea/Vomiting: Administer antiemetics (e.g., meclizine) if needed; repeat LNG dose if vomiting within 2 hours.

Menstrual Changes: Expect earlier or delayed menses; counsel on follow-up if no menses within 3 weeks.

Copper IUD

Cramping: Manage with NSAIDs (e.g., ibuprofen).

Bleeding: Reassure if transient; evaluate if persistent.

Rare Risks: Expulsion (<5%), perforation (<1/1,000), infection (early post-insertion).

Special Populations

Adolescents: Ensure confidentiality; LNG and UPA are safe; copper IUD suitable if long-term contraception desired.

Breastfeeding

LNG: Safe; no interruption in breastfeeding needed.

UPA: Avoid breastfeeding for 36 hours post-dose.

Copper IUD: Preferred non-hormonal option.

Obese Patients (BMI >30 kg/m^2)

UPA and copper IUD preferred; LNG less effective.

Postpartum: Safe for all EC methods; copper IUD can be inserted immediately postpartum if no infection.

Non-Contraceptive Benefits

STI Prevention: EC does not protect against STIs; recommend condoms and STI testing if indicated.

Clinical Management

Initiation

ECPs: Administer as soon as possible; no medical exam required.

Copper IUD: Perform pelvic exam, screen for infection; insert under sterile conditions.

Follow-Up

ECPs: Advise pregnancy test if no menses within 3 weeks; discuss regular contraception.

Copper IUD: Confirm placement (string check) at 4–6 weeks; monitor for complications.

Backup Contraception

After ECPs: Use condoms or abstain until regular contraception initiated (e.g., start COCs/POPs same day as ECP).

After Copper IUD: Immediate contraception provided; no backup needed.

Complications

ECPs: Manage nausea/vomiting; evaluate persistent bleeding.

Copper IUD: Ultrasound for suspected expulsion; antibiotics for infection; removal if complications occur.

Conclusion

Emergency contraception is a vital tool in reproductive health, offering effective options to prevent unintended pregnancy after unprotected intercourse. The copper IUD is the most effective method, followed by ulipristal acetate and levonorgestrel ECPs.

References

World Health Organization. (2020). Medical Eligibility Criteria for Contraceptive Use, 5th Edition.

American College of Obstetricians and Gynecologists. (2021). Practice Bulletin: Emergency Contraception.

Cleland, K., et al. (2014). Emergency contraception review: Evidence-based recommendations for clinicians. Clinical Obstetrics and Gynecology, 57(4), 741–750.

Trussell, J., et al. (2018). Emergency contraception: A last chance to prevent unintended pregnancy. Contraceptive Technology, 21st Edition.

Contraception in Unani Medicine

Contraception in Unani medicine, referred to as "*Tadbeer-e-Hamal*" (prevention of pregnancy), is addressed through plants, mineral and animal-derived drugs, dietary modifications and regimental therapies, aligning with the system's holistic approach.

Contraceptive methods in Unani are primarily natural, relying on herbal drug formulations, physical techniques and lifestyle adjustments to prevent conception. These methods are individualized to an individual's temperament (*mizaj*) and humoral constitution to ensure efficacy and minimize adverse effects. Unani texts, such as Avicenna's *Al-Qanun fi al-Tibb* (The Canon of Medicine) and *Al-Razi's Kitab al-Hawi*, document various contraceptive practices, reflecting centuries-old knowledge adapted to modern contexts.

The Unani approach to contraception is integrated into the broader framework of *Ilaj-bil-Tadbeer* (regimental therapy), *Ilaj-bil-Dawa* (pharmacotherapy) and *Ilaj-bil-Ghiza* (dietotherapy), emphasizing prevention over cure.

Contraceptive Methods in Unani Medicine

Unani contraception includes pharmacotherapy (herbal, mineral and animal origin), regimental therapies and dietary modifications. These methods are primarily reversible and aim to prevent conception by altering reproductive physiology or creating an unfavorable environment for fertilization or implantation.

Pharmacotherapy (Ilaj-bil-Dawa)

Unani pharmacotherapy employs single drugs (*Mufrad Advia)* and compound formulations (*Murakkab Advia*) to achieve contraceptive effects. These remedies are derived from plants, minerals and animal sources. These are classified by their temperament and potency (*Darjat-e-Advia*) into four degrees based on efficacy and safety.

Oral Contraceptives

1. *Khaksi* (Sisymbrium irio): A cold and dry drug used to reduce uterine receptivity to implantation. It is administered as a decoction or powder. (https://www.researchgate.net/publication/321386220_FUNDAMENTALS_OF_UNANI_SYSTEM_OF_MEDICINE-A_REVIEW)

2. *Neem* (Azadirachta indica): Seeds or oil taken orally to reduce sperm motility due to its cold and dry temperament.

3. *Habb-e-Mumsik*: A compound formulation containing ingredients like opium (in controlled doses), musk and saffron, believed to alter uterine conditions to prevent conception.

4. *Majoon-e-Falasifa*: A polyherbal preparation with hot and dry properties, used to regulate humoral balance and reduce fertility temporarily. https://www.researchgate.net/publication/322655260_Introduction_and_Principles_of_Unani_Medicine)

Mechanism: These dugs work by altering cervical mucus viscosity, reducing sperm motility, or creating an unfavorable endometrial environment. For example, cold and dry drugs counteract the hot and moist conditions needed for conception.

Administration: Typically taken as decoctions, powders or pastes (majoon), post-coitally or during specific menstrual cycle phases.

Efficacy: Limited clinical studies exist; efficacy is based on traditional use and varies by patient temperament and adherence.

Side Effects: Potential digestive upset, irregular bleeding or humoral imbalance if not according to patient *mizaj*. Correctives (*Muslehat*) like honey or ghee are used to minimize side effects. (https://pmc.ncbi.nlm.nih.gov/articles/PMC3038517/)

Vaginal Suppositories and Pessaries

1. Suppositories with Alum (*Phitkari*): Alum mixed with herbal oils (e.g., sesame oil) is used as a vaginal pessary to create a spermicidal environment.

2. *Myrrh* (Commiphora myrrha): Applied vaginally to reduce sperm viability due to its astringent and drying properties.

3. Pomegranate Seed Paste: Used as a pessary to alter vaginal pH and impair sperm function.

Mechanism: These act as local spermicides or alter the vaginal environment to prevent sperm penetration or survival.

Administration: Inserted vaginally before or after intercourse; often combined with herbal oils for ease of application.

Topical Applications

Herbal pastes (e.g., henna, neem) applied to the lower abdomen or genitalia to reduce reproductive heat (*hararat*) and fertility.

Mechanism: Alter local humoral balance to create an unfavorable environment for conception.

Efficacy: Less studied; used as an adjunct to other methods.

Regimental Therapies (*Ilaj-bil-Tadbeer*)

Regimental therapies involve physical or lifestyle interventions to prevent conception, often used in conjunction with pharmacotherapy.

Coital Techniques

Withdrawal (*Azl*): Practiced as a behavioral method, where the male partner withdraws before ejaculation. Described by Al-Razi, as a natural contraceptive method.

Efficacy: Similar to modern withdrawal (96% perfect use; 78% typical use), but user-dependent.

Advantages: Non-invasive, no cost.

Disadvantages: High failure rate, no STI protection.

Vaginal Irrigation (*Nutool)*

Method: Post-coital vaginal douching with herbal decoctions (e.g., chamomile, vinegar) to flush out semen or alter vaginal pH.

Mechanism: Creates a hostile environment for sperm survival.

Efficacy: Low; not recommended as a primary method due to inconsistent results.

Side Effects: Risk of vaginal infections, if not sterile.

Cupping (*Hijama*)

Method: Applied to pelvic regions to regulate blood flow and humoral balance, believed to reduce fertility temporarily.

Efficacy: Limited evidence; used as an adjunct therapy.

Exercise and Regimens

Specific physical activities or postures post-coitus to prevent sperm migration (e.g., elevating pelvis in specific ways).

Efficacy: Anecdotal, low reliability.

Emergency Contraception in Unani Medicine

Unani texts describe post-coital remedies to prevent pregnancy, analogous to modern emergency contraception. Some of them are mentioned below.

1. Decoction of *Rue* (Ruta graveolens): Taken within 24–48 hours post-coitus to alter endometrial receptivity.
2. Tamarind Seed Paste: Applied vaginally or taken orally to disrupt implantation.
3. Myrrh and Alum Combination: Used as a pessary or oral remedy to prevent conception.

Proposed Mechanisms of Action

Unani contraceptive methods operate within the humoral framework:

Sperm Motility Inhibition: Herbs like neem or alum create a spermicidal effect or alter cervical mucus to block sperm penetration.

Endometrial Alteration: Cold and dry remedies (e.g., *khaksi*, myrrh) reduce uterine receptivity to implantation.

Humoral Modulation: Cooling or drying interventions counteract the hot and moist conditions needed for conception.

Physical Barriers: Pessaries and irrigation mechanically prevent sperm from reaching the ovum.

Clinical Considerations

Patient Assessment

Temperament Evaluation: Assess patient's mizaj (e.g., hot and moist, cold and dry) via pulse examination (*Moain-e-Nabdh*) and history to select compatible remedies. (https://pmc.ncbi.nlm.nih.gov/articles/PMC3038517/)

Humoral Status: Evaluate dominant humors (e.g., blood, phlegm) to tailor interventions.

Medical History: Screen for contraindications (e.g., pregnancy, liver disease, allergies).

Reproductive Goals: Confirm desire for temporary contraception; discuss reversibility.

Efficacy

Pharmacotherapy: Moderate efficacy based on traditional use; modern clinical trials are sparse.

Regimental Therapies: Low to moderate efficacy; withdrawal and pessaries are user-dependent.

Dietotherapy: Supportive, not primary; enhances other methods.

Emergency Methods: Limited data; likely less effective than modern EC (e.g., levonorgestrel, copper IUD).

Counseling

Informed Choice: Discuss efficacy, side effects, and need for adherence; clarify that Unani methods are complementary to modern options.

Cultural Sensitivity: Respect patient beliefs, especially in regions where Unani is widely practiced (e.g., India). (https://pmc.ncbi.nlm.nih.gov/articles/PMC4253292/)

Combination with Modern Methods: Advise integration with condoms or modern EC for higher efficacy and STI protection.

Follow-Up: Monitor for side effects, irregular bleeding, or pregnancy; advise pregnancy testing if menses delayed.

Side Effects and Safety

Herbal drugs: Potential for gastrointestinal upset, allergic reactions, or toxicity (e.g., rue in high doses).

Pessaries/Irrigation: Vaginal irritation, infections if non-sterile.

Correctives (*Muslehat*): Used to mitigate side effects (e.g., honey to counter alum's astringency). (https://www.ncbi.nlm.nih.gov/pmc/articles/PMC3038517/)

Pharmacovigilance: Limited modern data on safety; emphasize proper preparation and dosing per Unani formularies. (https://pmc.ncbi.nlm.nih.gov/articles/PMC3038517/)

Contraindications

Pregnancy (ineffective, potential fetal risk with some drugs).

Known allergies to herbal/mineral components.

Chronic conditions (e.g., liver disease, renal impairment) requiring careful remedy selection.

Breastfeeding (avoid potent herbs like rue; use safer options like neem).

Integration with Modern Contraception

Complementary Use: Unani methods can be combined with modern barrier methods (e.g., condoms) for enhanced efficacy and STI protection.

Limitations: Lower efficacy compared to modern hormonal methods (e.g., COCs, IUDs); advise patients seeking high reliability to consider modern options.

Conclusion

Contraception in the Unani system of medicine offers a unique, holistic approach rooted in humoral theory and natural remedies. While drug formulations, regimental therapies and dietary modifications provide culturally relevant options, their efficacy is less established compared to modern methods like hormonal contraceptives or IUDs. By combining traditional wisdom with scientific rigor, clinicians can offer personalized, culturally sensitive contraceptive care.

Key References

1. World Health Organization. (2020). Medical Eligibility Criteria for Contraceptive Use, 5th Edition.

   Central Council for Research in Unani Medicine (CCRUM). (2024). Unani Medicine Formularies. (https://ccrum.res.in/UserView/index?mid=1804)

2. Ansari, A. P., et al. (2017). Fundamentals of Unani System of Medicine – A Review. European Journal of Biomedical and Pharmaceutical Sciences. (https://www.researchgate.net/publication/321386220_FUNDAMENTALS_OF_UNANI_SYSTEM_OF_MEDICINE-A_REVIEW)

3. Ahmad, S., et al. (2019). Importance of Pharmacovigilance in Unani System of Medicine. PMC. [](https://pmc.ncbi.nlm.nih.gov/articles/PMC3038517/)
4. Bhat, S. A., Fatima, S., & Raza, A. (2020). A Handbook for Gynecology in Unani Medicine.[] (https://www.amazon.com/Handbook-Gynecology-Unani-Medicine/dp/8193563670)

Mechanism of Action of Contraceptive Methods

Barrier	**Hormonal**	**IUCD**	**Natural**
Blocks sperm	Inhibits ovulation	Prevents implantation	Avoids fertile window
Prevents entry	Alters cervical mucus	Foreign body reaction	Abstinence

15

Urogynecology

(Masalik-i-Bawliya nisayiyah)

15.1 *Ta'diya Majra-i-Bawl* (Urinary Tract Infection)
15.2 *Salas-al-bawl* (Incontinence)
15.3 *Mutalazima Waja'-i-Mathana* (Painful Bladder Syndrome)

Learning Objective (At the end of the session, the students should be able to)-

Describe and discuss the causes, diagnosis, complications and management of UTI.
Define Urinary Incontinence and explain its etiopathogenesis, types, diagnosis, management and complications .
Explain Painful Bladder Syndrome.

15.1 Urinary Tract Infection

(*Ta'diya Majra-i-Bawl*)

Definition

A urinary tract infection (UTI) is an infection involving any part of the urinary system, including the kidneys, ureters, bladder and urethra. UTIs are significant due to their high prevalence in women, association with pelvic anatomy and impact on reproductive health. UTIs are classified as:

Lower UTI: Involving the bladder (cystitis) or urethra (urethritis).

Upper UTI: Involving the kidneys (pyelonephritis) or ureters (ureteritis, rare).

Uncomplicated UTI: Occurs in healthy, non-pregnant women with a structurally and functionally normal urinary tract.

Complicated UTI: Occurs in patients with structural or functional abnormalities, pregnancy, diabetes, immunosuppression or male sex.

Epidemiology

Prevalence: UTIs are among the most common bacterial infections, affecting approximately 50–60% of women. Women are 50 times more likely to develop UTIs than men due to anatomical factors.

Age Distribution: Peak incidence occurs in women aged 18–24 years (sexually active) and post-menopause due to changes in vaginal flora and urogenital atrophy.

Recurrence: 20–30% of women with a UTI will experience recurrence within 6 months, with 3–5% developing recurrent UTIs (≥3 episodes per year).

UTIs are common differential diagnosis in women presenting with pelvic pain, dysuria or vaginal symptoms and they may complicate pregnancy or gynecological procedures.

Etiology

UTIs are primarily bacterial, though fungal and viral causes are rare. Common pathogens include:

Escherichia coli (E. coli): Accounts for 70–95% of uncomplicated UTIs. Originates from the gastrointestinal tract and ascends via the urethra.

Other Gram-Negative Bacteria: Klebsiella pneumoniae (5–10%), Proteus mirabilis (5%), Enterobacter spp., and Pseudomonas aeruginosa (more common in complicated UTIs).

Gram-Positive Bacteria: Staphylococcus saprophyticus (5–15%, common in young women), Enterococcus faecalis and Streptococcus agalactiae (Group B Streptococcus, significant in pregnancy).

Fungal Causes: Candida albicans (in catheterized or immunocompromised patients).

Viral Causes: Rare, e.g., adenovirus in immunocompromised patients.

Atypical Organisms: Ureaplasma urealyticum, Mycoplasma hominis (associated with urethritis).

Risk Factors

UTIs in women are influenced by anatomical, behavioral and physiological factors:

1. Anatomical

Short urethra (3-4 cm in women vs. 20 cm in men), facilitating bacterial ascent.

Proximity of the urethra to the anus, increasing risk of fecal contamination.

Urogenital atrophy in post-menopausal women reduces protective vaginal flora.

2. Behavioral

Sexual intercourse (increases bacterial introduction into the urethra).

Poor hygiene practices (e.g., wiping back-to-front).

Delayed voiding or incomplete bladder emptying.

Use of spermicides or diaphragms, which alter vaginal flora.

3. Physiological

Pregnancy (increased urinary stasis due to progesterone-induced ureteral dilation and uterine compression).

Estrogen deficiency in menopause, reducing lactobacilli and increasing vaginal pH.

Diabetes mellitus (glucosuria promotes bacterial growth).

4. Iatrogenic

Catheterization (introduces bacteria, common in hospitalized patients).

Gynecological procedures (e.g., hysterectomy, cystoscopy).

5. Genetic/Host Factors

Genetic predisposition

Immunosuppression or comorbidities.

Pathophysiology

UTIs typically result from the ascending spread of bacteria from the periurethral area to the bladder and in some cases, the kidneys. The process involves:

1. Colonization

Pathogens colonize the periurethral area, often from the gut flora.

Virulence factors (e.g., E. coli fimbriae) enable adhesion to uroepithelial cells.

2. Invasion

Bacteria ascend the urethra to the bladder, causing cystitis.

In severe cases, bacteria ascend the ureters to the kidneys, causing pyelonephritis.

3. Host Response

The urinary tract's natural defence include urinary flow, bladder emptying and antimicrobial peptides (e.g., defensins).

Inflammation triggered by bacterial invasion leads to symptoms like dysuria and urgency.

Inadequate host defences (e.g., low estrogen, urinary stasis) increase susceptibility.

4. Complications

Recurrent infections may lead to biofilm formation, particularly in catheter-associated UTIs.

Pyelonephritis can progress to sepsis or renal abscesses if untreated.

Clinical Features

Symptoms vary depending on the site of infection:

1. Cystitis (Lower UTI)

Dysuria (burning or pain during urination).

Increased urinary frequency and urgency.

Suprapubic pain or discomfort.

Cloudy or foul-smelling urine.

Hematuria (gross or microscopic, in 30–50% of cases).

Absence of fever or systemic symptoms in uncomplicated cases.

2. Pyelonephritis (Upper UTI)

Fever (>38°C), chills and rigors.

Flank pain or costovertebral angle tenderness.

Nausea, vomiting or generalized malaise.

Symptoms of cystitis may be present.

3. Urethritis

Dysuria and urethral discharge.

Often associated with sexually transmitted infections (e.g., Chlamydia trachomatis, Neisseria gonorrhoeae).

4. Asymptomatic Bacteriuria (ASB)

Positive urine culture (>10^5 CFU/mL) without symptoms.

Common in pregnancy and elderly women; treatment is indicated only in specific cases (e.g., pregnancy, prior to urologic procedures).

Diagnosis

Accurate diagnosis is critical to differentiate UTIs from other gynecological or urological conditions (e.g., vaginitis, interstitial cystitis).

1. History

Assess symptoms, duration and recurrence.

Identify risk factors (sexual activity, hygiene, pregnancy, menopause, catheter use).

Rule out differential diagnoses (e.g., vaginitis, pelvic inflammatory disease).

2. Physical Examination

Suprapubic tenderness in cystitis.

Costovertebral angle tenderness in pyelonephritis.

Pelvic examination to rule out gynecological causes (e.g., vaginitis, cervicitis).

3. Laboratory Tests

Urinalysis

Pyuria (>10 WBCs/HPF in unspun urine or >5 WBCs/HPF in spun urine).

Hematuria, nitrites (indicating E. coli or other nitrate-reducing bacteria), or leukocyte esterase.

pH >7 may suggest Proteus infection (urease-producing).

Urine Culture

Gold standard for diagnosis.

Significant bacteriuria: $\geq 10^5$ CFU/mL for uncomplicated UTI; $\geq 10^3$ CFU/mL in symptomatic patients or catheterized patients.

Identifies the pathogen and antibiotic sensitivity.

Blood Tests (for pyelonephritis or complicated UTI):

Complete blood count (leukocytosis).

C-reactive protein or erythrocyte sedimentation rate (elevated in systemic infection).

Blood cultures in suspected sepsis.

4. Imaging (indicated in complicated UTI or recurrent infections):

Ultrasound: To detect hydronephrosis, renal abscess or structural abnormalities.

CT scan: For suspected pyelonephritis complications (e.g., perinephric abscess).

Cystoscopy: In recurrent UTIs to evaluate for bladder abnormalities.

5. Differential Diagnosis

Vaginitis (e.g., Candida, bacterial vaginosis).

Sexually transmitted infections (e.g., chlamydia, gonorrhea).

Interstitial cystitis or overactive bladder.

Urethral syndrome or pelvic floor dysfunction.

Treatment

Treatment depends on the type of UTI, patient characteristics and local antibiotic resistance patterns.

1. Uncomplicated Cystitis

First-Line: Antibiotics (3–5 days)

Nitrofurantoin: 100 mg BID for 5 days (safe in pregnancy after first trimester).

Fosfomycin: 3 g single dose (effective for multidrug-resistant E. coli).

Trimethoprim-sulfamethoxazole (TMP-SMX): 160/800 mg BID for 3 days (avoid if resistance >20% or in pregnancy).

Second-Line: Fluoroquinolones (e.g., ciprofloxacin 250 mg BID for 3 days; reserved due to resistance and side effects). Beta-lactams (e.g., amoxicillin-clavulanate, cefuroxime for 5–7 days).

Supportive Measures

Increase fluid intake to promote diuresis.

Analgesics (e.g., phenazopyridine) for dysuria relief (use <48 hours due to side effects).

2. Uncomplicated Pyelonephritis

Outpatient (mild cases)

Ciprofloxacin 500 mg BID or levofloxacin 750 mg daily for 5–7 days.

TMP-SMX 160/800 mg BID for 14 days (if susceptible).

Inpatient (severe cases or pregnancy):

IV ceftriaxone 1–2 g daily or gentamicin (with monitoring for nephrotoxicity).

Transition to oral antibiotics once afebrile for 48 hours (total 10–14 days).

Supportive Care: IV fluids, antipyretics.

3. Complicated UTI

Treat for 7–14 days based on severity and underlying condition.

Broad-spectrum antibiotics (e.g., IV ceftriaxone, piperacillin-tazobactam) until culture results guide therapy.

Address underlying factors (e.g., remove catheters, correct anatomical abnormalities).

4. Asymptomatic Bacteriuria

Treatment is indicated in:

Pregnant women (to prevent pyelonephritis and preterm labor).

Patients undergoing urologic procedures.

Immunocompromised patients.

Use culture-guided antibiotics for 3–7 days.

5. Recurrent UTIs

Non-Antibiotic Prophylaxis

Cranberry products (reduce E. coli adhesion, evidence mixed).

Vaginal estrogen in postmenopausal women (restores lactobacilli, reduces vaginal pH).

Behavioral modifications (post-coital voiding, adequate hydration).

Antibiotic Prophylaxis

Continuous low-dose: Nitrofurantoin 50–100 mg daily or TMP-SMX 40/200 mg daily for 6–12 months.

Post-coital: Single-dose nitrofurantoin or TMP-SMX after intercourse.

6. Pregnancy

Screen for asymptomatic bacteriuria at 12–16 weeks gestation.

Avoid fluoroquinolones and TMP-SMX in the first trimester.

Preferred agents: Nitrofurantoin, amoxicillin or cephalosporins.

Treat pyelonephritis aggressively to prevent maternal and fetal complications.

Complications

Acute: Sepsis, renal abscess, perinephric abscess or papillary necrosis.

Chronic: Recurrent UTIs, chronic kidney disease (rare) or antimicrobial resistance.

Pregnancy: Preterm labor, low birth weight or maternal sepsis.

Prevention

1. Lifestyle Modifications

Adequate hydration (2–3 L/day).

Regular and complete bladder emptying.

Post-coital voiding to flush bacteria.

Avoid spermicides or diaphragms in women prone to UTIs.

Proper perineal hygiene (wipe front-to-back).

2. Medical Interventions

Vaginal estrogen therapy in postmenopausal women.

Prophylactic antibiotics for recurrent UTIs.

Vaccination (e.g., investigational E. coli vaccines, not yet widely available).

3. Catheter Care

Minimize catheter use and duration.

Use aseptic insertion techniques and closed drainage systems.

Vaginal Flora: Estrogen promotes lactobacilli, which produce lactic acid and maintain low vaginal pH, inhibiting uropathogen growth. Menopause or hormonal contraception may disrupt this balance.

Pregnancy: Increased risk due to urinary stasis and glucosuria. UTIs in pregnancy require prompt treatment to prevent adverse outcomes.

Gynecological Procedures: Procedures like hysterectomy or sling placement increase UTI risk due to catheterization or tissue trauma.

Differential Diagnosis

UTIs must be distinguished from vaginitis, cervicitis or pelvic inflammatory disease, as symptoms overlap (e.g., dysuria, pelvic discomfort).

Conclusion

UTIs are a cornerstone of gynecological practice due to their prevalence and impact on women's health. Understanding their etiology, risk factors and management is essential for gynecologist. Prompt diagnosis, appropriate antibiotic therapy and preventive strategies planned according to the patient's risk profile are critical to reducing morbidity and preventing complications, particularly in high-risk groups such as pregnant or postmenopausal women.

Definitions

UTI (Urinary Tract Infection) ➤ Infection of urinary tract, commonly by E. coli; presents with dysuria, frequency, urgency.

Stress Incontinence ➤ Leakage of urine during physical exertion due to pelvic floor weakness.

Urge Incontinence ➤ Sudden, intense urge to urinate followed by involuntary leakage; often due to detrusor overactivity.

Painful Bladder Syndrome (PBS) ➤ Chronic pelvic pain with urinary urgency/frequency; also called interstitial cystitis.

Uterine Prolapse ➤ Descent of uterus into or beyond vaginal canal due to pelvic support failure.

Types of Urinary Incontinence **Mnemonic: "SUOFM" (Stress, Urge, Overflow, Functional, Mixed)**			
S	Stress	Leakage on coughing/sneezing	Weak pelvic floor muscles
U	Urge	Sudden urge + involuntary leakage	Detrusor overactivity
O	Overflow	Dribbling + incomplete emptying	Bladder outlet obstruction
F	Functional	Normal bladder, but can't reach toilet	Cognitive/mobility impairment
M	Mixed	Combo of stress + urge symptoms	Multiple contributing factors

15.2 Incontinences

(*Salas-al-bawl*)

Definition

Urinary incontinence (UI) is the involuntary loss of urine, resulting in social or hygienic problems. It is a common condition in women, significantly impacting quality of life and is an important topic in gynecology due to its association with pelvic floor disorders, pregnancy, childbirth and menopause. UI is classified into several types based on pathophysiology and clinical presentation:

1. Stress Urinary Incontinence (SUI): Urine leakage due to increased intra-abdominal pressure (e.g., coughing, sneezing, exercise).
2. Urge Urinary Incontinence (UUI): Urine leakage associated with a sudden, uncontrollable urge to void, often linked to detrusor overactivity.
3. Mixed Urinary Incontinence (MUI): Combination of SUI and UUI symptoms.
4. Overflow Incontinence: Leakage due to incomplete bladder emptying, often from bladder outlet obstruction or detrusor underactivity.
5. Functional Incontinence: Leakage due to physical or cognitive impairments preventing timely voiding (e.g., mobility issues, dementia).
6. Other Types: Transient incontinence (reversible causes like infection or medication) and continuous incontinence (e.g., due to fistulae).

Epidemiology

Prevalence: UI affects 25–45% of women, with prevalence increasing with age. Approximately 10–20% of women under 65 and 35–50% over 65 experience UI.

Types: SUI is the most common type in younger women (50–70% of cases), while UUI and MUI predominate in older women.

UI is frequently encountered in gynecology due to its association with pregnancy, childbirth, pelvic floor trauma and menopausal changes.

Risk Factors: Childbirth (especially vaginal delivery), obesity, menopause, pelvic surgery and aging significantly increase risk.

Etiology and Risk Factors

UI results from a complex interplay of anatomical, physiological and lifestyle factors, particularly those affecting the pelvic floor and lower urinary tract.

1. Anatomical Factors

Pelvic Floor Muscle Weakness: Damage to levator ani muscles or connective tissues from childbirth or aging reduces urethral support.

Urethral Hypermobility: Weakened pelvic support allows the urethra to descend during increased intra-abdominal pressure, leading to SUI.

Intrinsic Sphincter Deficiency (ISD): Impaired urethral sphincter function, often due to surgery, trauma or neurological conditions, contributes to SUI.

Bladder Neck Dysfunction: Impaired closure mechanisms exacerbate leakage.

2. Physiological Factors

Detrusor Overactivity: Involuntary bladder contractions cause UUI, often idiopathic or associated with neurological disorders (e.g., stroke, Parkinson's).

Detrusor Underactivity: Reduced bladder contractility leads to overflow incontinence, common in diabetes or spinal cord injury.

Estrogen Deficiency: Post-menopausal hypoestrogenism weakens pelvic tissues and reduces urethral mucosal coaptation, increasing UI risk.

3. Gynecological and Obstetric Factors

Pregnancy and Childbirth: Vaginal delivery, especially with prolonged labor, forceps or episiotomy, damages pelvic floor muscles and nerves.

Pelvic Organ Prolapse (POP): Prolapse of the bladder (cystocele) or uterus can distort anatomy, contributing to SUI or overflow incontinence.

Surgery: Hysterectomy or pelvic reconstructive surgery may disrupt pelvic floor innervation or support structures.

4. Lifestyle and Other Factors

Obesity (increases intra-abdominal pressure).

Chronic cough (e.g., from smoking or COPD).

Constipation (straining weakens pelvic floor).

Medications (e.g., diuretics, alpha-blockers, sedatives).

Neurological disorders (e.g., multiple sclerosis, spinal cord injury).

Genetic predisposition (e.g., collagen disorders like Ehlers-Danlos syndrome).

Pathophysiology

UI arises from dysfunction in the bladder, urethra, pelvic floor or neurological control mechanisms:

1. Stress Urinary Incontinence

Increased intra-abdominal pressure exceeds urethral closure pressure due to weakened pelvic floor support or intrinsic sphincter deficiency.

Urethral hypermobility or loss of mucosal coaptation (due to low estrogen) reduces resistance to leakage.

2. Urge Urinary Incontinence

Detrusor overactivity causes involuntary bladder contractions, triggered by sensory input or neurological dysfunction.

Common causes include idiopathic detrusor instability, neurogenic conditions or bladder irritants (e.g., infection, stones).

3. Overflow Incontinence

Bladder overdistension from outlet obstruction (e.g., prolapse, stricture) or detrusor underactivity leads to leakage of small volumes.

4. Functional Incontinence

Physical or cognitive limitations prevent timely voiding, despite normal bladder function.

5. Gynecological factor

Childbirth-related nerve damage (e.g., pudendal nerve) impairs pelvic floor and sphincter function.

Estrogen deficiency in menopause reduces vascularity and elasticity of urogenital tissues, exacerbating SUI and UUI.

Clinical Features

Symptoms vary by type of incontinence:

1. Stress Urinary Incontinence

Leakage during activities that increase intra-abdominal pressure (e.g., coughing, sneezing, laughing, exercise). Small to moderate volume loss. No urgency or nocturia (unless mixed with UUI).

2. Urge Urinary Incontinence

Sudden, intense urge to urinate followed by involuntary leakage. Frequent urination (>8 times/day), nocturia and large-volume loss. May be triggered by running water, cold or stress.

3. Mixed Incontinence

Combination of SUI and UUI symptoms, often with one predominating.

4. Overflow Incontinence

Frequent or constant dribbling, weak stream or sensation of incomplete emptying. Associated with pelvic organ prolapse or neurological conditions.

5. Functional Incontinence

Leakage due to inability to reach the toilet in time (e.g., arthritis, dementia).

6. Associated Symptoms

Pelvic pressure or pain (if prolapse present). Recurrent UTIs (due to incomplete emptying). Impact on quality of life (e.g., social withdrawal, depression).

Diagnosis

Accurate diagnosis requires a systematic approach to identify the type of UI and underlying causes.

1. History

Symptom Assessment: Type, frequency, volume and triggers of leakage (e.g., cough for SUI, urgency for UUI).

Voiding Diary: Record fluid intake, urination frequency and leakage episodes over 3–7 days.

Obstetric History: Number of deliveries, mode (vaginal vs. cesarean), complications (e.g., forceps, tears).

Medical History: Neurological disorders, diabetes, medications or prior pelvic surgery.

Quality of Life: Impact on daily activities, sexual function or mental health.

2. Physical Examination

General: Assess mobility, cognition and BMI.

Pelvic Examination

Evaluate for pelvic organ prolapse (using POP-Q system).

Assess pelvic floor muscle strength (e.g., Oxford scale 0–5).

Check for vaginal atrophy or masses.

Stress Test: Observe leakage with coughing or Valsalva (full bladder).

Neurological Exam: Assess sacral reflexes (e.g., bulbocavernosus reflex) for neurogenic causes.

3. Laboratory Tests

Urinalysis: Rule out infection, hematuria or glucosuria.

Urine Culture: If infection suspected.

Post-Void Residual (PVR): Measure via ultrasound or catheterization (<50 mL normal; >200 mL suggests overflow).

4. Urodynamic Testing (indicated for complex or refractory cases):

Cystometry: Assesses bladder pressure, capacity and detrusor activity.

Uroflowmetry: Measures flow rate and voiding patterns.

Urethral pressure profilometry: Evaluates sphincter function (for ISD).

Electromyography: Assesses pelvic floor muscle activity.

5. Imaging

Ultrasound: To assess bladder, kidneys or prolapse.

Cystoscopy: To rule out bladder lesions or fistulae.

MRI/CT: For suspected neurological or structural abnormalities.

6. Differential Diagnosis

Urinary tract infection (UTI).

Pelvic organ prolapse or gynecological masses.

Vesicovaginal or ureterovaginal fistula (post-surgical or obstetric).

Interstitial cystitis or bladder malignancy.

Overactive bladder (OAB) without incontinence.

Treatment

Treatment is planned according to the type of UI, severity and patient preferences, with a stepwise approach from conservative to surgical options.

1. Conservative Management

Lifestyle Modifications

Weight loss (reduces intra-abdominal pressure).

Fluid management (avoid excessive intake, limit bladder irritants like caffeine).

Smoking cessation and treatment of chronic cough.

Timed voiding or bladder training (gradual increase in voiding intervals).

Pelvic Floor Muscle Training (PFMT)

Kegel exercises to strengthen pelvic floor (effective for SUI and MUI).

Supervised by physiotherapist for optimal outcomes (8–12 weeks).

Biofeedback or Electrical Stimulation: Enhances PFMT efficacy in patients with weak pelvic muscles.

Vaginal Estrogen: Improves urogenital atrophy in postmenopausal women, reducing SUI and UUI symptoms.

2. Pharmacological Therapy

Urge Urinary Incontinence

Anticholinergics: Oxybutynin (2.5–5 mg BID), tolterodine (1–2 mg BID). Side effects: dry mouth, constipation, cognitive impairment.

Beta-3 Agonists: Mirabegron (25–50 mg daily), fewer side effects, improves detrusor relaxation.

Tricyclic Antidepressants: Imipramine (10–25 mg at night) for mixed UI (rarely used due to side effects).

Stress Urinary Incontinence

Limited pharmacological options; duloxetine (SNRI, 20–40 mg BID) may improve sphincter tone but is not FDA-approved for SUI.

Transient Incontinence: Treat underlying causes (e.g., antibiotics for UTI, adjust medications).

3. Minimally Invasive Interventions

SUI: Urethral Bulking Agents: Injection of collagen or synthetic materials to enhance urethral closure (temporary, less effective than surgery).

Pessaries: Support pelvic organs in women with prolapse-related SUI.

UUI: Intravesical Botulinum Toxin A: Inhibits detrusor overactivity (for refractory UUI). Requires repeat injections every 6–12 months.

Sacral Neuromodulation: Implanted device modulates bladder nerve activity (for refractory UUI or MUI).

Percutaneous Tibial Nerve Stimulation (PTNS): Non-invasive nerve stimulation for UUI.

4. Surgical Management

SUI: Midurethral Sling: Synthetic mesh (e.g., tension-free vaginal tape, TVT) is gold standard (90–95% success rate). Complications: mesh erosion, voiding dysfunction.

Colposuspension: Burch procedure (open or laparoscopic) elevates bladder neck (used if mesh contraindicated).

Autologous Fascial Sling: For severe ISD or failed mesh surgery.

UUI: Augmentation Cystoplasty: Increases bladder capacity (rare, for severe refractory cases).

Overflow Incontinence

Address outlet obstruction (e.g., prolapse repair, urethrolysis).

Fistulae: Surgical repair (e.g., vesicovaginal fistula repair).

5. Gynecological Causes

Treat concurrent prolapse with procedures like anterior colporrhaphy or sacrocolpopexy.

Avoid unnecessary hysterectomy unless uterine pathology is present.

Pregnancy-related UI often resolves postpartum; PFMT is first-line during pregnancy.

Complications

Physical: Recurrent UTIs, skin irritation or pressure ulcers from chronic leakage.

Psychosocial: Depression, anxiety, social isolation or sexual dysfunction.

Surgical: Mesh complications (erosion, pain), voiding dysfunction or recurrence of incontinence.

Prevention

1. Lifestyle Modifications

Maintain healthy weight (BMI <30).

Avoid bladder irritants (caffeine, alcohol, spicy foods).

Regular pelvic floor exercises, especially post-childbirth.

2. Obstetric Care

Minimize pelvic floor trauma during vaginal delivery (e.g., avoid prolonged second stage, judicious use of forceps).

Encourage PFMT during and after pregnancy.

3. Menopause Management

Vaginal estrogen to maintain urogenital health.

Regular screening for prolapse or atrophy.

4. Screening and Education

Educate women on UI risk factors and early intervention.

Screen high-risk groups (postpartum, postmenopausal, obese women).

Special cases

Pregnancy and Postpartum: UI is common (30–50% during pregnancy), particularly SUI due to increased intra-abdominal pressure and pelvic floor strain. Most cases resolve within 6–12 months postpartum, but persistent UI requires evaluation.

Pelvic Organ Prolapse: Often coexists with SUI or overflow incontinence; addressing prolapse may resolve UI.

Menopause: Estrogen deficiency exacerbates UI; vaginal estrogen is a key adjunctive therapy.

Surgery: Procedures like hysterectomy or prolapse repair may aggravate or worsen UI, necessitating preoperative urodynamic evaluation.

Sexual Function: UI during intercourse (coital incontinence) is often SUI; treatment improves sexual quality of life.

Conclusion

Urinary incontinence is a prevalent condition in women, with significant gynecological implications due to its association with pelvic floor disorders, childbirth and menopause. Diagnosis involves a detailed history, physical examination and selective use of urodynamic testing. Treatment ranges from conservative measures (PFMT, lifestyle changes) to pharmacological and surgical interventions, according to the patient's needs and UI type. Preventive strategies and patient education are needed to reduce the burden of UI and improving quality of life.

Condition	**Management Strategy**
UTI	Antibiotics + hydration
Stress Incontinence	Pelvic floor exercises, surgery (sling)
Urge Incontinence	Anticholinergics, bladder training
Uterine Prolapse	Pessary, pelvic exercises, surgery
PBS	Diet changes, bladder instillation, pain control

15.3 Painful Bladder Syndrome

(*Mutalazima Waja'-i-Mathana*)

Definition

Painful Bladder Syndrome (PBS), often referred to as Interstitial Cystitis (IC), is a chronic condition characterized by bladder pain, pressure or discomfort associated with urinary symptoms (e.g., urgency, frequency) in the absence of infection or other identifiable causes. The term PBS/IC is used interchangeably, with IC often reserved for cases with specific cystoscopic or histological findings (e.g., Hunner's lesions). PBS/IC significantly impacts quality of life and is an important differential diagnosis in gynecology due to overlapping of symptoms with other pelvic disorders.

Epidemiology

Prevalence: Affects 2–7% of women, with a female-to-male ratio of approximately 5:1. Prevalence varies due to diagnostic challenges and underreporting.

Age: Peak onset is 30–50 years, though it can occur in adolescents and postmenopausal women.

Gynecological Relevance: PBS/IC is frequently encountered in gynecology due to its overlap with conditions like endometriosis, vulvodynia and pelvic floor dysfunction.

Comorbidities: Associated with fibromyalgia, irritable bowel syndrome (IBS), chronic fatigue syndrome and autoimmune disorders (e.g., lupus, Sjogren's syndrome).

Etiology and Risk Factors

The exact etiology of PBS/IC remains unclear, but it is likely multifactorial, involving bladder, pelvic and systemic factors. Proposed contributors include:

1. Bladder Factors

Urothelial Dysfunction: Defective glycosaminoglycan (GAG) layer allows urinary solutes (e.g., potassium) to penetrate the bladder wall, causing irritation and inflammation.

Mast Cell Activation: Increased mast cell degranulation in the bladder wall releases histamine and cytokines, contributing to pain and inflammation.

Neurogenic Inflammation: Hypersensitivity of bladder sensory nerves amplifies pain perception.

2. Pelvic Factors

Pelvic floor dysfunction or hypertonic pelvic floor muscles exacerbate symptoms.

Cross-sensitization with other pelvic organs (e.g., uterus, vagina) due to shared neural pathways.

3. Systemic Factors

Autoimmune or inflammatory dysregulation (e.g., association with lupus or allergies).

Central sensitization, leading to amplified pain perception (common in chronic pain syndromes).

4. Risk Factors

Gender: Higher prevalence in women, possibly due to hormonal or anatomical factors.

Prior Pelvic Trauma: Childbirth, pelvic surgery or recurrent urinary tract infections (UTIs).

Hormonal Influence: Symptoms may worsen with menstrual cycle or menopause, suggesting estrogen's role.

Psychosocial Stress: Stress and anxiety may exacerbate symptoms via neurogenic pathways.

Genetic Predisposition: Family history of PBS/IC or related pain syndromes.

Pathophysiology

PBS/IC involves a complex interplay of bladder, neurological and immune mechanisms:

1. Bladder Wall Abnormalities

Disruption of the GAG layer, a protective mucin coating, allows urinary irritants to penetrate the urothelium, triggering inflammation and pain.

Increased mast cell activity and release of inflammatory mediators (e.g., histamine, nerve growth factor) contribute to chronic inflammation.

In severe cases (classic IC), Hunner's lesions (ulcerative patches) or glomerulations (petechial hemorrhages) are seen on cystoscopy.

2. Neurogenic Mechanisms

Sensitization of bladder afferent nerves (C-fibers) leads to pain and urgency.

Adjacent bladder and pelvic nerves may cause referred pain to the pelvis, vagina or lower abdomen.

3. Pelvic Floor Dysfunction

Hypertonic pelvic floor muscles or myofascial trigger points amplify pain and urinary symptoms.

4. Central Sensitization

Chronic pain leads to altered pain processing in the central nervous system, increasing symptom severity.

5. Gynecological Causes

Shared innervation (e.g., pudendal nerve) and visceral cross-sensitization link PBS/IC with gynecological conditions like endometriosis or vulvodynia.

Estrogen deficiency may exacerbate urothelial thinning and sensory nerve hypersensitivity.

Clinical Features

PBS/IC presents with a spectrum of symptoms, often fluctuating in severity:

1. Bladder Symptoms

Pain or Discomfort: Suprapubic or pelvic pain, pressure or burning, often worse with bladder filling and relieved by voiding.

Urgency and Frequency: Urination >8 times/day, nocturia (≥2 times/night) and small-volume voids (50–200 mL).

Dysuria: Burning or pain during urination, mimicking UTI but without infection.

2. Pelvic Symptoms

Pain radiating to the vagina, urethra or lower back.

Dyspareunia (painful intercourse), particularly with a full bladder.

Symptoms may worsen premenstrually or with stress.

3. Associated Symptoms

Fatigue, depression or anxiety due to chronic pain and sleep disruption.

Gastrointestinal symptoms (e.g., IBS-like complaints).

Myofascial pain or pelvic floor tenderness.

4. Subtypes

Ulcerative IC: Presence of Hunner's lesions, seen in 5–10% of cases, associated with severe symptoms.

Non-Ulcerative PBS/IC: More common, with normal or subtle cystoscopic findings (e.g., glomerulations).

5. Gynecological symptoms

Symptoms mimic endometriosis, vulvodynia or chronic pelvic pain, requiring careful differentiation. Exacerbation during menstruation or menopause suggests hormonal influence.

Diagnosis

Diagnosing PBS/IC is challenging due to its variable presentation and lack of definitive biomarkers. It is primarily a diagnosis of exclusion, requiring a systematic approach.

1. History

Symptom Assessment: Chronic (>6 weeks) bladder pain, urgency, frequency or nocturia.

Voiding Diary: Documents frequency, volume and pain episodes over 3–7 days.

Medical History: Rule out prior UTIs, pelvic surgery, endometriosis or neurological disorders.

Gynecological History: Menstrual cycle patterns, obstetric history or menopausal status.

Psychosocial Factors: Assess stress, anxiety or impact on quality of life.

2. Physical Examination

Pelvic Examination: Assess for vaginal atrophy, pelvic floor tenderness or trigger points.

Bladder Palpation: Suprapubic tenderness suggests bladder involvement.

Neurological Exam: Evaluate for sacral nerve dysfunction or central neurological conditions.

3. Laboratory Tests

Urinalysis and Culture: Rule out infection (sterile pyuria may be present in PBS/IC).

Urine Cytology: If hematuria or risk factors for bladder cancer present (e.g., smoking, age >50).

Potassium Sensitivity Test: Instillation of potassium chloride into the bladder to provoke pain (as a part of study, not routine).

4. Cystoscopy

Indicated in suspected IC to identify Hunner's lesions or glomerulations.

Hydrodistension (filling bladder under anesthesia) may reveal reduced bladder capacity or petechial bleeding.

Not required for PBS diagnosis if other criteria are met.

5. Urodynamic Testing (select cases):

Assesses bladder capacity, detrusor overactivity or compliance.

Typically shows low bladder capacity (<300 mL) and pain with filling.

6. Imaging

Pelvic ultrasound or MRI to rule out structural causes (e.g., masses, prolapse).

Rarely needed, unless gynecological or urological pathology suspected.

7. Differential Diagnosis

Urological: UTI, bladder cancer, overactive bladder or urolithiasis.

Gynecological: Endometriosis, adenomyosis, vulvodynia or pelvic inflammatory disease.

Neurological: Multiple sclerosis, spinal cord injury.

Other: Chronic pelvic pain syndrome, irritable bowel syndrome.

8. Diagnostic Criteria (e.g., American Urological Association, European Society for the Study of IC):

Chronic pelvic pain, pressure or discomfort perceived to be related to the bladder, with at least one urinary symptom (urgency or frequency).

Exclusion of infection, malignancy or other identifiable causes.

Optional: Cystoscopic findings (Hunner's lesions for IC).

Treatment

PBS/IC treatment is multidisciplinary, individualized and often requires a trial-and-error approach due to variable response. Goals are symptom relief and improved quality of life.

1. Conservative Management

Lifestyle Modifications

Dietary changes: Avoid bladder irritants (e.g., caffeine, alcohol, spicy foods, acidic foods).

Fluid management: Balance hydration to avoid concentrated urine without exacerbating frequency.

Stress management: Cognitive-behavioral therapy (CBT) or relaxation techniques.

Pelvic Floor Physical Therapy

Treats hypertonic pelvic floor muscles with myofascial release, biofeedback or manual therapy.

Improves pain and urinary symptoms in 60–80% of patients.

Bladder Training

Timed voiding to increase bladder capacity and reduce urgency.

2. Pharmacological Therapy

Oral Medications

Pentosan Polysulfate Sodium (PPS): Only FDA-approved drug for IC (100 mg TID). Restores GAG layer; efficacy modest (20–40% response rate).

Amitriptyline: Tricyclic antidepressant (10–75 mg at night). Reduces pain and urgency via antihistaminic and anticholinergic effects.

Antihistamines: Hydroxyzine (25–50 mg at night) reduces mast cell activity.

Anticholinergics or Beta-3 Agonists: For urgency/frequency (e.g., oxybutynin, mirabegron), though less effective in PBS/IC.

Analgesics: NSAIDs or gabapentinoids (e.g., gabapentin, pregabalin) for pain management.

Intravesical Therapy

Dimethyl Sulfoxide (DMSO): Instilled weekly for 6–8 weeks; reduces inflammation and pain.

Heparin or Lidocaine: Intravesical instillation to restore GAG layer or provide local anesthesia.

Hyaluronic Acid or Chondroitin Sulfate: Agents to repair urothelium.

3. Minimally Invasive Interventions

Cystoscopy with Hydrodistension: Therapeutic in some patients (temporary relief, 6–12 months).

Botulinum Toxin A: Intravesical injection to reduce detrusor overactivity and pain (refractory cases).

Sacral Neuromodulation: Modulates bladder nerve activity for refractory urgency and pain.

4. Surgical Management (rare, for severe refractory cases):

Fulguration or Resection of Hunner's Lesions: For ulcerative IC, improves symptoms in 80–90% of cases.

Augmentation Cystoplasty: Increases bladder capacity (rare due to high morbidity).

Urinary Diversion: Last resort for intractable cases, with or without cystectomy.

5. Gynecological diseases

Local Estrogen: Improves urogenital atrophy in postmenopausal women, reducing irritation.

Endometriosis Evaluation: Laparoscopy, if endometriosis suspected, as it may coexist with PBS/IC.

Pelvic Floor Therapy: In women with dyspareunia or pelvic floor dysfunction.

Hormonal Influence: Symptoms may improve with menstrual cycle regulation or estrogen therapy.

6. Psychosocial Support

CBT or counseling to address depression, anxiety or sexual dysfunction.

Support groups (e.g., Interstitial Cystitis Association) improve coping and quality of life.

Complications

Physical: Chronic pain, recurrent UTIs, reduced bladder capacity or hydronephrosis (rare).

Psychosocial: Depression, social isolation, sexual dysfunction or reduced quality of life.

Iatrogenic: Medication side effects (e.g., PPS-associated maculopathy), surgical complications.

Prevention

Early Intervention: Prompt treatment of recurrent UTIs or pelvic trauma to prevent chronic sensitization.

Lifestyle: Avoid bladder irritants, maintain healthy pelvic floor function and manage stress.

Gynecological Care: Regular screening for urogenital atrophy or pelvic floor dysfunction in high-risk groups (e.g., postmenopausal, postpartum women).

Patient Education: Empower patients to recognize triggers and seek multidisciplinary care.

Specific Cases

Overlap with Pelvic Pain Disorders: PBS/IC mimics endometriosis, vulvodynia or chronic pelvic pain, necessitating a thorough gynecological evaluation.

Hormonal Influence: Estrogen deficiency exacerbates symptoms; vaginal estrogen is a key adjunctive therapy.

Childbirth and Pelvic Trauma: Vaginal delivery or pelvic surgery may trigger or worsen PBS/IC.

Sexual Dysfunction: Dyspareunia is common; treatment of PBS/IC and pelvic floor dysfunction improves sexual health.

Pregnancy: Symptoms may improve or worsen; avoid certain medications (e.g., PPS) in pregnancy.

Conclusion

Painful Bladder Syndrome/Interstitial Cystitis is a complex, chronic condition with significant gynecological implications due to its symptoms overlapping with pelvic pain disorders and hormonal imbalances. Diagnosis requires careful exclusion of other causes, with cystoscopy reserved for suspected IC. Management is multidisciplinary, combining lifestyle changes, pelvic floor therapy, pharmacological agents and in severe cases, surgical interventions.

Long Answer Questions

1. Define urinary tract infection (UTI) and describe its types, symptoms and management.
2. Discuss urinary incontinence—classification, causes and therapeutic options.
3. Explain painful bladder syndrome (PBS)/interstitial cystitis—pathophysiology, diagnosis and treatment.
4. Describe uterine prolapse—etiology, grading, symptoms and surgical management.
5. Elaborate on the role of pelvic floor muscles in urogynecological disorders.

Short Answer Questions

1. What is stress urinary incontinence?
2. Name two common pathogens causing UTI.
3. Define interstitial cystitis.
4. Mention one symptom of uterine prolapse.
5. What is the role of Kegel exercises?

Multiple Choice Questions (1 Mark Each)

1. Most common cause of UTI in women:

a) E. coli b) Candida c) Chlamydia d) Gonorrhea

Ans: a) E. coli

2. Stress urinary incontinence occurs due to:
a) Overactive bladder b) Weak pelvic floor c) UTI d) Neuropathy
Ans: b) Weak pelvic floor

3. Painful bladder syndrome is also called:
a) Cystitis b) Interstitial cystitis c) Pyelonephritis d) Urethritis
Ans: b) Interstitial cystitis

4. Uterine prolapse is graded based on:
a) Cervical length b) Descent of uterus c) Menstrual history d) Vaginal depth
Ans: b) Descent of uterus

5. Which test confirms UTI diagnosis?
a) Pap smear b) Urine culture c) USG pelvis d) Wet mount
Ans: b) Urine culture

6. Which therapy is used for urge incontinence?
a) Antibiotics b) Anticholinergics c) Estrogen d) NSAIDs
Ans: b) Anticholinergics

7. Pelvic organ prolapse may cause:
a) Amenorrhea b) Dyspareunia c) Vaginal dryness d) Menorrhagia
Ans: b) Dyspareunia

8. Which exercise strengthens pelvic floor muscles?
a) Squats b) Kegel c) Lunges d) Sit-ups
Ans: b) Kegel

9. Interstitial cystitis presents with:
a) Fever b) Hematuria c) Pelvic pain d) Vaginal discharge
Ans: c) Pelvic pain

10. Which device is used to support prolapsed uterus non-surgically?
a) IUCD b) Pessary c) Catheter d) Diaphragm
Ans: b) Pessary

16

Diagnostic & Therapeutic Procedures

(Tashkhisi wa Mualajati Amaliyat)

16.1 *Amrad-i Niswan wa Ilm-al-Qabalat mein mustamal Ilaj bi'l-Tadbir ke mukhtalif tariqe* (Various *Ilaj bit Tadbeer* methods uses in Gynecology & Obstetrics)
16.2 *Amaliyat-i-Tasfiya* (*Silar ka kashifa, Mas-ha mahbileya Aaliya)* (Screening Procedures: (VIA, Schiller's, High vaginal Swab)
16.3 *Imtehan-i-Khlawi* (Cytological Examinations: Pap smear *kashifah* (Pap's Smear test)
16.4 *Jarahat-i-tabridiya* (Cryosurgery)
16.5 Hormone *ki janch* (Hormone Assay)
16.6 *Amrad-i-Niswan me shuaayi tasveerkashi* (Imaging Techniques in Gynaecology)
16.7 *Imtehan-i-Nasij-i-Maradi* (Histopathological Examinations: Cervical & Endometrial Biopsy)
16.8 *Ittisa wa ijteraaf* (Dilatation & Curettage)
16.9 *Ambuba nigari Rahim* (Hysterosalpingography)
16.10Ambuba nigari (Sonosalpingography)
16.11Batn beeni hamrah rang beeni (Laparoscopy with Dye instillations)
16.12Tanzeer-ul-mahbil aur tanzeeeru-r-rahim (Colposcopy & Hysteroscopy)
16.13Tanzeer-al-Batn (Laparoscopy)
16.14Hawai amboob nigari (Tubal Insufflation Test)
16.15Shigaf-i-batn (Laparotomy)
16.16Shigaf-i-rahim (Hysterotomy)
16.17Sal'a 'Adali Lifi barari (Myomectomy)
16.18Rahim barari (Hysterectomy)

Learning Objective (At the end of the session, the students should be able to)-

Demonstrate the steps of aseptic precautions & interpret the diagnostic procedure.
Explore various *Ilaj bit Tadbeer* methods used in Gynecology & Obstetrics .
Describe VIA, schiller's, High Vaginal swab & demonstrate the Screening Procedures.
Describe *Imtihaan–e-Khalvi* (Pap's smear Test) & demonstrate the procedure of screening for cervical cancer.
Explain & interpret the Hormone Assay.
Explore the procedures of imaging techniques in Gynaecology & Obstetrics.
Explain *Imtihaan-e-Naseej-e-Marzi* (Histopathological Examinations: Cervical & Endometrial Biopsy).
Observe & assist procedure of Dilatation & Curettage and Dilatation & Evacuation.
Explain proper wound care including cleaning, dressing & packing and Demonstrate the steps of I&D.
Observe and describe the procedure of Cryosurgery.
Explain *Ambubi-Rahim Nigari* (Hysterosalpingography & Sonosalpingography).
Explain *Tanzeerul Mahbil wa Rahim, Tanzeer ul Batan & Batan Beeni Hamrah Rangbeeni* (Colposcopy & Hysteroscopy, Laparoscopy & Laparoscopy with Dye Instillations).
Explain *Hawai Amboob Nigari* (Tubal Insufflation Test).
Explain *Shigaf-e-Batan* (Laparotomy), *Shigaaf-e-Rahim* (Hysterotomy), *Salaa Azli Leefi Barari* (Myomectomy) & *Rahim Barari* (Hysterectomy).

16.1 *Amrad-i Niswan* wa *Ilm al-Qabalat* mien mustamal *Ilaj bi'l-Tadbir* ke mukhtalif tariqe

(Various *Ilaj bit Tadbeer* methods uses in Gynecology & Obstetrics)

Introduction to *Ilaj-bil-Tadbeer*

Ilaj-bil-Tadbeer, or regimental therapy, is one of the therapy or methods of the Unani system of medicine, focusing on non-pharmacological interventions to restore health by correcting imbalances in the body's humors (*Akhlat*) and temperament (*Mizaj*). Derived from the Arabic term "*Tadbeer*" (management or regimen), it encompasses a range of therapeutic modalities aimed at eliminating morbid humors, strengthening vital faculties (*Quwa*), and maintaining the six essential factors (*Asbab-e-Sittah Zaruriyyah*) of health: air, food and drink, bodily movement and repose, mental work and rest, sleep and wakefulness and retention and excretion.

Principles of *Ilaj-bil-Tadbeer*

Unani medicine views gynecological diseases as resulting from imbalances in the four humors (blood, phlegm, yellow bile, black bile) or abnormal temperament of the uterus (*Su'-i-Mizaj Rahim*), which is naturally cold and moist. *Ilaj-bil-Tadbeer* aims to:

1. Eliminate Morbid Humors (*Tanqiya*): Remove excess or pathological humors causing disease (e.g., phlegm in amenorrhea, blood in menorrhagia).
2. Correct Temperament (*Tadil-e-Mizaj*): Restore the uterus's balanced temperament using therapies with opposite qualities (*Ilaj-bil-Zid*).
3. Strengthen Uterine Faculties: Enhance the digestive (*Hadima*), retentive (*Masika*) and expulsive (*Dafi'a*) faculties of the uterus to support menstruation, conception and parturition.
4. Maintain *Asbab-e-Sittah Zaruriyyah*: Ensure balance in lifestyle factors to prevent recurrence.
5. Promote Holistic Healing: Address physical, psychological and environmental factors contributing to gynecological disorders.

Types of *Ilaj-bil-Tadbeer*

Ilaj-bil-Tadbeer includes a variety of therapeutic modalities, each selected based on the patient's temperament, humor imbalance and specific gynecological condition. The main types used in gynecological diseases are:

1. *Hijama* (Cupping Therapy)

Application of suction cups to specific body points to remove morbid humors or improve blood flow. It can be dry (without incision) or wet (with bloodletting).

Mechanism: Facilitates *Tanqiya* (evacuation of morbid humors), improves circulation and corrects temperamental imbalances (e.g., hot and dry or cold and moist).

Application in Gynecology

Used in amenorrhea (*Ihtibas-e-Tamth*) to remove phlegmatic or melancholic humors causing obstruction.

Indicated for dysmenorrhea (*Usr-e-Tamth*) to relieve pelvic congestion.

Applied to lower back, sacral region or thighs to target uterine disorders.

Types

Wet cupping (*Hijama bil Shurt*): For blood or bile dominance (e.g., menorrhagia).

Dry cupping (*Hijama bila Shurt*): For pain relief or stimulation in cold temperament disorders.

Precautions: Avoid in anemia, pregnancy or severe debilitation.

2. *Nutool* (Irrigation or Medicated Pouring)

Pouring or dripping lukewarm herbal drug decoctions over affected areas to correct temperament or to disperse morbid matter.

Mechanism: Softens tissues, reduces inflammation and restores uterine temperament (e.g., cooling in hot temperament disorders).

Application in Gynecology

Used in vaginitis (*Waram-e-Mahbil*) or leucorrhoea (*Sailan-ur-Rahim*) with decoctions of astringent drugs (e.g., Acacia nilotica, chamomile).

Indicated for dysmenorrhea to relieve cervical obstruction or spasms.

Applied over the lower abdomen or pelvic region.

Drugs: Rose water, myrrh (Commiphora myrrha), or neem for cooling and anti-inflammatory effects.

Precautions: Ensure decoctions are at a safe temperature to avoid burns.

3. *Fasd* (Venesection)

Controlled bloodletting from specific veins to remove excess blood or morbid humors.

Mechanism: Reduces blood humor (*Dam*) dominance in conditions like menorrhagia or hot and moist temperament.

Application in Gynecology

Rarely used, reserved for severe menorrhagia (*Kasrat-e-Haiz*) due to blood humor excess.

Performed on veins like the saphenous or basilic vein.

Precautions: Contraindicated in anemia, pregnancy or debilitated patients; requires skilled practitioners.

4. *Dalk* (Massage Therapy)

Therapeutic massage with medicated oils or crude drug pastes to improve circulation, relieve pain or correct temperament.

Mechanism: Warms cold temperament, disperses morbid humors and strengthens uterine faculties.

Application in Gynecology

Indicated for amenorrhea or dysmenorrhea to stimulate uterine blood flow.

Used in infertility to enhance uterine receptivity.

Applied to the lower abdomen, back or thighs with hot temperament oils (e.g., sesame oil, *Roghan-e-Babuna* [chamomile oil]).

Types

Dalk-e-Layyin (soft massage): For relaxation and pain relief.

Dalk-e-Sulb (hard massage): To disperse morbid humors in chronic conditions.

Precautions: Avoid vigorous massage in pregnancy or acute inflammation.

5. *Takmeed* (Fomentation)

Application of warm or cold compresses (dry or wet) to the affected area.

Application in Gynecology

Warm fomentation for dysmenorrhea or amenorrhea to promote blood flow and relieve spasms.

Cold fomentation for vaginitis or hot temperament disorders to reduce inflammation.

Uses herbal drug decoctions (e.g., fennel, chamomile) or plain water.

Precautions: Avoid extreme temperatures to prevent tissue damage.

6. *Abzan* (Sitz Bath)

Immersion of the pelvic region in medicated or plain water (warm or cold) to treat local disorders.

Mechanism: Improves circulation, reduces inflammation and corrects temperament (e.g., warming in cold and moist conditions).

Application in Gynecology

Indicated for leucorrhoea, vaginitis or pelvic inflammatory disease (*Waram-e-Rahim*).

Used for post-partum care to promote uterine involution.

Medicated with astringent or anti-inflammatory drugs (e.g., myrrh, neem, rose).

Precautions: Ensure hygiene to prevent infections; avoid in acute pelvic infections.

7. *Bukhoor* (Vaginal Fumigation)

Exposure of the vaginal or pelvic area to fumes of burning herbs or medicated vapors.

Mechanism: Dries excessive moisture, corrects cold and moist temperament and has antimicrobial effects.

Application in Gynecology

Used for leucorrhoea, vaginitis or cervical infections to reduce discharge and inflammation.

Drugs: Myrrh, frankincense (Boswellia serrata) or sandalwood.

Avoid in pregnancy or in hypersensitivity to fumes; ensure proper ventilation.

8. *Hammam* (Steam Bath or Sauna)

Exposure to steam or warm environments to promote sweating and humor evacuation.

Mechanism: Warms cold temperament, enhances metabolism and expels morbid humors through perspiration.

Application in Gynecology

Indicated for amenorrhea or infertility due to cold and moist temperament.

Used post-partum to promote uterine cleansing and involution.

Precautions: Contraindicated in fever, dehydration or cardiac disorders.

9. *Riyazat* (Exercise)

Moderate physical activity according to the patient's condition improve circulation and humor balance.

Mechanism: Enhances uterine blood flow, strengthens faculties and prevents phlegm accumulation.

Application in Gynecology

Indicated for amenorrhea, PCOD or obesity-related disorders.

Examples: Walking, yoga or light aerobic exercises.

Precautions: Avoid strenuous exercise in pregnancy, acute pain or debilitation.

10. *Taleeq* (Leech Therapy)

Application of medicinal leeches to remove localized morbid blood or humors.

Mechanism: Reduces blood or bilious humor excess, relieves pelvic congestion.

Application in Gynecology

Used in menorrhagia or pelvic inflammatory conditions to reduce blood stasis.

Applied to sacral or lower abdominal regions.

Precautions: Contraindicated in anemia, bleeding disorders or pregnancy.

Specific Applications in Gynecological Diseases

Ilaj-bil-Tadbeer is done according to the specific gynecological disorder, humor imbalance and uterine temperament. Common applications include:

1. Amenorrhea (*Ihtibas-e-Tamth*)

Cause: Cold and moist temperament, phlegm dominance or uterine obstruction (*Sudda*).

Therapies: *Hijama* (dry or wet) on the sacral region to stimulate blood flow.

Nutool with hot temperament drugs (e.g., cinnamon, fennel) to disperse phlegm.

Takmeed (warm fomentation) to promote menstruation.

Riyazat (moderate exercise) to enhance circulation.

Goal: Warm the uterus and expel viscous humors.

2. Dysmenorrhea (*Usr-e-Tamth*)

Cause: Cold temperament, cervical obstruction or bilious irritation.

Therapies: *Dalk* with warming oils (e.g., *Roghan-e-Babuna*) to relieve spasms.

Abzan (sitz bath) with chamomile or myrrh to reduce inflammation.

Takmeed (warm compresses) to alleviate pain.

Goal: Relieve obstruction and reduce pain.

3. Leucorrhoea (*Sailan-ur-Rahim*)

Cause: Cold and moist temperament, phlegm or blood humor excess.

Therapies: *Bukhoor* with astringent herbs (e.g., myrrh, neem) to dry excessive discharge.

Abzan with antimicrobial herbs to treat infections.

Nutool with drying decoctions to correct temperament.

Goal: Dry the uterus and eliminate morbid humors.

4. Menorrhagia (*Kasrat-e-Haiz*)

Cause: Hot and moist temperament, blood humor dominance.

Therapies: *Fasd* (venesection) in severe cases to reduce blood excess.

Taleeq (leech therapy) to relieve pelvic congestion.

Nutool with cooling herbs (e.g., rose water, sandalwood) to balance temperament.

Goal: Cool and dry the uterus, reduce bleeding.

5. Infertility (*Uqr*)

Cause: Cold and dry or hot and dry temperament, weak uterine faculties.

Therapies: *Dalk* with warming and moistening oils to enhance uterine receptivity.

Hammam to improve systemic circulation and humor balance.

Riyazat to strengthen reproductive organs.

Goal: Restore uterine temperament and faculty strength.

6. Polycystic Ovarian Disease (PCOD)

Cause: Cold and moist temperament, phlegm dominance, obesity.

Therapies: *Hijama* to remove phlegmatic humors.

Riyazat (exercise) to reduce obesity and improve metabolism.

Nutool with hot and dry herbs to correct temperament.

Goal: Reduce phlegm and promote ovulation.

7. Hysteria (*Ikhtinaq-ur-Rahim*)

Cause: Cold temperament, retained humors (e.g., seminal fluid, putrefied matter).

Therapies: *Bukhoor* with sedative herbs to calm the nervous system.

Dalk with relaxing oils to reduce pelvic tension.

Hammam to promote systemic relaxation.

Goal: Expel retained humors and alleviate psychological symptoms.

8. Uterine Inflammation (*Waram-e-Rahim*)

Cause: Hot and dry temperament, bilious humor excess.

Therapies: *Nutool* with cold temperament drugs (e.g., rose, chamomile).

Abzan with anti-inflammatory drugs to reduce swelling.

Avoid warming therapies like *Hammam*.

Goal: Cool the uterus and reduce inflammation.

Indications and Contraindications

Indications

Chronic gynecological disorders resistant to medications.

Conditions with humor or temperament imbalances (e.g., amenorrhea, leucorrhoea).

Adjunct to dietotherapy and pharmacotherapy for holistic management.

Preventive care to maintain uterine health post-partum or in high-risk groups (e.g., obesity, PCOS).

Contraindications

Pregnancy (except gentle therapies like *Abzan* in specific cases).

Acute infections or malignancies (e.g., endometrial cancer, severe pelvic inflammatory disease).

Severe anemia, bleeding disorders or debilitation (contraindicates *Fasd, Taleeq*).

Hypersensitivity to herbal fumes (*Bukhoor*) or oils (*Dalk*).

Advantages of Ilaj-bil-Tadbeer

Non-invasive and holistic, addressing both local and systemic imbalances.

Complements pharmacotherapy and dietotherapy, enhancing treatment efficacy.

Minimal side effects when performed correctly.

Promotes patient involvement through lifestyle and environmental modifications.

Cost-effective and accessible in resource-limited settings.

Limitations

Requires skilled practitioners for procedures like *Fasd* or *Taleeq*.

Limited scientific validation compared to modern medicine, necessitating further research.

May not suffice for severe structural abnormalities (e.g., large uterine tumors) or malignancies, requiring surgical intervention.

Patient compliance may be challenging due to time-intensive therapies or lifestyle changes.

Complications

Infections: Improper hygiene during *Abzan, Bukhoor or Taleeq* may introduce infections.

Burns or Irritation: Overheated *Nutool* or *Takmeed* solutions can cause tissue damage.

Bleeding: Excessive *Fasd* or *Taleeq* may lead to anemia or hypotension.

Allergic Reactions: Herbal drug fumes or oils may cause hypersensitivity in susceptible individuals.

Prognosis

Favorable: Early intervention with *Ilaj-bil-Tadbeer* effectively resolves mild to moderate gynecological disorders (e.g., amenorrhea, leucorrhoea) by correcting temperament and humor imbalances.

Variable: Chronic conditions (e.g., PCOD, infertility) require prolonged therapy and lifestyle changes for optimal outcomes.

Poor: Advanced structural or malignant conditions (e.g., endometrial cancer) may not respond to regimental therapy alone, necessitating surgical or modern interventions.

Prevention

Maintain *Asbab-e-Sittah Zaruriyyah*: Ensure balanced diet, exercise, sleep and emotional well-being to prevent humor imbalances.

Regular Regimental Therapy: Periodic *Abzan* or *Dalk* in high-risk groups (e.g., obese women, PCOS patients) to maintain uterine health.

Early Intervention: Address mild temperamental imbalances with *Nutool* or *Riyazat* to prevent progression to chronic disorders.

Hygiene: Maintain genital hygiene to prevent infections that exacerbate temperament imbalances.

Key Points

Ilaj-bil-Tadbeer is a non-pharmacological treatment approach in Unani medicine, using therapies like *Hijama, Nutool, Dalk* and *Abzan* to correct humor and temperament imbalances in gynecological diseases.

Common gynecological conditions treated include amenorrhea, dysmenorrhea, leucorrhoea, menorrhagia, infertility, PCOD and hysteria, each linked to specific uterine temperament abnormalities.

Therapies are selected based on the principle of *Ilaj-bil-Zid*, counteracting the abnormal temperament (e.g., hot therapies for cold temperament).

Key modalities include *Hijama* for humor evacuation, *Nutool* for temperament correction, *Dalk* for pain relief and *Abzan* for infections or post-partum care.

Integration with modern diagnostics (e.g., ultrasound) and treatments enhances efficacy and safety.

Contraindications include pregnancy, acute infections and severe debilitation; skilled practitioners are essential for safe application.

16.2 Screening Procedures: VIA, Schiller's, High vaginal Swab

(*Amaliyat-i-Tasfiya: Silar ka kashifa, Mas-ha mahbileya Aaliya*)

1. Visual Inspection with Acetic Acid (VIA)

Definition

Visual Inspection with Acetic Acid (VIA) is a simple, cost-effective screening method used to detect cervical abnormalities, particularly precancerous lesions or early cervical cancer, by applying 3–5% acetic acid to the cervix and observing for characteristic changes.

Indications

Screening for cervical intraepithelial neoplasia (CIN) or cervical cancer in low-resource settings where Pap smear or HPV testing is unavailable.

Women aged 30–65 years, particularly in high-risk populations (e.g., high HPV prevalence, limited access to healthcare).

Alternative to Pap smear in resource-limited settings, as recommended by the World Health Organization (WHO).

Technique

1. Preparation

Perform in a well-lit setting with the patient in the lithotomy position.

Insert a sterile speculum to visualize the cervix.

Ensure no active vaginal infection or menstruation, as these may interfere with visualization.

2. Procedure

Apply 3–5% acetic acid to the cervix using a cotton swab or spray.

Wait 1–2 minutes to allow acetowhitening to develop.

Observe the cervix with the naked eye or low-power magnification (e.g., colposcope, if available).

3. Observation

Normal: No color change or faint whitening.

Abnormal: Dense, opaque white lesions (acetowhitening) in the transformation zone, suggestive of CIN or cancer.

Suspicious for Cancer: Raised, irregular lesions, ulceration or bleeding on touch.

4. Documentation: Note the location, size and extent of acetowhite areas.

Interpretation

Negative: No acetowhitening or transient, faint whitening.

Positive: Dense, well-defined acetowhite areas in the transformation zone, persisting >1 minute.

Suspicious for Cancer: Irregular, raised lesions or visible growths.

Sensitivity: ~80–90%; Specificity: ~80–85% (varies with operator experience).

Clinical Significance

VIA is a practical, low-cost alternative to Pap smear or HPV testing in low-resource settings.

Allows immediate results and "see-and-treat" approaches (e.g., cryotherapy for positive cases).

Limitations: Operator-dependent, lower specificity than HPV testing and less effective for detecting glandular lesions.

Complications

Mild discomfort or burning sensation during acetic acid application.

False positives due to inflammation or metaplasia.

Rarely, minor bleeding if the cervix is friable.

2. Schiller's Test

Definition

Schiller's Test is a diagnostic procedure that involves applying Lugol's iodine solution to the cervix to identify abnormal epithelial areas, as healthy glycogen-rich cervical epithelium stains dark brown, while abnormal areas do not.

Indications

Screening or evaluation of cervical abnormalities during colposcopy.

Adjunct to VIA or Pap smear to delineate suspicious areas for biopsy.

Identification of vaginal or vulvar lesions in rare cases.

Technique

1. Preparation

Performed in the lithotomy position with a speculum to expose the cervix. Ensure the cervix is clean and free of mucus or blood.

2. Procedure

Apply Lugol's iodine (2–5% iodine-potassium iodide solution) to the cervix using a cotton swab or spray. Observe the staining pattern immediately.

3. Observation

Normal: Healthy squamous epithelium (glycogen-rich) stains dark brown or mahogany.

Abnormal: Dysplastic or cancerous epithelium (glycogen-poor) appears mustard yellow, pale or unstained.

Metaplasia or Inflammation: May show partial or patchy staining.

4. Documentation: Record staining patterns and guide biopsy to non-staining areas.

Interpretation

Positive: Non-staining or yellow areas in the transformation zone, suggesting CIN or cancer.

Negative: Uniform dark brown staining, indicating healthy epithelium.

Sensitivity: ~60–80%; Specificity: ~60–70% (lower than VIA or colposcopy).

Clinical Significance

Useful as an adjunct to colposcopy to guide biopsies in suspected CIN or cervical cancer.

Less sensitive and specific than VIA or HPV testing, so rarely used alone.

Helps to differentiate squamous epithelium from columnar epithelium or metaplasia.

Enhances visualization of abnormal cervical areas during colposcopy.

Limited use in modern practice due to availability of more accurate methods (e.g., HPV testing, colposcopy-directed biopsy).

May be used in resource-limited settings as part of a comprehensive screening protocol.

Complications

Mild stinging or discomfort during iodine application.

Allergic reactions to iodine (rare).

False positives in cases of inflammation, atrophy or metaplasia.

3. High Vaginal Swab (HVS)

Definition

A High Vaginal Swab (HVS) is a diagnostic procedure involving the collection of vaginal secretions from the posterior fornix to identify infectious or microbial causes of vaginal symptoms.

Indications

Evaluation of vaginal discharge (e.g., abnormal color, odor or consistency).

Suspected vaginitis (bacterial vaginosis, candidiasis, trichomoniasis).

Screening for sexually transmitted infections (e.g., Chlamydia, Gonorrhea).

Recurrent vaginal infections or pelvic inflammatory disease (PID).

Pre- or postoperative assessment in gynecological surgery.

Technique

1. Preparation

Perform in the lithotomy position with a sterile speculum.

Avoid douching, vaginal medications or intercourse for 24-48 hours prior.

Do not perform during menstruation unless urgent indicated.

2. Procedure

Insert a sterile speculum to visualize the vaginal vault and cervix.

Use a sterile cotton or Dacron swab to collect secretions from the posterior fornix.

Avoid touching the vaginal walls or cervix to minimize contamination.

Place the swab in appropriate transport medium (e.g., Amies or Stuart's medium) for bacterial culture or PCR testing.

3. Sample Processing

Wet Mount: Saline microscopy to detect clue cells (bacterial vaginosis), trichomonads or yeast.

Gram Stain: Identifies bacterial morphology and clue cells.

Culture: For aerobic/anaerobic bacteria, yeast or specific pathogens.

PCR: For Chlamydia trachomatis, Neisseria gonorrhoeae or Trichomonas vaginalis.

pH Testing: Vaginal pH >4.5 suggests bacterial vaginosis or trichomoniasis.

Interpretation

Normal: Predominance of lactobacilli, pH 3.8–4.5, no pathogens.

Bacterial Vaginosis: Clue cells, pH >4.5, fishy odor (positive whiff test), Gardnerella vaginalis or mixed anaerobes.

Candidiasis: Budding yeast or pseudohyphae, normal pH (4.0–4.5).

Trichomoniasis: Motile trichomonads, pH >4.5, inflammatory cells.

STIs: Positive PCR or culture for Chlamydia, Gonorrhea or other pathogens.

Clinical Significance

Essential for diagnosing vaginal infections, which may mimic or coexist with other gynecological conditions (e.g., cervicitis, PID).

Guides targeted antimicrobial therapy, reducing unnecessary antibiotic use.

Identifies asymptomatic infections (e.g., Group B Streptococcus in pregnancy).

Critical in evaluating vaginal discharge, a common gynecological complaint.

Differentiates infectious causes from non-infectious conditions (e.g., atrophic vaginitis, cervical ectropion).

Important in pregnancy to screen for infections that may cause preterm labor or neonatal complications.

Complications

Mild discomfort during speculum insertion or swabbing.

Rare risk of vaginal wall trauma or bleeding.

Definitions

Hysteroscopy ➤ Endoscopic visualization of uterine cavity via cervix; diagnostic and operative.

Laparoscopy ➤ Minimally invasive abdominal procedure using CO_2 insufflation and camera.

Colposcopy ➤ Magnified inspection of cervix after acetic acid application; detects precancerous lesions.

Pap Smear ➤ Cytological screening for cervical dysplasia and carcinoma.

D&C (Dilatation & Curettage) ➤ Cervical dilation followed by scraping of endometrial lining; diagnostic or therapeutic.

16.3 Cytological Examinations: Pap's Smear test

(*Imtehan-i-Khlawi*: Pap smear *kashifah*)

Definition

The Pap Smear (Papanicolaou test) is a screening method to detect cervical abnormalities, including precancerous lesions (CIN) and cervical cancer, by collecting and examining cervical cells.

Indications

Routine cervical cancer screening in women aged 21–65 years (per ACOG guidelines).

Evaluation of abnormal vaginal bleeding, discharge or pelvic pain.

Follow-up after abnormal Pap or HPV test results.

Monitoring after treatment for CIN or cervical cancer.

Technique

1. Preparation

Perform in the lithotomy position with a sterile speculum.

Avoid intercourse, douching or vaginal medications for 48 hours prior.

Not done in days of menses, for optimal cell collection.

2. Procedure

Insert a speculum to visualize the cervix.

Use a cytobrush or spatula to collect cells from the transformation zone and endocervical canal.

Spread cells on a slide (conventional Pap) or place in liquid-based medium (LBC).

Send to cytology laboratory for staining and microscopic evaluation.

3. Screening Guidelines (ACOG, 2023)

Age 21–29: Pap smear every 3 years.

Age 30–65: Co-testing (Pap + HPV) every 5 years or Pap alone every 3 years.

Stop screening at age >65, if adequate prior negative screens and no high-risk factors.

Interpretation (Bethesda System)

Negative for Intraepithelial Lesion or Malignancy (NILM): Normal cells.

Atypical Squamous Cells (ASC)

ASC-US (undetermined significance): Mild atypia, often HPV-related.

ASC-H (cannot exclude HSIL): Suggests high-grade lesion.

Low-Grade Squamous Intraepithelial Lesion (LSIL): Mild dysplasia (CIN1).

High-Grade Squamous Intraepithelial Lesion (HSIL): Moderate/severe dysplasia (CIN2/3).

Squamous Cell Carcinoma: Invasive cancer.

Atypical Glandular Cells (AGC): Endocervical or endometrial abnormalities.

HPV Testing: Co-testing identifies high-risk HPV types (e.g., 16, 18).

Clinical Significance

Gold standard for cervical cancer screening, reducing incidence and mortality.

High sensitivity (~70–80%) and specificity (~90–95%) for detecting CIN2+.

Liquid-based cytology (LBC) allows reflex HPV testing and improves accuracy.

Limitations: False negatives (sampling errors), limited detection of glandular lesions.

Complications

Mild discomfort or spotting post-procedure.

Rare risk of infection or significant bleeding.

Patient Presents with Gynecological Complaint

↓

Step 1: History Taking

(Menstrual, sexual, obstetric, medical, surgical)

↓

Step 2: Physical Examination

(General + Pelvic + Speculum + Bimanual)

↓

Step 3: Basic Investigations

↓ ↓ ↓

USG Pelvis Pap Smear CBC, Hormones

↓

Step 4: Specialized Tests

↓ ↓ ↓

HSG → Tubal Patency

Hysteroscopy → Uterine Cavity

Laparoscopy → Pelvic Organs

↓

Step 5: Biopsy / Cytology

(Endometrial, Cervical, Vulvar)

↓

Step 6: Diagnosis → Treatment Planning

16.4 Cryosurgery

(*Jarahat-i-tabridiya*)

Definition

Cryosurgery (or cryotherapy) is a therapeutic procedure that uses extreme cold (liquid nitrogen or carbon dioxide) to destroy abnormal cervical tissue, such as CIN or benign lesions, by freezing and inducing necrosis.

Indications

Treatment of CIN1–2 (if biopsy-confirmed, small lesions).

Management of benign cervical conditions (e.g., ectropion, chronic cervicitis).

Used in "see-and-treat" protocols following positive VIA in low-resource settings.

Contraindications: CIN-3, suspected invasive cancer, pregnancy or large lesions (>75% of cervix).

Technique

1. Preparation

Confirm diagnosis with colposcopy and biopsy (except in VIA-based settings).

Perform in the lithotomy position with a speculum.

Counsel patient on post-procedure discharge and abstinence (2–4 weeks).

2. Procedure

Apply a cryoprobe (cooled to -50°C to -70°C) to the cervix, covering the transformation zone and lesion. Use a "double-freeze" technique: Freeze for 3 minutes, thaw for 5 minutes, freeze for 3 minutes. Ensure a 5–7 mm ice ball margin beyond the lesion.

3. Post-Procedure

Expect watery discharge for 2–4 weeks as necrotic tissue sloughs.

Follow-up with Pap smear or HPV testing at 6–12 months.

Outcomes

Success Rate: ~85–90% for CIN1–2; lower for larger or high-grade lesions.

Recurrence Rate: ~5–10%, requiring repeat treatment or alternative therapy (e.g., LEEP).

Clinical Significance

Minimally invasive, outpatient procedure with low cost and high efficacy.

Preferred in low-resource settings due to simplicity and no need for anesthesia.

Limitations: Not suitable for CIN3 or invasive cancer; cannot provide tissue for histology.

Key component of cervical cancer prevention in resource-limited settings.

Often combined with VIA in single-visit "see-and-treat" programs.

Requires follow-up to confirm lesion resolution and rule out recurrence.

Complications

Watery discharge or mild cramping (common).

Rare: Cervical stenosis, infection or incomplete lesion treatment.

16.5 Hormone Assay

(*Hormone ki janch*)

Definition

Hormone assay involves measuring levels of reproductive and related hormones in blood, urine or saliva to assess endocrine function, diagnose gynecological disorders and guide treatment.

Indications

Evaluation of menstrual irregularities (e.g., amenorrhea, oligomenorrhea, PCOS).

Infertility workup (e.g., ovulation assessment, ovarian reserve).

Menopause or perimenopause evaluation.

Diagnosis of endocrine disorders (e.g., hyperandrogenism, hypothyroidism).

Monitoring hormonal therapy (e.g., IVF, HRT).

Suspected gynecological tumors (e.g., estrogen-secreting ovarian tumors).

Technique

1. Sample Collection

Blood: Most common; collected via venipuncture, timed to menstrual cycle phase (e.g., Day 2–3 for FSH, LH; mid-luteal for progesterone).

Urine: Used for metabolites (e.g., pregnanediol for progesterone).

Saliva: Emerging for cortisol or sex hormones (less common).

2. Key Hormones Assessed

Follicle-Stimulating Hormone (FSH): Ovulation, ovarian reserve (Day 2–3).

Luteinizing Hormone (LH): Ovulation trigger, PCOS (LH:FSH ratio >2).

Estradiol (E2): Follicular development, endometrial health.

Progesterone: Confirms ovulation, luteal phase adequacy (mid-luteal >10 ng/mL).

Testosterone/Androgens: Hyperandrogenism (e.g., PCOS, hirsutism).

Prolactin: Amenorrhea, galactorrhea, pituitary disorders.

Thyroid Hormones (TSH, Free T4): Menstrual irregularities, infertility.

Anti-Mullerian Hormone (AMH): Ovarian reserve, PCOS.

Cortisol/DHEAS: Adrenal disorders, Cushing’s syndrome.

3. Laboratory Methods

Immunoassays (e.g., ELISA, chemiluminescence) for high sensitivity.

Liquid chromatography-mass spectrometry (LC-MS) for precision (e.g., androgens).

4. Timing

Follicular phase (Day 2–3): FSH, LH, estradiol.

Mid-cycle: LH surge (ovulation).

Luteal phase (Day 21): Progesterone.

Random: AMH, thyroid hormones, prolactin.

Interpretation

Amenorrhea

Primary: High FSH/LH (ovarian failure), low E2; normal/low FSH/LH (hypothalamic-pituitary dysfunction).

Secondary: High prolactin (pituitary adenoma), high androgens (PCOS).

Infertility

Low AMH (<1 ng/mL): Poor ovarian reserve.

Low progesterone (<10 ng/mL): Luteal phase defect.

PCOS: Elevated LH: FSH ratio, high testosterone, high AMH.

Menopause: High FSH (>25 IU/L), low E2 (<30 pg/mL).

Endocrine Tumors: Elevated E2 (granulosa cell tumors), high testosterone (Sertoli-Leydig tumors).

Clinical Significance

Essential for diagnosing and managing endocrine-related gynecological disorders.

Guides ovulation induction, IVF protocols or hormone replacement therapy.

Identifies systemic conditions (e.g., thyroid dysfunction) impacting reproductive health.

Essential for infertility, PCOS and menopause management.

Hormonal imbalances often underlie common gynecological complaints (e.g., irregular menses, hirsutism).

Serial assays monitor response to therapy (e.g., clomiphene, gonadotropins).

Complications

Minimal; related to venipuncture (e.g., bruising, infection).

False results due to improper timing, medications (e.g., oral contraceptives) or assay interference.

16.6 Imaging Techniques in Gynaecology

(*Amrad-i-Niswan me shuaayi tasveerkashi*)

Imaging plays a pivotal role in gynecology for the diagnosis, management and follow-up of conditions affecting the female reproductive tract, including the uterus, ovaries, fallopian tubes, cervix and vagina. The choice of imaging modality depends on the clinical question, patient characteristics and resource availability.

1. Ultrasound (US)

Definition

Ultrasound uses high-frequency sound waves to create detailed images of pelvic organs. It is the cornerstone of gynecological imaging due to its safety, accessibility and versatility. Transabdominal ultrasound (TAUS) and transvaginal ultrasound (TVUS) are the primary approaches, with TVUS offering superior resolution for pelvic structures.

Principles

Sound waves reflect off tissues, creating echoes that form images based on tissue density and interfaces. Doppler ultrasound assesses blood flow, helps in the evaluation of vascular structures (e.g., ovarian masses, endometrial pathology).

Indications

Gynecological

Evaluation of pelvic pain, abnormal uterine bleeding or palpable masses.

Assessment of uterine abnormalities (e.g., fibroids, adenomyosis, endometrial pathology).

Characterization of ovarian cysts or masses (benign vs. malignant).

Monitoring follicular development in infertility treatment.

Diagnosis of ectopic pregnancy or miscarriage.

Evaluation of pelvic inflammatory disease (PID) or tubo-ovarian abscess.

Obstetrical

Early pregnancy assessment (gestational sac, fetal viability).

Screening for congenital anomalies or placental abnormalities.

Technique

1. Transabdominal Ultrasound (TAUS)

Preparation: Full bladder to displace bowel and improve visualization of pelvic organs.

Procedure: A 3–5 MHz probe is used over the lower abdomen.

Indications: Large masses, pediatric patients or when TVUS is contraindicated (e.g., virgo intacta).

2. Transvaginal Ultrasound (TVUS)

Preparation: Empty bladder for patient comfort and optimal imaging.

Procedure: A 5–9 MHz probe is inserted into the vagina, providing high-resolution images of the uterus, ovaries, and adnexa.

Indications: Detailed evaluation of endometrium, ovaries or early pregnancy.

3. Doppler Ultrasound

Assess vascular flow in ovarian masses, endometrial lesions or ectopic pregnancies.

4. 3D/4D Ultrasound

Provides volumetric images for complex uterine anomalies (e.g., septate uterus) or fetal anomalies.

Findings

Uterus

Fibroids: Hypoechoic, well-defined masses; may show calcifications or cystic degeneration.

Adenomyosis: Thickened myometrium with hypoechoic streaks or cysts; “Swiss cheese” appearance.

Endometrial pathology: Thickened endometrium (>5 mm postmenopausal, >15 mm premenopausal) suggests hyperplasia or carcinoma.

Ovaries

Functional cysts: Simple, unilocular, thin-walled.

Complex masses: Septations, solid components or increased vascularity suggest malignancy.

Polycystic ovaries: ≥12 follicles (2–9 mm) or ovarian volume >10 cm^3.

Fallopian Tubes: Visible if dilated (hydrosalpinx) or with tubo-ovarian abscess.

Ectopic Pregnancy: Adnexal mass with “ring of fire” on Doppler (increased vascularity).

Advantages

Non-invasive, radiation-free and safe in pregnancy.

Real-time imaging allows dynamic assessment (e.g., sliding sign for adhesions).

Cost-effective and widely available.

TVUS provides high-resolution images of pelvic structures.

Limitations

Operator-dependent; requires skilled interpretation.

Limited by body image(obesity), bowel gas or retroverted uterus.

Poor visualization of deep pelvic or extrapelvic structures.

Less specific for characterizing complex masses compared to MRI.

Gynecological Relevance

First-line imaging for most gynecological conditions due to accessibility and safety.

Essential in infertility workup (e.g., antral follicle count, endometrial thickness).

Guides interventions (e.g., cyst aspiration, embryo transfer).

Critical in early pregnancy evaluation and emergency settings (e.g., ectopic pregnancy).

2. Magnetic Resonance Imaging (MRI)

Definition

MRI uses magnetic fields and radio waves to produce detailed images of pelvic organs, offering superior soft-tissue contrast and multiplanar imaging. It is a second-line modality in gynecology, used when ultrasound is inconclusive or further characterization is needed.

Principles

T1- and T2-weighted sequences provide anatomical detail and tissue characterization.

Contrast-enhanced MRI (gadolinium) assesses vascularity and lesion enhancement.

Diffusion-weighted imaging (DWI) and apparent diffusion coefficient (ADC) maps aid in malignancy detection.

Indications

Characterization of indeterminate adnexal masses (benign vs. malignant).

Evaluation of complex uterine anomalies (e.g., Mullerian duct anomalies).

Diagnosis and staging of gynecological malignancies (e.g., endometrial, cervical or ovarian cancer).

Assessment of deep endometriosis or adenomyosis.

Pre-surgical planning for fibroids, prolapse or malignancy.

Evaluation of pelvic floor dysfunction or fistulae.

Technique

1. Preparation

Screen for contraindications (e.g., metal implants, claustrophobia).

Administer anti-peristaltic agents (e.g., hyoscine) to reduce bowel motion artifacts.

Optional bladder filling for pelvic floor assessment.

2. Procedure

Perform in a 1.5T or 3T MRI scanner with pelvic coil.

Standard sequences: T1-weighted (fat-sensitive), T2-weighted (fluid-sensitive) and contrast-enhanced T1.

Additional sequences: DWI for malignancy, fat-suppression for endometriosis.

Multiplanar imaging (axial, sagittal, coronal) for comprehensive evaluation.

3. Contrast: Gadolinium enhances vascular lesions; contraindicated in renal impairment or pregnancy.

Findings

Uterus

Fibroids: Well-defined, hypointense on T2, variable enhancement.

Adenomyosis: Thickened junctional zone (>12 mm), T2 hypointense foci or cystic areas.

Endometrial cancer: T2 hyperintense lesion invading myometrium; enhances with contrast.

Ovaries

Benign cysts: T2 hyperintense, thin-walled, no enhancement.

Malignant tumors: Solid components, irregular septations, restricted diffusion on DWI.

Endometriomas: “T1 bright, T2 shading” (hemorrhagic content).

Cervix: Cervical cancer shows T2 hyperintensity, myometrial invasion or lymph node involvement.

Pelvic Floor: Dynamic MRI (during Valsalva) assesses prolapse or levator ani defects.

Advantages

Superior soft-tissue contrast for characterizing complex lesions.

No ionizing radiation, safe in pregnancy (non-contrast).

Multiplanar imaging for precise anatomical mapping.

Highly accurate for staging malignancies and assessing endometriosis.

Limitations

Expensive and less accessible than ultrasound.

Longer scan times (20–40 minutes) and patient discomfort (claustrophobia).

Gadolinium contraindicated in pregnancy or severe renal impairment.

Limited real-time capability compared to ultrasound.

Gold standard for characterizing indeterminate adnexal masses or deep endometriosis.

Essential for preoperative planning in gynecological cancers or complex uterine surgeries.

Preferred for evaluating congenital uterine anomalies (e.g., septate vs. bicornuate uterus).

Increasing role in pelvic floor disorders and dynamic imaging.

3. Computed Tomography (CT)

Definition

CT uses X-rays to produce cross-sectional images of the pelvis, primarily used in gynecology for staging malignancies, evaluating complications or assessing non-gynecological pathology mimicking pelvic disease.

Principles

X-ray beams create detailed images based on tissue density.

Intravenous contrast enhances vascular structures and lesions.

Multi-detector CT (MDCT) provides high-resolution, multiplanar reconstructions.

Indications

Staging of gynecological malignancies (e.g., ovarian, cervical, or endometrial cancer).

Evaluation of acute pelvic pain (e.g., ovarian torsion, tubo-ovarian abscess).

Assessment of postoperative complications (e.g., abscess, hematoma).

Detection of distant metastases or lymph node involvement.

Differential diagnosis of non-gynecological conditions (e.g., appendicitis, diverticulitis).

Technique

1. Preparation

Screen for contrast allergies or renal impairment.

Administer oral contrast for bowel delineation in some cases.

Fast for 4–6 hours if contrast is used.

2. Procedure

Perform with a multi-detector CT scanner, typically in axial, sagittal and coronal planes.

Use intravenous iodinated contrast for enhanced imaging (unless contraindicated).

Thin-slice (1–3 mm) imaging for detailed pelvic evaluation.

3. Protocol

Non-contrast CT for initial assessment (e.g., calcifications, hemorrhage).

Contrast-enhanced CT for vascularity and lesion characterization.

Findings

Uterus: Fibroids appear as well-defined, enhancing masses; endometrial cancer shows myometrial invasion.

Ovaries: Complex masses with solid components or ascites suggest malignancy; torsion shows enlarged ovary with absent flow.

Lymph Nodes: Enlarged (>1 cm) or necrotic nodes indicate metastasis.

Complications: Abscesses (rim-enhancing collections), hematomas (hyperdense on non-contrast).

Advantages

Rapid imaging (minutes), ideal for emergencies.

Excellent for detecting metastases, lymph nodes or extrapelvic pathology.

Widely available compared to MRI.

Limitations

Ionizing radiation, limiting use in pregnancy and young patients.

Inferior soft-tissue contrast compared to MRI.

Limited role in characterizing adnexal masses or early-stage gynecological conditions.

Contrast risks (allergy, nephrotoxicity).

Primarily used for cancer staging or acute pelvic emergencies.

Less common in routine gynecological evaluation due to radiation exposure and limited soft-tissue detail.

Valuable for detecting complications (e.g., post-hysterectomy abscess) or non-gynecological mimics.

4. Hysterosalpingography (HSG)

Definition

Hysterosalpingography (HSG) is a fluoroscopic imaging technique that uses contrast to evaluate the uterine cavity and fallopian tubes, primarily for infertility or recurrent miscarriage workup.

Principles

Radiopaque contrast injected into the uterine cavity outlines its shape and assesses tubal patency under real-time fluoroscopy.

X-ray images capture contrast flow and spillage into the peritoneal cavity.

Indications

Infertility evaluation (assess tubal patency, uterine anomalies).

Investigation of recurrent miscarriage (e.g., uterine septum, synechiae).

Post-surgical assessment (e.g., tubal ligation, myomectomy).

Suspected Asherman's syndrome or intrauterine adhesions.

Technique

1. Preparation

Perform in the follicular phase (Days 7–12) to avoid pregnancy.

Screen for pelvic infection or contrast allergy.

Administer prophylactic antibiotics (e.g., doxycycline) if infection risk is high.

Premedicate with NSAIDs for pain relief.

2. Procedure

Position patient in lithotomy position; insert a speculum and cannula into the cervical os.

Inject 5–10 mL of water-soluble iodinated contrast (e.g., iohexol) under fluoroscopy.

Capture serial X-ray images to visualize uterine cavity and tubal spillage.

Document filling defects, tubal patency or peritoneal spillage.

3. Post-Procedure: Monitor for cramping or rare allergic reactions.

Findings

Uterus

Normal: Smooth, triangular cavity.

Abnormal: Filling defects (polyps, fibroids, synechiae), unicornuate or septate uterus.

Asherman's syndrome: Irregular filling defects or obliterated cavity.

Fallopian Tubes

Patent: Contrast spills freely into the peritoneal cavity.

Obstructed: No spillage, proximal or distal block (e.g., hydrosalpinx).

Peritubal adhesions: Loculated contrast spillage.

Advantages

Gold standard for assessing tubal patency and uterine cavity abnormalities.

Relatively low cost and widely available.

Therapeutic benefit in some cases (contrast may clear minor tubal blockages).

Limitations

Ionizing radiation, contraindicated in pregnancy.

Risk of pain, infection or contrast allergy (rare). Limited evaluation of extrauterine structures (e.g., ovaries, endometriosis).

Less accurate for uterine anomalies compared to MRI or 3D ultrasound.

Essential in infertility workup to identify tubal factor infertility or uterine anomalies.

Guides management (e.g., hysteroscopy for synechiae, IVF for tubal occlusion).

Complements ultrasound or MRI for comprehensive evaluation.

5. Other Imaging Modalities

a. X-ray

Role: Limited in gynecology; used for detecting calcifications (e.g., calcified fibroids, ovarian teratomas) or skeletal abnormalities in pelvic pain.

Findings: Calcified fibroids appear as "popcorn" calcifications; teratomas may show teeth or bone.

Limitations: Minimal role due to radiation and poor soft-tissue detail.

b. Positron Emission Tomography (PET)

Definition: Combines CT with radioactive tracers (e.g., 18F-FDG) to assess metabolic activity, primarily for gynecological cancer staging.

Indications

Staging or restaging of ovarian, cervical or endometrial cancer.

Detection of recurrence or metastases.

Findings: Hypermetabolic lesions suggest malignancy or recurrence.

Advantages: High sensitivity for detecting metastatic disease.

Limitations: Expensive, limited availability and radiation exposure.

Uses: In oncology to guide treatment planning and monitor response.

c. Saline Infusion Sonohysterography (SIS)

Definition: Ultrasound with saline infusion into the uterine cavity to evaluate endometrial abnormalities.

Indications: Abnormal uterine bleeding, suspected polyps or submucosal fibroids.

Technique: Inject 5–10 mL saline via a catheter during TVUS to outline the endometrial cavity.

Findings: Polyps (echogenic masses), fibroids (hypoechoic), or synechiae (irregular bands).

Advantages: Enhances endometrial visualization; no radiation.

Limitations: Invasive, risk of infection or discomfort.

Choosing the Right Modality

Ultrasound is the first-line modality for most gynecological conditions due to its safety and versatility.

MRI is preferred for complex masses, endometriosis or cancer staging.

CT is reserved for emergencies or oncology staging.

HSG is specific for infertility-related tubal and uterine evaluation.

Pregnancy: Avoid radiation-based modalities (CT, HSG, X-ray); ultrasound and non-contrast MRI are safe.

Cost and Access: Ultrasound and HSG are cost-effective and widely available, while MRI and PET are resource-intensive.

Conclusion

Imaging techniques are integral to gynecological practice, enabling accurate diagnosis and management of conditions ranging from benign uterine abnormalities to gynecological malignancies. Ultrasound is the first-line modality due to its safety, accessibility and versatility, while MRI provides superior soft-tissue detail for complex cases. CT and HSG have specific roles in oncology and infertility respectively, while emerging modalities like PET and SIS expand diagnostic capabilities.

16.7 Histopathological Examinations: Cervical & Endometrial Biopsy

(*Imtehan-i-Nasij-i-Maradi*)

Cervical Biopsy

Definition

A cervical biopsy involves the removal of a small sample of cervical tissue for histopathological examination to diagnose abnormalities such as cervical intraepithelial neoplasia (CIN), cervical cancer or inflammatory conditions. It is typically performed during colposcopy when abnormalities are identified via screening tests (e.g., Pap smear, HPV testing, or VIA).

Indications

Abnormal Pap smear results (e.g., ASC-US with positive HPV, LSIL, HSIL, AGC).

Positive visual inspection with acetic acid (VIA) or Schiller's test suggesting precancerous or cancerous lesions.

Suspicious cervical lesions (e.g., visible growths, ulcers, or persistent bleeding).

Evaluation of chronic cervicitis or suspected infections (e.g., HPV, herpes).

Follow-up after treatment for CIN or cervical cancer to assess recurrence.

Technique

1. Preparation

Perform in an outpatient setting, typically during colposcopy.

Obtain informed consent; explain potential discomfort and risks.

Schedule outside menstruation for optimal visualization.

Ensure no active pelvic infection; treat if present.

2. Procedure

Position: Patient in lithotomy position with a speculum to visualize the cervix.

Colposcopy: Apply 3–5% acetic acid or Lugol's iodine to identify abnormal areas (acetowhite or non-staining regions).

Biopsy Types

a. Punch Biopsy: Most common; uses biopsy forceps to remove 2–3 mm tissue samples from suspicious areas (transformation zone or lesions).

b. Cone Biopsy (Conization): Removes a cone-shaped portion of the cervix using a cold knife (CKC) or loop electrosurgical excision procedure (LEEP/LLETZ). Indicated for deeper lesions or microinvasive cancer.
c. Endocervical Curettage (ECC): Scrapes the endocervical canal to sample tissue, often combined with punch biopsy for HSIL or AGC.

Hemostasis: Apply Monsel's solution or silver nitrate to control minor bleeding.

Specimen Handling: Place tissue in 10% formalin for histopathological analysis.

3. Post-Procedure

Advise on mild cramping or spotting for 1–2 days.

Recommend avoiding intercourse, tampons or douching for 1–2 weeks.

Histopathological Findings

Normal Cervix: Stratified squamous epithelium (ectocervix) or columnar epithelium (endocervix) with no atypia.

Cervical Intraepithelial Neoplasia (CIN)

CIN1: Mild dysplasia; atypical cells in the lower third of the epithelium.

CIN2: Moderate dysplasia; atypical cells in the lower two-thirds.

CIN3: Severe dysplasia/carcinoma in situ; full-thickness atypia without stromal invasion.

Invasive Cervical Cancer

Squamous cell carcinoma: Keratinizing or non-keratinizing; stromal invasion.

Adenocarcinoma: Glandular atypia with invasion.

Inflammatory Conditions: Chronic cervicitis with lymphocytic infiltration or koilocytes (HPV-related changes).

Other: Endocervical polyps, metaplasia or rare tumors (e.g., sarcoma).

Interpretation (Bethesda System Correlation)

CIN1 correlates with LSIL; CIN2/3 with HSIL.

Atypical glandular cells (AGC) may indicate endocervical adenocarcinoma or endometrial pathology.

Pathologist reports nuclear atypia, mitotic activity and stromal invasion to guide management.

Clinical Significance

Confirms or rules out precancerous or cancerous lesions, guiding treatment (e.g., observation for CIN1, excision for CIN2/3).

Differentiates benign (e.g., metaplasia, cervicitis) from malignant conditions.

Provides prognostic information for cervical cancer staging.

Sensitivity: ~90–95% for detecting CIN or cancer; specificity depends on biopsy site selection.

Complications

Common: Mild pain, spotting or vaginal discharge.

Rare: Heavy bleeding, infection or cervical stenosis (post-conization).

Cone biopsy risks: Cervical incompetence, preterm delivery in future pregnancies.

Uses

Essential for cervical cancer screening and management, complementing Pap smear, HPV testing and VIA.

Guides therapeutic decisions (e.g., LEEP, cryotherapy, or hysterectomy).

Critical in high-risk populations (e.g., HPV-positive, immunocompromised women).

Endocervical curettage enhances detection of occult endocervical lesions.

Endometrial Biopsy

Definition

An endometrial biopsy involves sampling the endometrial lining of the uterus for histopathological examination to diagnose conditions such as endometrial hyperplasia, cancer or benign disorders causing abnormal uterine bleeding.

Indications

Abnormal uterine bleeding (AUB):

Postmenopausal bleeding.

Heavy menstrual bleeding or intermenstrual bleeding in premenopausal women.

Suspected endometrial hyperplasia or cancer (e.g., thickened endometrium on ultrasound, >4 mm postmenopausal).

Infertility workup (e.g., luteal phase defect, recurrent miscarriage).

Evaluation of endometrial response to hormonal therapy (e.g., tamoxifen, HRT).

Suspected endometritis or chronic infections (e.g., tuberculosis).

Technique

1. Preparation

Perform in an outpatient setting; obtain informed consent.

Screen for pregnancy (contraindicated) and active pelvic infection.

Schedule in proliferative phase (premenopausal) or anytime (postmenopausal).

Administer NSAIDs or local anesthesia (paracervical block) for pain relief.

2. Procedure

Position: Lithotomy position with speculum insertion.

Pipelle Biopsy (most common)

Insert a flexible, plastic Pipelle catheter (3–4 mm diameter) through the cervix into the uterine cavity.

Apply suction via a syringe to aspirate endometrial tissue.

Rotate and move the catheter to sample multiple areas (fundus, anterior/posterior walls).

Alternative Methods

Endometrial Curettage: Uses a metal curette; performed during D&C or hysteroscopy.

Hysteroscopy-Guided Biopsy: Targeted sampling of suspicious areas under direct visualization.

Specimen Handling: Place tissue in 10% formalin for histopathology.

3. Post-Procedure

Monitor for cramping or spotting (1–2 days).

Advise avoiding intercourse or tampons for 3–5 days.

Histopathological Findings

Normal Endometrium

Proliferative phase: Tubular glands, compact stroma, mitotic activity.

Secretory phase: Coiled glands, glycogen vacuoles, decidualized stroma.

Postmenopausal: Atrophic endometrium (thin, inactive glands).

Endometrial Hyperplasia

Simple hyperplasia: Increased gland-to-stroma ratio, no atypia.

Complex hyperplasia: Crowded glands, branching, no atypia.

Atypical hyperplasia: Nuclear atypia, increased risk of progression to cancer.

Endometrial Cancer

Endometrioid adenocarcinoma: Glandular atypia, stromal invasion.

Non-endometrioid (e.g., serous, clear cell): High-grade, aggressive features.

Benign Conditions

Endometrial polyps: Glandular overgrowth with fibrous stroma.

Endometritis: Plasma cells, inflammatory infiltrates.

Subinvolution: Retained placental or decidual tissue.

Other: Tuberculosis (granulomas), gestational trophoblastic disease.

Interpretation

Hyperplasia with atypia has a 20–30% risk of progression to endometrial cancer.

Endometrial cancer staging requires hysterectomy for complete histopathological assessment.

Hormonal effects (e.g., tamoxifen) may mimic hyperplasia; clinical correlation is essential.

Clinical Significance

Gold standard for diagnosing endometrial pathology, particularly cancer and hyperplasia.

Sensitivity: ~90–95% for detecting endometrial cancer with Pipelle; higher with hysteroscopy-guided biopsy.

Guides management (e.g., hormonal therapy for hyperplasia, hysterectomy for cancer).

Differentiates benign (e.g., polyps) from malignant causes of AUB.

Complications

Common: Mild cramping, spotting or discomfort.

Rare: Uterine perforation, infection or heavy bleeding.

Vasovagal reaction in sensitive patients.

Uses

Critical for evaluating AUB, a common gynecological complaint.

Essential in postmenopausal bleeding to rule out malignancy (endometrial cancer risk increases with age).

Complements ultrasound (endometrial thickness >4 mm in postmenopausal women warrants biopsy).

Guides infertility treatment by assessing endometrial receptivity.

16.8 Dilatation & Curettage

(*Ittisa wa ijteraaf*)

Definition

Dilatation and Curettage (D&C) is a therapeutic and diagnostic procedure involving dilation of the cervix and scraping of the endometrial lining to remove tissue for histopathology or to treat conditions such as heavy uterine bleeding or retained products of conception.

Indications

Diagnostic

Abnormal uterine bleeding unresponsive to medical management.

Suspected endometrial hyperplasia or cancer (when biopsy is inadequate).

Evaluation of recurrent miscarriage or retained products of conception.

Investigation of endometrial infections (e.g., tuberculosis).

Therapeutic

Management of heavy menstrual bleeding or postpartum hemorrhage.

Removal of retained products of conception (miscarriage, abortion).

Treatment of endometrial polyps or submucosal fibroids.

Evacuation of molar pregnancy (gestational trophoblastic disease).

Technique

1. Preparation

Perform in an operating room under general or regional anesthesia.

Obtain informed consent; screen for pregnancy, infection, or bleeding disorders.

Administer prophylactic antibiotics (e.g., doxycycline) if infection risk is high.

Perform preoperative ultrasound to assess endometrial thickness or retained tissue.

2. Procedure

Position: Lithotomy position with speculum insertion.

Cervical Dilatation

Use graduated dilators (e.g., Hegar or Pratt) to dilate the cervix to 6–10 mm, depending on the curette size.

Misoprostol (400 mcg vaginally, 4–6 hours prior) may be used to soften the cervix, especially in nulliparous or postmenopausal women.

Curettage

Insert a sharp or suction curette into the uterine cavity.

Systematically scrape the endometrial lining (anterior, posterior, lateral walls, and fundus).

Suction curettage is preferred for retained products of conception to minimize trauma.

Specimen Handling: Collect tissue in 10% formalin for histopathology.

Optional Hysteroscopy: Performed concurrently to guide curettage or visualize abnormalities.

3. Post-Procedure

Monitor for bleeding, pain, or signs of infection.

Advise avoiding intercourse, tampons or douching for 1–2 weeks.

Follow-up with histopathology results and ultrasound if indicated.

Histopathological Findings

Additional findings in therapeutic D&C

Retained products of conception: Chorionic villi, decidual tissue.

Molar pregnancy: Hydropic villi, trophoblastic proliferation.

Submucosal fibroids or polyps: Fibrous or glandular tissue.

Pathologist assesses for malignancy, hormonal effects, or infection.

Clinical Significance

Diagnostic D&C provides larger tissue samples than Pipelle biopsy, improving sensitivity for diffuse endometrial pathology.

Therapeutic D&C effectively controls acute bleeding or removes retained tissue.

Sensitivity: ~95–98% for detecting endometrial cancer or hyperplasia when combined with hysteroscopy.

Limitations: Blind procedure; may miss focal lesions (polyps, small cancers) without hysteroscopy.

Complications

Common: Cramping, spotting or mild bleeding.

Rare

Uterine perforation (0.1–1%), risking bowel or bladder injury.

Cervical laceration or stenosis.

Intrauterine adhesions (Asherman's syndrome, 10–20% risk after multiple D&Cs).

Infection (endometritis, pelvic abscess).

Anesthesia-related risks.

Uses

Widely used for both diagnostic and therapeutic purposes in AUB and pregnancy-related complications.

Complements ultrasound and endometrial biopsy in evaluating postmenopausal bleeding.

Preferred for evacuating retained products or molar pregnancies.

Increasingly replaced by hysteroscopy-guided procedures for focal lesions due to higher precision.

Clinical relevance

1. Cervical Biopsy

Essential in cervical cancer screening and management pathways, bridging screening (Pap smear, HPV) to treatment (LEEP, conization).

Requires colposcopic expertise to target abnormal areas accurately.

Critical for confirming CIN or cancer before definitive therapy.

2. Endometrial Biopsy

First-line for evaluating AUB, especially in postmenopausal women.

Less invasive than D&C; preferred in outpatient settings.

Guides hormonal or surgical management of hyperplasia and cancer.

3. Dilatation and Curettage

Reserved for cases where biopsy is inadequate or therapeutic intervention is needed.

Hysteroscopy-guided D&C improves diagnostic yield and reduces complications.

Avoid overuse due to risk of Asherman's syndrome, especially in reproductive-age women.

Combined Approach

Ultrasound or MRI often precedes biopsy or D&C to guide sampling.

Histopathology results correlate with clinical and imaging findings for comprehensive diagnosis.

Multidisciplinary management (gynecologist, pathologist, oncologist) is critical for malignant findings.

Conclusion

Histopathology examination of cervical and endometrial biopsies, along with dilatation and curettage, are cornerstone procedures in gynecology for diagnosing and managing conditions ranging from precancerous lesions to endometrial cancer and pregnancy-related complications. Cervical biopsy is critical in cervical cancer screening pathways, while endometrial biopsy and D&C are essential for evaluating abnormal uterine bleeding and pregnancy outcomes.

16.9 Hysterosalpingography

(*Ambuba nigari Rahim*)

Definition

Hysterosalpingography (HSG) is a fluoroscopic imaging technique that uses radiopaque contrast to evaluate the uterine cavity and fallopian tubes for structural abnormalities and tubal patency. It is a key diagnostic tool in the infertility workup, providing detailed visualization of the uterine shape and tubal lumen.

Indications

Infertility evaluation to assess tubal patency (e.g., primary or secondary infertility).

Investigation of recurrent pregnancy loss (e.g., uterine anomalies, intrauterine adhesions).

Evaluation of suspected uterine abnormalities (e.g., fibroids, polyps, synechiae).

Post-surgical assessment (e.g., tubal ligation, myomectomy, or tubal recanalization).

Suspected Asherman's syndrome or congenital uterine anomalies (e.g., septate uterus).

Technique

1. Preparation

Perform during the follicular phase (Days 7–12 of the menstrual cycle) to avoid pregnancy and ensure a thin endometrium for optimal visualization.

Obtain informed consent; explain risks (e.g., pain, radiation, infection).

Screen for pregnancy, active pelvic infection, or contrast allergy.

Administer prophylactic antibiotics (e.g., doxycycline 100 mg BID for 5 days) if infection risk is high (e.g., history of pelvic inflammatory disease).

Premedicate with NSAIDs (e.g., ibuprofen 400–800 mg) 30–60 minutes prior to reduce cramping.

2. Procedure

Position: Patient in lithotomy position with a speculum to expose the cervix.

Cervical Cannulation: Insert a sterile cannula (e.g., HSG catheter with balloon or tenaculum) into the cervical os.

Contrast Injection: Slowly inject 5–10 mL of water-soluble iodinated contrast (e.g., iohexol or iopamidol) under real-time fluoroscopy.

Imaging: Capture serial X-ray images to visualize:

Uterine cavity filling (early phase).

Contrast flow through fallopian tubes (tubal phase).

Spillage into the peritoneal cavity (indicating tubal patency).

Documentation: Record uterine contour, tubal patency, and any abnormalities.

3. Post-Procedure

Monitor for cramping, spotting, or signs of allergic reaction.

Advise avoiding intercourse or tampons for 24–48 hours to reduce infection risk.

Provide follow-up instructions for reviewing results and planning further management.

Findings

Uterus Normal: Smooth, triangular cavity with no filling defects.

Uterus Abnormal

Filling defects: Endometrial polyps (smooth, round), submucosal fibroids (irregular), or synechiae (irregular bands, Asherman's syndrome).

Congenital anomalies: Septate uterus (partial division), bicornuate uterus (two horns), unicornuate uterus (single horn).

Fallopian Tubes

Patent: Free spillage of contrast into the peritoneal cavity bilaterally.

Obstructed:

Proximal obstruction: No contrast beyond the cornual region (e.g., tubal spasm, scarring).

Distal obstruction: Dilated tubes with no peritoneal spillage (e.g., hydrosalpinx).

Peritubal Adhesions: Loculated contrast spillage or abnormal tubal course.

Other: Extravasation of contrast (e.g., venous intravasation) may occur with excessive pressure.

Clinical Significance

Gold standard for assessing tubal patency and uterine cavity abnormalities in infertility evaluation.

Sensitivity: ~85–90% for detecting tubal occlusion; specificity: ~80–85%.

Therapeutic benefit: Contrast injection may dislodge minor tubal blockages, improving fertility in some cases.

Guides management: IVF for tubal occlusion, hysteroscopy for synechiae, or surgery for uterine anomalies.

Advantages

Provides detailed visualization of the uterine cavity and fallopian tubes.

Relatively low cost and widely available compared to MRI or laparoscopy.

Real-time imaging allows dynamic assessment of contrast flow.

May have a therapeutic effect by clearing minor tubal obstructions.

Limitations

Ionizing radiation exposure (1–2 mSv), contraindicated in pregnancy.

Risk of pain, infection (1–3%), or contrast allergy (rare, <1%).

Limited evaluation of extrauterine structures (e.g., ovaries, endometriosis).

False positives for tubal occlusion due to spasm (mitigated by slow contrast injection or antispasmodics).

Less accurate for uterine anomalies compared to 3D ultrasound or MRI.

Complications

Common: Mild to moderate cramping, spotting or vaginal discharge.

Rare: Pelvic infection (endometritis, salpingitis), contrast allergy, uterine perforation or vasovagal reaction.

Gynecological Uses

Essential in the infertility workup to identify tubal factor infertility (15–20% of cases) or uterine abnormalities.

Complements ultrasound and laparoscopy for comprehensive evaluation.

Critical for planning interventions (e.g., tubal surgery, IVF, or hysteroscopic resection).

Useful in recurrent miscarriage to detect uterine anomalies or synechiae.

16.10 Sonosalpingography

(*Ambuba nigari*)

Definition

Sonosalpingography (SSG), also known as saline infusion sonohysterography with tubal assessment or hysterosonography, is an ultrasound-based technique that uses saline or other echogenic fluid to evaluate the uterine cavity and assess tubal patency. It is a less invasive alternative to HSG, avoiding radiation exposure.

Indications

Infertility evaluation to assess tubal patency and uterine cavity abnormalities.

Investigation of recurrent pregnancy loss (e.g., uterine septum, synechiae).

Evaluation of abnormal uterine bleeding (e.g., polyps, fibroids).

Post-surgical assessment of the uterine cavity (e.g., after myomectomy or adhesiolysis).

Preferred in patients with contrast allergies or those wishing to avoid radiation.

Technique

1. Preparation

Perform in the follicular phase (Days 7–12) to avoid pregnancy and optimize endometrial visualization.

Obtain informed consent; explain mild discomfort or cramping.

Screen for pregnancy or active pelvic infection.

Administer NSAIDs (e.g., ibuprofen 400 mg) 30–60 minutes prior if needed.

2. Procedure

Position: Patient in lithotomy position with a speculum to expose the cervix.

Transvaginal Ultrasound (TVUS): Insert a 5–9 MHz transvaginal probe to visualize the uterus and adnexa.

Cervical Cannulation: Insert a sterile catheter (e.g., HSG catheter or intrauterine insemination catheter) into the cervical os, with or without a balloon to prevent backflow.

Fluid Injection: Inject 10–20 mL of sterile saline (for uterine cavity assessment) or saline with air bubbles (for tubal patency) slowly into the uterine cavity.

Optional: Use echogenic contrast (e.g., Echovist, Levovist) for enhanced visualization of tubal flow.

Imaging

Uterine cavity: Observe for filling defects (polyps, fibroids) or contour abnormalities (septum).

Fallopian tubes: Visualize saline or air bubbles flowing through the tubes and spilling into the peritoneal cavity (seen as free fluid in the cul-de-sac). Doppler ultrasound may assess tubal flow dynamics.

Documentation: Record uterine and tubal findings in real-time.

3. Post-Procedure

Monitor for mild cramping or spotting.

Advise avoiding intercourse or tampons for 24–48 hours to reduce infection risk.

Findings

Uterus

Normal: Smooth, triangular cavity with no filling defects.

Abnormal:

Polyps: Hyperechoic, pedunculated masses.

Submucosal fibroids: Hypoechoic, intramural extension.

Synechiae: Irregular bands disrupting the cavity (Asherman's syndrome).

Congenital anomalies: Septate or bicornuate uterus.

Fallopian Tubes

Patent: Saline or air bubbles flow through the tubes, with free fluid in the cul-de-sac.

Obstructed: No flow beyond the cornual region (proximal block) or dilated tubes with no spillage (distal block, e.g., hydrosalpinx).

Adhesions: Limited free fluid or abnormal tubal course.

Clinical Significance

Highly sensitive (~90%) and specific (~85–90%) for detecting uterine abnormalities; slightly less accurate than HSG for tubal patency.

Preferred in low-risk patients or settings where radiation avoidance is prioritized (e.g., young women, early infertility workup).

Guides infertility treatment (e.g., IVF for tubal occlusion, hysteroscopy for polyps).

Complements HSG or laparoscopy for comprehensive evaluation.

Advantages

No ionizing radiation, safe for women of reproductive age.

Performed with ultrasound, which is widely available and cost-effective.

Real-time imaging with dynamic assessment of the uterine cavity and tubes.

High resolution for endometrial abnormalities compared to HSG.

Minimal discomfort and lower infection risk compared to HSG.

Limitations

Operator-dependent; requires skilled ultrasonographer.

Less accurate than HSG for distal tubal pathology or subtle adhesions.

Limited visualization of tubal lumen compared to fluoroscopy.

May miss small filling defects or complex uterine anomalies without 3D ultrasound.

Complications

Common: Mild cramping, spotting or fluid leakage.

Rare: Infection (endometritis, <1%), uterine perforation, or vasovagal reaction.

Gynecological uses

Preferred alternative to HSG in early infertility evaluation or radiation-sensitive patients.

Enhances endometrial assessment in abnormal uterine bleeding or infertility.

Useful in low-resource settings with ultrasound availability but no fluoroscopy.

Complements hysteroscopy for preoperative planning of uterine abnormalities.

16.11 Laparoscopy with Dye instillations

(Batn beeni hamrah rang beeni)

Introduction

Laparoscopy with dye instillation, also known as chromopertubation, is a minimally invasive surgical procedure widely used in gynecology to evaluate the patency of the fallopian tubes and diagnose pelvic pathologies. This technique combines diagnostic laparoscopy with the instillation of a dye, typically methylene blue or indigo carmine, through the cervix to assess tubal function, particularly in the context of infertility evaluations. It is commonly performed as part of a comprehensive fertility workup or to diagnose conditions such as endometriosis, pelvic adhesions or tubal occlusions.

Indications

Laparoscopy with dye instillation is indicated for:

1. Infertility Evaluation: To assess fallopian tube patency in women with unexplained infertility or suspected tubal factor infertility.
2. Pelvic Pain: To diagnose conditions like endometriosis, pelvic inflammatory disease (PID) or adhesions.
3. Suspected Tubal Pathology: To confirm or rule out tubal occlusion, hydrosalpinx or peritubal adhesions.
4. Preoperative Assessment: Before fertility-enhancing procedures, such as tubal reconstructive surgery.
5. Ectopic Pregnancy Evaluation: To assess tubal integrity in cases of suspected ectopic pregnancy or previous tubal surgery.

Contraindications

1. Absolute Contraindications

Unstable hemodynamic status (e.g., shock).

Severe cardiopulmonary disease precluding general anesthesia.

Known hypersensitivity to the dye used (e.g., methylene blue or indigo carmine).

2. Relative Contraindications

Active pelvic infection or untreated PID.

Severe obesity or extensive abdominal adhesions, which may complicate access.

Pregnancy, unless clinically justified (e.g., suspected ectopic pregnancy).

Procedure

1. Preoperative Preparation

Patient Evaluation: Includes a thorough history, physical examination and relevant imaging (e.g., ultrasound) to rule out contraindications.

Informed Consent: Discuss risks, benefits and alternatives, including potential complications like dye allergies or infection.

Antibiotic Prophylaxis: May be administered to reduce infection risk.

Anesthesia: General anesthesia is typically used due to the need for pneumoperitoneum and patient comfort.

2. Surgical Technique

Positioning: The patient is placed in the lithotomy position with a slight Trendelenburg tilt to facilitate pelvic visualization.

Access: A small incision (5–10 mm) is made at the umbilicus to insert a laparoscope. Additional 5-mm ports may be placed in the lower abdomen for accessory instruments.

Pneumoperitoneum: The abdominal cavity is insufflated with carbon dioxide (CO_2) to create a working space, maintaining intra-abdominal pressure at 12–15 mmHg.

The laparoscope is used to inspect the pelvic organs, including the uterus, ovaries, fallopian tubes and surrounding structures, for abnormalities like endometriosis, fibroids or adhesions.

Dye Instillation (Chromopertubation)

A cannula (e.g., Cohen or Hulka cannula) is inserted transcervically into the uterine cavity.

A dilute solution of methylene blue or indigo carmine (typically 5–10 mL) is injected slowly through the cannula.

The surgeon observes the fallopian tubes laparoscopically for dye spillage from the fimbrial ends, indicating tubal patency.

Absence of spillage suggests tubal occlusion, which may be proximal (near the uterus) or distal (e.g., hydrosalpinx).

Documentation: Findings are recorded, including tubal patency, presence of adhesions or other pathologies. Photographs or videos may be taken for records.

Closure: Ports are removed, CO_2 is evacuated and incisions are closed with sutures or adhesive strips.

3. Postoperative Care

Recovery: Patients are monitored for 2–4 hours post-procedure in a recovery unit. Most are discharged the same day.

Pain Management: Mild analgesics (e.g., NSAIDs) are prescribed for postoperative discomfort.

Follow-Up: A postoperative visit is scheduled within 1–2 weeks to discuss findings and plan further management (e.g., fertility treatments or additional surgery).

Complications to Monitor: Include infection, bleeding or organ injury (e.g., bowel, bladder, or vascular injury), though these are rare (<1%).

Findings and Interpretation

Normal Findings: Dye spills freely from both fimbrial ends, indicating patent fallopian tubes. Pelvic organs appear normal without adhesions or endometriosis.

Abnormal Findings

Proximal Tubal Occlusion: No dye passage through the tubes, often due to scarring, PID, or congenital anomalies.

Distal Tubal Occlusion: Dye fills the tube but does not spill, indicating a blockage (e.g., hydrosalpinx).

Adhesions or Endometriosis: May restrict tubal mobility or cause partial occlusion.

Uterine Anomalies: May be noted during dye instillation or visualization (e.g., bicornuate uterus).

Complications

Laparoscopy with dye instillation is generally safe, with a complication rate of <2%. Potential complications include:

1. Anesthetic Risks: Reactions to general anesthesia.

2. Surgical Risks

Injury to bowel, bladder or blood vessels during trocar insertion (<0.5%).

Infection or abscess formation.

3. Dye-Related Risks

Allergic reactions to methylene blue or indigo carmine (rare).

Transient blue-green discoloration of urine (benign).

4. Pneumoperitoneum-Related Risks: CO_2 embolism (extremely rare) or shoulder pain from residual gas.

Advantages

Minimally Invasive: Small incisions reduce recovery time and scarring compared to open surgery.

Diagnostic and Therapeutic: Allows simultaneous diagnosis (e.g., tubal occlusion) and treatment (e.g., adhesiolysis or endometriosis ablation).

High Accuracy: Provides direct visualization of tubal patency and pelvic anatomy, superior to hysterosalpingography (HSG) in detecting peritubal adhesions or endometriosis.

Limitations

Invasive Nature: Requires anesthesia and carries surgical risks, unlike non-invasive tests like HSG.

Limited Therapeutic Scope: Cannot correct all tubal pathologies (e.g., severe proximal occlusion may require IVF).

Cost and Availability: More expensive and resource-intensive than HSG, requiring specialized equipment and trained personnel.

Dye Availability: Indigo carmine shortages (noted in recent years) may limit use in some settings.

Comparison

1. Hysterosalpingography (HSG): A non-invasive alternative using X-ray and contrast to assess tubal patency. HSG is less costly but cannot visualize pelvic adhesions or endometriosis and has a higher false-positive rate for tubal occlusion.

2. Hysterosalpingo-Contrast Sonography (HyCoSy): Uses ultrasound and saline or contrast to assess tubal patency. It avoids radiation but is less accurate for pelvic pathology.

3. Laparoscopy with Dye: The gold standard for assessing tubal patency and pelvic anatomy, offering direct visualization and therapeutic potential.

Clinical Relevance

Laparoscopy with dye instillation is a cornerstone in the infertility workup when tubal or pelvic factors are suspected. It guides management decisions, such as:

Patent Tubes: Proceed with ovulation induction or intrauterine insemination (IUI).

Tubal Occlusion: Consider tubal surgery (e.g., salpingostomy) or in vitro fertilization (IVF).

Endometriosis or Adhesions: Perform ablation or adhesiolysis during the procedure to improve fertility outcomes.

Conclusion

Laparoscopy with dye instillation remains a vital diagnostic and therapeutic tool in gynecology, particularly for infertility and pelvic pathology evaluation. Its ability to directly visualize tubal patency and pelvic structures makes it indispensable in cases where non-invasive tests are inconclusive. While associated with low risks, proper patient selection and surgical expertise are critical to maximizing its benefits.

Key Points

Chromopertubation assesses fallopian tube patency and pelvic pathology.

It is the gold standard for tubal evaluation but is more invasive than HSG or HyCoSy.

Common dyes include methylene blue and indigo carmine.

Complications are rare but include organ injury and dye allergies.

The procedure guides infertility treatment decisions, such as IVF or surgical correction.

Therapeutic Gynecological Procedures

Mnemonic: "HELP CURE"

Letter	Procedure	Application
H	Hysterectomy	Uterine fibroid, cancer, AUB
E	Endometrial ablation	Menorrhagia, contraindicated in cancer
L	LEEP	Cervical dysplasia
P	Polypectomy	Uterine/cervical polyps
C	Cryotherapy	Cervical ectopy, low-grade lesions
U	Uterosacral ligament plication - Prolapse correction	
R	Repair procedures	Fistula, incontinence (sling)
E	Electrosurgery	Ablation or excision of lesions

16.12 Colposcopy & Hysteroscopy

(*Tanzeer-ul-mahbil aur tanzeeeru-r-rahim*)

Colposcopy

Introduction

Colposcopy is a diagnostic procedure used in gynecology to closely examine the cervix, vagina and vulva for signs of disease, particularly cervical intraepithelial neoplasia (CIN) and cervical cancer. It involves the use of a colposcope, a low-power stereoscopic microscope with magnification (typically 5–20x) and illumination, to visualize epithelial and vascular changes not visible to the naked eye. Colposcopy is necessary in the evaluation of abnormal cervical screening results, such as atypical Pap smears or positive human papillomavirus (HPV) tests, and plays a critical role in the early detection and management of cervical pathology.

Indications

Colposcopy is indicated for:

1. Abnormal Cervical Screening Results

Atypical squamous cells of undetermined significance (ASC-US) with high-risk HPV positivity.

Low-grade squamous intraepithelial lesion (LSIL) or high-grade squamous intraepithelial lesion (HSIL).

Atypical glandular cells (AGC) or adenocarcinoma in situ (AIS).

2. Persistent HPV Infection: High-risk HPV positivity persisting beyond 1–2 years.

3. Visible Cervical Abnormalities: Suspicious lesions, polyps, or ulceration noted during speculum examination.

4. Post-Treatment Surveillance: Follow-up after treatment for CIN (e.g., loop electrosurgical excision procedure [LEEP] or cone biopsy).

5. Unexplained Vaginal Bleeding: Postcoital or intermenstrual bleeding suggestive of cervical pathology.

6. Vulvar or Vaginal Lesions: To evaluate suspicious lesions or HPV-related changes in the lower genital tract.

7. Sexual Assault Evaluation: To document traumatic lesions or collect forensic evidence.

Contraindications

Colposcopy is a low-risk procedure with few contraindications:

1. Absolute Contraindications

Active pelvic infection (e.g., cervicitis or pelvic inflammatory disease) until treated.

Uncooperative patient unable to tolerate the procedure.

2. Relative Contraindications

Heavy menstrual bleeding, which may obscure visualization (reschedule after menses).

Pregnancy, unless high-grade lesions or malignancy are suspected, due to increased cervical vascularity.

Recent cervical surgery (e.g., within 6–8 weeks), as healing may obscure findings.

Procedure

1. Preoperative Preparation

Patient Counseling: Explain the procedure, its purpose and possible outcomes (e.g., need for biops). Obtain informed consent.

Timing: Ideally performed during the non-menstrual phase of the cycle to optimize visualization.

Medications: No routine antibiotics or anesthesia are required. Analgesics (e.g., ibuprofen) may be offered for discomfort, especially if biopsies are anticipated.

Equipment: A colposcope with adjustable magnification (5–20x), a speculum, acetic acid (3–5%), Lugol's iodine (optional), biopsy forceps, endocervical curette and hemostatic agents (e.g., Monsel's solution or silver nitrate).

2. Technique

Positioning: The patient is placed in the lithotomy position.

Speculum Insertion: A bivalve speculum is inserted to expose the cervix.

Initial Inspection: The cervix is examined under low magnification for gross abnormalities (e.g., erosions, masses or leukoplakia).

Acetic Acid Application

A 3–5% acetic acid solution is applied to the cervix using a cotton swab or spray.

Acetic acid causes dehydration of epithelial cells, highlighting abnormal areas (e.g., CIN) as acetowhite lesions due to increased nuclear density.

Normal epithelium appears pink, while abnormal areas turn white within 30–60 seconds.

Green Filter Use: A green filter on the colposcope enhances visualization of vascular patterns (e.g., mosaicism or punctation).

Lugol's Iodine (Optional)

Applied to the cervix to assess glycogen content.

Normal squamous epithelium (glycogen-rich) stains dark brown (Schiller test positive).

Abnormal areas (glycogen-poor, e.g., CIN or cancer) remain unstained or mustard-yellow (Schiller test negative).

Grading of Findings: Lesions are graded using systems like the Reid Colposcopic Index, which evaluates margins, color, vascularity, and iodine staining to predict severity (e.g., CIN 1–3).

Biopsy

Suspicious areas (e.g., acetowhite lesions, mosaicism, or irregular vessels) are biopsied using Tischler or Kevorkian forceps.

Endocervical curettage (ECC) is performed if the transformation zone is not fully visible or glandular abnormalities are suspected.

Hemostasis is achieved with Monsel's solution or silver nitrate if bleeding occurs.

Documentation: Findings are recorded using standardized terminology (e.g., International Federation for Cervical Pathology and Colposcopy [IFCPC] nomenclature). Diagrams or photographs may be used.

3. Postoperative Care

Immediate Care: Patients may experience mild cramping or spotting, especially if biopsies were taken.

Instructions: Avoid tampons, douching or intercourse for 1–2 weeks if biopsies were performed to reduce infection risk.

Follow-Up: Results are discussed within 1–2 weeks, with management based on biopsy findings (e.g., observation, LEEP, or cone biopsy).

Complications: Rare but include bleeding, infection, or cervical stenosis (<1%).

Colposcopic Findings

1. Normal Findings

Smooth, pink squamous epithelium.

Uniform transformation zone with columnar epithelium and squamocolumnar junction.

No acetowhite changes or abnormal vascular patterns.

Dark brown staining with Lugol's iodine.

2. Abnormal Findings

Acetowhite Lesions: Indicate increased nuclear density, suggestive of HPV-related changes or CIN.

Vascular Patterns

Punctation: Pinpoint blood vessels, often seen in low-grade lesions.

Mosaicism: Tile-like vascular patterns, suggestive of high-grade CIN.

Atypical Vessels: Irregular, corkscrew-shaped vessels, concerning for invasive cancer.

Irregular Margins: Raised or rolled edges may indicate CIN 2/3 or carcinoma.

Non-Staining with Lugol's Iodine: Suggests glycogen-poor epithelium (e.g., CIN or cancer).

Leukoplakia: White patches visible before acetic acid, often due to hyperkeratosis or HPV.

Erosion or Ulceration: May indicate infection, trauma, or malignancy.

3. Transformation Zone Types (IFCPC Classification)

Type 1: Fully visible squamocolumnar junction, easiest to assess.

Type 2: Partially visible, extends into the endocervical canal.

Type 3: Not fully visible, requiring ECC or further evaluation (common in postmenopausal women).

Complications

Colposcopy is a safe outpatient procedure with a complication rate of <1%. Potential complications include:

1. Bleeding: Minor spotting after biopsy, rarely requiring intervention.
2. Infection: Rare, minimized with sterile technique.
3. Pain: Mild cramping during or after the procedure, managed with NSAIDs.
4. Cervical Stenosis: Rare, associated with extensive biopsies or ECC.
5. Allergic Reactions: Extremely rare with acetic acid or Lugol's iodine.

Advantages

High Sensitivity: Detects subtle epithelial and vascular changes not visible on routine examination.

Targeted Biopsies: Allows precise sampling of abnormal areas, improving diagnostic accuracy.

Outpatient Procedure: Performed in 10–20 minutes with minimal recovery time.

Limitations

Operator-Dependent: Requires training to interpret findings accurately.

Incomplete Visualization: Type 3 transformation zones may necessitate additional procedures (e.g., cone biopsy).

False Negatives: Subtle or endocervical lesions may be missed, especially in inexperienced hands.

Discomfort: Biopsies or ECC may cause mild pain or cramping.

Cost: More resource-intensive than Pap smears or HPV testing, though cost-effective for high-risk cases.

Comparison with Other Modalities

Pap Smear: A screening tool with lower specificity; colposcopy is diagnostic and confirmatory.

HPV Testing: Identifies high-risk HPV but cannot localize lesions; colposcopy visualizes abnormalities.

Cervical Biopsy without Colposcopy: Blind biopsies have lower yield compared to colposcopy-guided sampling.

Hysterosalpingography (HSG): Used for tubal patency, not cervical pathology; unrelated to colposcopy.

Clinical Relevance in Cervical Cancer Prevention

Colposcopy is integral to the cervical cancer screening and prevention pathway

Triage of Abnormal Screens: Confirms or rules out high-grade lesions (CIN 2/3) in patients with abnormal Pap or HPV results.

Management: Directs treatment (e.g., LEEP for CIN 2/3) or surveillance for low-grade lesions (CIN 1).

Early Detection: Identifies precancerous lesions, reducing progression to invasive cervical cancer.

Post-Treatment Monitoring: Ensures clearance of lesions after excisional procedures.

Conclusion

Colposcopy is an important diagnostic tool in gynecology, bridging cervical screening and definitive management of precancerous and cancerous lesions. Its ability to provide magnified visualization and targeted biopsies ensures accurate diagnosis and guides treatment, significantly reducing cervical cancer morbidity and mortality.

Key Points

Colposcopy evaluates the cervix, vagina and vulva for abnormalities following abnormal Pap or HPV tests.

Acetic acid and Lugol's iodine highlight abnormal epithelium and vascular patterns.

Biopsies and ECC confirm histologic diagnoses (e.g., CIN 1–3 or cancer).

The procedure is safe, outpatient and operator-dependent, requiring training for accuracy.

Colposcopy is central to cervical cancer prevention, guiding triage and treatment.

Hysteroscopy

Introduction

Hysteroscopy is a minimally invasive procedure that allows direct visualization of the uterine cavity using a hysteroscope, a thin, lighted endoscope. It is widely used in gynecology for both diagnostic and therapeutic purposes, particularly in evaluating and treating conditions affecting the endometrium, uterine cavity and endocervix. Hysteroscopy is a cornerstone in the management of abnormal uterine bleeding, infertility, and other gynecologic conditions, offering high diagnostic accuracy and the ability to perform targeted interventions in an outpatient or inpatient setting.

Indications

Hysteroscopy is indicated for

1. Diagnostic Purposes

Abnormal Uterine Bleeding (AUB): Evaluation of heavy menstrual bleeding, intermenstrual bleeding or postmenopausal bleeding to identify causes such as endometrial polyps, submucosal fibroids or malignancy.

Infertility and Recurrent Pregnancy Loss: To assess uterine cavity abnormalities (e.g., septa, adhesions, or polyps) that may impair implantation or pregnancy maintenance.

Suspected Endometrial Pathology: To investigate endometrial hyperplasia, carcinoma or chronic endometritis via direct visualization and biopsy.

Lost Intrauterine Devices (IUDs): To locate and retrieve displaced or embedded IUDs.

Congenital Uterine Anomalies: To diagnose conditions like septate or bicornuate uterus.

2. Therapeutic Purposes

Polypectomy: Removal of endometrial polyps.

Myomectomy: Resection of submucosal fibroids.

Adhesiolysis: Lysis of intrauterine adhesions (Asherman's syndrome).

Septum Resection: Correction of uterine septa to improve fertility outcomes.

Endometrial Ablation: Destruction of the endometrial lining for heavy menstrual bleeding in patients not desiring future fertility.

Tubal Sterilization: Placement of sterilization devices (e.g., Essure, though less common now).

Removal of Foreign Bodies: Extraction of retained products of conception or foreign objects.

Contraindications

1. Absolute Contraindications

Acute Pelvic Infection: Including cervicitis, endometritis, or pelvic inflammatory disease (PID), due to risk of spreading infection.

Known Cervical or Endometrial Cancer: Unless performed for staging or biopsy under controlled conditions, due to risk of tumor dissemination.

Pregnancy: Except in rare cases (e.g., removal of retained products of conception).

Uncontrolled Bleeding Disorders: Due to risk of significant hemorrhage.

2. Relative Contraindications

Heavy Uterine Bleeding: May obscure visualization, requiring rescheduling or preoperative treatment (e.g., GnRH agonists).

Severe Cervical Stenosis: May prevent hysteroscope insertion, though dilation may be attempted.

Severe Comorbidities: Conditions precluding anesthesia or prolonged procedures.

Procedure

1. Preoperative Preparation

Patient Evaluation: Includes history, physical examination and imaging (e.g., transvaginal ultrasound) to identify indications and rule out contraindications.

Informed Consent: Discuss risks, benefits and alternatives, including potential complications like uterine perforation or fluid overload.

Timing: Preferably performed in the early follicular phase (days 5–10 of the menstrual cycle) for optimal endometrial visualization, unless urgent (e.g., postmenopausal bleeding).

Medications

Misoprostol (200–400 µg vaginally or orally) may be used 4–12 hours pre-procedure to soften the cervix, especially in nulliparous or postmenopausal patients.

Antibiotic prophylaxis (e.g., doxycycline) may be given if infection risk is high (e.g., history of PID).

Analgesics (e.g., NSAIDs) or local anesthesia (e.g., paracervical block) for office-based procedures; general or regional anesthesia for operative hysteroscopy.

Equipment

Hysteroscope: Rigid (2–4 mm for diagnostic, 5–10 mm for operative) or flexible, with a light source and camera.

Distension Media: Saline for diagnostic procedures; electrolyte-free solutions (e.g., glycine, sorbitol) for operative procedures using monopolar energy.

Instruments: Scissors, graspers, resectoscopes, or morcellators for therapeutic procedures.

2. Surgical Technique

Positioning: The patient is placed in the lithotomy position.

Cervical Preparation: A speculum is inserted to visualize the cervix, which is cleaned with antiseptic. Cervical dilation may be required for larger hysteroscopes (e.g., Hegar dilators).

Hysteroscope Insertion

The hysteroscope is inserted through the cervical canal into the uterine cavity under direct visualization or video guidance.

The uterine cavity is distended with fluid (saline or electrolyte-free solution) or gas (CO_2, less common) to a pressure of 40–100 mmHg for visualization.

Diagnostic Hysteroscopy

The endocervix, uterine cavity and tubal ostia are systematically inspected.

Findings (e.g., polyps, fibroids, adhesions or septa) are documented using standardized terminology.

Targeted biopsies may be taken if endometrial pathology is suspected.

Operative Hysteroscopy

Performed using resectoscopes, morcellators or specialized instruments.

Examples: Resection of polyps or fibroids, lysis of adhesions or endometrial ablation.

Bipolar energy is preferred for safety with saline distension; monopolar energy requires electrolyte-free media.

Fluid Management

Fluid input and output are closely monitored to prevent fluid overload, especially with electrolyte-free solutions (risk of hyponatremia).

Maximum fluid deficit: ~1,000 mL for saline, ~750 mL for glycine/sorbitol.

Closure and Recovery: No sutures are required. Patients are monitored for 1–4 hours post-procedure, depending on anesthesia and intervention.

3. Postoperative Care

Recovery: Most patients are discharged the same day for diagnostic procedures; operative cases may require overnight observation.

Pain Management: NSAIDs for mild cramping; stronger analgesics rarely needed.

Instructions: Avoid tampons, douching, or intercourse for 1–2 weeks if operative intervention was performed.

Follow -Up: Scheduled within 1–2 weeks to discuss findings, biopsy results, or further management (e.g., fertility planning or repeat hysteroscopy).

Complications to Monitor: Include infection, bleeding, uterine perforation or fluid overload symptoms (e.g., dyspnea, confusion).

Findings and Interpretation

Normal Findings

Uniform, thin endometrium (in follicular phase).

Patent cervical canal and tubal ostia.

No structural abnormalities (e.g., septa, adhesions, or masses).

Abnormal Findings

Endometrial Polyps: Pedunculated or sessile growths, often benign but may cause bleeding or infertility.

Submucosal Fibroids: Protrude into the cavity, causing AUB or infertility.

Intrauterine Adhesions (Asherman's Syndrome): Fibrous bands, often post-surgical or post-inflammatory, leading to amenorrhea or infertility.

Uterine Septum: Congenital anomaly associated with recurrent pregnancy loss.

Endometrial Hyperplasia or Cancer: Thickened, irregular endometrium or mass-like lesions; biopsy confirms diagnosis.

Chronic Endometritis: Erythematous or micropapillary endometrium, often requiring biopsy for confirmation.

Complications

Hysteroscopy has a low complication rate (<1–2%), but potential risks include:

1. Uterine Perforation: (<1%) Occurs during cervical dilation or hysteroscope insertion, especially in stenotic cervices. May require laparoscopy or laparotomy if severe.

2. Fluid Overload: Due to excessive absorption of distension media, leading to hyponatremia, pulmonary edema, or cerebral edema (more common with glycine/sorbitol).

3. Infection: Endometritis or PID, minimized with sterile technique and antibiotics.

4. Bleeding: Usually mild; significant hemorrhage is rare but may require hemostatic agents or uterine tamponade.

5. Cervical Trauma: Laceration or stenosis from dilation, particularly in nulliparous or postmenopausal patients.

6. Anesthetic Risks: Related to general or regional anesthesia in operative cases.

Advantages

Direct Visualization: Provides high-resolution imaging of the uterine cavity, superior to ultrasound or hysterosalpingography (HSG) for intracavitary pathology.

Diagnostic and Therapeutic: Allows simultaneous diagnosis and treatment (e.g., polypectomy, adhesiolysis).

Minimally Invasive: Outpatient procedure with rapid recovery and minimal scarring.

Improved Outcomes: Enhances fertility by correcting structural abnormalities and guides management of AUB.

Limitations

Operator-Dependent: Requires training for accurate diagnosis and safe intervention.

Limited Scope: Cannot address extrauterine pathology (e.g., adnexal masses) or deep myometrial fibroids.

Fluid Risks: Electrolyte-free media require strict fluid monitoring to prevent overload.

Cost: More expensive than ultrasound or HSG, though cost-effective for targeted indications.

Cervical Stenosis: May prevent access, requiring alternative approaches (e.g., ultrasound-guided dilation).

Comparison with Other Modalities

Transvaginal Ultrasound (TVUS): Non-invasive, first-line for AUB or infertility but less specific for intracavitary lesions.

Hysterosalpingography (HSG): Assesses tubal patency and uterine cavity contour but cannot visualize endometrial pathology or perform interventions.

Saline Infusion Sonography (SIS): Enhances ultrasound visualization of the uterine cavity but is less precise than hysteroscopy for small lesions or biopsies.

MRI: Useful for deep myometrial or adnexal pathology but not routine for intracavitary evaluation.

Clinical Relevance

Hysteroscopy is integral to gynecological practice for

Abnormal Uterine Bleeding: Identifies and treats causes like polyps, fibroids, or hyperplasia, reducing the need for hysterectomy.

Infertility: Improves pregnancy rates by correcting uterine abnormalities (e.g., septa, adhesions).

Endometrial Cancer: Facilitates early diagnosis via biopsy, especially in postmenopausal bleeding.

Recurrent Pregnancy Loss: Corrects structural causes like septa or adhesions to improve outcomes.

Conclusion

Hysteroscopy is a versatile and essential tool in gynecology, offering unparalleled diagnostic and therapeutic capabilities for uterine cavity disorders. Its minimally invasive nature, combined with the ability to address conditions like AUB, infertility, and endometrial pathology, makes it a cornerstone of modern gynecologic practice.

Key Points

Hysteroscopy visualizes the uterine cavity for diagnosis (e.g., AUB, infertility) and treatment (e.g., polypectomy, septal resection).

Distension media (saline or glycine) and fluid monitoring are critical to prevent overload.

Common findings include polyps, fibroids, adhesions, and septa; biopsies confirm malignancy.

Complications (e.g., perforation, fluid overload) are rare but require vigilance.

Hysteroscopy is superior to HSG or ultrasound for intracavitary pathology and therapeutic interventions.

Role of Endoscopy in Gynecology

Endoscopic Techniques
↓
Type of Access
↓ ↓
Cervical Abdominal
↓ ↓
Hysteroscopy Laparoscopy
↓ ↓
Visualize Uterine Cavity Visualize Pelvic Organs
↓ ↓
Diagnostic Therapeutic
↓ ↓
Polyps, AUB, Septa Fibroids, Endometriosis, Adhesions

16.13 Laparoscopy

(*Tanzeer-al-Batn*)

Introduction

Laparoscopy is a minimally invasive surgical technique that uses a laparoscope—a thin, fiber-optic telescope with a camera—to visualize and treat conditions within the pelvic and abdominal cavities. In gynecology, it is a cornerstone for both diagnostic and therapeutic purposes, offering high-resolution visualization of pelvic organs (e.g., uterus, ovaries, fallopian tubes) with minimal morbidity compared to open surgery.

Indications

Laparoscopy is indicated for a wide range of gynecologic conditions:

1. Diagnostic Purposes

Infertility Evaluation: To assess tubal patency (via chromopertubation), endometriosis or pelvic adhesions.

Pelvic Pain: To diagnose causes such as endometriosis, ovarian cysts, or adhesions.

Pelvic Mass Evaluation: To characterize adnexal masses (e.g., ovarian cysts, tumors) or rule out malignancy.

Suspected Ectopic Pregnancy: To confirm location and guide management.

Congenital Anomalies: To evaluate Müllerian anomalies or pelvic organ abnormalities.

2. Therapeutic Purposes

Endometriosis: Excision or ablation of endometriotic lesions.

Ovarian Cysts: Cystectomy or oophorectomy for benign or suspicious masses.

Myomectomy: Removal of uterine fibroids, particularly subserosal or intramural types.

Hysterectomy: Total or subtotal laparoscopic hysterectomy for benign or malignant conditions.

Tubal Surgery: Salpingectomy (e.g., for ectopic pregnancy or hydrosalpinx) or tubal ligation for sterilization.

Adhesiolysis: Lysis of pelvic or intrauterine adhesions to restore anatomy or fertility.

Pelvic Organ Prolapse: Procedures like sacrocolpopexy for uterine or vaginal prolapse.

Oncologic Procedures: Staging for endometrial, cervical, or early ovarian cancer, or lymph node dissection.

Contraindications

1. Absolute Contraindications

Hemodynamic Instability: E.g., shock from ruptured ectopic pregnancy or severe bleeding, requiring urgent laparotomy.

Severe Cardiopulmonary Disease: Precluding general anesthesia or pneumoperitoneum tolerance.

Generalized Peritonitis: Due to risk of worsening infection with insufflation.

2. Relative Contraindications

Extensive Prior Abdominal Surgery: Dense adhesions may complicate access or visualization.

Severe Obesity: Increases technical difficulty, though not an absolute barrier.

Advanced Pregnancy: Beyond the first trimester, due to risk to the fetus and limited working space.

Coagulopathy: Increases bleeding risk, requiring correction pre-procedure.

Procedure

1. Preoperative Preparation

Patient Evaluation: Includes history, physical examination, imaging (e.g., ultrasound, MRI) and laboratory tests (e.g., CBC, coagulation profile).

Informed Consent: Discuss risks (e.g., organ injury, bleeding), benefits and alternatives (e.g., laparotomy or medical management).

Bowel Preparation: Optional; may involve a watery or liquid diet or enema for better visualization in complex cases.

Antibiotic Prophylaxis: Administered (e.g., cefazolin) for operative procedures to reduce infection risk.

Anesthesia: General anesthesia is standard due to pneumoperitoneum and patient comfort.

2. Surgical Technique

Positioning: The patient is placed in the lithotomy position with a slight Trendelenburg tilt (15–30°) to displace intestines cephalad and improve pelvic visualization.

Access

Primary Port: A 5–10 mm incision is made at the umbilicus for laparoscope insertion.

Veress Needle or Open (Hasson) Technique: Used to create pneumoperitoneum with carbon dioxide (CO_2) to a pressure of 12–15 mmHg in adults.

Additional Ports: 1–3 accessory ports (5–12 mm) are placed in the lower abdomen (e.g., suprapubic or iliac fossae) for instruments like graspers, scissors, or energy devices.

Visualization

The laparoscope (5–10 mm, 0° or 30° angled) provides high-definition imaging of the pelvic organs, peritoneum, and abdominal cavity.

Systematic inspection includes the uterus, ovaries, fallopian tubes, bladder, rectosigmoid, and peritoneal surfaces for abnormalities (e.g., endometriosis, adhesions, masses).

Diagnostic Procedures

Chromopertubation: Dye (e.g., methylene blue or indigo carmine) is injected transcervically to assess tubal patency (see Laparoscopy with Dye Instillation chapter).

Biopsy: Sampling of suspicious lesions (e.g., peritoneal implants or ovarian masses).

Therapeutic Procedures

Endometriosis Treatment: Excision or ablation of endometriotic implants using laser, monopolar, or bipolar energy.

Cystectomy/Myomectomy: Dissection of ovarian cysts or fibroids with preservation of healthy tissue.

Hysterectomy: Dissection of uterine attachments, ligation of vessels, and removal via morcellation or vaginal extraction.

Adhesiolysis: Cutting adhesions with scissors or energy devices to restore anatomy.

Energy Devices: Bipolar, monopolar, or ultrasonic (e.g., Harmonic scalpel) devices are used for cutting, coagulation, or hemostasis.

Closure

Ports are removed, and CO2 is evacuated to prevent postoperative shoulder pain.

Incisions are closed with absorbable sutures or adhesive strips. Fascial closure is required for ports >10 mm to prevent hernias.

3. Postoperative Care

Recovery: Patients are monitored for 2–6 hours (outpatient) or 1–2 days (inpatient, e.g., hysterectomy). Most diagnostic procedures allow same-day discharge.

Pain Management: NSAIDs or opioids for incisional pain or referred shoulder pain from residual CO2.

Instructions: Avoid heavy lifting or intercourse for 1–2 weeks (longer for major procedures like hysterectomy).

Follow-Up: Scheduled within 1–2 weeks to discuss pathology results and further management.

Complications to Monitor: Include infection, bleeding, organ injury, or venous thromboembolism (VTE).

Findings and Interpretation

Normal Findings

Smooth, pink uterus with normal size and shape.

Patent fallopian tubes (if chromopertubation performed).

Normal ovaries without cysts or masses.

No adhesions or endometriotic implants.

Abnormal Findings

Endometriosis: Chocolate cysts (endometriomas), peritoneal implants, or adhesions.

Adnexal Masses: Ovarian cysts (e.g., functional, dermoid, or malignant), hydrosalpinx, or paratubal cysts.

Adhesions: Fibrous bands restricting organ mobility, often from prior surgery or PID.

Uterine Anomalies: Septate or bicornuate uterus, often associated with infertility.

Ectopic Pregnancy: Tubal mass or rupture with hemoperitoneum.

Pelvic Inflammatory Disease: Tubo-ovarian abscess or pyosalpinx.

Complications

Laparoscopy is safe, with a complication rate of <2%. Potential complications include:

1. Access-Related

Vascular Injury: Damage to major vessels (e.g., aorta, iliac vessels) during Veress needle or trocar insertion (<0.1%).

Bowel or Bladder Injury: Rare (<0.5%), typically during entry or adhesiolysis; may require repair via laparoscopy or laparotomy.

2. Pneumoperitoneum-Related

CO2 Embolism: Extremely rare but life-threatening; presents with sudden cardiovascular collapse.

Subcutaneous Emphysema: From improper CO2 insufflation, usually self-limiting.

3. Procedure-Related

Bleeding: From vessel injury or incomplete hemostasis, managed with energy devices or sutures.

Infection: Wound infection or pelvic abscess, minimized with antibiotics.

4. Anesthetic Risks: Reactions to general anesthesia, including respiratory complications.

5. Postoperative

Shoulder Pain: From residual CO2 irritating the diaphragm, resolving within 1–2 days.

Hernia: At port sites, particularly >10 mm, if fascial closure is inadequate.

Advantages

Minimally Invasive: Small incisions (5–12 mm) reduce pain, scarring, and recovery time compared to laparotomy.

Diagnostic and Therapeutic: Allows simultaneous diagnosis and treatment (e.g., endometriosis excision, myomectomy).

Improved Visualization: Magnified, high-definition imaging enhances detection of subtle pathology.

Reduced Hospital Stay: Most procedures are outpatient or require 1–2 days of hospitalization.

Lower Complication Rates: Compared to open surgery, with less blood loss and infection risk.

Limitations

Operator-Dependent: Requires specialized training for safe and effective performance.

Technical Challenges: Dense adhesions, obesity, or large masses may necessitate conversion to laparotomy (<5% of cases).

Cost: Higher initial costs due to equipment and training, though offset by shorter hospital stays.

Limited Access: Not suitable for all patients (e.g., those with severe cardiopulmonary disease).

Anesthesia Requirement: General anesthesia carries risks, unlike some office-based procedures (e.g., hysteroscopy).

Comparison with Other Modalities

Ultrasound: Non-invasive, first-line for pelvic masses or AUB but lacks therapeutic capability and specificity for subtle pathology (e.g., endometriosis).

Hysterosalpingography (HSG): Assesses tubal patency but cannot visualize pelvic organs or treat pathology.

Hysteroscopy: Evaluates the uterine cavity but not extrauterine structures; often combined with laparoscopy for infertility workups.

Laparotomy: More invasive, reserved for cases unsuitable for laparoscopy (e.g., large fibroids, advanced malignancy).

MRI/CT: Useful for preoperative planning but not diagnostic or therapeutic for most gynecologic conditions.

Clinical Relevance

Infertility: Diagnoses and treats tubal factors, endometriosis, or adhesions, improving pregnancy rates.

Pelvic Pain: Identifies and manages endometriosis or adhesions, often alleviating symptoms.

Oncology: Facilitates staging and debulking in early gynecologic cancers.

Benign Conditions: Offers definitive treatment for fibroids, cysts or prolapse with minimal morbidity.

Emergency Settings: Manages ectopic pregnancy or ovarian torsion with precision and speed.

Conclusion

Laparoscopy is a transformative technique in gynecology, offering unparalleled diagnostic and therapeutic capabilities for a wide range of conditions. Its minimally invasive nature, combined with high accuracy and versatility, makes it indispensable for managing infertility, pelvic pain and benign or malignant gynecologic disorders.

Key Points

Laparoscopy visualizes and treats pelvic and abdominal pathology with minimal invasiveness.

Indications include infertility, pelvic pain, adnexal masses and gynecologic cancers. Chromopertubation assesses tubal patency during infertility evaluations.

Complications (e.g., organ injury, bleeding) are rare but require prompt recognition.

Laparoscopy is superior to imaging for direct visualization and intervention, with faster recovery than laparotomy.

16.14 Tubal Insufflation Test

(*Hawai amboob nigari*)

Definition

The tubal insufflation test, also known as Rubin's test, is a historical procedure that assesses fallopian tube patency by insufflating carbon dioxide (CO_2) gas through the cervix and monitoring for its passage into the peritoneal cavity. It has largely been replaced by HSG and SSG due to its lower accuracy and lack of imaging.

Indications

Historically used for infertility evaluation to assess tubal patency.

Rarely performed today; reserved for settings lacking access to HSG or SSG.

Investigation of suspected tubal occlusion in infertility or recurrent pregnancy loss.

Technique

1. Preparation

Perform in the follicular phase (Days 7–12) to avoid pregnancy.

Obtain informed consent; explain potential discomfort or shoulder pain (from CO_2).

Screen for pregnancy, active pelvic infection, or recent uterine surgery.

Administer NSAIDs for pain relief if needed.

2. Procedure

Position: Patient in lithotomy position with a speculum to expose the cervix.

Cervical Cannulation: Insert a Rubin's cannula or similar device into the cervical so, secured with a tenaculum if necessary.

Gas Insufflation

Slowly insufflate CO_2 gas (100–200 mL) at a controlled pressure (<200 mmHg) using a kymograph or insufflation device.

Monitor pressure changes to assess tubal patency.

Assessment

Patent Tubes: Gas passes freely, causing a drop in pressure and audible hissing or bubbling in the peritoneal cavity (heard via stethoscope).

Obstructed Tubes: Sustained high pressure (>200 mmHg) or no gas flow.

Shoulder Pain: Referred pain from diaphragmatic irritation by CO_2 indicates peritoneal spillage (patent tubes).

Documentation: Note pressure readings, gas flow and patient symptoms.

3. Post-Procedure

Monitor for cramping, shoulder pain or vasovagal symptoms.

Advise rest for 1–2 hours and avoidance of intercourse for 24–48 hours.

Findings

Patent Tubes

Pressure drops below 100 mmHg with gas flow.

Audible bubbling or shoulder pain confirms peritoneal spillage.

Obstructed Tubes

Persistent high pressure (>200 mmHg) or no gas flow.

Unilateral obstruction may show partial pressure drop.

Uterine Abnormalities

Cannot assess uterine cavity contour (no imaging component).

False Positives/Negatives

Tubal spasm may mimic obstruction (false positive).

Partial patency may be missed (false negative).

Clinical Significance

Historically significant but obsolete in modern practice due to low sensitivity (~70%) and specificity (~60–70%) compared to HSG or SSG.

Provides no imaging of the uterine cavity or tubal anatomy.

Rarely used except in extremely resource-limited settings without ultrasound or fluoroscopy.

Advantages

Simple, low-cost procedure requiring minimal equipment.

No radiation exposure or contrast use.

Can be performed in outpatient settings with basic facilities.

Limitations

Lack of imaging limits visualization of uterine or tubal anatomy.

High rate of false positives (tubal spasm) and false negatives (partial patency).

Risk of discomfort or complications from gas insufflation.

Cannot differentiate proximal vs. distal tubal obstruction or detect adhesions.

Largely replaced by HSG, SSG or laparoscopy due to superior accuracy.

Complications

Common: Cramping, shoulder pain (from CO_2 irritation), or vasovagal reaction.

Rare: Infection (endometritis, <1%), uterine perforation or air embolism (extremely rare with CO_2).

Gynecological Uses

Historical role in infertility evaluation but rarely used today due to advancements in imaging (HSG, SSG, laparoscopy).

Limited to settings with no access to modern diagnostic tools.

Does not provide sufficient diagnostic detail for comprehensive infertility management.

HSG and SSG complement ultrasound, MRI, or laparoscopy for comprehensive infertility evaluation.

Laparoscopy with chromotubation (dye injection) is the definitive method for tubal patency but is invasive and reserved for surgical person.

Patient Factors

Radiation exposure (HSG) is a concern in young women; SSG is safer.

Contrast allergies or infection risk guide the choice of procedure.

Infertility Management

Tubal occlusion (proximal or distal) may necessitate IVF or tubal surgery.

Uterine abnormalities (e.g., septum, synechiae) require hysteroscopic correction.

Findings guide counseling on fertility prognosis and treatment options.

Conclusion

Hysterosalpingography, sonosalpingography and tubal insufflation are diagnostic procedures used to evaluate tubal patency and uterine cavity abnormalities in the context of infertility and recurrent pregnancy loss. HSG remains the gold standard due to its detailed imaging, while SSG offers a radiation-free alternative with excellent endometrial visualization. The tubal insufflation test is largely obsolete due to its lack of imaging and lower accuracy.

16.15 Laparotomy

(*Shigaf-i-batn*)

Introduction

Laparotomy is an open surgical procedure involving a large abdominal incision to access the pelvic and abdominal cavities for diagnostic or therapeutic purposes in gynecology. While minimally invasive techniques like laparoscopy have become the preferred approach for many gynecologic conditions, laparotomy remains essential for complex cases, emergencies or situations where laparoscopy is contraindicated or technically unfeasible. It provides direct access to pelvic organs (uterus, ovaries, fallopian tubes) and surrounding structures, allowing comprehensive evaluation and management of benign and malignant gynecologic conditions.

Indications

Laparotomy is indicated for

1. Diagnostic Purposes

Uncertain Pelvic Mass: To evaluate large, complex or potentially malignant adnexal masses not adequately assessed by imaging or laparoscopy.

Staging of Gynecological Malignancies: To assess the extent of ovarian, endometrial or cervical cancer, including lymph node sampling.

Unexplained Pelvic Pain: When laparoscopy is inconclusive or contraindicated.

2. Therapeutic Purposes

Hysterectomy: Total or radical hysterectomy for large uterine fibroids, advanced endometriosis or gynecologic cancers (e.g., endometrial or cervical cancer).

Myomectomy: Removal of large or multiple uterine fibroids, particularly intramural or subserosal, not amenable to laparoscopic resection.

Ovarian Surgery: Oophorectomy or cystectomy for large ovarian masses, suspected malignancy or torsion.

Endometriosis: Excision of deep infiltrating endometriosis or large endometriomas not manageable laparoscopically.

Pelvic Adhesiolysis: Lysis of extensive adhesions from prior surgeries, pelvic inflammatory disease (PID) or endometriosis.

Emergency Conditions: Management of ruptured ectopic pregnancy, ovarian torsion or tubo-ovarian abscess with hemodynamic instability.

Oncologic Debulking: Cytoreductive surgery for advanced ovarian cancer to remove tumor burden.

Uterine Rupture or Trauma: Repair in cases of obstetric or traumatic emergencies.

Pelvic Organ Prolapse: Open procedures like abdominal sacrocolpopexy for severe prolapse.

Contraindications

1. Absolute Contraindications

None, as laparotomy is often a fallback procedure when other approaches are unsafe or inadequate.

2. Relative Contraindications

Patient Preference for Minimally Invasive Surgery: If laparoscopy is feasible and equally effective.

Severe Cardiopulmonary Disease: Increases anesthesia risks, though laparotomy may still be necessary in emergencies.

Morbid Obesity: Complicates wound healing and increases infection risk, though not an absolute barrier.

Procedure

1. Preoperative Preparation

Patient Evaluation: Includes a detailed history, physical examination, imaging (e.g., ultrasound, CT, MRI) and laboratory tests (e.g., CBC, coagulation profile, CA-125 for suspected malignancy).

Informed Consent: Discuss risks (e.g., bleeding, infection, prolonged recovery), benefits and alternatives (e.g., laparoscopy or expectant management).

Bowel Preparation: Often required (e.g., clear liquid diet, enema, or oral laxatives) to reduce intraoperative bowel content and improve visualization.

Antibiotic Prophylaxis: Administered 30–60 minutes pre-incision (e.g., cefazolin) to reduce surgical site infection risk.

Thromboprophylaxis: Sequential compression devices and/or heparin to prevent venous thromboembolism (VTE), especially in prolonged or oncologic procedures.

Anesthesia: General anesthesia is standard; epidural analgesia may be used for postoperative pain control.

2. Surgical Technique

Positioning: The patient is placed supine; a slight Trendelenburg tilt may be used to access the pelvis. A urinary catheter is inserted to decompress the bladder.

Incision Types

Midline Vertical: From pubis to umbilicus (or above for oncologic procedures), providing wide access for complex cases or malignancies.

Pfannenstiel: Low transverse incision, cosmetically favorable, used for benign conditions (e.g., hysterectomy, myomectomy).

Maylard or Cherney: Transverse muscle-cutting incisions for broader pelvic exposure.

Abdominal Entry

Skin, subcutaneous tissue, fascia and peritoneum are incised layer by layer.

The rectus muscles are separated (midline) or divided (transverse) to access the peritoneal cavity.

Exploration

Systematic inspection of the uterus, ovaries, fallopian tubes, bladder, ureters, bowel and peritoneum for abnormalities (e.g., masses, adhesions, metastases).

Peritoneal washings may be collected for cytology in suspected malignancy.

Therapeutic Procedures

Hysterectomy: Ligation of uterine vessels, dissection of attachments and removal of the uterus (total or subtotal).

Myomectomy: Enucleation of fibroids with preservation of the uterus, often requiring multilayer closure.

Oophorectomy/Salpingectomy: Removal of ovaries or fallopian tubes for masses, torsion or prophylaxis.

Debulking: Removal of tumor implants, omentum or lymph nodes in ovarian cancer.

Adhesiolysis: Dissection of adhesions using sharp or blunt techniques.

Energy Devices: Monopolar, bipolar or ultrasonic devices for cutting and hemostasis.

Hemostasis and Closure

Meticulous hemostasis using sutures, clips or energy devices.

The peritoneum (optional), fascia and skin are closed with absorbable or non-absorbable sutures. Subcutaneous drains may be placed for large procedures.

3. Postoperative Care

Recovery: Hospital stay ranges from 2–7 days, depending on the procedure (e.g., 2–3 days for hysterectomy, longer for oncologic debulking).

Pain Management: Patient-controlled analgesia (PCA), epidural or oral/IV analgesics (e.g., opioids, NSAIDs) for incisional pain.

Wound Care: Monitor for infection, dehiscence or hematoma; keep incision dry for 48 hours.

Mobilization: Early ambulation (within 24 hours) to reduce VTE risk.

Instructions: Avoid heavy lifting or strenuous activity for 6–8 weeks; refrain from intercourse for 4–6 weeks post-hysterectomy.

Follow-Up: Scheduled 1–2 weeks post-discharge to assess recovery and discuss pathology results.

Complications to Monitor: Include infection, wound dehiscence, VTE, ileus or organ injury.

Findings and Interpretation

Normal Findings

Normal-sized uterus, ovaries and fallopian tubes without adhesions or masses.

Clear peritoneal surfaces and no evidence of metastatic disease.

Abnormal Findings

Fibroids: Subserosal, intramural or pedunculated masses on the uterus.

Ovarian Pathology: Cysts (functional, dermoid, or malignant), endometriomas or torsion.

Endometriosis: Peritoneal implants, endometriomas or deep infiltrating lesions.

Adhesions: Fibrous bands from prior surgery, PID or endometriosis.

Malignancy: Tumor implants, ascites, or lymph node enlargement in ovarian, endometrial, or cervical cancer.

Ectopic Pregnancy: Tubal or abdominal pregnancy with possible hemoperitoneum.

Complications

Laparotomy has a higher complication rate (5–15%) than laparoscopy due to its invasiveness:

1. Intraoperative

Bleeding: From major vessels (e.g., uterine, ovarian) or incomplete hemostasis.

Organ Injury: Bowel, bladder or ureter injury (1–2%), requiring repair.

2. Postoperative

Wound Infection: Occurs in 3–5% of cases, higher in obese patients or diabetics.

Wound Dehiscence: Partial or complete separation of incision layers (<1%).

Incisional Hernia: Long-term risk (5–10%) at incision sites.

VTE: Deep vein thrombosis or pulmonary embolism, mitigated with prophylaxis.

Ileus: Delayed bowel function, usually resolving within 3–5 days.

Adhesions: Postoperative scarring, potentially causing pain or infertility.

3. Anesthetic Risks: Related to general anesthesia, including respiratory or cardiovascular complications.

Advantages

Wide Access: Provides unrestricted exposure for large or complex pathology (e.g., massive fibroids, advanced cancer).

Versatility: Allows comprehensive exploration and management of multiple organ systems.

Tactile Feedback: Enables direct palpation of tissues, critical for oncologic staging or complex dissections.

Feasibility in Emergencies: Preferred for hemodynamically unstable patients (e.g., ruptured ectopic pregnancy).

No Pneumoperitoneum: Avoids CO_2-related complications, suitable for patients with cardiopulmonary limitations.

Limitations

Invasive: Larger incisions lead to increased pain, longer recovery (4–8 weeks) and higher complication rates compared to laparoscopy.

Cosmesis: Larger scars, particularly with midline incisions, are less aesthetically favorable.

Hospital Stay: Prolonged compared to laparoscopy (2–7 days vs. 0–2 days).

Adhesion Risk: Higher likelihood of postoperative adhesions, potentially causing pain or infertility.

Cost: Higher due to longer hospitalization and recovery, though offset in cases where laparoscopy is not feasible.

Comparison with Other Modalities

Laparoscopy: Preferred for most gynecological procedures due to minimal invasiveness, faster recovery and lower complications. Laparotomy is reserved for cases where laparoscopy is inadequate (e.g., large masses, extensive adhesions).

Ultrasound: Non-invasive, first-line for imaging but lacks therapeutic capability.

Hysterosalpingography (HSG): Assesses tubal patency but cannot address extrauterine pathology or perform interventions.

Hysteroscopy: Evaluates the uterine cavity but not the pelvis; often combined with laparotomy for comprehensive management.

MRI/CT: Useful for preoperative planning but not diagnostic or therapeutic.

Clinical Relevance

Laparotomy remains critical in gynecology for

Complex Benign Conditions: Manages large fibroids, severe endometriosis or extensive adhesions not amenable to laparoscopy.

Gynecologic Oncology: Facilitates debulking and staging for ovarian, endometrial or cervical cancer.

Emergencies: Essential for life-threatening conditions like ruptured ectopic pregnancy or ovarian torsion with instability.

Fertility Preservation: Allows myomectomy or adhesiolysis in patients desiring future fertility.

Prolapse Repair: Offers durable outcomes for procedures like sacrocolpopexy in severe cases.

Conclusion

Laparotomy remains an indispensable technique for complex, emergent or oncologic cases where laparoscopy is insufficient. Despite its invasiveness, it provides unmatched access and tactile feedback, making it critical for managing large masses, advanced malignancies or emergencies.

Key Points

Laparotomy is an open surgical approach for complex gynecologic conditions, emergencies or when laparoscopy is not feasible.

Indications include large fibroids, advanced cancer or ruptured ectopic pregnancy.

Common incisions are midline vertical or Pfannenstiel, chosen based on pathology and cosmesis.

Complications (e.g., infection, adhesions) are higher than laparoscopy, requiring careful postoperative care.

Laparotomy is less preferred than laparoscopy but remains essential for specific scenarios.

16.16 Hysterotomy

(*Shigaf-i-rahim*)

Introduction

Hysterotomy is a surgical procedure involving an incision into the uterus to access its contents, typically performed in specific obstetric or gynecologic scenarios. Unlike hysterectomy, which removes the uterus, hysterotomy involves entering the uterine cavity while preserving the organ, often to deliver a fetus or remove intrauterine contents. It is most commonly associated with cesarean section (C-section) in obstetrics but has distinct gynecologic applications, such as in cases of failed medical abortion or complex fetal anomalies.

Indications

Hysterotomy is indicated in the following scenarios

1. Obstetric Indications

Cesarean Section: The most common form of hysterotomy, performed to deliver a fetus when vaginal delivery is contraindicated or unsafe (e.g., fetal distress, placenta previa, breech presentation).

Late-Term Pregnancy Termination: For fetal anomalies or maternal health risks, when medical induction fails or is not feasible (typically second trimester).

Failed Medical Abortion: Removal of retained products of conception or fetus after unsuccessful medical termination.

Intrauterine Fetal Demise (IUFD): When induction of labor fails or is contraindicated, particularly in the second trimester.

Uterine Rupture Repair: To deliver the fetus and repair the uterus in cases of spontaneous or traumatic rupture.

2. Gynecologic Indications

Removal of Retained Products of Conception (RPOC): When dilation and curettage (D&C) or medical management fails, particularly in cases of adherent placenta or incomplete miscarriage.

Access to Intrauterine Pathology: Rarely, to remove large or deeply embedded intrauterine foreign bodies (e.g., impacted IUDs) or tumors not accessible via hysteroscopy.

3. Rare Indications

Fetal Surgery: Hysterotomy to access the fetus for in-utero interventions (e.g., repair of congenital anomalies like spina bifida).

Emergency Access: In extreme cases, where rapid uterine access is needed (e.g., severe postpartum hemorrhage unresponsive to other measures).

Contraindications

1. Absolute Contraindications

None in emergencies where hysterotomy is life-saving (e.g., uterine rupture, severe hemorrhage).

2. Relative Contraindications

Active Uterine or Pelvic Infection: Increases risk of postoperative infection or sepsis; treat infection first unless urgent.

Maternal Coagulopathy: Uncorrected bleeding disorders increase hemorrhage risk, requiring preoperative optimization.

Desire for Non-Surgical Management: If medical induction or D&C is feasible and preferred (e.g., early pregnancy loss).

Severe Maternal Comorbidities: Cardiopulmonary instability may contraindicate surgery unless emergent.

Procedure

1. Preoperative Preparation

Patient Evaluation: Includes history, physical examination, imaging (e.g., ultrasound to confirm fetal position, placental location or RPOC) and laboratory tests (e.g., CBC, coagulation profile, blood typing).

Informed Consent: Discuss risks (e.g., hemorrhage, infection, future pregnancy complications), benefits, and alternatives (e.g., medical induction, D&C). Address implications for future fertility, especially in obstetric cases.

Antibiotic Prophylaxis: Administered 30–60 minutes pre-incision (e.g., cefazolin) to reduce infection risk.

Thromboprophylaxis: Sequential compression devices and/or heparin for high-risk patients (e.g., prolonged surgery, obesity) to prevent venous thromboembolism (VTE).

Anesthesia

General anesthesia for most cases, particularly emergencies or fetal surgery.

Regional anesthesia (spinal or epidural) preferred for elective cesarean sections to reduce maternal risks and allow patient participation.

Bowel Preparation: Rarely needed; may include a clear liquid diet for elective cases.

2. Surgical Technique

Positioning: Supine with a left lateral tilt (15–30°) in obstetric cases to prevent aortocaval compression by the gravid uterus. A urinary catheter is placed to decompress the bladder.

Incision

Abdominal Incision

Pfannenstiel: Low transverse incision, cosmetically favorable, commonly used for cesarean section or elective hysterotomy.

Midline Vertical: Preferred for emergencies (e.g., uterine rupture) or when extensive access is needed (e.g., fetal surgery, large RPOC).

Uterine Incision

Low Transverse: Most common for cesarean section, made in the lower uterine segment to minimize bleeding and optimize future pregnancy outcomes.

Classical (Vertical): Used in preterm deliveries (<32 weeks), anterior placenta previa or fetal surgery; higher risk of rupture in future pregnancies.

T- or J-Shaped: Rarely used, for complex cases requiring extended access.

Procedure Steps

Abdominal Entry: Skin, subcutaneous tissue, fascia and peritoneum are incised layer by layer. Rectus muscles are separated (midline) or divided (transverse).

Uterine Exposure: The uterus is identified, and the vesicouterine peritoneum is incised to reflect the bladder inferiorly, reducing injury risk.

Uterine Incision

For cesarean section: A low transverse incision is made and the fetus is delivered (head or breech extraction). The placenta is removed manually or spontaneously.

For hysterotomy: The incision (transverse or vertical) is made to access RPOC, foreign bodies, or pathology, followed by curettage or excision.

Hemostasis: Uterine vessels are clamped or ligated; oxytocin (10–40 IU IV) is administered to promote uterine contraction and reduce bleeding.

Closure

Uterus: Closed in 1–2 layers with absorbable sutures (e.g., chromic catgut or polyglactin). Double-layer closure is preferred for low transverse incisions to reduce future rupture risk.

Peritoneum: Closure is optional; often left open to reduce adhesion formation.

Fascia and Skin: Closed with absorbable or non-absorbable sutures; drains may be placed for complex cases.

3. Postoperative Care

Recovery: Hospital stay of 2–5 days for cesarean section or gynecologic hysterotomy; longer for complications or fetal surgery.

Pain Management: Patient-controlled analgesia (PCA), epidural or oral/IV analgesics (e.g., NSAIDs, opioids) for incisional and uterine pain.

Wound Care: Monitor for infection, dehiscence or hematoma; keep incision dry for 48 hours.

Mobilization: Early ambulation (within 24 hours) to reduce VTE risk.

Instructions

Avoid heavy lifting or strenuous activity for 6–8 weeks.

Refrain from intercourse for 4–6 weeks to allow healing.

For cesarean patients, monitor for signs of endometritis or wound complications.

Follow-Up

Scheduled 1–2 weeks post-discharge to assess recovery and discuss pathology results (if applicable). For cesarean patients, a 6-week postpartum visit is standard.

Complications to Monitor: Include hemorrhage, infection, VTE or uterine scar complications (e.g., dehiscence).

Findings and Interpretation

Obstetric Hysterotomy (Cesarean Section)

Normal: Healthy fetus delivered, normal placenta and intact uterine anatomy.

Abnormal: Placenta previa, accreta or uterine anomalies (e.g., bicornuate uterus); may require additional interventions (e.g., hysterectomy for accreta).

Gynecologic Hysterotomy

Normal: No residual pathology post-removal of RPOC or foreign bodies.

Abnormal: Adherent placenta, uterine synechiae or unexpected malignancy (requires biopsy or further resection).

Complications

Hysterotomy has a complication rate of 5–15%, higher in emergent or complex cases:

1. Intraoperative

Hemorrhage: From uterine atony, placenta accreta, or vessel injury; managed with uterotonics, sutures, or hysterectomy (<5%).

Bladder/Ureter Injury: Rare (<1%), from dissection near the vesicouterine space; requires repair.

Bowel Injury: Extremely rare, typically in adhered pelvis.

2. Postoperative

Infection: Endometritis (2–5%, higher post-cesarean), wound infection, or pelvic abscess.

Wound Dehiscence: Partial or complete incision separation (<1%).

VTE: Deep vein thrombosis or pulmonary embolism (1–2%), higher in postpartum or high-risk patients.

Uterine Scar Complications

Dehiscence/Rupture: Higher risk with classical incisions (4–9% in future pregnancies vs. <1% for low transverse).

Adhesions: May cause chronic pain or infertility.

Ileus: Delayed bowel function, resolving within 3–5 days.

3. Long-Term

Future Pregnancy Risks: Increased risk of placenta accreta, previa, or uterine rupture in subsequent pregnancies, especially with classical incisions.

Incisional Hernia: 5–10% with midline incisions.

Fertility Impact: Adhesions or synechiae may impair future fertility.

Advantages

Direct Access: Provides rapid and effective access to the uterine cavity for delivery or removal of pathology.

Life-Saving: Critical for emergencies like fetal distress, uterine rupture, or severe haemorrhage.

Versatile: Applicable in obstetric (cesarean) and gynecologic (e.g., RPOC) contexts.

Preserves Uterus: Unlike hysterectomy, allows potential for future pregnancies (with increased risks).

Limitations

Invasive: Requires abdominal surgery, with longer recovery (6–8 weeks) and higher morbidity than D&C or medical management.

Scar-Related Risks: Classical incisions increase future pregnancy complications (e.g., rupture).

Cost: Higher than non-surgical options due to hospitalization and surgical resources.

Anesthesia Risks: General or regional anaesthesia carries cardiopulmonary risks, especially in emergencies.

Adhesion Formation: Higher risk than minimally invasive procedures (e.g., hysteroscopy).

Comparison with Other Modalities

Dilation and Curettage (D&C): Less invasive for early pregnancy loss or RPOC but inadequate for late-term or complex cases.

Medical Management: Prostaglandins (e.g., misoprostol) or mifepristone for pregnancy termination or IUFD; less effective in second trimester or with adherent tissue.

Hysteroscopy: Minimally invasive for intrauterine pathology (e.g., polyps, RPOC) but limited by uterine size or accessibility in pregnancy.

Hysterectomy: Definitive for severe haemorrhage or malignancy but sacrifices fertility; reserved when hysterotomy is insufficient.

Laparoscopy: Rarely used for uterine access but may complement hysterotomy in complex cases (e.g., ectopic pregnancy with uterine involvement).

Clinical Relevance

Hysterotomy is critical in

Obstetrics: Cesarean section is the most common indication, ensuring safe delivery in high-risk pregnancies (e.g., fetal distress, placenta previa).

Gynaecology: Addresses failed medical abortions or complex intrauterine pathology, preserving fertility when possible.

Emergencies: Life-saving for maternal or fetal indications (e.g., rupture, haemorrhage).

Fetal Surgery: Enables rare in-utero interventions for congenital anomalies, improving neonatal outcomes.

Conclusion

Hysterotomy is a vital surgical procedure in gynaecology and obstetrics, primarily used for cesarean delivery, late-term terminations or removal of complex intrauterine pathology. Its invasive nature necessitates careful patient selection and meticulous technique to minimize complications, particularly in preserving future fertility.

Key Points

Hysterotomy involves a uterine incision, most commonly for cesarean section or removal of RPOC.

Indications include fetal distress, failed medical abortion, IUFD or rare fetal surgery.

Low transverse incision is preferred for cesarean; classical incision carries higher future rupture risk.

Complications include haemorrhage, infection and future pregnancy risks (e.g., rupture, accreta).

Hysterotomy preserves the uterus, unlike hysterectomy, but is more invasive than D&C or medical management.

16.17 Myomectomy

(*Sal'a 'Adali Lifi barari*)

Introduction

Myomectomy is a surgical procedure to remove uterine fibroids (leiomyomas) while preserving the uterus, making it a key fertility-sparing option for women with symptomatic fibroids who desire future pregnancies. Uterine fibroids are benign smooth muscle tumours, common in reproductive-age women, and can cause heavy menstrual bleeding, pelvic pain or infertility. Myomectomy can be performed via abdominal (laparotomy), laparoscopic, robotic-assisted or hysteroscopic approaches, done according to the fibroid's size, number, location, and patient factors.

Indications

Myomectomy is indicated for

1. Symptomatic Fibroids

Abnormal Uterine Bleeding (AUB): Heavy or prolonged menstrual bleeding (menorrhagia) unresponsive to medical therapy (e.g., tranexamic acid, hormonal treatments).

Pelvic Pain or Pressure: Due to fibroid size or location, causing symptoms like dysmenorrhea, dyspareunia, or bladder/bowel compression.

Infertility or Recurrent Pregnancy Loss: Submucosal or intramural fibroids distorting the uterine cavity, impairing implantation or pregnancy maintenance.

Obstructive Symptoms: Fibroids causing urinary frequency/retention, constipation or hydronephrosis from ureteral compression.

2. Desire for Uterine Preservation: In women wishing to maintain fertility or avoid hysterectomy for personal reasons.

3. Rapid Fibroid Growth: Suggestive of potential malignancy (e.g., leiomyosarcoma, though rare <1%), requiring surgical evaluation.

4. Recurrent Symptoms Post-Conservative Treatment: When medical therapies (e.g., GnRH agonists) or minimally invasive procedures (e.g., uterine artery embolization) fail to control symptoms.

Contraindications

1. Absolute Contraindications

Suspected Uterine Malignancy: Leiomyosarcoma or endometrial cancer requires hysterectomy or oncologic evaluation rather than myomectomy.

Severe Medical Comorbidities: Uncontrolled cardiopulmonary disease or coagulopathy precluding surgery.

2. Relative Contraindications

No Desire for Future Fertility: Hysterectomy may be preferred for definitive treatment in women not seeking pregnancy.

Extensive Fibroid Burden: Numerous or large fibroids may make myomectomy technically challenging, increasing risks (e.g., bleeding, hysterectomy conversion).

Active Pelvic Infection: Increases postoperative infection risk; treat infection first.

Patient Preference for Non-Surgical Options: If medical or interventional radiology treatments (e.g., UAE) are viable.

Types of Myomectomy

1. By Approach

Abdominal Myomectomy (via Laparotomy): Open surgery for large, multiple or deep intramural fibroids.

Laparoscopic Myomectomy: Minimally invasive for subserosal or intramural fibroids, suitable for smaller or fewer fibroids.

Robotic-Assisted Myomectomy: Uses robotic systems for enhanced precision, ideal for complex cases (e.g., multiple fibroids, obesity).

Hysteroscopic Myomectomy: For submucosal fibroids protruding into the uterine cavity, performed via the cervix.

2. By Fibroid Location

Submucosal: Inside the uterine cavity, often causing AUB or infertility.

Intramural: Within the myometrium, potentially causing pain or pressure.

Subserosal: On the outer uterine surface, often causing bulk symptoms.

Pedunculated: Fibroids on a stalk, subserosal or submucosal, amenable to resection.

Procedure

1. Preoperative Preparation

Patient Evaluation

History and physical examination to assess symptoms and fertility goals.

Imaging: Transvaginal ultrasound, MRI or saline infusion sonography (SIS) to map fibroid number, size, location, and relation to the endometrium.

Endometrial biopsy if AUB is present to rule out hyperplasia or malignancy.

Laboratory tests: CBC (assess anemia from menorrhagia), coagulation profile and blood typing.

Informed Consent: Discuss risks (e.g., bleeding, adhesion formation, hysterectomy risk), benefits and alternatives (e.g., UAE, medical therapy). Emphasize fertility implications and recurrence risk (10–30%).

Preoperative Optimization

Anemia Correction: Iron supplementation or blood transfusion for severe menorrhagia.

GnRH Agonists: May be used 2–3 months preoperatively to shrink fibroids and reduce bleeding risk, though they increase tissue friability.

Antibiotic Prophylaxis: Administered 30–60 minutes, pre-incision (e.g., cefazolin) to reduce infection risk.

Thromboprophylaxis: Sequential compression devices and/or heparin for high-risk patients to prevent VTE.

Anesthesia: General anaesthesia for abdominal, laparoscopic or robotic approaches; local or regional anaesthesia (e.g., paracervical block) may suffice for hysteroscopic myomectomy.

2. Surgical Techniques

Abdominal Myomectomy (Laparotomy)

Incision: Midline vertical (for large/multiple fibroids) or Pfannenstiel (transverse, cosmetically favorable).

Procedure: Entry into the peritoneal cavity, exposure of the uterus, and identification of fibroids. Uterine incision (often transverse or vertical) over the fibroid, enucleation using blunt/sharp dissection, and removal while preserving healthy myometrium.

Vasoconstrictive agents (e.g., vasopressin diluted 20 IU/100 mL saline) injected into the myometrium to reduce bleeding. Multilayer closure of the myometrium with absorbable sutures to restore uterine integrity and minimize adhesion formation. Anti-adhesion barriers (e.g., Seprafilm) may be applied.

Closure: Fascia and skin closed with sutures; drains may be placed for large dissections.

Laparoscopic Myomectomy

Access: 3–4 small incisions (5–12 mm) for laparoscope and instruments; CO_2 insufflation to 12–15 mmHg.

Procedure

Fibroid enucleation using laparoscopic graspers, scissors, or morcellators (for large fibroids). Myometrial closure with barbed or absorbable sutures, often challenging due to limited tactile feedback. Fibroids removed via morcellation (in a bag to prevent tissue dissemination) or through a larger port.

Advantages: Reduced pain, shorter recovery (2–4 weeks vs. 6–8 weeks for laparotomy), and smaller scars.

Hysteroscopic Myomectomy

Access: Via the cervix, no abdominal incisions; uses a hysteroscope (5–10 mm).

Procedure: Uterine cavity distended with saline (diagnostic) or electrolyte-free fluid (e.g., glycine for monopolar resection). Submucosal fibroids resected using a resectoscope, morcellator or loop electrode. Fluid management critical to prevent overload (deficit limit: ~1,000 mL saline, ~750 mL glycine).

Advantage: Outpatient, minimal recovery (1–2 days), ideal for submucosal fibroids.

3. Postoperative Care

Recovery

Abdominal: Hospital stay of 2–5 days, full recovery in 6–8 weeks.

Laparoscopic/Robotic: Hospital stay of 0–2 days, recovery in 2–4 weeks.

Hysteroscopic: Outpatient, recovery in 1–2 days.

Pain Management: NSAIDs or opioids for incisional/cramping pain; less for hysteroscopic approach.

Wound Care: Monitor for infection, dehiscence, or hematoma (abdominal/laparoscopic).

Instructions

Avoid heavy lifting or intercourse for 4–6 weeks (abdominal/laparoscopic) or 1–2 weeks (hysteroscopic).

Delay pregnancy for 3–6 months post-myomectomy to allow uterine healing, especially for deep intramural fibroids.

Follow-Up: Scheduled 1–2 weeks post-discharge to assess recovery and discuss pathology (to rule out malignancy).

Complications to Monitor: Include bleeding, infection, adhesion formation, or uterine rupture in future pregnancies.

Findings and Interpretation

Intraoperative Findings

Fibroid Characteristics: Number, size, location (submucosal, intramural, subserosal), and consistency (firm, calcified, or degenerated).

Unexpected Pathology: Leiomyosarcoma (<1%) or endometrial pathology, requiring frozen section or further resection.

Pathological Findings

Benign: Leiomyomas with typical smooth muscle histology.

Malignant (Rare): Leiomyosarcoma or endometrial stromal sarcoma, necessitating oncologic consultation.

Complications

Myomectomy has a complication rate of 5–20%, varying by approach:

1. Intraoperative

Bleeding: Significant risk (5–10%), especially with large or intramural fibroids; may require transfusion or hysterectomy (<2%).

Organ Injury: Bladder, ureter or bowel (<1%), more common in abdominal approach with adhesions.

Uterine Perforation: Rare in hysteroscopic myomectomy, managed with observation or repair.

2. Postoperative

Infection: Wound infection (2–5% abdominal, <1% laparoscopic/hysteroscopic) or endometritis.

Adhesions: Common (10–20%) after abdominal or laparoscopic myomectomy, potentially causing infertility or pain.

Fluid Overload: In hysteroscopic myomectomy, due to excessive absorption of distension media (e.g., hyponatremia with glycine).

VTE: Rare (<1%) but higher in abdominal approach or prolonged surgery.

Uterine Rupture: Rare (<1%) in subsequent pregnancies, higher with deep intramural fibroids or inadequate closure.

3. Long-Term

Fibroid Recurrence: 10–30% within 5–10 years, requiring repeat intervention or hysterectomy.

Infertility: Adhesions or synechiae may impair fertility despite uterine preservation.

Incisional Hernia: 5–10% with abdominal approach.

Advantages

Fertility Preservation: Maintains the uterus for future pregnancies, unlike hysterectomy.

Symptom Relief: Effective for AUB, pain or pressure caused by fibroids.

Minimally Invasive Options: Laparoscopic, robotic or hysteroscopic approaches reduce recovery time and morbidity.

Limitations

Recurrence Risk: Fibroids may regrow, requiring further treatment.

Surgical Risks: Higher bleeding risk than hysterectomy, especially for large or intramural fibroids.

Technical Complexity: Laparoscopic or robotic approaches require advanced training; hysteroscopy limited to submucosal fibroids.

Fertility Uncertainty: While fertility-sparing, adhesions or synechiae may reduce pregnancy success.

Cost: Varies by approach; robotic is most expensive, followed by laparoscopic, abdominal and hysteroscopic.

Comparison with Other Modalities

Hysterectomy: Definitive for fibroids but sacrifices fertility; preferred when fertility is not desired.

Uterine Artery Embolization (UAE): Minimally invasive, reduces fibroid size but may impair fertility; not suitable for submucosal fibroids.

Medical Therapy: GnRH agonists, progestins or tranexamic acid for symptom control; temporary and less effective for large fibroids.

Focused Ultrasound Surgery (FUS): Non-invasive, MRI-guided ablation for select fibroids; limited availability and long-term data.

Hysteroscopy: Limited to submucosal fibroids; cannot address intramural or subserosal fibroids.

Clinical Relevance

Myomectomy is pivotal in gynaecology for:

Fertility Preservation: Improves pregnancy outcomes in women with submucosal or cavity-distorting fibroids.

Symptom Management: Relieves AUB, pain or pressure, improving quality of life.

Alternative to Hysterectomy: Offers a uterine-sparing option for women not desiring definitive surgery.

Diagnostic Role: Confirms benign pathology and rules out malignancy in rapidly growing fibroids.

Conclusion

Myomectomy is a critical fertility-sparing procedure for women with symptomatic uterine fibroids, offering relief from bleeding, pain or infertility while preserving the uterus. Its multiple approaches-abdominal, laparoscopic, robotic and hysteroscopic -allow treatment based on fibroid characteristics and patient needs.

Key Points

Myomectomy removes fibroids while preserving the uterus, ideal for fertility preservation.

Approaches include abdominal (large fibroids), laparoscopic/robotic (minimally invasive), and hysteroscopic (submucosal fibroids).

Complications include bleeding, adhesions and rare uterine rupture in pregnancy.

Fibroid recurrence (10–30%) may necessitate repeat intervention.

Myomectomy balances symptom relief with fertility goals, unlike hysterectomy or UAE.

16.18 Hysterectomy

(*Rahim barari*)

Introduction

Hysterectomy, the surgical removal of the uterus, is one of the most common gynecologic procedures worldwide. It is performed for a variety of benign and malignant conditions, offering definitive treatment for issues such as abnormal uterine bleeding, fibroids or gynecologic cancers.

Hysterectomy can be performed via multiple approaches—abdominal (laparotomy), vaginal, laparoscopic or robotic-assisted—each with specific indications, advantages and risks.

Indications

Hysterectomy is indicated for

1. Benign Conditions

Uterine Fibroids (Leiomyomas): For symptomatic fibroids causing heavy menstrual bleeding, pelvic pain or pressure, unresponsive to medical therapy (e.g., GnRH agonists) or minimally invasive procedures (e.g., uterine artery embolization).

Abnormal Uterine Bleeding (AUB): When refractory to hormonal therapy, endometrial ablation or other interventions.

Endometriosis/Adenomyosis: Severe cases with debilitating pain or bleeding not managed conservatively.

Pelvic Organ Prolapse: Symptomatic uterine prolapse, often combined with vaginal repair procedures (e.g., colporrhaphy).

Chronic Pelvic Pain: When attributable to uterine pathology and other causes (e.g., adhesions, PID) are excluded.

Pelvic Inflammatory Disease (PID): For refractory tubo-ovarian abscesses or chronic infection unresponsive to antibiotics.

2. Malignant Conditions

Endometrial Cancer: Primary treatment for early-stage disease, typically with bilateral salpingo-oophorectomy (BSO).

Cervical Cancer: Radical hysterectomy for early-stage disease (e.g., stage IA2–IB1), often with lymphadenectomy.

Ovarian Cancer: As part of cytoreductive surgery, often including the uterus and adnexa.

Uterine Sarcoma: For confirmed or suspected cases, often requiring extensive resection.

3. Emergency Indications

Postpartum Haemorrhage: Uncontrolled bleeding unresponsive to uterotonics or uterine-sparing procedures (e.g., balloon tamponade).

Uterine Rupture: Obstetric or traumatic emergency requiring immediate surgery.

Severe Infection: Refractory endometritis or septic abortion.

4. Prophylactic Indications

Risk-reducing hysterectomy in patients with hereditary cancer syndromes (e.g., Lynch syndrome, BRCA mutations), often with BSO.

Contraindications

1. Absolute Contraindications

None, as hysterectomy may be life-saving in emergencies (e.g., uncontrollable haemorrhage).

2. Relative Contraindications

Desire for Future Fertility: Uterine-sparing options (e.g., myomectomy, endometrial ablation) should be prioritized.

Uncontrolled Comorbidities: Severe cardiopulmonary disease or coagulopathy, requiring preoperative optimization.

Acute Pelvic Infection: Should be treated before elective surgery to minimize complications.

Types of Hysterectomy

1. By Extent

Total Hysterectomy: Removal of the uterus and cervix; most common for benign and malignant conditions.

Subtotal (Supracervical) Hysterectomy: Removal of the uterine body, preserving the cervix; less common, used in selective benign cases to reduce surgical time or preserve pelvic floor support.

Radical Hysterectomy: Removal of the uterus, cervix, upper vagina and parametrial tissues; indicated for early-stage cervical cancer, often with pelvic lymphadenectomy.

2. By Approach

Abdominal Hysterectomy (via Laparotomy): Open surgery for large uteri, malignancy or extensive adhesions.

Vaginal Hysterectomy: Performed through the vaginal canal, ideal for prolapse or smaller uteri in multiparous women.

Laparoscopic Hysterectomy: Minimally invasive, including total laparoscopic hysterectomy (TLH) or laparoscopic-assisted vaginal hysterectomy (LAVH).

Robotic-Assisted Hysterectomy: Uses robotic systems for enhanced precision, often for complex cases (e.g., malignancy or obesity).

Procedure

1. Preoperative Preparation

Patient Evaluation: Includes history, physical examination, imaging (e.g., transvaginal ultrasound, MRI), and laboratory tests (e.g., CBC, coagulation profile, CA-125 for suspected malignancy).

Endometrial Sampling: Mandatory for AUB or postmenopausal bleeding to rule out hyperplasia or cancer.

Informed Consent: Discuss risks (e.g., bleeding, infection, organ injury), benefits and alternatives (e.g., medical management, myomectomy). Address fertility loss and menopausal implications if BSO is planned.

Bowel Preparation: Optional; may include liquid diet or enema for abdominal approaches to improve visualization.

Antibiotic Prophylaxis: Administered 30–60 minutes pre-incision (e.g., cefazolin) to reduce infection risk.

Thromboprophylaxis: Sequential compression devices and/or heparin to prevent venous thromboembolism (VTE), especially in oncologic or prolonged surgeries.

Anesthesia: General anaesthesia for abdominal, laparoscopic or robotic approaches; spinal or epidural anaesthesia may be used for vaginal hysterectomy.

2. Surgical Techniques

Abdominal Hysterectomy (Laparotomy)

Incision: Midline vertical (for large uteri or malignancy) or Pfannenstiel (transverse, cosmetically favorable).

Procedure:

Entry into the peritoneal cavity, retraction of bowel, and identification of pelvic organs.

Ligation of round ligaments, ovarian ligaments (if preserving ovaries), or infundibulopelvic ligaments (if BSO).

Dissection of vesicouterine and rectouterine spaces, ligation of uterine arteries and cardinal ligaments.

Removal of the uterus (± cervix) through the incision; vaginal cuff closure with absorbable sutures.

For radical hysterectomy, additional removal of parametria, upper vagina and pelvic lymph nodes.

Closure: Peritoneum (optional), fascia and skin closed with sutures; drains may be placed for oncologic cases.

Vaginal Hysterectomy

Access: Through the vaginal canal, no abdominal incisions.

Procedure: Circumferential incision around the cervix, entry into the peritoneal cavity via anterior/posterior cul-de-sacs. Sequential ligation of uterine ligaments and vessels, removal of the uterus and vaginal cuff closure. Ideal for prolapse or smaller uteri in multiparous women; limited by restricted visualization.

Laparoscopic Hysterectomy (TLH or LAVH):

Access: 3–4 small incisions (5–12 mm) for laparoscope and instruments; CO2 insufflation to 12–15 mmHg.

Procedure: Similar steps to abdominal hysterectomy but performed with laparoscopic instruments (e.g., graspers, bipolar energy devices). Uterus removed via morcellation (for larger uteri) or vaginal extraction. Vaginal cuff closed laparoscopically or vaginally (LAVH).

Advantages: Reduced recovery time, less pain, and smaller scars compared to laparotomy.

Additional Cases

Bilateral Salpingo-Oophorectomy (BSO): May accompany hysterectomy for malignancy, prophylaxis, or benign adnexal pathology.

Lymphadenectomy: Performed in oncologic cases to stage cancer (e.g., pelvic or para-aortic nodes).

3. Postoperative Care

Recovery

Abdominal: Hospital stay of 2–5 days, full recovery in 6–8 weeks.

Vaginal/Laparoscopic/Robotic: Hospital stay of 0–2 days, recovery in 2–4 weeks.

Pain Management: Patient-controlled analgesia (PCA), epidural or oral/IV analgesics (e.g., NSAIDs, opioids).

Wound Care: Monitor for infection, dehiscence or hematoma; keep incisions dry for 48 hours (abdominal approach).

Mobilization: Early ambulation (within 24 hours) to reduce VTE risk.

Instructions: Avoid heavy lifting, strenuous activity or intercourse for 4–6 weeks; longer (6–8 weeks) for abdominal hysterectomy.

Hormone Replacement Therapy (HRT): Considered if BSO induces surgical menopause in premenopausal patients, balancing risks (e.g., VTE) and benefits (e.g., symptom relief).

Follow-Up: Scheduled 1–2 weeks post-discharge to assess recovery, discuss pathology results, and plan adjuvant therapy (e.g., radiation for malignancy).

Complications to Monitor: Include infection, bleeding, VTE, bowel obstruction or vaginal cuff dehiscence.

Findings and Interpretation

Pathological Findings

Benign: Leiomyomas, adenomyosis, endometrial hyperplasia, or benign ovarian pathology (if BSO performed).

Malignant: Endometrial adenocarcinoma, cervical squamous cell carcinoma or sarcoma; staging confirmed by lymph node and peritoneal findings.

Intraoperative Findings

Adhesions, endometriosis or unexpected malignancy may necessitate procedure modification (e.g., conversion to laparotomy).

Frozen section analysis may guide intraoperative decisions in suspected malignancy.

Complications

Hysterectomy has a complication rate of 5–15%, varying by approach:

1. Intraoperative

Bleeding: From uterine or ovarian vessels; managed with sutures, clips or energy devices (1–3%).

Organ Injury: Bladder (1–2%), ureter (0.5–1%) or bowel (<1%), requiring repair.

Uterine Perforation: Rare in vaginal hysterectomy, more common with adhesions or inexperienced operators.

2. Postoperative

Infection: Surgical site infection (3–5% abdominal, <2% vaginal/laparoscopic) or pelvic abscess.

Vaginal Cuff Dehiscence: Partial or complete separation of the vaginal cuff (<1%), often presenting with vaginal bleeding or discharge.

VTE: Deep vein thrombosis or pulmonary embolism (1–2%), higher in oncologic cases.

Bowl Dysfunction: Ileus (common in abdominal approach) or obstruction (rare).

Urinary Dysfunction: Retention or incontinence, often transient; ureteral injury may cause fistulae.

Lymphocele/Lymphedema: After lymphadenectomy in oncologic cases.

Menopausal Symptoms: If BSO performed in premenopausal patients, it causes hot flashes, vaginal dryness or osteoporosis risk.

3. Long-Term

Adhesions: May cause chronic pain or bowel obstruction.

Incisional Hernia: More common with abdominal approach (5–10%).

Pelvic Floor Dysfunction: Altered anatomy may exacerbate prolapse or incontinence.

Advantages

Definitive Treatment: Resolves AUB, fibroid-related symptoms or early-stage malignancy.

Versatile Approaches: Options (vaginal, laparoscopic, robotic) allow tailoring to patient needs and pathology.

Improved Quality of Life: Relieves pain, bleeding or prolapse symptoms.

Oncologic Benefit: Curative for early endometrial or cervical cancer; debulking improves survival in ovarian cancer.

Limitations

Fertility Loss: Permanent, necessitating thorough counselling for reproductive-age patients.

Invasiveness: Abdominal approach has longer recovery, higher pain and increased complications compared to vaginal/laparoscopic.

Cost: Varies by approach; robotic is most expensive, followed by laparoscopic, abdominal and vaginal.

Surgical Risks: Higher with abdominal approach or in patients with comorbidities (e.g., obesity, diabetes).

Menopausal Impact: BSO in premenopausal patients requires long-term HRT consideration.

Comparison with Other Modalities

Medical Management: Hormonal therapy (e.g., levonorgestrel IUD, GnRH agonists) or NSAIDs for AUB or fibroids; less invasive but may be less effective.

Endometrial Ablation: Uterine-sparing option for AUB, unsuitable for malignancy or large fibroids.

Myomectomy: Preserves fertility for fibroids but may not address AUB or recurrence risk.

Uterine Artery Embolization (UAE): Minimally invasive for fibroids, not suitable for malignancy or prolapse.

Laparoscopy vs. Laparotomy: Laparoscopic approaches (TLH, LAVH, robotic) preferred for faster recovery and fewer complications unless contraindicated (e.g., large uterus, malignancy).

Clinical Relevance

Hysterectomy is pivotal in gynaecology for:

Benign Conditions: Definitive treatment for AUB, fibroids or endometriosis, improving quality of life.

Gynecological Cancers: Curative for early-stage endometrial or cervical cancer; part of multimodal therapy for ovarian cancer.

Emergencies: Life-saving in postpartum haemorrhage or uterine rupture.

Prophylaxis: Reduces cancer risk in high-risk genetic syndromes.

Pelvic Reconstruction: Addresses prolapse, often combined with other repairs.

Conclusion

Hysterectomy remains a cornerstone of gynaecological surgery, offering definitive management for a spectrum of benign and malignant conditions. Its multiple approaches—abdominal, vaginal, laparoscopic and robotic—allow treatment based on patient and disease factors.

Key Points

Hysterectomy removes the uterus for benign (e.g., fibroids, AUB) or malignant (e.g., endometrial cancer) indications.

Approaches include abdominal (laparotomy), vaginal, laparoscopic or robotic, with vaginal/ laparoscopic preferred for lower morbidity.

Complications include bleeding, infection, organ injury and VTE; risks are higher with abdominal approach.

BSO may induce surgical menopause, requiring HRT consideration in premenopausal patients.

Thorough counselling is necessary, especially regarding fertility loss and long-term implications.

Long Answer Questions

1. Describe the diagnostic procedures used in gynaecology including imaging, biopsy and endoscopy.
2. Discuss hysteroscopy—indications, technique and complications.
3. Explain laparoscopy in gynaecology—uses, advantages and limitations.
4. Describe therapeutic procedures for abnormal uterine bleeding.
5. Elaborate on cervical biopsy and colposcopy—technique and interpretation.

Short Answer Questions

1. What is the role of transvaginal ultrasound in gynaecology?
2. Name two indications for laparoscopy.
3. Define hysteroscopy.
4. Mention one therapeutic use of D&C.
5. What is the purpose of colposcopy?

Multiple Choice Questions (1 Mark Each)

1. Gold standard for evaluating tubal patency:

a) USG b) HSG c) CT scan d) MRI

Ans: b) HSG

2. Hysteroscopy is used to visualize:

a) Cervix b) Uterine cavity c) Ovaries d) Fallopian tubes

Ans: b) Uterine cavity

3. Which procedure is minimally invasive and uses CO_2 insufflation?

a) Laparotomy b) Laparoscopy c) Hysteroscopy d) D&C

Ans: b) Laparoscopy

4. Endometrial biopsy is indicated in:

a) Amenorrhea b) Menorrhagia c) Dysmenorrhea d) Dyspareunia

Ans: b) Menorrhagia

5. Which imaging is preferred for ovarian cyst evaluation in young women?

a) CT scan b) Mammogram c) Ultrasound d) MRI

Ans: c) Ultrasound

6. Which procedure is used to treat retained products of conception?

a) Colposcopy b) D&C c) HSG d) Pap smear

Ans: b) D&C

7. Which test uses acetic acid and magnification to assess cervical lesions?

a) Pap smear b) Colposcopy c) Biopsy d) Hysteroscopy

Ans: b) Colposcopy

8. Which procedure allows direct visualization of pelvic organs?

a) Laparoscopy b) HSG c) USG d) Pap smear

Ans: a) Laparoscopy

9. Which therapeutic procedure is used for fibroid removal via hysteroscopy?

a) Myomectomy b) Polypectomy c) Ablation d) Hysterectomy

Ans: a) Myomectomy

10. Which test is used to screen for cervical cancer?

a) Colposcopy b) Pap smear c) Biopsy d) Hysteroscopy

Ans: b) Pap smear

Common Drugs in Unani Gynecology

Unani gynecology covers a range of single (*mufrad*) and compound (*murakkab*) drugs to address menstrual and gynecological disorders. These drugs are selected based on their pharmacological actions, such as emmenagogue (*mudirr-e-haiz*), uterine tonic (*muqawwi rahim*), hemostatic (*habis al-dam*), astringent (*qabid*), resolvent (*muhallil*), or antimicrobial properties. Below is a detailed list of common drugs, their properties, and applications, drawn from the National Formulary of Unani Medicine and some clinical studies.

a. Single Drugs (*Mufrad*)

1. **Zingiber officinale (Ginger/*Zanjabeel)***   Properties: Emmenagogue, analgesic, anti-inflammatory.   Uses: Dysmenorrhea, amenorrhea; reduces prostaglandin-induced pain (Sultana et al., 2014).   Dosage: 1–2 g powder or decoction daily.
2. **Foeniculum vulgare (Fennel/*Badiyan)***   Properties: Emmenagogue, antispasmodic, analgesic.   Uses: Dysmenorrhea, amenorrhea; promotes menstrual flow (Jenabi & Fereidoony, 2018).   Dosage: 2–3 g seeds in tea or decoction.
3. **Matricaria chamomilla (Chamomile/*Babuna*)**   Properties: Analgesic, anti-inflammatory, emmenagogue.   Uses: Dysmenorrhea, PMS; reduces uterine spasms (Jenabi & Fereidoony, 2018).   Dosage: 1–2 cups of tea daily.
4. **Pimpinella anisum (Anise/*Anisoon*)**   Properties: Emmenagogue, uterine tonic.   Uses: Amenorrhea, infertility; stimulates ovulation (Sultana & Rahman, 2011).   Dosage: 2–3 g powder or decoction.
5. **Trigonella foenum-graecum (Fenugreek/*Hulba*)**   Properties: Emmenagogue, insulin-sensitizing.   Uses: Amenorrhea, PCOS; reduces ovarian cysts (Sultana et al., 2020).   Dosage: 2–5 g seeds or extract (Furocyst).
6. **Withania somnifera (Ashwagandha/*Asgand*)**   Properties: Uterine tonic, ovulation inducer, adaptogenic.   Uses: Infertility, amenorrhea; strengthens reproductive system (Sultana & Rehman, 2017).   Dosage: 3–6 g root powder daily.

7. **Asparagus racemosus (Shatavari/*Satawar*)**

Properties: Uterine tonic, emmenagogue.

Uses: Infertility, uterine prolapse, stress urinary incontinence; strengthens pelvic muscles (CCRUM, 2009).

Dosage: 3–5 g root powder.

8. **Quercus infectoria (Oak Gall/*Mazu*)**

Properties: Astringent, hemostatic.

Uses: Menorrhagia, leucorrhoea, uterine prolapse; tones tissues (Sultana et al., 2015).

Dosage: 1–2 g powder or in pessaries.

9. **Symplocos racemosa (*Lodhra*)**

Properties: Astringent, hemostatic.

Uses: Menorrhagia, leucorrhoea; reduces excessive bleeding (Sultana et al., 2015).

Dosage: 2–3 g bark powder.

10. **Azadirachta indica (*Neem*/Nim)**

Properties: Antimicrobial, anti-inflammatory.

Uses: PID, cervicitis, leucorrhoea; treats infections (Sultana et al., 2013).

Dosage: 1–2 g leaf paste or decoction.

11. **Boswellia serrata (Frankincense/*Kundur*)**

Properties: Anti-inflammatory, resolvent.

Uses: PID, uterine cancer, metritis; reduces inflammation (CCRUM, 2009).

Dosage: 1–2 g resin powder.

12. **Curcuma longa (Turmeric/*Haldi*)**

Properties: Anti-inflammatory, antimicrobial, resolvent.

Uses: PID, cervicitis, uterine cancer; supports tissue healing (Sultana et al., 2010).

Dosage: 1–3 g powder or decoction.

13. **Aloe barbadensis (Aloe Vera/*Sibr*)**

Properties: Healing, anti-inflammatory.

Uses: Cervicitis, cervical erosion; promotes tissue repair (Sultana et al., 2020).

Dosage: Gel applied topically or 1–2 g orally.

b. Compound Drugs (*Murakkab*)

1. ***Majoon Dabidul Ward***

Composition: Rose petals (Rosa damascena), saffron (Crocus sativus), and other herbs.

Uses: Dysmenorrhea, PMS; relieves pain and regulates flow (Sultana et al., 2014).

Dosage: 5–10 g with water daily.

2. ***Majoon Muqawwi Rahim***

Composition: Withania somnifera, Asparagus racemosus, Pimpinella anisum.

Uses: Amenorrhea, infertility, uterine prolapse; strengthens uterus (Sultana & Rahman, 2011).

Dosage: 5–10 g daily for 3 cycles.

3. ***Qurs-i-Shibb***

Composition: Acacia arabica gum, Cinnamomum camphora.

Uses: Menorrhagia; hemostatic and astringent (Sultana et al., 2021).

Dosage: 2–3 tablets or vaginal suppositories daily.

4. ***Sufoofe Sailan***

Composition: Quercus infectoria, Symplocos racemosa.

Uses: Leucorrhoea, cervicitis; reduces discharge and tones tissues (Sultana et al., 2019).

Dosage: 3–5 g powder daily for 21 days.

5. ***Habbe Hamal***

Composition: Withania somnifera, Barleria prionitis, Nymphaea alba.

Uses: Infertility; induces ovulation and supports conception (Sultana & Rehman, 2017).

Dosage: 1–2 pills daily from day 5 of cycle.

6. ***Majoon Ushba***

Composition: Smilax china, Santalum album.

Uses: PID, cervicitis; antimicrobial and anti-inflammatory (CCRUM, 2009).

Dosage: 5–10 g daily.

7. ***Marham-i-Basaliqoon***

Composition: Aloe barbadensis, Azadirachta indica, beeswax.

Uses: Cervicitis, cervical erosion; promotes healing (Sultana et al., 2020).

Dosage: Applied as vaginal ointment for 14 days.

References

CCRUM. (2009). National Formulary of Unani Medicine. Central Council for Research in Unani Medicine, New Delhi.

Breast Carcinoma – Quick Revision

Definition
Malignant tumor of breast tissue, most commonly arising from ductal epithelial cells.
Most Common Type
- Invasive Ductal Carcinoma (IDC) → ~80% cases
Other types: Lobular, Medullary, Mucinous, Paget's disease, Inflammatory carcinoma

Risk Factors

Mnemonic: "BREAST CARE"

B	BRCA1/BRCA2 mutation
R	Radiation exposure
E	Early menarche
A	Age > 40
S	Smoking / Alcohol
T	Late menopause
C	Nulliparity
A	Atypical hyperplasia
R	Recent OC/hormone therapy
E	Estrogen excess

Flash Facts
- Most common cancer in women worldwide
- Common metastasis sites: bone, lung, liver
- Triple-negative cancers are more aggressive
- Tamoxifen is used in ER+ tumors

Clinical Features

- Hard, irregular, fixed mass
- Painless lump (upper outer quadrant)
- Nipple retraction or discharge
- Skin changes: dimpling, peau d'orange
- Axillary lymphadenopathy

Diagnosis Tools
- Clinical Breast Exam
- Mammography – microcalcifications
- Ultrasound – younger patients
- FNAC / Core Biopsy – confirm histology
- ER/PR/HER2 status – guide treatment

Staging – TNM System
- T – Tumor size
- N – Node involvement
- M – Metastasis

Treatment Modalities

Type	Option
Local	Surgery (Lumpectomy/Mastectomy)
Regional	Radiotherapy
Systemic	Chemotherapy, Hormonal therapy
Targeted	HER2 blockers (e.g., trastuzumab)

Cervical Cancer – Quick Revision

Definition
Malignancy of the cervical epithelium, commonly originating from the transformation
Most Common Type
- Squamous Cell Carcinoma (~80%)
- Other types: Adenocarcinoma, adenosquamous, small cell, neuroendocrine

Risk Factors – Mnemonic: "SAFE HPV"
S Smoking
A Age at early sexual activity
F Frequent STIs
E Early childbearing
H HPV 16 & 18 infection
P Poor hygiene / parity
V Vaccination not received (HPV)

Flash Facts
- Most preventable female cancer with screening & HPV vaccine
- HPV vaccine recommended before sexual debut (ages 9–14)
- Regular Pap tests reduce mortality significantly
- WHO advocates elimination as a public health problem

Symptoms

- Postcoital bleeding
- Foul-smelling vaginal discharge
- Pelvic pain, leg swelling (late stage)
- Weight loss, cachexia

Diagnosis
- Screening: Pap smear, HPV DNA test
- Confirmatory: Cervical biopsy
- Staging: FIGO system
- Imaging: MRI pelvis, chest X-ray, cystoscopy if advanced

FIGO Staging Highlights
I Confined to cervix
II Invades vagina, parametria
III Extends to pelvic wall or lower third of vagina
IV Involves bladder, rectum, distant sites

Treatment Overview
Early (I) Surgery (LEEP, hysterectomy)
Mid (II-III) Radiotherapy + chemotherapy
Advanced (IV) Palliative care + systemic therapy
Precancer (CIN) Cryotherapy, LEEP, close monitoring

Endometrial Cancer – Quick Revision

Definition
Malignancy of the uterine lining (endometrium), most common gynecological cancer in developed countries.
Most Common Type
- Endometrioid Adenocarcinoma
Other types: Serous, Clear Cell, Mucinous, Carcinosarcoma

Risk Factors – Mnemonic: "UNOPPOSED"
U Unopposed estrogen therapy
N Nulliparity
O Obesity
P PCOS
P Postmenopausal age
O Ovarian tumors secreting estrogen
S Sequential tamoxifen use
E Early menarche
D Diabetes mellitus
Estrogen exposure without progesterone opposition plays a central role.

Symptoms
- Postmenopausal bleeding (hallmark)
- Abnormal heavy menstrual bleeding
- Pelvic pain or pressure
- White/yellow discharge (rare)

Diagnosis
- Transvaginal USG: Thickened endometrial stripe (>4 mm postmenopause)
- Endometrial biopsy: Gold standard
- Hysteroscopy/D&C: Confirm and stage
- MRI pelvis: Assess myometrial & cervical invasion
FIGO Staging Highlights (2023)
I Confined to uterus
II Involves cervix
III Extends beyond uterus (serosa, vagina, lymph nodes)
IV Bladder, bowel or distant metastasis

Flash Facts
- Estrogen-driven cancer; obesity is major modifiable risk
- Lynch syndrome (HNPCC) increases lifetime risk
- Often detected early due to postmenopausal bleeding
- Endometrial biopsy is both diagnostic & screening in high-risk women

Treatment Overview
I Total hysterectomy + BSO
II Radical hysterectomy + lymphadenectomy
III–IV Surgery + radiotherapy ± chemotherapy
Hormone-sensitive Progesterone therapy (in select young cases)

Ovarian Cancer – Quick Revision

Definition
Malignancy originating from ovarian tissue, often diagnosed late due to vague symptoms and deep pelvic location.

Most Common Type
- Epithelial Ovarian Cancer (especially Serous cystadenocarcinoma)

Others: Germ cell tumors (young age), Sex cord-stromal tumors, Metastatic (Krukenberg tumor)

Flash Facts
- Called the "Silent Killer" due to vague symptoms
- BRCA mutation screening recommended in high-risk cases
- CA-125 may be raised in TB, PID, endometriosis—interpret carefully
- OCPs reduce risk by suppressing ovulation

Risk Factors – Mnemonic: "NASTY BODIES"

N Nulliparity
A Age > 50
S Smoking
T Talc powder use (controversial)
Y Young age → Germ cell tumors
B BRCA1/BRCA2 mutation
O Obesity
D Delay in childbirth
I Infertility / Ovulation excess
E Endometriosis
S Sister/FH of ovarian/breast cancer

Familial and ovulation-related **risks dominate.**

Symptoms (Often Silent)
- Abdominal distension or bloating
- Pelvic pain
- Early satiety / appetite loss
- Irregular menstruation
- Ascites (in advanced stages)

Diagnosis
- Transvaginal Ultrasound (TVS)
- CA-125 – Marker in epithelial type (↑ in postmenopausal women)
- CT / MRI Abdomen-Pelvis – Staging
- Histopathology – After surgical removal
- Risk of Malignancy Index (RMI) used pre-op

FIGO Staging Highlights

Stage	Extent
I	Confined to ovaries
II	Extension to pelvis
III	Peritoneal metastasis or lymph nodes
IV	Distant metastasis (liver, lungs)

Treatment Overview

Stage	Management
Early (I)	Surgery (TAH + BSO + staging)
Advanced	Cytoreductive surgery + chemotherapy
Chemo agents	Paclitaxel + Carboplatin
Follow-up	CA-125 monitoring
Fertility-sparing	Unilateral salpingo-oophorectomy (select cases)

List of Books for further reading- As per mentioned in the syllabus.

S.No	Books Name
1	Masihi A. Me'ate Maseehi. Vol. I. New Delhi: Central Council for Research in Unani Medicine; 2008.
2	Arzani MA. Mizanuttib. New Delhi: Qaumi Council bray-e-Froghe Urdu Zaban; 2002.
3	Jurjani AH. Zkhira-e Kwarizam Shahi (Urdu translation). Delhi: Idara Kitabush Shifa; 2010.
4	Kabeeruddin Byaz-e-Kabeer. New Delhi: Central Council for Research in Unani Medicine; 2008.
5	Razi ABMZ. Kitabul-Mansoori (Urdu translation). New Delhi: Central Council for Research in Unani Medicine; 1991.
6	Razi ABMZ. Kitabul-Hawi Fit-Tib. Vol. VII. New Delhi: Central Council for Research in Unani Medicine; 2000.
7	Razi ABMZ. Kitabul-Hawi Fit-Tib. Vol. IX. New Delhi: Central Council for Research in Unani Medicine; 2001.
8	Razi ABMZ. Kitabul-Hawi Fit-Tib. Vol. X. New Delhi: Central Council for Research in Unani Medicine; 2002.
9	Khan MA. Beyaz-e-Ajmal. New Delhi: Ejaz Publishing House; 1995.
10	Khan MA. Haziq. Delhi: Idara Kitabush Shifa; 2002.
11	Khan MA. Akseer-e-Azam (Urdu translation). Delhi: Idara Kitabush Shifa; 2011.
12	Baghdadi AH. Kitabul Murakhtarat fit-Tib (Urdu translation). Vol. III. New Delhi: Central Council for Research in Unani Medicine; 2004.
13	Baker PN, Kenny L, editors. Obstetrics by ten teachers. CRC Press; 2011 Mar 25.
14	Baghdadi AH. Kitabul Murakhtarat fit-Tib (Urdu translation). Vol. I. New Delhi: Central Council for Research in Unani Medicine; 2005.
15	Qamri AM. Ghina Muna (Urdu translation). New Delhi: Central Council for Research in Unani Medicine; 2008.
16	Tabari A. Firdaus al-Ḥikmafi'l Ṭibb (Urdu translation). New Delhi: Central Council for Research in Unani Medicine; 2010.
17	Majoosi AA. Kamilus-Sana, Vol. II. New Delhi: Central Council for Research in Unani Medicine; 2010.
18	Ibn Sina. Al-Qānūnfi'l Ṭibb (Urdu translation). Vols. I–IV. Delhi: Idara Kitabush Shifa; YNM.
19	Kumar P, Malhotra N. Jeffcoate's Principle of Gynaecology. 7th International ed. New Delhi: Jaypee Medical Publisher (P) Ltd; 2008.
20	Rashid LK. Five Teachers Textbook of Gynaecology. New Delhi: CBS Publisher and Distributor; 2013.
21	Jonathan sB. Novak's Gynaecology. Maryland (UsA): Williams & Wilkins, Baltimore; 2021.
22	Howkins J, Bourne G. shaw's Textbook of Gynaecology. 17th ed. Elsevier; 2023.
23	Wilson JR. Obstetrics & Gynaecology. Mosby; YNM.
24	Dutta DC. Textbook of Gynaecology. New Delhi: Jaypee B. Medical Publisher; 2023.
25	Dutta DC. Textbook of Obstetrics. New Delhi: Jaypee B. Medical Publisher; 2019.

S.No	Books Name
26	Williams JW. Gynaecology. New York: McGraw-Hill Professional; 2021.
27	Williams JW. Obstetrics. New York: McGraw-Hill Professional; 2010.
28	Dewhurst J. Textbook of Obstetrics & Gynaecology. Oxford: Blackwell Publishing; 2007.
29	Seshadri L, Arjun G. Essentials of obstetrics. Wolters kluwer india Pvt Ltd; 2020.
30	Seshadri L. Essentials of gynaecology. Wolters kluwer india Pvt Ltd; 2021.
31	Masihi A. kitab ul umda fil jarahat (urdu translation).Vol.I, New Delhi:CCRUM.
32	Kabiruddin H. Bayaz Kabir kamil. Lahore: Siddiqui publication.
33	Khan HMA. Ramooze Aazam (Persian translation). Vol.1&2. New Delhi: CCRUM; 2006.
34	Qarshi HMH. Jamiul Hikmat. Vol 1 & 2. New Delhi: Idara kitab us shifa; 2011.
35	Ibne Zuhr AMAM. Kitab al Taiseer fil Madawa wal tadbeer (urdu translation). New Delhi: CCRUM; 1986.
36	Razi ABMZ. Kitab al Fakhir fil tib (urdu translation). Vol I. New Delhi:CCRUM; 2008.

List of Practicals for Examination

S.No.	Practical Activity details
1	General & Systemic Examination
2	Examination of Breast
3	Pelvic Examination
4	Writing a gynecological case report
5	Case report writing for obstetric cases
6	Patient's discharge summary
7	Gradation of Uterine Prolapse
8	Pelvic floor exercises
9	Pessary Insertion techniques
10	Polypectomy
11	Technique to insert & remove IUCDs, use of cervical cap and diaphragm
12	Various Ilaj bit Tadbeer methods used in Gynecology & Obstetrics
13	VIA, schiller's, High Vaginal swab & their screening Procedures.
14	*Imtihaan–e-Khalvi* (Pap's smear Test) & procedure of screening for cervical cancer
15	Dilatation & Curettage (D&C) and Dilatation & Evacuation (D&E)
16	Proper wound care (Cleaning, Dressing & Packing), and steps of I&D.
17	Cryosurgery

www.ingramcontent.com/pod-product-compliance
Lightning Source LLC
LaVergne TN
LVHW060012210926
848481LV00013B/3691